CURRENT CLINICAL PATHOLOGY

ANTONIO GIORDANO, MD, PHD
SERIES EDITOR

For further volumes:
http://www.springer.com/series/7632

Michael J. Murphy
Editor

Diagnostic and Prognostic Biomarkers and Therapeutic Targets in Melanoma

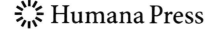

Editor
Michael J. Murphy, M.D.
Department of Dermatology
University of Connecticut Health Center
Farmington, CT, USA
drmichaelmurphy@netscape.net

ISBN 978-1-60761-432-6   e-ISBN 978-1-60761-433-3
DOI 10.1007/978-1-60761-433-3
Springer New York Dordrecht Heidelberg London

Library of Congress Control Number: 2011941011

© Springer Science+Business Media, LLC 2012
All rights reserved. This work may not be translated or copied in whole or in part without the written permission of the publisher (Humana Press, c/o Springer Science+Business Media, LLC, 233 Spring Street, New York, NY 10013, USA), except for brief excerpts in connection with reviews or scholarly analysis. Use in connection with any form of information storage and retrieval, electronic adaptation, computer software, or by similar or dissimilar methodology now known or hereafter developed is forbidden.
The use in this publication of trade names, trademarks, service marks, and similar terms, even if they are not identified as such, is not to be taken as an expression of opinion as to whether or not they are subject to proprietary rights.
While the advice and information in this book are believed to be true and accurate at the date of going to press, neither the authors nor the editors nor the publisher can accept any legal responsibility for any errors or omissions that may be made. The publisher makes no warranty, express or implied, with respect to the material contained herein.

Printed on acid-free paper

Humana Press is part of Springer Science+Business Media (www.springer.com)

To Aileen, with love

Preface

Developments in genomic and proteomic technologies are shedding light on the molecular pathobiology of melanoma, and uncovering diagnostic and prognostic biomarkers and therapeutic targets for this deadly disease. In this book, experts review recent major advances in melanoma biomarker research. The clinical applications of a wide range of genetic, epigenetic and protein biomarkers are outlined. The integration of these biomarkers with traditional prognostic and predictive indicators in the management of patients with melanoma is described.

I would like to thank all my colleagues in Australia, Germany, Italy, Japan, the Netherlands, the United Kingdom, and the United States of America for contributing chapters to this endeavor.

Michael J. Murphy
Farmington, CT, USA

Contents

1 **Introduction to Diagnostic and Prognostic Biomarkers and Therapeutic Targets in Melanoma** 1
Michael J. Murphy

2 **Diagnostic and Prognostic Biomarkers in Melanoma: Current State of Play** 9
Jochen Utikal, Jürgen C. Becker, and Selma Ugurel

3 **Molecular Pathogenesis of Melanoma: Established and Novel Pathways** 19
Paolo Antonio Ascierto, Maria Libera Ascierto, Mariaelena Capone, Zendee Elaba, Michael J. Murphy, and Giuseppe Palmieri

4 **Staging of Melanoma** 39
Zendee Elaba, Michael J. Murphy, Philip Kerr, and Jane M. Grant-Kels

5 **Clinical and Histopathological Parameters in Melanoma** 49
Cheryl Bilinski, Avery LaChance, and Michael J. Murphy

6 **Genetic/Epigenetic Biomarkers: Distinction of Melanoma from Other Melanocytic Neoplasms** 69
Minoru Takata

7 **mRNA Biomarkers in Melanoma** 79
Giovanna Chiorino and Maria Scatolini

8 **Epigenetic Biomarkers in Melanoma** 89
Suhu Liu, Suping Ren, Paul M. Howell Jr., and Adam I. Riker

9 **MicroRNA Biomarkers in Melanoma** 113
Jim Kozubek, Faseeha Altaf, and Soheil Sam Dadras

10 **MicroRNAs as Biomarkers and Therapeutic Targets in Melanoma** 127
Daniel W. Mueller and Anja K. Bosserhoff

11 **Mitochondrial DNA Biomarkers in Melanoma** 145
Mark L. Steinberg

12	**Tissue-Based Protein Biomarkers in Melanoma: Immunohistochemistry: (A) Diagnosis** 159
	Steven J. Ohsie, Basil A. Horst, Alistair Cochran, and Scott W. Binder
13	**Tissue-Based Protein Biomarkers in Melanoma: Immunohistochemistry: (B) Prognostication** 177
	Basil A. Horst, Steven J. Ohsie, Alistair Cochran, and Scott W. Binder
14	**Tissue-Based Protein Biomarkers in Melanoma: Mass Spectrometry-Based Strategies** 189
	Michael J. Murphy, Karim Rezaul, and David K. Han
15	**Serological Biomarkers in Melanoma** 195
	Mel Ziman, Michael Millward, Robert Pearce, and Mark Lee
16	**Molecular Markers of Lymph Node Disease in Melanoma** 209
	Sandro Pasquali, Augustinus P.T. van der Ploeg, and Simone Mocellin
17	**Melanoma Cell Propagation: Cancer Stem Cell, Clonal Evolution and Interconversion Models of Tumorigenicity** 227
	Qiuzhen Liu, Marianna Sabatino, David F. Stroncek, Ping Jin, Francesco M. Marincola, and Ena Wang
18	**Surgical Management of Melanoma: Concept of Field Cancerization and Molecular Evaluation of Tissue Margins** 243
	Amanda Phelps and Michael J. Murphy
19	**Chemotherapy for Melanoma** 247
	Hedwig Stanisz, Thomas Vogt, and Knuth Rass
20	**Molecular-Targeted Therapy for Melanoma** 265
	Alessia E. Russo, Ylenia Bevelacqua, Andrea Marconi, Andrea Veronesi, and Massimo Libra
21	**Anti-Angiogenesis Therapy for Melanoma** 281
	Roberta Ferraldeschi and Paul Lorigan
22	**Immunological Biomarkers and Immunotherapy for Melanoma** 295
	Jochen T. Schaefer
23	**Diagnostic and Prognostic Biomarkers and Therapeutic Targets in Melanoma: An Overview** 305
	Ahmad A. Tarhini and John M. Kirkwood

Index 319

Contributors

Faseeha Altaf, BS University of Connecticut (Storrs campus), Storrs, CT, USA

Maria Libera Ascierto, PhD Unit of Medical Oncology and Innovative Therapy, Istituto Nazionale Tumori Fondazione "G. Pascale", Naples, Italy

Paolo Antonio Ascierto, MD Unit of Medical Oncology and Innovative Therapy, Istituto Nazionale Tumori Fondazione "G. Pascale", Naples, Italy

Jürgen C. Becker, MD, PhD Department of Dermatology, Medical University of Graz, Graz, Austria

Ylenia Bevelacqua, MD Department of Biomedical Sciences, University of Catania, Catania, Italy

Cheryl Bilinski, BA University of Connecticut Medical School, Farmington, CT, USA

Scott W. Binder, MD Department of Pathology and Laboratory Medicine, David Geffen School of Medicine at the University of California, Los Angeles, CA, USA

Anja K. Bosserhoff, PhD Institute of Pathology, Molecular Pathology, University of Regensburg, Regensburg, Germany

Mariaelena Capone, PhD Unit of Medical Oncology and Innovative Therapy, Istituto Nazionale Tumori Fondazione "G. Pascale", Naples, Italy

Giovanna Chiorino, PhD Cancer Genomics Laboratory, "Edo ed Elvo Tempia" Foundation, Biella, Italy

Alistair Cochran, MD Departments of Pathology and Laboratory Medicine and Surgery, David Geffen School of Medicine at the University of California, Los Angeles, CA, USA

Soheil Sam Dadras, MD, PhD Departments of Dermatology and Genetics and Developmental Biology, University of Connecticut Health Center, Farmington, CT, USA

Zendee Elaba, MD Department of Pathology, Hartford Hospital, Hartford, CT, USA

Roberta Ferraldeschi, MD Department of Medical Oncology, The Christie Hospital NHS Foundation Trust, Withington, Manchester, UK

Jane M. Grant-Kels, MD Department of Dermatology, University of Connecticut Health Center, Farmington, CT, USA

David K. Han, PhD Department of Cell Biology, Center for Vascular Biology, University of Connecticut Health Center, Farmington, CT, USA

Basil A. Horst, MD Departments of Dermatology, Pathology and Cell Biology, Columbia University Medical Center, New York, NY, USA

Paul M. Howell Jr., BS Mitchell Cancer Institute, University of South Alabama, Mobile, AL, USA

Ping Jin, PhD Cell Processing Section, Department of Transfusion Medicine, Clinical Center, National Institutes of Health, Bethesda, MD, USA

Philip Kerr, MD Department of Dermatology, University of Connecticut Health Center, Farmington, CT, USA

John M. Kirkwood, MD Department of Medicine/Division of Hematology/Oncology, UPMC Cancer Pavilion, University of Pittsburgh Cancer Institute, Pittsburgh, PA, USA

Jim Kozubek, MS Department of Genetics and Developmental Biology, University of Connecticut Health Center, Farmington, CT, USA

Avery LaChance, BA University of Connecticut Medical School, Farmington, CT, USA

Mark Lee, MD Plastic Surgery, Sir Charles Gairdner Hospital, Perth, WA, Australia

Massimo Libra, MD, PhD Department of Biomedical Sciences, University of Catania, Catania, Italy

Suhu Liu, MD, PhD Harvard University, Dana-Farber Cancer Institute, Boston, MA, USA

Qiuzhen Liu, MD, PhD Infectious Disease and Immunogenetics Section (IDIS), Clinical Center, National Institutes of Health, Bethesda, MD, USA

Paul Lorigan, MD Department of Medical Oncology, The Christie Hospital NHS Foundation Trust, Withington, Manchester, UK

Andrea Marconi, MD Department of Biomedical Sciences, University of Catania, Catania, Italy

Francesco M. Marincola, MD Infectious Disease and Immunogenetics Section (IDIS), Clinical Center, National Institutes of Health, Bethesda, MD, USA

Michael Millward, MD School of Medicine and Pharmacology, University of Western Australia, Perth, WA, Australia

Simone Mocellin, MD, PhD Surgery Branch, Department of Oncological and Surgical Sciences, University of Padova, Padova, Italy

Daniel W. Mueller, PhD Institute of Pathology, Molecular Pathology, University of Regensburg, Regensburg, Germany

Michael J. Murphy, MD Department of Dermatology, University of Connecticut Health Center, Farmington, CT, USA

Steven J. Ohsie, MD Affiliated Pathologists Medical Group/Pathology, Inc., Torrence, CA, USA

Giuseppe Palmieri, MD, PhD Unit of Cancer Genetics, Institute of Biomolecular Chemistry, National Research Council (CNR), Sassari, Italy

Sandro Pasquali, MD Surgery Branch, Department of Oncological and Surgical Sciences, University of Padova, Padova, Italy

Robert Pearce, MD School of Exercise, Biomedical and Health Science, Edith Cowan University, Joondalup, WA, Australia

Amanda Phelps, BA Central Connecticut State University, New Britain, CT, USA

Knuth Rass, MD Department of Dermatology, Venerology and Allergology, University Hospital of the Saarland, Homburg/Saar, Germany

Suping Ren, MD, PhD Mitchell Cancer Institute, University of South Alabama, Mobile, AL, USA

Karim Rezaul, PhD Department of Cell Biology, Center for Vascular Biology, University of Connecticut Health Center, Farmington, CT, USA

Adam I. Riker, MD Department of Surgery, Ochsner Medical Center, Ochsner Cancer Institute, Ochsner Health System, New Orleans, LA, USA

Alessia E. Russo, MD Department of Biomedical Sciences, University of Catania, Catania, Italy

Marianna Sabatino, MD Cell Processing Section, Department of Transfusion Medicine, Clinical Center, National Institutes of Health, Bethesda, MD, USA

Maria Scatolini, PhD Cancer Genomics Laboratory, "Edo ed Elvo Tempia" Foundation, Biella, Italy

Jochen T. Schaefer, MD Department of Dermatology, University of Connecticut Health Center, Farmington, CT, USA

Hedwig Stanisz, MD Department of Dermatology, Venerology and Allergology, University Hospital of the Saarland, Homburg/Saar, Germany

Mark L. Steinberg, PhD Department of Chemistry, The City College of New York, New York, NY, USA

David F. Stroncek, MD Cell Processing Section, Department of Transfusion Medicine, Clinical Center, National Institutes of Health, Bethesda, MD, USA

Minoru Takata, MD, PhD Department of Dermatology, Okayama University Postgraduate School of Medical, Dentistry and Pharmaceutical Sciences, Okayama, Japan

Ahmad A. Tarhini, MD, MSc Department of Medicine/Division of Hematology/Oncology, UPMC Cancer Pavilion, University of Pittsburgh Cancer Institute, Pittsburgh, PA, USA

Selma Ugurel, MD Department of Dermatology, Medical University of Graz, Graz, Austria

Jochen Utikal, MD Department of Dermatology, University Medical Center Mannheim, Mannheim, Germany

Augustinus P.T. van der Ploeg, MSc Erasmus University Medical Center, Daniel den Hoed Cancer Center, Rotterdam, The Netherlands

Andrea Veronesi, MD Division of Medical Oncology C, National Cancer Institute, IRCCS, Aviano, Italy

Thomas Vogt, MD Department of Dermatology, Venerology and Allergology, University Hospital of the Saarland, Homburg/Saar, Germany

Ena Wang, MD Infectious Disease and Immunogenetics Section (IDIS), Clinical Center, National Institutes of Health, Bethesda, MD, USA

Mel Ziman, PhD School of Pathology and Laboratory Medicine, University of Western Australia, Joondalup, WA, Australia

School of Exercise, Biomedical and Health Science, Edith Cowan University, Joondalup, WA, Australia

Introduction to Diagnostic and Prognostic Biomarkers and Therapeutic Targets in Melanoma

Michael J. Murphy

The aim of this book is to discuss both the technologies used in the discovery of melanoma biomarkers and the clinical application of these biomarkers for diagnosis and staging of disease, determination of prognosis, prediction of drug response, monitoring the efficacy of therapy, identification of novel therapeutic targets, and drug development. A broad range of biomarkers [described as any measurable molecular alteration within a cancer cell (i.e., DNA/chromosomal, mRNA, microRNA, mitochondrial DNA, epigenetic and protein)] is outlined. Of note, individual/panels or patterns of molecular markers may now be employed to stratify microscopically-similar melanocytic tumors into subsets with different biological behaviors and outcomes [1, 2]. In addition, with the more widespread use of molecular-targeted melanoma therapies, it has become increasingly necessary to evaluate putative drug targets in order to predict clinical response [3]. An important goal is the enhancement of both safety and efficacy of melanoma management by facilitating the tailoring of treatment(s) to individual patients ("personalized medicine"). Novel biomarkers could be used to distinguish patients with melanomas requiring targeted intervention from those individuals who require no further therapy. Some of these biomarkers may also have a role in cancer screening, early detection and/or risk assessment. In this regard, current high-throughput laboratory technologies have facilitated the discovery and validation of biomarkers in patients with melanoma; although, efforts are still hampered by some of the limitations of currently available methodologies. The ideal biomarker should be sensitive, specific, rapidly analyzable, reliable, cost-effective, and demonstrate clinical relevance beyond traditional "gold-standard" clinical and histopathological data available at the time of diagnosis and/or follow-up. Despite some notable discoveries, the translation from "bench-to-bedside" has been slow and the number of biomarkers validated for use in the management of patients with melanoma remains limited. It is likely that further advances in genomic and proteomic technologies and bioinformatics will lead to the identification of additional clinically-useful biomarkers for disease classification, staging, prognostication, treatment selection, and monitoring of therapeutic response, in addition to novel drug target discovery and facilitation of drug development.

Melanoma is considered an epidemic cancer as its worldwide incidence has increased 697% between 1950 and 2000, faster than that of any other cancer subtype; although, recent evidence suggests that this rise may have peaked [4]. The American Cancer Society now estimates that the lifetime risk of developing melanoma is

M.J. Murphy, M.D. (✉)
Department of Dermatology, University of Connecticut Health Center, Farmington, CT, USA
e-mail: drmichaelmurphy@netscape.net

approximately 1 in 50 for Caucasians, 1 in 200 for Hispanics and 1 in 1,000 for African-Americans [4]. In the United States, invasive melanoma is the 6th most common cancer in men and the 7th in women; the lifetime probability of developing this tumor is 1 in 37 for males and 1 in 56 for females. An estimated 68,130 new cases of cutaneous melanoma were diagnosed in 2010, with 8,700 estimated deaths from this disease [4]. While representing <7% of all skin malignancies, melanoma is the most lethal cutaneous malignancy and accounts for ~75% of all deaths from skin tumors.

The TNM staging categories and groupings of the updated 2009 American Joint Committee on Cancer (AJCC) Melanoma Staging System are outlined in Tables 4.1 and 4.2 of this book [5]. "*T*" parameters are defined by primary tumor thickness, ulceration, and mitotic status; "*N*" parameters by the number of lymph nodes with metastatic disease and extent of metastatic burden; and "*M*" parameters by the site(s) of metastases and serum lactate dehydrogenase (LDH) levels. For patients with melanoma, the formal TNM system currently provides the basis for tumor staging, prediction of survival, treatment selection and stratification of patients in clinical trials. Approximately 84% of cutaneous melanomas are locally confined; 8% of patients are diagnosed after the tumor has spread regionally; and 4% are diagnosed with distant metastasis. In the remaining 4% of patients, the staging information is unknown. For patients with invasive melanoma, the single best indicator of prognosis is the stage at first clinical presentation, which for AJCC stages I, II, and III is determined by histopathological findings. Specifically, primary tumor depth (Breslow thickness), the presence or absence of ulceration, the presence or absence of microscopic metastases [either peritumoral microsatellites or regional sentinel lymph node (SLN) disease], and the number of regional lymph nodes involved are key to the correct staging of early- and intermediate-stage melanoma. The 5-year survival rate is ~90% for AJCC stage I melanoma and ~70% for AJCC stage II melanoma, but decreases significantly to 25–50% for AJCC stage III melanoma (depending on the number of lymph nodes involved), and ~10% for stage IV disease [1, 2]. Because the identification of metastatic disease is a major prognostic factor for melanoma recurrence and outcome, accurate tumor staging is important for optimal management of these patients. However, the clinical and histopathological features cannot accurately predict the behavior of melanoma in all cases [1, 2]. Individuals at identical clinical and/or pathological stages can exhibit different survival probabilities. A small subset of patients with thin melanomas will develop metastases and die from their disease, while many patients with thick melanomas never develop recurrent disease after excision of the primary tumor. The discovery of biomarkers that could predict which patients are likely to develop metastasis is one approach that would allow earlier therapeutic intervention for those individuals identified to be at high risk for relapse. A major drawback with the current TNM staging system is that it does not easily allow for the integration of newly discovered pathobiological concepts, data revealed by ancillary diagnostic techniques, and/or novel tumor biomarkers. Therefore, a need exists for biomarkers which would help to identify patients at risk for disease progression, in addition to those individuals whose disease has already progressed subclinically [1, 2].

Research is on-going into the molecular mechanisms that underlie the malignant transformation of melanocytes to melanoma and the progression of primary cutaneous tumors to invasive and metastatic disease. Significant progress has been made in our understanding of the cellular, molecular and genetic basis for melanoma. The traditional classification of melanoma into four subtypes (i.e., acral lentiginous, superficial spreading, nodular, and lentigo maligna), which is based on clinical-histopathological features, is now being challenged by the results of molecular studies [1, 2, 6]. The identification of key melanoma-associated somatic gene mutations (i.e., BRAF, NRAS, and KIT) is likely to play a significant role in the development of a future molecular classification scheme for this tumor. Furthermore, the integration of clinical, morphologic and genomic data may help to characterize each individual melanoma and guide the selection of novel target-oriented drugs in clinical trials. Unfortunately, the number of melanoma-related deaths continues to increase and results of cytotoxic and immunologic therapy for metastatic disease have remained largely disappointing. Tumor heterogeneity hinders the optimal use of currently available therapeutic modalities in patients with melanoma. In addition, for patient cohorts grouped by established TNM clinical staging systems, response to treatment and corresponding survival rates never approach 100% concordance. Poor treatment results in some patients could be partly due to imprecise staging at the time of diagnosis, inappropriate selection of therapy, or a combination thereof. Subgroups of patients with melanoma may not be given the opportunity to receive necessary therapeutic intervention, while others may be subjected to inappropriate and potentially harmful treatment. There have been several significant breakthroughs in the past decade with regard to the management of patients with melanoma [3]. Again these advances are based on the recognition of discrete subsets of melanoma; each with distinct chromosomal aberrations, gene mutations and oncogenic pathway activation. Several obvious benefits may be realized from recent molecular discoveries. Firstly, melanomas can be classified into cohorts that have potentially similar clinical course and treatment responses. Secondly, if the pathogenic mechanisms within a distinct subgroup of melanomas are well understood, targeted therapies could be potentially developed. Pharmacogenetic and pharmacogenomic strategies in melanoma are reviewed elsewhere [3].

As stated previously, numerous molecular biomarkers, which highlight the mechanisms of melanoma pathogenesis and progression, have been identified [1, 2]. The clinical utility of a number of these biomarkers, for improving upon routine histopathological methods in the staging and prognostication of melanoma patients, has also been investigated [1, 2]. In this regard, the role of molecular diagnostic techniques in the detection of both SLN and circulating melanoma cells is an area of active research and warrants further discussion. Although molecular analysis of melanocyte-related markers has also been undertaken in bone marrow specimens and biological fluids (effusions and cerebrospinal fluid), the most commonly performed assays in melanoma patients have been on SLN and peripheral blood specimens [2]. The detection of tumor cells in specimens from melanoma patients with early-stage disease could identify those at high risk for metastasis. The amplification of tumor-related DNA or mRNA sequences, by techniques such as standard reverse transcription-polymerase chain reaction (RT-PCR) and quantitative real-time polymerase chain reaction (qRT), has been undertaken in SLNs and peripheral blood of melanoma patients in an effort to detect the presence of occult tumor cells [2]. A review of tumor biomarkers used in this setting is provided in Chaps. 15 and 16. Of note, amplification of melanocyte-specific transcripts by standard RT-PCR allows for the detection of one melanoma cell among 10^6–10^7 non-tumor cells. The use of qRT may increase this sensitivity of detection to 1 melanoma cell per 10^7–10^8 background cells. This is in contrast with the lower detection sensitivities for laboratory techniques more routinely employed in SLN analysis. Immunohistochemistry can detect 1 melanoma cell in a background of 10^5–10^6 non-tumor cells. This sensitivity further decreases to 1 tumor cell per 10^4–10^5 non-tumor cells by light microscopic review alone (i.e., hematoxylin and eosin [H+E] stained sections) of SLNs. Routine molecular testing could have diagnostic utility in the detection of subclinical and/or submicroscopic metastases in SLNs and/or peripheral blood of patients with melanoma [2]. Molecular technologies may also have utility in the microstaging of primary melanoma and the differentiation of second primary tumors from cutaneous metastases [1, 2].

The alkylating agent dacarbazine (DTIC) is the only FDA-approved chemotherapeutic agent for treatment of metastatic melanoma; although, responses are infrequently seen (5–10% of patients) and are generally short-lived [3]. Other chemotherapeutic agents, such as carmustine (BCNU), temozolomide, taxanes and platinum-analogs, have equally poor efficacy in this setting. In addition, there are two FDA-approved biological response modifiers for metastatic melanoma, interleukin-2 (IL-2) and interferon-α2b (IFN-α2b) [3]. Studies report that high-dose IL-2 results in durable responses in only 10–20% of stage IV melanoma patients, and is associated with severe, albeit short-lived, toxicities. IFN-α2b is an approved adjuvant immunotherapy for stage III melanoma, and while demonstrating a 10–20% improvement in relapse-free survival, no clear effect on melanoma-related mortality is seen [3]. A large set of genes are found to be differentially regulated in IFN-sensitive and IFN-resistant melanoma cell lines, identifying both sensitivity- and resistance-associated genomic signatures [3]. A recent study explored the impact of cytokine gene polymorphisms on clinical outcome for stage IV melanoma patients treated with biochemotherapy (cisplatin, vinblastine, and DTIC; combined with IL-2 and IFN-α) [3]. The IFN-γ +874 single nucleotide polymorphism (SNP) was found to be significantly associated with treatment response, progression-free survival, and overall survival [3]. When three gene polymorphisms (IFN-γ +874, IL-10 -1082G>A, and ERCC1 codon 118) were combined, four distinct groups of patients with significantly different outcomes were identified [3]. Another study reported that a 32 bp deletion polymorphism in the chemokine receptor 5 gene (CCR5Δ32) was significantly associated with decreased survival in stage IV melanoma patients receiving immunotherapy (IFN, IL-2, or vaccination) [3]. Because current therapy for advanced melanoma utilizes cytotoxic agents and biological response modifiers that mediate tumor regression by different mechanisms, combined testing for multiple genetic polymorphisms could potentially generate more accurate pharmacogenomic information than single SNP analysis.

The mitogen-activated protein kinase (MAPK) signaling pathway (RAS/RAF/MEK/ERK) has been found to be constitutively activated in up to 80–90% of melanomas [1–3]. The two most common mechanisms for this activation are gain-of-function mutations in either NRAS (15–30% of melanomas) or BRAF (50–70% of melanomas) (Fig. 3.1). Therefore, drugs that target this pathway are of considerable interest (see Chap. 20). Since the discovery of BRAF mutations in melanoma, several oral targeted multi-kinase inhibitors which decrease BRAF activity have been developed [3]. For example, the broad-spectrum multi-kinase inhibitor sorafenib (BAY 43-9006) targets BRAF, vascular endothelial growth factor receptor (VEGFR)-2, VEGFR-3, platelet-derived growth factor receptor (PDGFR)-β, FMS-like tyrosine kinase 3, and KIT. Unfortunately, early clinical studies using sorafenib in melanoma patients, as a single agent or in combination with chemotherapy, demonstrated little benefit beyond disease stabilization [3]. Clinical trials are now ongoing with second generation selective and non-selective RAF inhibitors, such as PLX4032 (vemurafenib), SB-590885/GSK2118436, XL-281, and RAF-265 (www.clinicaltrials.gov). In recent Phase I-III trials, XL-281 (ARAF, BRAF, and CRAF inhibitor) and PLX4032 (BRAF^{V600E} inhibitor) were shown to have single-agent antitumor activity in patients with melanoma, with the achievement of objective responses [3, 7]. These studies indicate the potential therapeutic value of single-agent therapy against a mutated oncogene in melanoma. However, not all patients respond to this treatment, and dose-limiting toxicities, primary and secondary drug resistance, and the development of therapy-related cutaneous squamous cell carcinomas/keratoacanthomas (in up to 30% of patients) represent issues that must be addressed. While PLX4032 selectively inhibits downstream MEK/ERK signaling and cellular activation in BRAF^{V600E} mutant cells, it paradoxically activates this signaling pathway in cells with wild-type BRAF. It therefore has the potential to induce carcinogenesis in cells lacking the BRAF^{V600E} mutation. These findings emphasize the requirement for current and future clinical studies of BRAF inhibitors to select for patients who have BRAF-mutant melanomas. In addition, MEK, which is directly activated by BRAF, is another potential drug target in patients with melanoma [3].

Imatinib mesylate, a tyrosine kinase inhibitor of BCR-ABL, KIT and PDGFR, is an FDA-approved treatment for both chronic myelogenous leukemias (which harbor the BCR-ABL fusion protein) and gastrointestinal stromal tumors (GISTs; which harbor oncogenic KIT and/or PDGFRA mutations) [3]. There is a strong association between specific activating mutations of KIT with clinical responses to imatinib in GISTs and mastocytosis [3]. In a study of 102 primary melanomas, KIT mutations were identified in 17% of chronic sun-damaged cutaneous, 11% of acral, and 21% of mucosal melanomas, but not in any melanomas on skin without chronic sun damage; supporting a role for KIT as an oncogene in a subset of tumors [1]. In addition, KIT gene amplification has been found to be present in 6% of chronic sun-damaged, 7% of acral, and 8% of mucosal melanomas [1]. Similar rates of KIT alterations in acral and mucosal melanomas, but lower rates (~2%) in chronic sun-damaged cutaneous tumors are reported by other studies [1]. Point mutations in KIT result in constitutive activation of the c-KIT protein in melanoma cells, and the activation of downstream proliferative and pro-survival signaling pathways. At the protein level, immunohistochemical studies have shown c-KIT expression in 81% of mucosal and acral melanomas [3]. Interestingly, cases with activating mutations are commonly positive for c-KIT protein expression; although, this is not uniformly the case. Furthermore, many tumors that do not have detectable gene mutation or amplification show high expression levels of c-KIT protein [3]. Inhibition of KIT signaling has been shown *in vitro* to inhibit proliferation of cultured melanoma cells [3]. In addition, several anecdotal case reports have noted remarkable responses to small molecule KIT inhibitors (imatinib, sorefenib, and dasatinib) in patients with widely metastatic melanoma [3]. However, recent Phase II trials using imatinib reported that, among 63 patients with melanoma, only one clinical response was seen (in a patient with an acral tumor) [3]. Importantly, these patients' melanomas were not tested for the presence of a KIT (or PDGFRA) mutation, with only c-KIT (and PDGFRA) immunohistochemical testing (for protein expression) being performed. C-KIT receptor protein expression, in the absence of downstream signaling activity, has not been shown to be highly predictive of clinical response to imatinib [3]. More specifically, KIT mutations, and not gene amplifications, appear to be associated with drug response in melanoma patients [3]. These findings clearly illustrate the importance of proper patient selection prior to imatinib treatment, including KIT and PDGFRA gene mutational analysis. With this in mind, a number of multicenter Phase II clinical trials, using imatinib, in addition to sunitinib, nilotinib, and dasatanib, for the treatment of metastatic melanomas with KIT genomic aberrations (i.e., from acral, mucosal, and chronically sun-damaged sites) have been initiated.

Many treatment-responsive patients ultimately relapse as a result of acquired resistance to selective kinase-targeted therapies. This may be due to a number of factors, including re-establishment of negative feedback and/or alternative activation of MAPK signaling, other BRAF mutations or amplifications, mutations in RAS (HRAS, KRAS, or NRAS) or MEK1 genes, or activation of alternative pathways that drive proliferation, resistance to apoptosis or tumor escape (PI3K-AKT, CMET, KIT, FGFR, and EGFR) [3]. As a result of the intrinsic redundancy in the multiple genetic pathways that are activated in melanoma, it is likely that the use of synergistic combinations of mutation-targeted agents will be required to achieve optimal outcomes and overcome potential drug resistance in patients with metastatic disease [3]. In addition to MAPK-related mechanisms, other possible therapeutic targets in melanoma include GNAQ, CDK4, ERBB4, and ETV_1, as well as PI3K AKT, apoptosis, DNA repair, angiogenesis, ubiquitin-proteosome and epigenetic pathways [3]. Clinical trials evaluating novel drugs directed against some of these targets are currently underway [3].

Melanoma tumors can demonstrate spontaneous immune-mediated regression [3]. In addition, tumor-specific cytotoxic T-cells and antibodies may be found in the peripheral blood of patients with melanoma [3]. Therefore, immunotherapy is a potentially effective treatment strategy for individuals with this disease [3]. One approach is the enhancement of anti-melanoma immune responses through the optimization of T-cell activation. The latter involves interactions between the T-cell receptor (TCR), the co-stimulatory receptor CD28, and the ligands CD80 and CD86 [3]. T-cell inhibition is mediated by the inhibitory receptor, cytotoxic T lymphocyte-associated antigen-4 (CTLA-4), a molecule that shares 30% structural homology with CD28, and is expressed by activated T-cells and T-regulatory cells (Tregs). CTLA-4 binds CD80/CD86 with greater affinity than CD28 does, thereby inhibiting CD28-mediated T-cell activation and IL-2 production [3]. CTLA-4 is critical in maintaining immune tolerance to self-antigens, but may also limit host responses to tumor antigens and the efficacy of vaccine therapy. CTLA-4 blockade, either alone or in combination with melanoma-specific vaccines, has been explored as a potential strategy to treat advanced-stage melanoma [3]. A recent Phase III clinical trial found that patients with previously treated metastatic melanoma who received ipilimumab (MDX-010, a monoclonal antibody targeting CTLA-4), with or without a gp100 peptide vaccine, showed improved overall survival compared with those who received gp100 alone [8]. Importantly, this clinical trial was the first randomized study to show an improvement in overall survival in patients with advanced disease [8]. In march 2011, the FDA approved ipilimumab for the treatment of unresectable or metastatic melanoma. However, not all patients have responded well to CTLA-4 blockade, and some have developed severe autoimmune reactions [3]. Of note, the presence of serum antibodies against the cancer-associated antigen, NY-ESO-1, has been found to be associated with efficacy of anti-CTLA-4 therapy [3]. In addition, metastatic tumors at different sites in an individual patient can demonstrate distinct immunological signatures and local microenvironmental changes, possibly explaining the variable responses to immunotherapy seen in some patients. Variations in the CTLA-4 gene could also influence the response to its inhibition in patients with metastatic melanoma. In a recent study, three SNPs in this gene were found to be associated with responses to CTLA-4 blockade: proximal promoter SNPs, rs4553808 and rs11571327, and the nonsynonymous SNP rs231775 [3]. A haplotype analysis, that included seven SNPs, suggested that the common haplotype TACCGGG is associated with no response, whereas the haplotype TGCCAGG predicts treatment outcome. Unfortunately, no specific haplotype or SNP predicts which patients will develop the severe autoimmune reactions triggered by CTLA-4 blockade therapy [3]. Other potential immunological approaches in melanoma patients include the use of Toll-like receptor antagonists (i.e., imiquimod) and a HLA-B7/β2-microglobulin gene transfer product [3].

In the future, molecular technologies could be used to determine pathway activation and indicate which combinations of drugs would be most effective in an individual patient with melanoma. For example, the employment of laser capture-microdissection to isolate both melanoma cells and "normal-appearing" surrounding tissue would facilitate gene expression profiling and genotyping for both germline aberrations and somatic mutations (i.e., those acquired by melanoma cells) in routine surgical specimens. Disease outcome may depend on a combination of both the inherited germline and tumor genomes. Determination of germline DNA alterations could be used to assess the host baseline pharmacogenomic profile. This strategy could have important consequences for clinical trial design, with the incorporation of pharmacogenomics into inclusion (and exclusion) criteria. Previous studies of targeted drugs may have failed in part because of inadequate melanoma characterization, resulting in the inclusion of few to no potentially treatment-responsive patients.

It is envisioned that newer technologies, such as SNP-based arrays, DNA sequencing methods and mass spectrometry-based proteomic strategies (see Chap. 14), will be increasingly employed in the evaluation of melanocytic tumors, with results of molecular studies incorporated into current morphological-based diagnostic and prognostic classification systems (i.e., clinical findings and light microscopic changes). In addition to the wider use and acceptance of comparative genomic hybridization (CGH), fluorescence in situ hybridization (FISH), DNA microarray and epigenetic profiling tools, these genomic/

proteomic technologies will: (1) facilitate more accurate diagnosis and classification of melanocytic tumors; (2) improve on current staging criteria and lead to better stratification of melanoma patients into prognostically relevant groups; and (3) promote the individualization of therapy ("personalized medicine"), based on a patient's germline genetic variation, somatic genomic aberrations that arise during tumor development, and protein abundance, structure, stability, and function in established tumors. Melanoma management is currently moving toward prospective profiling of tumors at diagnosis for patterns/panels of genomic aberrations and protein changes relevant to both the sensitivity and resistance of targeted therapies.

References

1. Gerami P, Gammon B, Murphy MJ. Melanocytic neoplasms I: molecular diagnosis. In: Murphy MJ, editor. Molecular diagnostics in dermatology and dermatopathology, Current clinical pathology and oncology. New York: Humana Press/Springer; 2011. p. 73–103.
2. Murphy MJ, Carlson JA. Melanocytic neoplasms II: molecular staging. In: Murphy MJ, editor. Molecular diagnostics in dermatology and dermatopathology, Current clinical pathology and oncology. New York: Humana Press/Springer; 2011. p. 105–30.
3. Murphy MJ, Pincelli C, Hoss DM, Borroni R. Pharmacogenetics and pharmacogenomics I: linking diagnostic classification to therapeutic decisions. In: Murphy MJ, editor. Molecular diagnostics in dermatology and dermatopathology, Current clinical pathology and oncology. New York: Humana Press/Springer; 2011. p. 419–41.
4. American Cancer Society. Available at http://www.cancer.org/Cancer/SkinCancer-Melanoma/DetailedGuide/melanoma-skin-cancer-key-statistics. Accessed June 26, 2011.
5. Balch CM, Gershenwald JE, Soong SJ, et al. Final version of 2009 AJCC melanoma staging and classification. J Clin Oncol. 2009;27:6199–206.
6. Curtin JA, Fridlyand J, Kageshita T, et al. Distinct sets of genetic alterations in melanoma. N Engl J Med. 2005;353:2135–47.
7. Chapman PB, Hauschild A, Robert C, the BRIM-3 Study Group, et al. Improved Survival with Vemurafenib in Melanoma with BRAF V600E Mutation. N Engl J Med. 2011;364:2507–16.
8. Hodi FS, O'Day SJ, McDermott DF, et al. Improved survival with ipilimumab in patients with metastatic melanoma. N Engl J Med. 2010;363:711–23.

Diagnostic and Prognostic Biomarkers in Melanoma: Current State of Play

Jochen Utikal, Jürgen C. Becker, and Selma Ugurel

Introduction

Melanoma is the most deadly skin cancer. The incidence and mortality rates of this tumor have been increasing over the last number of decades. Besides clinical and histopathological characteristics (i.e., anatomic site and subtype of the primary tumor, Breslow thickness, ulceration, vascular invasion, mitotic index), an increasing variety of molecular markers have been identified, providing the possibility of a more detailed diagnostic and prognostic categorization of melanoma. Recently published gene expression and proteomic profiling data indicate new candidate molecules involved in melanoma pathogenesis, which are currently being validated. This ongoing process of biomarker identification and validation is resulting in a rapidly changing molecular view of cutaneous melanoma, which holds the promise of improving our diagnostic and prognostic classification systems, as well as identifying therapeutic targets. In this chapter, we provide a comprehensive overview of the currently known serological and immunohistochemical biomarkers in melanoma.

J. Utikal, M.D.
Department of Dermatology, University Medical Center Mannheim, Mannheim, Germany

J.C. Becker, M.D., Ph.D. (✉) • S. Ugurel, M.D.
Department of Dermatology, Medical University of Graz, Graz, Austria
e-mail: juergen.becker@meduni-graz.at

Tumor Tissue-Based Biomarkers

Cutaneous melanoma develops in three sequential stages (i.e., radial growth phase, vertical growth phase and metastases). The prognosis in any stage is only partially explained by morphological and histopathological parameters, such as primary tumor localization, patient gender and age, mitotic rate, tumor thickness and ulceration. Moreover, while some parameters seem to reflect merely the tumor burden, others, such as ulceration, appear to be intrinsically related to tumor biology. Additional technologies that help to assign patients to specific risk groups include immunohistochemistry, gene expression profiling, comparative genomic hybridization, and gene mutational analysis.

For diagnostic purposes, a small panel of melanocytic lineage markers (i.e., S100, MART-1, and gp100/HMB45) is sufficient to discriminate melanoma from non-melanocytic skin cancer. However, no marker has proven useful in distinguishing spindle cell/desmoplastic melanoma from other tumors. Ki-67 remains the most useful adjunct in distinguishing benign from malignant melanocytic tumors [1].

For prognostic classification, the situation is more complex. The transformation from benign melanocytes to metastatic melanoma results from a combination of genetic alterations contributing to the hallmarks of cancer (i.e., uncontrolled proliferation, unlimited replicative potential, apoptosis resistance, invasion, and angiogenesis). Several marker molecules involved in these genetic alterations have been identified, and their expression in primary melanoma has been studied and correlated with prognosis. Table 2.1 summarizes the most important tissue biomarkers known for melanoma, whose abnormal expression is associated with patient prognosis. It is likely that the most detailed prognostic classification for melanoma will not result from analysis of one biomarker, but rather from a panel of multiple biomarkers in this list.

In a recent retrospective study, primary melanomas (for which long-term clinical follow-up was available) were analyzed using a cDNA expression microarray [22]. The authors described a signature of 174 genes that identified patients at risk of developing distant metastasis. From these 174 genes, 141 were underexpressed and 33 overexpressed in tumors whose host remained free of metastasis for 4 years. Thirty of these 174 genes had already been studied in melanoma; these genes are involved in cell cycle regulation (CKS2, CDC2, CCNB1, CENPF, and DHFR), mitosis

Table 2.1 Immunohistochemical markers of melanoma associated with impaired prognosis

	Association with impaired prognosis	References
Melanocyte lineage/differentiation antigens		
gp100/HMB45	Increased expression	Niezabitowski et al. [2]
Tumor suppressors/oncogenes/signal transducers		
AP-2 (activator protein-2alpha) transcription factor	Loss of nuclear AP-2 expression	Berger et al. [3]
bcl-6	Expression	Alonso et al. [4]
c-Kit	Expression	Janku et al. [5]
c-met	Expression	Cruz et al. [6]
c-myc	Increased expression	Kraehn et al. [7]
CYLD	Decreased expression	Massoumi et al. [8]
EGFR (epidermal growth factor receptor)	Increased expression	Udart et al. [9]
ERK (extracellular signal-regulated kinase)	Absence of cytoplasmic ERK activation	Jovanovic et al. [10]
HER3	Increased expression	Reschke et al. [11]
HDM2 (human homologue of murine mdm2)	Increased expression	Polsky et al. [12]
ING3/ING4	Decreased nuclear expression	Wang et al. [13]
MITF (microphthalmia-associated transcription factor)	Gene amplification	Ugurel et al. [14]
P16^{INK4A}	Decreased expression	Mihic-Probst et al. [15] Alonso et al. [4]
p-Akt (activated serine-threonine protein kinase B)	Increased expression	Dai et al. [16]
pRb (retinoblastoma protein)	Inactivation due to protein phosphorylation	Roesch et al. [17]
PTEN	Decreased expression	Mikhail et al. [18]
SNF5	Loss of expression	Lin et al. [19]
Cell cycle-associated proteins		
Cyclin A, B, D, E	Increased expression	Florenes et al. [20] Florenes et al. [21]
Geminin	Increased expression	Winnepenninckx et al. [22]
Ki-67 (detected by MIB-1)	Increased expression	Gimotty et al. [23] Alonso et al. [4] Ostmeier et al. [24]
P21^{CIP1}	Decreased expression	Alonso et al. [4]
PCNA (proliferating cell nuclear antigen)	Increased expression	Winnepenninckx et al. [22]

(continued)

Table 2.1 (continued)

	Association with impaired prognosis	References
Regulators of apoptosis		
APAF-1 (Apoptotic protease activating factor-1)	Decreased expression	Fujimoto et al. [25]
Bak	Decreased expression	Fecker et al. [26]
Bax	Decreased expression	Fecker et al. [26]
bcl-2	Increased expression	Tas et al. [27]
Survivin	Increased expression	Tas et al. [27]
Molecules involved in angiogenesis		
LYVE-1 (lymphatic vascular endothelial hyaluronan receptor-1)	Increased expression	Dadras et al. [28]
PTN (pleiotrophin)	Increased expression	Wu et al. [29]
Molecules involved in cell adhesion and motility		
Beta-catenin	Loss of nuclear staining	Bachmann et al. [30]
CEACAM1 (carcinoembryonic-antigen-related cell-adhesion molecule 1)	Increased expression	Thies et al. [31]
Dysadherin	Increased expression	Nishizawa et al. [32]
E-cadherin	Decreased expression	Andersen et al. [33]
Integrins beta1 and beta3	Increased expression	Saalbach et al. [34]
MMPs (matrix metalloproteinases)	Increased expression	Redondo et al. [35]
Osteonectin [also termed BM40 or SPARC (secreted protein, acidic and rich in cysteine)]	Increased expression	Massi et al. [36]
P-cadherin	Strong cytoplasmic expression	Bachmann et al. [30]
Immunoregulators		
HLA allele frequency	Specific expression	Luongo et al. [37]
		Ostmeier et al. [24]
Others		
ALCAM/CD166 (Activated leukocyte cell adhesion molecule)	Increased expression	Swart et al. [38]
CXCR4 receptor	Increased expression	Scala et al. [39]
HSP90 (heat shock protein 90)	Increased expression	McCarthy et al. [40]
MCM4 and MCM6 (minichromosome maintenance complex component 4 and 6)	Increased expression	Winnepenninckx et al. [22]
Melastatin	Decreased expression	Duncan et al. [41]
Metallothionein	Increased expression	Weinlich et al. [42]
NCOA3 (nuclear receptor coactivator 3)	Increased expression	Kashani-Sabet et al. [43]
Nestin	Increased expression	Bakos et al. [44]
		Piras et al. [45]
Nodal	Increased expression	Strizzi et al. [46]
Nuclear 8-hydroxy-2'-deoxyguanosine	Increased expression	Murtas et al. [47]
Osteopontin (OPN, SPP1)	Increased expression	Rangel et al. [48]
		Kashani-Sabet et al. [43]
RGS1 (regulator of G-protein signaling 1)	Increased expression	Kashani-Sabet et al. [43]
Sox9 (sex determining region Y-box 9)	Increased expression	Bakos et al. [44]
TA (telomerase activity)	Increased expression	Carvalho et al. [49]

(HCAP-G and STK6), mitotic spindle checkpoint (BUB1), inhibition (BIRC5) or stimulation (GPR105) of apoptosis, DNA replication (TOP2A, RRM2, TYMS, PCNA, MCM4, and MCM6), stress response (GLRX2, DNAJA1, HSPA4, HSPA5, HSPD1, and TXNIP), ubiquitin cycle (SIP), actin and calmodulin binding (CNN3), intracellular signaling (STMN2), negative regulation of the Wnt signaling pathway (CTNNBIP1), inhibition of MITF expression (EMX2), regulation of proteolysis (TNA), testis cancer (CML66), and metastasis suppression (NME1). The authors speculated that the use of immunohistochemistry with antibodies directed against corresponding encoded proteins would facilitate improved prognostication of melanoma patients, and thereby allow for treatment stratification. In particular, determination of karyopherin-alpha2, MCMs (minichromosome maintenance proteins), geminin and PCNA could be used to screen for melanoma patients with poor clinical outcome.

In another recent study, Gould Rothberg et al. used a multimarker prognostic assay to help triage patients at increased risk of recurrent melanoma [50]. Protein expression for 38 candidate biomarkers relevant to melanoma oncogenesis was evaluated, using an automated quantitative analysis (AQUA) method for immunofluorescence-based testing in formalin-fixed paraffin-embedded (FFPE) specimens. A favorable prognosis was predicted by the expression of ATF2, p21(WAF1), p16(INK4A), beta-catenin and fibronectin. Primary tumors that met at least four of these five conditions were considered a low-risk group, and those that met three or fewer conditions formed a high-risk group for metastasis development.

Similarly, genetic abnormalities have recently been recognized to influence the prognosis of cancer patients. Indeed, a new classification system for melanoma that combines genetic aberrations with histomorphological characteristics has been proposed by Bastian et al. [51–53]. Of note, MITF gene copy number in tumor cells seems to be a useful prognostic marker in metastatic melanoma [14].

Moreover, it has recently been shown that an *in vitro* ATP-based chemosensitivity assay helps to differentiate between chemosensitive and chemoresistant melanoma patients, and can be used as a biomarker of chemotherapy response and survival outcome. A phase II study evaluating this assay in 53 patients with metastatic melanoma, followed by sensitivity-directed individualized chemotherapy, demonstrated that the chemosensitivity profile of an individual patient (reflected by the best individual chemosensitivity index [BICSI]) correlated with therapeutic outcome [54]. A surprisingly high proportion (~40%) of the investigated patient cohort were classified as chemosensitive, the remaining (~60%) classified as chemoresistant. Objective response was reported as 36.4% in chemosensitive patients compared to 16.1% in chemoresistant patients ($p=0.114$); progression arrest (CR+PR+SD) was 59.1% versus 22.6% ($p=0.01$). Chemosensitive patients showed an increased overall survival of 14.6 months compared to 7.4 months in their chemoresistant counterparts ($p=0.041$).

Serological Markers

Despite a large research effort, the prognosis of metastasized melanoma is still poor, and best results have been achieved in cases when the tumor is still amendable to surgical intervention. Thus, the search for reliable methods to detect early metastases and identify patients with high risk of disease progression who should undergo more vigorous follow-up is of major importance. Serological markers for tumor progression combine several advantages, such as the ease of obtaining serum samples and the availability of numerous methods to detect small molecules or proteins that correlate with tumor burden. Accordingly, several serological biomarkers have been established. In a number of European countries, the melanocyte lineage/differentiation antigens S100-beta and melanoma inhibitory activity (MIA) are routinely used for early detection of tumor relapse or metastasis during follow-up of melanoma patients (Table 2.2). Both

Table 2.2 Serologic markers of melanoma

	Serologic marker	References
Melanocyte lineage/ differentiation antigens	S100-beta	Guo et al. [55] Schultz et al. [56] Hauschild et al. [57] Krahn et al. [58] Garbe et al. [59]
	MIA (melanoma inhibitory activity)	Bogdahn et al. [60] Blesch et al. [61] Bosserhoff et al. [62] Stahlecker et al. [63] Garbe et al. [59]
	Tyrosinase	Agrup et al. [64]
	5-S-Cysteinyldopa	Wimmer et al. [65]
	L-dopa/L-tyrosine	Stoitchkov et al. [66]
Proangiogenic factors	VEGF (vascular endothelial growth factor)	Ugurel et al. [67]
	BFGF (basic fibroblast growth factor)	Ugurel et al. [67]
	IL-8 (interleukin-8)	Ugurel et al. [67]
Molecules involved in cell adhesion and motility	sICAM-1 (soluble intracellular adhesion molecule 1)	Hirai et al. [68] Vuoristo et al. [69]
	sVCAM (soluble vascular cell adhesion molecule 1)	Franzke et al. [70] Vuoristo et al. [69]
	Matrix metalloproteinases (MMP-1 and MMP-9)	Nikkola et al. [71]
	Tissue inhibitor of metalloproteinases (TIMP-1 and TIMP-2)	Yoshino et al. [72]
Cytokines and cytokine receptors	IL-6 (interleukin-6)	Mouawad et al. [73]
	IL-10 (interleukin-10)	Dummer et al. [74]
	sIL-2R (soluble interleukin-2-receptor)	Nemunaitis et al. [75] Boyano et al. [76]
HLA molecules	sHLA-DR (soluble HLA-DR)	Rebmann et al. [77]
	sHLA-class-I (soluble HLA-class I)	Westhoff et al. [78]
Others	LDH (lactate dehydrogenase)	Sirott et al. [79]
	CRP (C-reactive protein)	Deichmann et al. [80]
	Albumin	Sirott et al. [79]
	TuM2-PK (tumor pyruvate kinase type M2)	Ugurel et al. [81]
	CD95 (Fas)	Ugurel et al. [82]
	YKL-40	Schmidt et al. [83] Schmidt et al. [84]
	CYT-MAA (cytoplasmic melanoma-associated antigen)	Vergilis et al. [85]
	HMW-MAA (high-molecular-weight melanoma-associated antigen)	Vergilis et al. [85]
	sULBP2 (soluble UL16 binding protein 2)	Paschen et al. [86]
	TA90IC (tumor-associated antigen 90 immune complex)	Faries et al. [87]
	Serum amyloid A	Findeisen et al. [88]
	anti HERV-K antibodies	Hahn et al. [89]

proteins show high (but not exclusive) specificity for melanoma cells, and both correlate with the patient's tumor load.

The S100 protein is a 21-kd thermo-labile acidic dimeric protein which was originally isolated from the central nervous system. It consists of two subunits, alpha and beta in any pairing (i.e., alpha/alpha, alpha/beta, and beta/beta). It affects the assembly and disassembly of microtubules and also interacts in a calcium-dependent manner with p53, the product of a tumor suppressor gene. The beta subunit is expressed by cells of the central nervous system as well as cells of melanocytic lineage. Initially, the presence of S100-beta in the cerebrospinal fluid was used as a marker of central nervous system damage [90]. More recently, it was observed that S100-beta was elevated in the serum of melanoma patients [55].

MIA was originally detected in melanoma cell culture supernatants [60], and has been shown to exert an important role in cell-matrix-interaction and metastasis [61].

Studies comparing both these serum markers have demonstrated that S100-beta is superior to MIA as an early indicator of tumor progression, relapse or metastasis [58, 91]; hence, S100-beta is more often used in this setting [92]. Both markers have been shown to be useful prognostic markers in melanoma patients with distant metastases [56, 57], but have failed to provide prognostic significance in early stages of melanoma, especially in patients who are tumor-free after surgical excision [63]. Moreover, S100-beta fails to identify patients with lymph node micrometastases detected by sentinel lymph node biopsy [93]. Nonetheless, the correlation of serum S100 concentration with tumor load makes it a useful marker for monitoring therapeutic response in patients with advanced metastatic melanoma [57].

The strongest prognostic serum biomarker in advanced metastatic melanoma is lactate dehydrogenase (LDH), a nonspecific marker that indicates high tumor load in a variety of human tumors, including melanoma. Studies comparing LDH, S100-beta and MIA, using multivariate data analysis, showed that LDH was the strongest independent prognostic factor in stage IV melanoma patients [91]. Due to its high prognostic significance, in addition to its easy and cost-efficient detection, serum LDH is the only molecular marker that has been incorporated into the current melanoma staging and classification system of the American Joint Committee on Cancer (AJCC) [94]. In fact, it serves as a stratification parameter in most randomized clinical trials that test therapeutic interventions in advanced melanoma, and may also be used to monitor therapeutic response in these patients.

Other potential serum biomarkers have been reported to correlate with tumor load and disease progression in melanoma. These are related to different characteristic features of melanoma, such as melanocytic differentiation (i.e., tyrosinase), tumor angiogenesis (i.e., VEGF, bFGF, IL-8), cell adhesion and motility (i.e., ICAM-1, MMPs), cytokines and their receptors (i.e., IL-6, IL-10), antigen presentation (i.e., HLA molecules), tumor cell metabolism (i.e., TuM2-PK), apoptosis (i.e., Fas/CD95), and many others (Table 2.2). However, none of these markers has been demonstrated to be superior to S100-beta or LDH in reflecting the prognosis of patients with advanced stage disease. Moreover, these markers have also failed to be of prognostic relevance in early-stage tumor-free patients.

An innovative approach to identify novel, potentially better serological biomarkers in melanoma patients is serum proteomic profiling. This methodology offers the possibility of screening the whole serum proteome for markers which correlate with different criteria, such as prognostic significance and prediction of therapeutic response. Using this technology, marker proteins from thematic fields, that are different to those mentioned above, might be found and subsequently validated for their clinical utility. Studies have shown that stage I and stage IV melanoma patients can be differentiated by their serum proteomic profiles [95]. Another recent proteomic profiling study reported the identification of serum amyloid A as a new prognostic serum biomarker in melanoma patients [88].

Perspective

Melanoma is a highly aggressive form of skin cancer which is difficult to treat once the tumor has metastasized beyond the locoregional area. Established biomarkers include the morphological and histopathological characteristics of the primary tumor. More recently, molecular biomarkers have been identified, facilitating more detailed diagnostic and prognostic categorization of melanoma patients and allowing for stratified or even personalized therapy.

References

1. Ohsie SJ, Sarantopoulos GP, Cochran AJ, Binder SW. Immunohistochemical characteristics of melanoma. J Cutan Pathol. 2008;35:433–44.
2. Niezabitowski A, Czajecki K, Rys J, Kruczak A, Gruchała A, Wasilewska A, Lackowska B, Sokołowski A,

Szklarski W. Prognostic evaluation of cutaneous malignant melanoma: a clinicopathologic and immunohistochemical study. J Surg Oncol. 1999;70:150–60.
3. Berger AJ, Davis DW, Tellez C, Prieto VG, Gershenwald JE, Johnson MM, Rimm DL, Bar-Eli M. Automated quantitative analysis of activator protein-2alpha subcellular expression in melanoma tissue microarrays correlates with survival prediction. Cancer Res. 2005;65:11185–92.
4. Alonso SR, Ortiz P, Pollan M, Perez-Gomez B, Sanchez L, Acuna MJ, Pajares R, Martinez-Tello FJ, Hortelano CM, Piris MA, Rodriguez-Peralto JL. Progression in cutaneous malignant melanoma is associated with distinct expression profiles: a tissue microarray-based study. Am J Pathol. 2004;164:193–203.
5. Janku F, Novotny J, Julis I, Julisova I, Pecen L, Tomancova V, Kocmanova G, Krasna L, Krajsova I, Stork J, Petruzelka L. KIT receptor is expressed in more than 50% of early-stage malignant melanoma: a retrospective study of 261 patients. Melanoma Res. 2005;15:251–6.
6. Cruz J, Reis-Filho JS, Silva P, Lopes JM. Expression of c-met tyrosine kinase receptor is biologically and prognostically relevant for primary cutaneous malignant melanomas. Oncology. 2003;65:72–82.
7. Kraehn GM, Utikal J, Udart M, Greulich KM, Bezold G, Kaskel P, Leiter U, Peter RU. Extra c-myc oncogene copies in high risk cutaneous malignant melanoma and melanoma metastases. Br J Cancer. 2001;84:72–9.
8. Massoumi R, Kuphal S, Hellerbrand C, Haas B, Wild P, Spruss T, Pfeifer A, Fässler R, Bosserhoff AK. Down-regulation of CYLD expression by snail promotes tumor progression in malignant melanoma. J Exp Med. 2009;206:221–32.
9. Udart M, Utikal J, Krahn GM, Peter RU. Chromosome 7 aneusomy. A marker for metastatic melanoma? Expression of the epidermal growth factor receptor gene and chromosome 7 aneusomy in nevi, primary malignant melanomas and metastases. Neoplasia. 2001;3:245–54.
10. Jovanovic B, Kröckel D, Linden D, Nilsson B, Egyhazi S, Hansson J. Lack of cytoplasmic ERK activation is an independent adverse prognostic factor in primary cutaneous melanoma. J Invest Dermatol. 2008;128:2696–704.
11. Reschke M, Mihic-Probst D, van der Horst EH, Knyazev P, Wild PJ, Hutterer M, Meyer S, Dummer R, Moch H, Ullrich A. HER3 is a determinant for poor prognosis in melanoma. Clin Cancer Res. 2008;14:5188–97.
12. Polsky D, Melzer K, Hazan C, Panageas KS, Busam K, Drobnjak M, Kamino H, Spira JG, Kopf AW, Houghton A, Cordon-Cardo C, Osman I. HDM2 protein overexpression and prognosis in primary malignant melanoma. J Natl Cancer Inst. 2002;94:1803–6.
13. Wang Y, Dai DL, Martinka M, Li G. Prognostic significance of nuclear ING3 expression in human cutaneous melanoma. Clin Cancer Res. 2007;13:4111–6.
14. Ugurel S, Houben R, Schrama D, Voigt H, Zapatka M, Schadendorf D, Bröcker EB, Becker JC. Microphthalmia-associated transcription factor gene amplification in metastatic melanoma is a prognostic marker for patient survival, but not a predictive marker for chemosensitivity and chemotherapy response. Clin Cancer Res. 2007;13:6344–50.
15. Mihic-Probst D, Mnich CD, Oberholzer PA, Seifert B, Sasse B, Moch H, Dummer R. p16 expression in primary malignant melanoma is associated with prognosis and lymph node status. Int J Cancer. 2006;118:2262–8.
16. Dai DL, Martinka M, Li G. Prognostic significance of activated Akt expression in melanoma: a clinicopathologic study of 292 cases. J Clin Oncol. 2005;23:1473–82.
17. Roesch A, Becker B, Meyer S, Hafner C, Wild PJ, Landthaler M, Vogt T. Overexpression and hyperphosphorylation of retinoblastoma protein in the progression of malignant melanoma. Mod Pathol. 2005;18:565–72.
18. Mikhail M, Velazquez E, Shapiro R, Berman R, Pavlick A, Sorhaindo L, Spira J, Mir C, Panageas KS, Polsky D, Osman I. PTEN expression in melanoma: relationship with patient survival, Bcl-2 expression, and proliferation. Clin Cancer Res. 2005;11:5153–7.
19. Lin H, Wong RP, Martinka M, Li G. Loss of SNF5 expression correlates with poor patient survival in melanoma. Clin Cancer Res. 2009;15:6404–11.
20. Florenes VA, Faye RS, Maelandsmo GM, Nesland JM, Holm R. Levels of cyclin D1 and D3 in malignant melanoma: deregulated cyclin D3 expression is associated with poor clinical outcome in superficial melanoma. Clin Cancer Res. 2000;6:3614–20.
21. Florenes VA, Maelandsmo GM, Faye R, Nesland JM, Holm R. Cyclin A expression in superficial spreading malignant melanomas correlates with clinical outcome. J Pathol. 2001;195:530–6.
22. Winnepenninckx V, Lazar V, Michiels S, Dessen P, Stas M, Alonso SR, Avril MF, Ortiz Romero PL, Robert T, Balacescu O, Eggermont AM, Lenoir G, Sarasin A, Tursz T, van den Oord JJ, Spatz A, Melanoma Group of the European Organization for Research and Treatment of Cancer. Gene expression profiling of primary cutaneous melanoma and clinical outcome. J Natl Cancer Inst. 2006;98:472–82.
23. Gimotty PA, Van Belle P, Elder DE, Murry T, Montone KT, Xu X, Hotz S, Raines S, Ming ME, Wahl P, Guerry D. Biologic and prognostic significance of dermal Ki67 expression, mitoses, and tumorigenicity in thin invasive cutaneous melanoma. J Clin Oncol. 2005;23:8048–56.
24. Ostmeier H, Fuchs B, Otto F, Mawick R, Lippold A, Krieg V, Suter L. Prognostic immunohistochemical markers of primary human melanomas. Br J Dermatol. 2001;145:203–9.
25. Fujimoto A, Takeuchi H, Taback B, Hsueh EC, Elashoff D, Morton DL, Hoon DS. Allelic imbalance of 12q22-23 associated with APAF-1 locus correlates with poor disease outcome in cutaneous melanoma. Cancer Res. 2004;64:2245–50.

26. Fecker LF, Geilen CC, Tchernev G, Trefzer U, Assaf C, Kurbanov BM, Schwarz C, Daniel PT, Eberle J. Loss of proapoptotic Bcl-2-related multidomain proteins in primary melanomas is associated with poor prognosis. J Invest Dermatol. 2006;126:1366–71.
27. Tas F, Duranyildiz D, Argon A, et al. Serum bcl-2 and survivin levels in melanoma. Melanoma Res. 2004;14:543–6.
28. Dadras SS, Paul T, Bertoncini J, et al. Tumor lymphangiogenesis: a novel prognostic indicator for cutaneous melanoma metastasis and survival. Am J Pathol. 2003;162:1951–60.
29. Wu H, Barusevicius A, Babb J, et al. Pleiotrophin expression correlates with melanocytic tumor progression and metastatic potential. J Cutan Pathol. 2005;32:125–30.
30. Bachmann IM, Straume O, Puntervoll HE, Kalvenes MB, Akslen LA. Importance of P-cadherin, beta-catenin, and Wnt5a/frizzled for progression of melanocytic tumors and prognosis in cutaneous melanoma. Clin Cancer Res. 2005;11:8606–14.
31. Thies A, Moll I, Berger J, et al. CEACAM1 expression in cutaneous malignant melanoma predicts the development of metastatic disease. J Clin Oncol. 2002;20:2530.
32. Nishizawa A, Nakanishi Y, Yoshimura K, et al. Clinicopathologic significance of dysadherin expression in cutaneous malignant melanoma: immunohistochemical analysis of 115 patients. Cancer. 2005;103:1693–700.
33. Andersen K, Nesland JM, Holm R, Florenes VA, Fodstad O, Maelandsmo GM. Expression of S100A4 combined with reduced E-cadherin expression predicts patient outcome in malignant melanoma. Mod Pathol. 2004;17:990–7.
34. Saalbach A, Wetzel A, Haustein UF, Sticherling M, Simon JC, Anderegg U. Interaction of human Thy-1 (CD90) with the integrin $\alpha_v\beta_3$ (CD51/CD61): an important mechanism mediating melanoma cell adhesion to activated endothelium. Oncogene. 2005;24:4710–20.
35. Redondo P, Lloret P, Idoate M, Inoges S. Expression and serum levels of MMP-2 and MMP-9 during human melanoma progression. Clin Exp Dermatol. 2005;30:541–5.
36. Massi D, Franchi A, Borgognoni L, Reali UM, Santucci M. Osteonectin expression correlates with clinical outcome in thin cutaneous malignant melanomas. Hum Pathol. 1999;30:339–44.
37. Luongo V, Pirozzi G, Caraco C, Errico S, de Angelis F, Celentano E, Paino F, Chiofalo MG, Luongo M, Mozzillo N, Lombardi ML. HLA allele frequency and clinical outcome in Italian patients with cutaneous melanoma. Tissue Antigens. 2004;64:84–7.
38. Swart GW, Lunter PC, Kilsdonk JW, Kempen LC. Activated leukocyte cell adhesion molecule (ALCAM/CD166): signaling at the divide of melanoma cell clustering and cell migration? Cancer Metastasis Rev. 2005;24:223–36.
39. Scala S, Ottaiano A, Ascierto PA, et al. Expression of CXCR4 predicts poor prognosis in patients with malignant melanoma. Clin Cancer Res. 2005;11:1835–41.
40. McCarthy MM, Pick E, Kluger Y, Gould-Rothberg B, Lazova R, Camp RL, Rimm DL, Kluger HM. HSP90 as a marker of progression in melanoma. Ann Oncol. 2008;19:590–4.
41. Duncan LM, Deeds J, Hunter J, et al. Down-regulation of the novel gene melastatin correlates with potential for melanoma metastasis. Cancer Res. 1998;58:1515–20.
42. Weinlich G, Eisendle K, Hassler E, Baltaci M, Fritsch PO, Zelger B. Metallothionein - overexpression as a highly significant prognostic factor in melanoma: a prospective study on 1270 patients. Br J Cancer. 2006;94:835–41.
43. Kashani-Sabet M, Venna S, Nosrati M, Rangel J, Sucker A, Egberts F, Baehner FL, Simko J, Leong SP, Haqq C, Hauschild A, Schadendorf D, Miller 3rd JR, Sagebiel RW. A multimarker prognostic assay for primary cutaneous melanoma. Clin Cancer Res. 2009;15:6987–92.
44. Bakos RM, Maier T, Besch R, Mestel DS, Ruzicka T, Sturm RA, Berking C. Nestin and SOX9 and SOX10 transcription factors are coexpressed in melanoma. Exp Dermatol. 2010;19:e89–94.
45. Piras F, Perra MT, Murtas D, Minerba L, Floris C, Maxia C, Demurtas P, Ugalde J, Ribatti D, Sirigu P. The stem cell marker nestin predicts poor prognosis in human melanoma. Oncol Rep. 2010;23:17–24.
46. Strizzi L, Postovit LM, Margaryan NV, Lipavsky A, Gadiot J, Blank C, Seftor RE, Seftor EA, Hendrix MJ. Nodal as a biomarker for melanoma progression and a new therapeutic target for clinical intervention. Expert Rev Dermatol. 2009;4:67–78.
47. Murtas D, Piras F, Minerba L, Ugalde J, Floris C, Maxia C, Demurtas P, Perra MT, Sirigu P. Nuclear 8-hydroxy-2'-deoxyguanosine as survival biomarker in patients with cutaneous melanoma. Oncol Rep. 2010;23:329–35.
48. Rangel J, Nosrati M, Torabian S, Shaikh L, Leong SP, Haqq C, Miller 3rd JR, Sagebiel RW, Kashani-Sabet M. Osteopontin as a molecular prognostic marker for melanoma. Cancer. 2008;112:144–50.
49. Carvalho L, Lipay M, Belfort F, Santos I, Andrade J, Haddad A, Brunstein F, Ferreira L. Telomerase activity in prognostic histopathologic features of melanoma. J Plast Reconstr Aesthet Surg. 2006;59:961–8.
50. Gould Rothberg BE, Berger AJ, Molinaro AM, Subtil A, Krauthammer MO, Camp RL, Bradley WR, Ariyan S, Kluger HM, Rimm DL. Melanoma prognostic model using tissue microarrays and genetic algorithms. J Clin Oncol. 2009;27:5772–80.
51. Curtin JA, Fridlyand J, Kageshita T, Patel HN, Busam KJ, Kutzner H, Cho KH, Aiba S, Bröcker EB, LeBoit PE, Pinkel D, Bastian BC. Distinct sets of genetic alterations in melanoma. N Engl J Med. 2005;353:2135–47.

52. Curtin JA, Busam K, Pinkel D, Bastian BC. Somatic activation of KIT in distinct subtypes of melanoma. J Clin Oncol. 2006;24:4340–6.
53. Viros A, Fridlyand J, Bauer J, Lasithiotakis K, Garbe C, Pinkel D, Bastian BC. Improving melanoma classification by integrating genetic and morphologic features. PLoS Med. 2008;5:e120.
54. Ugurel S, Schadendorf D, Pfoehler C, Neuber K, Thoelke A, Ulrich J, Hauschild A, Spieth K, Kaatz M, Rittgen W, Delorme S, Tilgen W, Reinhold U. In vitro drug sensitivity predicts response and survival after individualized sensitivity-directed chemotherapy in metastatic melanoma: a multicenter phase II trial of the Dermatologic Cooperative Oncology Group. Clin Cancer Res. 2006;12:5454–63.
55. Guo HB, Stoffel-Wagner B, Bierwirth T, Mezger J, Klingmüller D. Clinical significance of serum S100 in metastatic malignant melanoma. Eur J Cancer. 1995; 31A:1898–902.
56. Schultz ES, Diepgen TL, Von Den Driesch P. Clinical and prognostic relevance of serum S-100 beta protein in malignant melanoma. Br J Dermatol. 1998;138: 426–30.
57. Hauschild A, Engel G, Brenner W, Glaeser R, Moenig H, Henze E, Christophers E. Predictive value of serum S100B for monitoring patients with metastatic melanoma during chemotherapy and/or immunotherapy. Br J Dermatol. 1999;140:1065–71.
58. Krahn G, Kaskel P, Sander S, Waizenhofer PJ, Wortmann S, Leiter U, Peter RU. S100 beta is a more reliable tumor marker in peripheral blood for patients with newly occurred melanoma metastases compared with MIA, albumin and lactate-dehydrogenase. Anticancer Res. 2001;21:1311–6.
59. Garbe C, Leiter U, Ellwanger U, Blaheta HJ, Meier F, Rassner G, Schittek B. Diagnostic value and prognostic significance of protein S-100beta, melanoma-inhibitory activity, and tyrosinase/MART-1 reverse transcription-polymerase chain reaction in the follow-up of high-risk melanoma patients. Cancer. 2003;97: 1737–45.
60. Bogdahn U, Apfel R, Hahn M, Gerlach M, Behl C, Hoppe J, Martin R. Autocrine tumor cell growth-inhibiting activities from human malignant melanoma. Cancer Res. 1989;49:5358–63.
61. Blesch A, Bosserhoff AK, Apfel R, Behl C, Hessdoerfer B, Schmitt A, Jachimczak P, Lottspeich F, Buettner R, Bogdahn U. Cloning of a novel malignant melanoma-derived growth-regulatory protein, MIA. Cancer Res. 1994;54:5695–701.
62. Bosserhoff AK, Kaufmann M, Kaluza B, et al. Melanoma-inhibitory activity, a novel serum marker for progression of malignant melanoma. Cancer Res. 1997;57:3149–53.
63. Stahlecker J, Gauger A, Bosserhoff A, Büttner R, Ring J, Hein R. MIA as a reliable tumor marker in the serum of patients with malignant melanoma. Anticancer Res. 2000;20:5041–4.
64. Agrup P, Carstam R, Wittbjer A, Rorsman H, Rosengren E. Tyrosinase activity in serum from patients with malignant melanoma. Acta Derm Venereol. 1989;69:120–4.
65. Wimmer I, Meyer JC, Seifert B, Dummer R, Flace A, Burg G. Prognostic value of serum 5-S-cysteinyldopa for monitoring human metastatic melanoma during immunochemotherapy. Cancer Res. 1997;57:5073–6.
66. Stoitchkov K, Letellier S, Garnier JP, et al. Evaluation of the serum L-dopa/L-tyrosine ratio as a melanoma marker. Melanoma Res. 2003;13:587–93.
67. Ugurel S, Rappl G, Tilgen W, Reinhold U. Increased serum concentration of angiogenic factors in malignant melanoma patients correlates with tumor progression and survival. J Clin Oncol. 2001;19:577–83.
68. Hirai S, Kageshita T, Kimura T, et al. Serum levels of sICAM-1 and 5-S-cysteinyldopa as markers of melanoma progression. Melanoma Res. 1997;7:58–62.
69. Vuoristo MS, Laine S, Huhtala H, et al. Serum adhesion molecules and interleukin-2 receptor as markers of tumour load and prognosis in advanced cutaneous melanoma. Eur J Cancer. 2001;37:1629–34.
70. Franzke A, Probst-Kepper M, Buer J, et al. Elevated pretreatment serum levels of soluble vascular cell adhesion molecule 1 and lactate dehydrogenase as predictors of survival in cutaneous metastatic malignant melanoma. Br J Cancer. 1998;78:40–5.
71. Nikkola J, Vihinen P, Vuoristo MS, Kellokumpu-Lehtinen P, Kahari VM, Pyrhonen S. High serum levels of matrix metalloproteinase-9 and matrix metalloproteinase-1 are associated with rapid progression in patients with metastatic melanoma. Clin Cancer Res. 2005;11:5158–66.
72. Yoshino Y, Kageshita T, Nakajima M, Funakubo M, Ihn H. Clinical relevance of serum levels of matrix metallopeptidase-2, and tissue inhibitor of metalloproteinase-1 and −2 in patients with malignant melanoma. J Dermatol. 2008;35:206–14.
73. Mouawad R, Benhammouda A, Rixe O, et al. Endogenous interleukin 6 levels in patients with metastatic malignant melanoma: correlation with tumor burden. Clin Cancer Res. 1996;2:1405–9.
74. Dummer W, Becker JC, Schwaaf A, Leverkus M, Moll T, Brocker EB. Elevated serum levels of interleukin-10 in patients with metastatic malignant melanoma. Melanoma Res. 1995;5:67–8.
75. Nemunaitis J, Fong T, Shabe P, Martineau D, Ando D. Comparison of serum interleukin-10 (IL-10) levels between normal volunteers and patients with advanced melanoma. Cancer Invest. 2001;19:239–47.
76. Boyano MD, Garcia-Vazquez MD, Lopez-Michelena T, et al. Soluble interleukin-2 receptor, intercellular adhesion molecule-1 and interleukin-10 serum levels in patients with melanoma. Br J Cancer. 2000;83:847–52.
77. Rebmann V, Ugurel S, Tilgen W, Reinhold U, Grosse-Wilde H. Soluble HLA-DR is a potent predictive indicator of disease progression in serum from early-stage melanoma patients. Int J Cancer. 2002;100:580–5.

78. Westhoff U, Fox C, Otto FJ. Soluble HLA class I antigens in plasma of patients with malignant melanoma. Anticancer Res. 1998;18:3789–92.
79. Sirott MN, Bajorin DF, Wong GY, Tao Y, Chapman PB, Templeton MA, Houghton AN. Prognostic factors in patients with metastatic malignant melanoma. A multivariate analysis. Cancer. 1993;72:3091–8.
80. Deichmann M, Kahle B, Moser K, Wacker J, Wust K. Diagnosing melanoma patients entering American Joint Committee on Cancer stage IV, C-reactive protein in serum is superior to lactate dehydrogenase. Br J Cancer. 2004;91:699–702.
81. Ugurel S, Bell N, Sucker A, Zimpfer A, Rittgen W, Schadendorf D. Tumor type M2 pyruvate kinase (TuM2-PK) as a novel plasma tumor marker in melanoma. Int J Cancer. 2005;117:825–30.
82. Ugurel S, Rappl G, Tilgen W, Reinhold U. Increased soluble CD95 (sFas/CD95) serum level correlates with poor prognosis in melanoma patients. Clin Cancer Res. 2001;7:1282–6.
83. Schmidt H, Johansen JS, Sjoegren P, Christensen IJ, Sorensen BS, Fode K, Larsen J, von der Maase H. Serum YKL-40 predicts relapse-free and overall survival in patients with American Joint Committee on Cancer stage I and II melanoma. J Clin Oncol. 2006;24:798–804.
84. Schmidt H, Johansen JS, Gehl J, Geertsen PF, Fode K, von der Maase H. Elevated serum level of YKL-40 is an independent prognostic factor for poor survival in patients with metastatic melanoma. Cancer. 2006;106:1130–9.
85. Vergilis IJ, Szarek M, Ferrone S, Reynolds SR. Presence and prognostic significance of melanoma-associated antigens CYT-MAA and HMW-MAA in serum of patients with melanoma. J Invest Dermatol. 2005;125:526–31.
86. Paschen A, Sucker A, Hill B, Moll I, Zapatka M, Nguyen XD, Sim GC, Gutmann I, Hassel J, Becker JC, Steinle A, Schadendorf D, Ugurel S. Differential clinical significance of individual NKG2D ligands in melanoma: soluble ULBP2 as an indicator of poor prognosis superior to S100B. Clin Cancer Res. 2009;15:5208–15.
87. Faries MB, Gupta RK, Ye X, Lee C, Yee R, Leopoldo Z, Essner R, Foshag LJ, Elashoff D, Morton DL. A Comparison of 3 tumor markers (MIA, TA90IC, S100B) in stage III melanoma patients. Cancer Invest. 2007;25:285–93.
88. Findeisen P, Zapatka M, Peccerella T, Matzk H, Neumaier M, Schadendorf D, Ugurel S. Serum amyloid A as a prognostic marker in melanoma identified by proteomic profiling. J Clin Oncol. 2009;27: 2199–208.
89. Hahn S, Ugurel S, Hanschmann KM, Strobel H, Tondera C, Schadendorf D, Löwer J, Löwer R. Serological response to human endogenous retrovirus K in melanoma patients correlates with survival probability. AIDS Res Hum Retroviruses. 2008;24: 717–23.
90. Persson L, Hårdemark HG, Gustafsson J, Rundström G, Mendel-Hartvig I, Esscher T, Påhlman S. S-100 protein and neuron-specific enolase in cerebrospinal fluid and serum: markers of cell damage in human central nervous system. Stroke. 1987;18: 911–8.
91. Deichmann M, Benner A, Bock M, Jäckel A, Uhl K, Waldmann V, Näher H. S100-Beta, melanoma-inhibiting activity, and lactate dehydrogenase discriminate progressive from nonprogressive American Joint Committee on Cancer stage IV melanoma. J Clin Oncol. 1999;17:1891–6.
92. Jury CS, McAllister EJ, MacKie RM. Rising levels of serum S100 protein precede other evidence of disease progression in patients with malignant melanoma. Br J Dermatol. 2000;143:269–74.
93. Acland K, Evans AV, Abraha H, Healy CM, Roblin P, Calonje E, Orchard G, Higgins E, Sherwood R, Russell-Jones R. Serum S100 concentrations are not useful in predicting micrometastatic disease in cutaneous malignant melanoma. Br J Dermatol. 2002;146:832–5.
94. Balch CM, Gershenwald JE, Soong SJ, et al. Final version of 2009 AJCC melanoma staging and classification. J Clin Oncol. 2009;27:6199–206.
95. Mian S, Ugurel S, Parkinson E, Schlenzka I, Dryden I, Lancashire L, Ball G, Creaser C, Rees R, Schadendorf D. Serum proteomic fingerprinting discriminates between clinical stages and predicts disease progression in melanoma patients. J Clin Oncol. 2005;23:5088–93.

Molecular Pathogenesis of Melanoma: Established and Novel Pathways

3

Paolo Antonio Ascierto, Maria Libera Ascierto, Mariaelena Capone, Zendee Elaba, Michael J. Murphy, and Giuseppe Palmieri

Introduction

Melanoma is the eighth most common malignancy in the USA and has shown a rapid increase in its incidence rate over the past two decades, especially for early-stage disease [1–4]. A recent analysis of data from the Surveillance Epidemiology and End Results (SEER) Program indicates that the incidence of melanoma increases with age, showing somewhat different patterns in men and women [3]. This cancer arises from melanocytes, which are specialized pigmented cells that are predominantly found in the skin and eyes, where they produce melanin, the pigment responsible for skin and hair color. Cutaneous melanocytes originate from highly motile neural crest progenitors that migrate to the skin during embryonic development. In the skin, melanocytes reside in the basal layer of the epidermis and hair follicles, and their homeostasis is regulated by epidermal keratinocytes [1]. In response to ultraviolet (UV) radiation, keratinocytes secrete factors that regulate melanocyte survival, differentiation, proliferation and motility, stimulating melanocytes to produce melanin and resulting in the tanning response. Accordingly, melanocytes play a key role in protecting our skin from the damaging effects of UV radiation and in preventing skin cancer. Individuals with pigmentary disorders, such as vitiligo and albinism, lack functional melanocytes and are hypersensitive to UV radiation vis-à-vis critical growth regulatory genes; the production of autocrine growth factors and the loss of adhesion receptors all contribute to disrupted intracellular signaling in melanocytes, allowing them to escape their tight regulation by keratinocytes [4]. Consequently, melanocytes can proliferate and migrate, leading to the formation of a nevus or common mole. Melanocytic proliferation can be restricted to the epidermis (junctional nevus), the

---

P.A. Ascierto, M.D. (✉) • M.L. Ascierto, Ph.D.
• M. Capone, Ph.D.
Unit of Medical Oncology and Innovative Therapy,
Istituto Nazionale Tumori Fondazione "G. Pascale",
Naples, Italy
e-mail: paolo.ascierto@gmail.com

Z. Elaba, M.D.
Department of Pathology, Hartford Hospital,
Hartford, CT, USA

M.J. Murphy, M.D.
Department of Dermatology, University
of Connecticut Health Center, Farmington, CT, USA

G. Palmieri, M.D., Ph.D.
Unit of Cancer Genetics, Institute
of Biomolecular Chemistry, National Research
Council (CNR), Sassari, Italy

dermis (intradermal nevus) or show combined components (compound nevus). Melanocytic nevi are benign, but can rarely show transformation to radial growth phase (RGP) melanoma, an intraepidermal lesion that may demonstrate focal microinvasion of the dermis. RGP cells can progress to vertical growth phase (VGP), with nodules or nests of malignant cells invading the dermis, a more dangerous stage in which the cells have metastatic potential. Not all melanomas pass through each of these individually distinct phases – RGP or VGP can both develop directly from isolated melanocytes or nevi, and both can progress directly to metastatic disease [5]. Exposure to UV radiation is an important causative factor for melanocytic transformation; although, the relationship between risk and exposure is complex. Intermittent sun exposure and sunburn history have been identified from epidemiological studies as important risk factors for the development of melanoma [5].

The pathogenic effects of sun exposure can involve genotoxic, mitogenic, or immunosuppressive responses to UVB- and/or UVA-induced damage in the skin [6, 7]. It is unclear whether the UVB or UVA component of solar radiation is more important in melanoma development [8, 9]. One of the major reasons for this uncertainty is that sunlight is a complex and changing mix of different UV wavelengths, so it is very difficult to accurately delineate the precise lifetime exposures of individuals and entire populations to UVB and UVA from available surrogates, such as latitude at diagnosis or exposure questionnaires [10]. A significant body of epidemiological evidence suggests that both UVB and UVA are involved in melanoma pathogenesis [11–13].

Molecular Pathways Involved in Melanoma

The clinical heterogeneity of melanoma has been historically explained by the existence of four distinct subtypes of this tumor with different susceptibilities to UV radiation: superficial spreading melanoma, nodular melanoma, acral lentiginous melanoma, and lentigo maligna melanoma [14].

However, melanoma is a complex genetic disease and notoriously resistant to current therapies. Therefore, the future successful management of this disease will require an in-depth understanding of the biology underlying its initiation and progression. This will allow improved staging and subtype classification, and will lead to the design of better therapeutic approaches and agents. Comprehensive testing strategies, such as comparative genomic hybridization and gene mutational analysis using DNA sequencing, have identified some of the crucial cell signaling pathways in melanoma, as discussed below (Table 3.1 and Figs. 3.1 and 3.2).

Table 3.1 Genetic aberrations in melanoma according to anatomical location (Adapted from Gerami et al. [2])

Melanoma subtype	Predominant histopathological subtype	BRAF mutation (%)	NRAS mutation (%)	KIT mutation/ amplification (%)	Chromosomal alterations
Melanoma on NCSD skin	SSM	59	22	0	Gain on 6p,7,8q,17q,20q Loss on 9p,10,21q
Melanoma on CSD skin	LMM	11	15	2–17	Gain on 6p,11q13,17q,20q Loss on 6q,8p,9p,13,21q
Acral melanoma	ALM	23	10	7–23	Gain on 6p,7,8q,17q,20q Amplification on 5p13,5p15,11q13,12q14 Loss on 6q,9p,10,11q,21q
Mucosal melanoma	Unspecified	11	5	8–21	Gain on 1q,6p,7,8q,11q13,17q,20q Amplification on 1q31,4q12,12q14 Loss on 3q,4q,6q,8p,9p,10,11p,11q,21q

NCSD non-chronic sun-damaged, *CSD* chronic sun-damaged, *SSM* superficial spreading melanoma, *LMM* lentigo maligna melanoma, *ALM* acral lentiginous melanoma

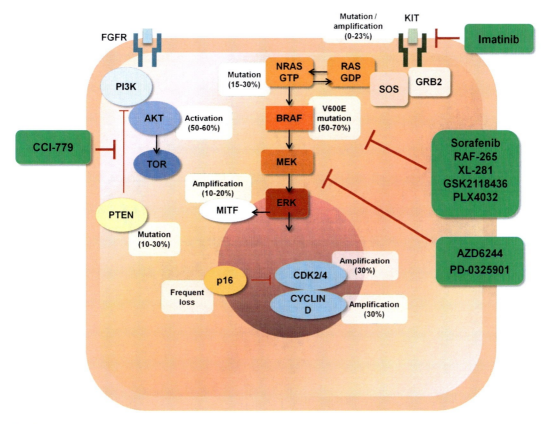

Fig. 3.1 Established molecular pathways in melanoma. The identification of recurrent aberrations in signaling pathways, such as mitogen-activated protein kinase (MAPK; RAS/RAF/MEK/ERK), KIT and PI3K-AKT, is promoting the development of targeted therapies for melanoma (*green boxes*) (Modified from Gerami et al. [2]. Reprinted with permission from Springer, Copyright © 2011)

Established Pathways

RAS/RAF/MEK/ERK Signaling

RAS and BRAF are two important molecules belonging to the mitogen-activated protein kinase (MAPK) signal transduction pathway, which regulates cell growth, survival, and invasion (Fig. 3.1). MAPK signaling is initiated at the cell membrane, either by the binding of receptor tyrosine kinases (RTKs) to ligand(s) or integrin adhesion to the extracellular matrix, with transmission of activation signals via RAS-GTPase on the inner surface of the cell membrane. Active, GTP-bound RAS binds to effector proteins, such as RAF serine-threonine kinase or phosphatidylinositol 3-kinase (PI3K) [15, 16].

The most commonly mutated component of this pathway is BRAF, one of the three human RAF genes (together with ARAF and CRAF). The most common mutation in the BRAF gene (~90% of cases) results in the substitution of valine with glutamic acid at position 600 (V600E) [17]. $BRAF^{V600E}$ induces constitutive ERK signaling, stimulating proliferation and survival, and providing essential tumor growth and maintenance functions [18]. $BRAF^{V600E}$ also contributes to neo-angiogenesis by stimulating autocrine vascular endothelial growth factor (VEGF) secretion [19]. Recent studies have identified several genes in melanoma that function downstream of BRAF. These include those encoding: the transcription factors MITF (microphthalmia-associated transcription factor) [20] and BRN-2 (POU domain class 3 transcription factor) [18]; the cell cycle regulators cyclin D1 [21] and $p16^{CDKN2A}$ [22, 23]; and the tumor maintenance enzymes, matrix

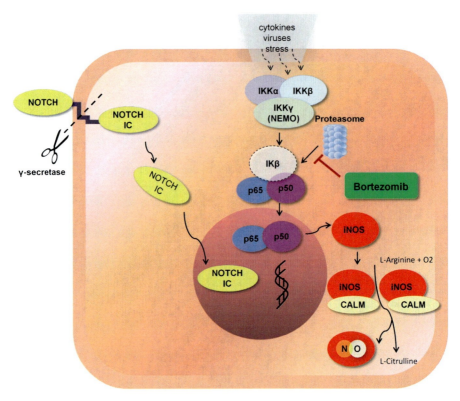

Fig. 3.2 Novel molecular pathways in melanoma. The identification of novel aberrations in signaling pathways, such as Notch, NF-κB and iNOS, is promoting the development of targeted therapies for melanoma (*green box*)

metalloproteinase-1 [24] and inducible nitric oxide synthase (iNOS) [25]. Thus, BRAF is implicated in several aspects of melanoma induction and progression; although, the presence of BRAF mutations in melanocytic nevi strongly suggests that BRAF activation is necessary, but not sufficient for the development of melanoma (also known as melanomagenesis). As evidence for a role of activated BRAF in melanocytic proliferation and transformation, a transgenic zebrafish expressing BRAF^{V600E} has been shown to develop patches of ectopic melanocytes (termed fish-nevi) [26].

Remarkably, the presence of activated BRAF in p53-deficient zebrafish leads to the formation of melanocytic lesions that rapidly develop into invasive melanomas, which resemble human melanomas in terms of histopathological features and biological behavior [27]. These data provide direct evidence that the p53 and BRAF pathways functionally interact to induce melanomagenesis.

BRAF also cooperates with the CDKN2A gene, which encodes two proteins: (1) the cyclin-dependent kinase inhibitor p16^{CDKN2A}, which is a component of the cyclin D1-RB pathway, and (2) the tumor suppressor p14^{ARF}, which has been functionally linked to the Murine Double Minute (MDM2)-p53 pathway (see below). Activating BRAF mutations are reported to constitutively induce up-regulation of p16^{CDKN2A}, leading to cell cycle arrest (this phenomenon appears to be a protective response to inappropriate mitogenic signals). In particular, mutant BRAF protein induces cellular senescence by increasing the expression levels of p16^{CDKN2A} protein, which in turn may limit the cellular proliferation caused by mutations of BRAF [23].

However, while BRAF mutation appears to be an early and important event in the development of melanocytic tumors, it is not sufficient for malignant transformation (i.e., melanoma). In this regard, up to 80% of benign melanocytic nevi may demonstrate mutations of BRAF. Recently, it has been demonstrated that other factors, such as those regulated by the IGFBP7 protein, may participate in the cell cycle arrest and cellular senescence caused by BRAF activation

[27–29]. As for p53 deficiency, genetic and/or epigenetic inactivation of the p16^{CDKN2A} gene and/or alterations of additional cell cycle-related factors may contribute to BRAF-driven melanocytic proliferation.

The first BRAF inhibitor used in clinical trials was sorafenib (BAY43-9006), an oral multikinase inhibitor that decreases the activity of not only RAF, but also VEGF receptor -1, -2 and -3, PDGFR, Flt-3, p38, c-KIT, and FGFR-1, theoretically inhibiting both tumor cell growth and angiogenesis (Fig. 3.1) [30]. However, while sorafenib inhibits the growth of melanoma xenografts in mice [20], it has shown little or no antitumor activity in advanced melanoma patients if used as a single agent [31]. To improve the efficacy of sorafenib in this setting, it has been combined with standard chemotherapeutic drugs; preliminary results of studies using sorafenib with carboplatin and paclitaxel were encouraging [32]. Clinical trials are now ongoing with second generation selective and non-selective RAF inhibitors, such as PLX4032 (vemurafenib), SB-590885/GSK2118436, XL-281, and RAF-265 (www.clinicaltrials.gov). In recent Phase I-III trials, XL-281 (ARAF, BRAF and CRAF inhibitor) and PLX4032 (BRAF^{V600E} inhibitor) were shown to have single-agent antitumor activity in melanoma patients with the achievement of objective responses [2]. These studies indicate the potential therapeutic value of single-agent therapy against a mutated oncogene in melanoma.

Recently, it has been shown that melanoma cell lines with mutant BRAF are also sensitive to MEK inhibition [33]. In BRAF-mutant tumors, MEK inhibition results in down-regulation of cyclin D1, up-regulation of p27, hypophosphorylation of the retinoblastoma-susceptibility tumor suppressor protein (RB), and growth arrest in the G$_1$ phase of the cell cycle [33]. MEK inhibition also induces differentiation and senescence of BRAF-mutant cells, in addition to apoptosis in some, but not all, BRAF^{V600E} mutant models. Two MEK inhibitors are currently being tested in clinical trials: PD-0325901 [34] and ARRY-142886 (AZD6244) [35].

Mutations in NRAS, another key regulator of the MAPK pathway upstream of BRAF, can also be found in melanoma (Fig. 3.1); although, at a significantly lower frequency than BRAF^{V600E} (Table 3.1). Overall, 15–30% of melanomas show activating NRAS mutations that are located predominantly within exon 1 (codons 12 and 13) or exon 2 [codons 59 and 61 (90%)] of the gene [2]. NRAS mutations have been identified in 22% of melanomas on non-chronic sun-damaged skin, 10% of acral lentiginous melanomas, 5% of mucosal melanomas, and 15% of melanomas from skin with chronic sun damage [2]. Similar to BRAF^{V600E}, it appears that NRAS mutations are infrequently found in melanomas on chronically sun-damaged skin, and are more commonly seen in melanomas on skin with intermittent sun exposure (i.e., trunk and extremities) [2]. In general, NRAS and BRAF mutations are mutually exclusive; although, rare double-mutant cases have been reported. Together, they account for MAPK pathway activation in >80% of melanomas [2]. However, in contrast to BRAF-mutant melanomas, which typically require a synchronous mutation in a member of the PI3K pathway, the upstream location of NRAS allows for mutant forms to simultaneously activate both MAPK and PI3K-AKT signaling. In melanomas lacking BRAF or NRAS mutations, the signaling cascade can be triggered by autocrine mechanisms, that include the down-regulation of RAF-1 or SPRY-2 (MAPK inhibitory proteins), or up-regulation of c-MET. Of note, mutations in the other RAS genes, KRAS and HRAS, occur in only ~2% and ~1% of melanomas, respectively [2].

KIT

Mutations of KIT (another RTK) have been identified in 17% of chronic sun-damaged cutaneous, 11% of acral and 21% of mucosal melanomas, but not in any melanomas on skin without chronic sun damage; supporting a role for KIT as an oncogene in a subset of tumors (Fig. 3.1 and Table 3.1) [2]. In addition, KIT gene amplification has been found to be present in 6% of chronic sun-damaged cutaneous, 7% of acral and 8% of mucosal melanomas [2]. Point mutations in KIT result in constitutive activation of the c-KIT protein (CD117) in melanoma cells, and the activation of downstream proliferative and pro-survival signaling pathways. At the protein level, immunohistochemical studies have shown c-KIT expression in 81% of mucosal and acral melanomas [2]. Interestingly, cases with activating mutations are commonly positive for c-KIT protein expression; however, many tumors that do not have detectable gene mutation or amplification also show high expression levels for this protein [2]. Several anecdotal case reports have noted remarkable responses to small molecule KIT inhibitors (imatinib, sorafenib and dasatinib) in patients with widely metastatic melanoma [2]. Of note, KIT mutations, and not gene amplifications, appear to be predictive of clinical response to imatinib in melanoma patients [2]. These findings clearly illustrate the importance of proper patient selection prior to imatinib treatment, including the performance of KIT (and PDGFRA) gene mutational analysis.

In summary, somatic BRAF, NRAS and KIT mutations are now recognized as frequent events associated with melanoma development (Table 3.1). Whereas KIT mutations are most common in acral, mucosal and chronically sun-damaged skin melanomas, BRAF and NRAS mutations seem to predominate in melanomas that arise on skin without chronic sun damage. The identification of somatic gene mutations in melanoma may serve as the basis for a future integrated genomic-morphologic classification scheme for this tumor, in addition to the rationale for drug development and more effective targeted therapy.

High-Risk Melanoma Susceptibility Genes (CDKN2A and CDK4)

Genetic risk factors for melanoma include germline mutations in (1) the cyclin-dependent kinase inhibitor 2 (CDKN2A, chromosome 9p21) gene, also called Multi-Tumor Suppressor MTS1 [36] and (2) the cyclin-dependent kinase 4 (CDK4, chromosome 12q14) gene. These are designated as "high-risk" melanoma susceptibility genes. The CDKN2A gene consists of four exons (1α, 1β, 2 and 3) and encodes for two proteins, p16^{CDKN2A} (including exons 1α, 2 and 3) and p14^{ARF} (a product of an alternative splicing that includes exons 1β and 2), which are known to function as tumor suppressors [37]. In particular, p16^{CDKN2A} is part of the G_1–S cell cycle checkpoint mechanism that involves RB. The p16^{CDKN2A} protein inhibits CDK4, which in turn phosphorylates RB and allows progression through the G_1–S checkpoint. The p14^{ARF} protein interacts with MDM2, which targets p53 for degradation [38].

Under normal conditions, the cellular expression level of p53 is low. In response to DNA damage, p53 accumulates and prevents cell division. Therefore, inactivation of the TP53 gene can result in an accumulation of genetic damage within cells, promoting tumor formation [39]. In the case of melanoma, such inactivation is predominantly due to functional gene silencing, since the frequency of TP53 mutation is low in this tumor [40].

The majority of melanomas are sporadic, but 5–10% of cases occur in familial clusters. Approximately 20–40% of highly penetrant familial melanoma is the result of germline alterations in the CDKN2A gene [2, 41, 42]. In addition, somatic mutations in CDKN2A (predominantly involving exons 1 and 2) and/or chromosomal deletions of 9p21 (where CDKN2A resides) are extremely frequent events in melanoma [2, 41, 42]. CDKN2A polymorphisms (C500G and C540T) and mutations in cyclin-dependent kinase inhibitor 2A/p14 alternate reading frame (CDKN2A/ARF) are also associated with increased melanoma risk [2, 41, 42].

The penetrance of CDKN2A mutations is influenced by UV radiation exposure [43] and varies according to the incidence rates of melanoma in different populations (indeed, the same factors that affect population incidence of melanoma may also mediate CDKN2A mutation penetrance). The penetrance of CDKN2A mutations is also greatly influenced by geographic location and ethnicity, with reported rates of 13% in Europe, 50% in the USA, and 32% in Australia by 50 years of age; and 58% in Europe, 76% in the USA, and 91% in Australia by age 80 [44]. In addition, clinical features including age at melanoma diagnosis, presence and number of dysplastic melanocytic nevi, and occurrence of pancreatic cancer vary significantly among CDKN2A mutation carriers [42–46]. It has been hypothesized that differences in CDKN2A penetrance could also be related to additional modifier factors, such as the co-existence of common genetic polymorphisms in DNA repair, apoptosis and immune response pathways, or other co-inherited predisposing genetic variants [i.e., melanocortin-1-receptor (MC1R)] [2].

CDKN2A mutations are more frequent in patients with a strong family history of melanoma (three or more affected family members; 35.5%) compared with patients without familial recurrence of the disease (8.2%) [47]. Although families with CDKN2A mutations display an average disease penetrance of 30% by 50 years of age and 67% by age 80, studies have shown that melanoma risk is greatly influenced by the geographic latitude in which an individual is born, levels of sun exposure, and other modifier genes [48].

The role of CDKN2A testing within melanoma genetics is controversial [2]. There are now at least five commercial laboratories which offer serum- or buccal swab-based testing for germline mutations in CDKN2A (http://www.genetests.org). Mutations in this gene are identified in only ~1% of unselected melanoma cases and routine genetic analysis in all melanoma patients is inappropriate. The incidence of CDKN2A mutation is quite low when using single criteria, such as the presence of clinically atypical melanocytic nevi (4%), two or more primary melanomas (2%), or early onset (<40 years old) melanomas (1%); although, combinations thereof may increase the rate of detection significantly. In a recent study, which reviewed the likelihood of finding CDKN2A germline mutations, it was proposed that in moderate-to-high melanoma incidence areas, (1) individuals with three or more primary cutaneous melanomas or (2) families with at least one invasive melanoma and two or more other diagnoses of melanoma and/or pancreatic cancer among first- or second-degree relatives on the same side of the family may be ideal candidates for evaluation [2]. Based on current evidence, CDKN2A testing of patients with clinically atypical nevi and/or dysplastic nevi does not appear to be useful. Currently, the primary benefit of testing for the presence of mutations in this gene is to identify patients and family members who may benefit from increased surveillance and intensive skin cancer screening, with the possible earlier detection of melanoma in carriers [2]. The patient's ethnicity, age at diagnosis, and other risk factors, such as sun exposure history, are important considerations. Useful resources for familial melanoma testing are GenoMEL, an international melanoma genetics research consortium (www.genomel.org), and the Huntsman Cancer Institute Melanoma and Skin Cancer Program (http://www.huntsmancancer.org/group/melanomaProgram/overview.jsp).

Recently, a meta-analysis was conducted to assess the modifier effect of MC1R allelic variants on the penetrance of CDKN2A mutations in melanoma-prone families. Data from seven independent populations [41, 49–53], including 96 melanoma families carrying CDKN2A mutations, clearly showed that MC1R variants doubled melanoma risk in CDKN2A mutation carriers. Moreover, the risk was more than tripled for carriers of MC1R-RHC variants, while carriers of multiple MC1R variants had almost four-fold risk of developing melanoma than wild-type MC1R subjects [49].

CDK4 is a rare high-penetrance melanoma predisposition gene [2, 54]. Indeed, only three melanoma families worldwide are known carriers of mutations in CDK4 (Arg24Cys and Arg24His) [55]. From a functional point of view, the Arg24Cys mutation, located in the $p16^{CDKN2A}$-binding domain of CDK4, makes the $p16^{CDKN2A}$ protein unable to inhibit the cyclin D1-CDK4 complex, resulting in a form of oncogenic activation of CDK4.

Low-Risk Melanoma Susceptibility Genes

Epidemiological studies have directly linked specific phenotypic traits, such as skin pigmentation, eye color, and tanning ability to melanoma predisposition [2]. MC1R, a gene involved in skin pigmentation, has been recently implicated in melanoma susceptibility [2]. Activation of MC1R, through α-melanocyte stimulating hormone (α-MSH) binding, results in increased cAMP production with up-regulation of downstream melanosomal enzymes, such as tyrosinase and tyrosinase-related protein (TYRP1). Activation of this pathway stimulates melanin synthesis and a switch from basal pheomelanogenesis to eumelanogenesis, resulting in darker skin pigmentation and increased protection from UV radiation. MC1R is extremely polymorphic, with over 60 variant alleles identified to date. Importantly, the MC1R allelotype can influence skin and hair color, as well as susceptibility to melanoma. One of the earliest studies noted a relative risk of 3.9 for melanoma in carriers of MC1R variants compared with normal homozygotes [2]. Interestingly, the influence of MC1R on melanoma susceptibility appears to go beyond its effect on pigmentary phenotype. As stated previously, MC1R may play a role as a modifier gene in melanoma risk among CDKN2A mutation carriers. One study has found that co-inheritance of CDKN2A mutations and MC1R red-hair variants increase the risk of melanoma from 50% to 80% [2]. Investigations have also suggested that MC1R variants increase the risk for development of BRAF-mutant melanomas [2].

Genome-wide association studies have identified single nucleotide polymorphisms (SNPs) or genetic variants of other pigmentation-related genes, including TPCN2, ASIP, KITLG, NCKX5, IRF4, OCA2, SLC24A4, TYR and TYRP1, that are associated with variable melanoma risk and confirming the importance of gene-environment interactions in tumor pathogenesis [2, 54]. BSM1, a vitamin D receptor variant, is also associated with elevated melanoma susceptibility. In addition, individuals with hereditary retinoblastoma (resulting from germline RB mutations) and xeroderma pigmentosum (resulting from defects in nucleotide excision repair) are at increased risk of melanoma development [2, 54].

PTEN and PI3K-AKT Pathways

Phosphatase and tensin homolog deleted in chromosome ten (PTEN), originally known as mutated in multiple advanced cancers or TGF-β-regulated and epithelial cell-enriched phosphatase 1, is a tumor suppressor gene that is mutated in a large fraction of human melanomas (Fig. 3.1) [56].

The PTEN protein has at least two biochemical functions: it demonstrates both lipid phosphatase and protein phosphatase activity. The lipid phosphatase activity of PTEN decreases intracellular phosphatidylinositols [3,4-bisphosphate (PIP2) and 3,4,5-triphosphate (PIP3)] that are produced during intracellular signaling via activation of the lipid kinase phosphatidylinositol 3-kinase (PI3K). PI3K activation results in increased PIP3 and a consequent conformational change leading to activation of AKT [57–59]. This latter protein is a serine/threonine kinase and belongs to the AKT protein kinase family: comprising AKT1, AKT2, and AKT3.

AKT activation stimulates cell cycle progression, survival, metabolism and migration via phosphorylation of many physiological substrates [57–62]. Based on its role as a key regulator of cell survival, AKT is emerging as a central player in tumorigenesis. Activated AKT appears to promote cell proliferation, possibly through the down-regulation of the cyclin-dependent kinase inhibitor p27, as well as the up-regulation and stabilization of cyclins E and D1 [63]. The activation of AKT also results in the suppression of apoptosis that may be induced by a variety of stimuli, including growth factor withdrawal, detachment of extracellular matrix, UV irradiation, cell cycle disturbance, and/or activation of FAS signaling [64–66]. Mechanisms associated with the ability of AKT to suppress apoptosis include the phosphorylation and inactivation of many pro-apoptotic proteins, such as BAD (Bcl-2 antagonist of cell death, a Bcl-2 family member) [66], caspase-9 [67], MDM2 (that leads to increased p53 degradation) [68–70], and the forkhead family of transcription factors [71], as well as the activation of NF-κB [72]. UV irradiation induces apoptosis in human keratinocytes both *in vitro* and *in vivo*, but also activates survival pathways including PIP3 kinase and its substrate AKT in order to limit the extent of cell death [73]. A direct correlation between radiation resistance and levels of PI3K activity has indeed been described. While activating mutations of AKT are rarely found in melanoma (<5%; although rare mutations in the AKT1 and AKT3 genes have been recently reported in a limited number of human melanomas and melanoma cell lines [74–76]), the silencing of AKT function via targeting of PI3K inhibits cell proliferation and reduces the sensitivity of melanoma cells to UV radiation [77]. Constitutive activation of AKT (preferentially AKT3) has been reported in >60% of melanomas.

The lipid phosphatase activity of PTEN protein is capable of degrading the products of PI3K [78], suggesting that PTEN may function to directly antagonize the activity of the PI3K-AKT pathway [79, 80]. As predicted by this model, genetic inactivation of PTEN in human cancer cells leads to constitutive activation of this AKT pathway and promotion of tumorigenesis. Numerous mutations and/or deletions in the PTEN gene have been found in human tumors, including lymphoma, thyroid, breast and prostatic carcinomas, and melanoma [81–83]. PTEN somatic mutations are found in 40–60% of melanoma cell lines and 10–20% of primary melanomas [84], with the majority of such mutations occurring in the phosphatase domain [82, 83]. The paradox between the detection of a low mutation frequency and a higher level of gene silencing in primary melanomas has led to speculation that PTEN inactivation may predominantly occur through epigenetic mechanisms [85]. Several distinct methylation sites have been found within the PTEN promoter and hypermethylation at these sites has been shown to reduce PTEN expression in melanoma [86]. Therefore, loss of PTEN function may result in aberrant cell growth, escape from apoptosis, and abnormal cell spreading and migration. In addition, alterations of the BRAF-MAPK pathway are frequently associated with PTEN-AKT impairment, with BRAF mutations and PTEN loss co-existing in >20% of melanomas [87]. In the case of melanoma, PTEN inactivation has been largely observed as a late event; although, a dose-dependent downregulation of PTEN expression has been implicated in the early stages of tumorigenesis [88]. The protein phosphatase activity of PTEN appears to be less important in tumorigenesis.

Therapeutic agents used to target the PI3K pathway include CCI-779 (Temsirolimus) and RAD001 (Everolimus) (Fig. 3.1). Both of these molecules target mTOR (mammalian target of rapamycin), a serine/threonine kinase downstream of AKT, which modulates protein synthesis, cell cycle progression, and angiogenesis. Since mTOR is a cytosolic protein expressed by all tissues, these inhibitors do not have high specificity in the targeting of melanoma tumor cells. Furthermore, it has been determined that the mTOR pathway has a complicated feedback loop that involves suppression of AKT; hence, mTOR inhibitors could potentially activate AKT in some cells [89]. The MAPK and PI3K signaling pathways play key roles in melanoma cell proliferation and survival, suggesting that parallel inhibition of targets in both pathways may result in synergistic inhibition of growth in melanomas.

MITF

Microphthalmia-associated transcription factor (MITF) is a basic helix–loop–helix leucine zipper transcription factor that is considered to be the master regulator of melanocyte biology, partly because it regulates the expression of melanogenic proteins such as tyrosinase, silver homologue (gp100) and melanoma-associated antigen recognized by T cells-1 (MART-1, also known as Melan-A) [90]. MITF also regulates melanoblast survival and melanocyte lineage commitment, and is a key player in melanoma pathobiology (Fig. 3.1) [90]. The connection between MITF and melanoma development is complex, as it is known to play the dual roles of both inducer and repressor of cellular proliferation [91]. High levels of MITF expression lead to G_1 cell cycle arrest and differentiation, through induction of the cell cycle inhibitors p16^{CDKN2A} and p21$^{Waf1/Cip}$ [92, 93], whereas very low or null expression levels predispose to apoptosis. Only intermediate levels promote cell proliferation. Therefore, it is thought that melanoma cells have developed strategies to maintain MITF levels in the range compatible with tumorigenesis. It has been shown that constitutive ERK activity, stimulated by BRAF^{V600E} in melanoma cells, is associated with ubiquitin dependent degradation of MITF [94]. Nevertheless, continued expression of MITF is necessary for both proliferation and survival of melanoma cells via regulation of CDK2 and bcl-2 genes, respectively [95, 96]. Furthermore, BRAF mutation is associated with MITF amplification in 10–15% of melanomas [97]. Since a low fraction of melanomas carrying BRAF mutations demonstrate MITF amplification, one could speculate that other mechanisms are likely to be involved in ERK-dependent proteosomal degradation of MITF.

MITF has also been recently shown to act downstream of the canonical WNT pathway, which includes cysteine-rich glycoproteins that play a critical role in cancer development [98]. In particular, the WNT gene family is found to be involved in the development of the neural crest during melanocyte differentiation from pluripotent cells among several species (from zebrafish to mammals) [98–101]. Moreover, several WNT proteins have been shown to be overexpressed in various human cancers; among them, the up-regulation of WNT2 appears to participate in inhibiting the normal apoptotic machinery in melanoma cells [102]. It has also been recently suggested that WNT2 protein expression levels may be useful in the distinction of melanocytic nevus from melanoma [103]. A key downstream effector of this pathway is β-catenin. In the absence of WNT signals, β-catenin is targeted for degradation through phosphorylation controlled by a complex consisting of glycogen synthase kinase-3-beta (GSK3β), axin, and adenomatous polyposis coli (APC) proteins. WNT signaling leads to inactivation of GSK3β, thereby stabilizing the intracellular levels of β-catenin and subsequently increasing the transcription of downstream target genes. Mutations in multiple components of the WNT pathway have been identified in many human cancers; all of these mutations induce nuclear accumulation of β-catenin [104]. In human melanoma, stabilizing mutations of β-catenin have been found in a significant fraction of established cell lines. Almost one third of these cell lines display aberrant nuclear accumulation of β-catenin, although few mutations have been classified as pathogenic variants [104, 105]. These observations support the hypothesis that this pathway contributes to the development and behavior of melanoma. Another mechanism could involve mutant BRAF; it has been recently shown that oncogenic BRAF controls MITF on two levels: it down-regulates the protein by stimulating its degradation, but then counteracts this by increasing MITF expression through the transcription factor BRN2 [106].

Novel Pathways

Notch1

Notch proteins are a family of single-pass type I transmembrane receptors of ~300 kDa that were first identified in *Drosophila melanogaster* (at this level, a mutated protein causes "notches" in the fly wing) [107].

These receptors are activated by specific transmembrane ligands which are expressed on an adjacent cell and activate Notch signaling through direct cell-cell interaction. The Notch signaling pathway plays a pivotal role in tissue homeostasis and regulation of cell fate, including self-renewal of adult stem cells and differentiation of precursors along specific cell lineages [108, 109]. Increasing evidence suggests its involvement in tumorigenesis, since deregulated Notch signaling is frequently observed in a variety of human cancers, including T-cell acute lymphoblastic leukemia [110], small cell lung carcinoma [111], neuroblastoma [112, 113], and cervical [114, 115] and prostatic carcinoma [116, 117]. Notch can act as either an oncogene or a tumor suppressor gene, depending on both the cellular and tissue context. Many studies suggest a tumor suppressor role for Notch1 in keratinocytes [118]. In such cells, Notch signaling induces growth arrest and differentiation (deletion of Notch1 in murine epidermis leads to epidermal hyperplasia and skin carcinoma) [119–121]. The anti-tumor effect of Notch1 in murine skin appears to be mediated by $p21^{Waf1/Cip}$ induction and repression of WNT signaling [117].

Unlike keratinocyte-derived squamous cell carcinoma and basal cell carcinoma, melanomas have significantly higher Notch activity in comparison with normal melanocytes (Fig. 3.2) [122, 123]. Investigations of the expression of Notch receptors and their ligands in benign and malignant cutaneous melanocytic lesions indicate that Notch and its ligands are significantly up-regulated in atypical nevi and melanomas compared to common melanocytic nevi [122, 123]. Furthermore, constitutively-induced gene activation in human melanocytes strongly suggests that Notch1 acts as a transforming oncogene in this cell type [124]. The versatile effects of Notch1 signaling on cell differentiation, proliferation, survival, and tumorigenesis may easily explain why Notch1 plays different roles in various types of skin cancer. Such different activities of Notch1 in skin cancer are probably determined by its interaction with the downstream β-catenin target. In murine skin carcinoma, β-catenin is functionally activated by Notch1 signaling and mediates tumor-suppressive effects [123]. In melanoma, β-catenin mediates oncogenic activity by also cross-talking with the WNT pathway or by regulating N-cadherin, with different effects on tumorigenesis depending on Notch1 activation [125].

Recent evidence suggests that Notch1 enhances the development of vertical growth phase (in melanoma) through activation of the MAPK and PI3K-AKT pathways; inhibition of either the MAPK or PI3K-AKT pathway reverses the tumor cell growth induced by Notch1 signaling [126]. Future studies aimed at identifying new targets of Notch1 signaling will allow the assessment of the mechanisms underlying the cross-talk between Notch1, MAPK, and PI3K-AKT pathways. Finally, Notch signaling can enhance cell survival by interacting with the transcriptional factor NF-κB (Notch1 seems to directly interact with NF-κB, leading to retention of NF-κB within the nucleus of T-cells) [127]. Nevertheless, it has been shown that Notch1 can directly regulate IFN-γ expression through the formation of complexes between NF-κB and the IFN-γ promoter [127]. Although there is a lack of consensus concerning the cross-talk between Notch1 and NF-κB, existing data suggest that two mechanisms of NF-κB activation may be present: (1) an early Notch-independent phase and (2) a late Notch-dependent phase [128]. Finally, RAS-mediated transformation requires the presence of intact Notch signaling; impairment of such Notch1 receptor signaling may significantly reduce the ability of RAS to transform cells [129, 130].

Nuclear Factor-κB

Nuclear factor-κB (NF-κB) plays an important role in inflammation, cell proliferation and survival, as well as in the regulation of virus replication. The NF-κB family (also known as the Rel/NF-κB family) of transcription factors consists of five members: p50, p52, RelA (also known as p65), RelB and c-Rel [131, 132]. All proteins carry a Rel Homology Domain (RHD), followed by a Nuclear Localization Signal (NLS). The RHD domain is involved in homo- or heteromeric dimer formation and interacts with the ankyrin repeat motifs present in the seven members of the IκB family: IκBα, IκBβ, IκBγ, IκBε, IκBζ, IκBNS and bcl-3. Among them, IκBζ, IκBNS and bcl-3 are nuclear proteins that regulate transcription by interacting with NF-κB family members in the nucleus. The remaining IκB family members interact with the RHD of NF-κB in the cytoplasm and mask the NLS, thereby sequestering NF-κB family members in the cytoplasm. Therefore, NF-κB family members are transcriptionally inactive when they form complexes with cytoplasmic IκB family proteins. A wide range of stimuli activate NF-κB, which upon activation must translocate to the nucleus to interact with κB-sites located in the regulatory regions of target genes. Nuclear translocation of NF-κB can be driven by three distinct signaling pathways: the classical activation pathway, the alternative activation pathway, and the atypical pathway [132].

The classical pathway (or canonical pathway) is triggered by pro-inflammatory cytokines, antigens, bacterial cell-wall components, viruses and genotoxic stress, which leads to the activation of the IκB kinase (IKK) complex, consisting of IKKα, IKKβ and NEMO (NF-κB essential modulator, also known as IKKγ). In the classical activation pathway, activated IKKβ phosphorylates specific serine residues of IκB in a NEMO-dependent manner, which results in polyubiquitination and subsequent degradation of IκB by 26S proteasomes. Then, released NF-κB, primarily the p50:RelA heterodimer, translocates to the nucleus, binds to the NF-κB site and activates gene transcription. This pathway, which mostly targets p50:RelA and p50:c-Rel dimers, is essential for innate immunity and responsible for the inhibition of apoptosis under most conditions.

The second pathway, the alternative or non-canonical pathway, leads to the selective activation of p52:RelB dimers by inducing the processing of p100 precursor protein. This pathway is triggered by certain members of the TNF cytokine family, such as lymphotoxin β, B-cell activating factor belonging to the TNF family (BAFF) and CD40 ligand through the selective activation of IKKα homodimers by NF-κB-inducing kinase. The alternative pathway is important for the development of secondary lymphoid organs and the adaptive immune response [132–136].

The third signaling pathway is classified as atypical because it is independent of IKK, and is activated by UV radiation and doxorubicin, both of which cause DNA damage.

It has become clear that aberrant regulation of NF-κB and the signaling pathways that control its activity are involved in cancer development and progression. Aberrant NF-κB regulation has been observed in many cancers, including both solid and hematopoietic malignancies. NF-κB can affect all six hallmarks of cancer through the transcriptional activation of genes associated with cell proliferation, angiogenesis, metastasis, tumor promotion, inflammation and suppression of apoptosis [137–142]. There is evidence that NF-κB plays an important role in melanoma pathobiology (Fig. 3.2) [143–146]. In fact, NF-κB is constitutively activated in melanoma [147], with expression levels greater in primary melanomas than in normal melanocytes [148, 149]. Evidence also suggests that IκB expression is significantly reduced in melanomas relative to melanocytic nevi [149]. These results suggest that increased expression and phosphorylation of NF-κB occur at the stage of the benign melanocytic nevus, but that there may be sufficient levels of the inhibitory protein IκB to sequester NF-κB in the cytoplasm. In contrast, melanomas have high RelA expression and high activation of the phosphoserine-529 form of RelA, but have reduced IκB expression [150].

A number of mechanisms have been proposed to explain the activation of NF-κB in melanoma. AKT/PKB increases IKK activity and also directly phosphorylates NF-κB [151, 152]. Activation of the RAS/RAF/MEK/ERK pathway, which occurs frequently in melanoma, can induce activation of NF-κB [153, 154]. The mechanisms through which this occurs are as yet unknown.

Since NF-κB seems to be frequently activated in melanoma, different therapeutic approaches aimed to inhibit this pathway have been proposed. One of these drugs, bortezomib (Velcade) also known as PS-341, is already FDA-approved for use in patients with multiple myeloma, and is capable of blocking the proteosomic degradation of IκB [155]. Unfortunately, no clinical responses were observed in a trial of 27 patients with metastatic melanoma using bortezomib as single-agent therapy [156]. However, in preclinical studies, bortezomib demonstrated dramatic synergy with temozolomide, suggesting that it may be effective when combined with cytotoxic chemotherapy [157]. Other therapeutic approaches undergoing clinical evaluation include the direct inhibition of IKK, which could similarly block activation of NF-κB. Some of these are small-molecule inhibitors that block NF-κB and induce apoptosis in melanoma cells both *in vitro* and *in vivo* [145, 146, 151]. One of the most problematic aspects of cancer therapy based on the inhibition of NF-κB activity is a lack of specificity. So far, the vast majority of investigated drugs also interfere with other NF-κB activities (i.e., immunity, inflammation, cellular homeostasis), thus resulting in a high frequency of toxic side effects. To this end, research efforts are now focused on identifying novel NF-κB targets that are specifically activated in tumors, but not in normal cells. The inhibition of such targets should theoretically block the oncogenic potential of NF-κB in cancer cells without affecting its role in normal tissues.

iNOS

Nitric oxide (NO) is a free radical that is largely synthesized by the NO synthase (NOS) enzyme. Recently, studies of NO function have focused on its role in tumor pathobiology. A majority of human and experimental tumors are stimulated by NO, which contributes to tumor growth and metastasis by promoting migratory, invasive, and angiogenic properties of tumor cells [158]. In one experiment, the scavenging of endogenous NO resulted in inhibition of melanoma cell growth; this was restored with the introduction of an NO donor [159].

An increasing number of publications support the notion that UV radiation stimulates the production of NO in human keratinocytes, resulting in a series of secondary downstream changes and release of cytokines and other molecules that are of critical importance in the maintenance of normal melanocyte homeostasis and in the modulation of melanocyte proliferation and melanin synthesis [160, 161]. Therefore, NO generation by keratinocytes is postulated to be involved in melanomagenesis and progression (Fig. 3.2).

NO can be produced by three NOS isoforms: (1) endothelial NOS (eNOS, NOS III) and (2) neuronal NOS (nNOS, NOS I), which are both constitutively expressed, and (3) inducible NOS (iNOS, NOS II), which is regulated at the transcriptional level by a variety of mediators (such as interferon regulatory factor-1 [157, 162], NF-κB [163, 164], TNF-α and INF-γ [165, 166]) and has been found to be frequently expressed in melanoma [167–170]. The iNOS gene is located at chromosome 17q11.2 and encodes a 131 kDa protein. Although the exact function of iNOS in tumorigenesis remains unclear, the overproduction of NO may influence the development and/or progression of melanoma. It has been shown that transfection of the iNOS gene into murine melanoma cells induces apoptosis, suppresses tumorigenicity, and abrogates metastasis [171, 172]. More generally, NO induces apoptosis by altering the expression and function of multiple apoptosis-related proteins (i.e., down-regulation of bcl-2, accumulation of p53, cleavage of PARP) [173–179].

The role of iNOS in melanoma progression remains controversial. Higher levels of iNOS have been found in subcutaneous and lymph node metastases as compared to distant metastases of melanoma patients [180]. However, iNOS is found to be expressed to a lesser extent in metastases as compared with melanocytic nevi and primary melanomas [181]. Nevertheless, the expression of iNOS in both lymph node deposits and in-transit metastases has been proposed as an indicator of poor prognosis in patients with melanoma [182].

Conclusion

Melanoma remains a prototype of solid cancers with an increasing incidence and extremely poor prognosis at advanced stages [183]. It demonstrates a plethora of genetic (gene mutation, deletion, amplification or translocation) and epigenetic [a heritable change other than in the DNA sequence, generally transcriptional modulation by DNA methylation, chromatin alterations (such as histone modification), and/or microRNA expression] alterations that contribute to the limited efficacy of current anti-cancer treatments [184, 185].

This scenario is further complicated by the fact that a significant percentage of melanomas do not seem to evolve from melanocytic nevi, with only ~50% of them associated with dysplastic nevi [186], strongly suggesting that melanoma often arises from "normal-appearing" skin without following a sequential accumulation of phenotypically evident molecular events, as seen for some other human tumors [161, 187].

Recently, it has been suggested that melanomas may be derived from transformed melanocytic stem cells, melanocyte progenitors, or de-differentiated mature melanocytes [188, 189]. In the very near future, the biologic and molecular characterization of melanoma stem cells will determine whether the well-known drug resistance of melanoma is a function of quiescent or drug-resistant cancer stem cells and whether the inhibition of self-renewing cancer stem cells prevents melanoma growth. What we can affirm with certainty is that the targeting of a single component in such complex signaling pathways is unlikely to yield significant anti-tumor responses in melanoma patients. For this reason, further evaluation of all known molecular targets along with the molecular characterization of melanoma tumors may be helpful in predicting those subsets of patients who would be expected to be more or less likely to respond to specific therapeutic interventions. Now is the time to successfully translate the knowledge from such research into clinical practice.

References

1. Beddingfield III FC. The melanoma epidemic: res ipsa loquitur. Oncologist. 2002;8:459–65.
2. Gerami P, Gammon B, Murphy M. Melanocytic neoplasms I: molecular diagnosis. In: Murphy MJ, editor. Molecular diagnostics in dermatology and dermatopathology. New York: Springer; 2011.
3. Dennis LK. Analysis of the melanoma epidemic, both apparent and real: data from the 1973 through 1994 surveillance, epidemiology, and end results program registry. Arch Dermatol. 1999;135:275–80.
4. Lipsker DM, Hedelin G, Heid E, Grosshans EM, Cribier BJ. Striking increases of thin melanomas contrasts with a stable incidence of thick melanomas. Arch Dermatol. 1999;135:1451–6.
5. Gandini S, Sera F, Cattaruzza MS, Pasquini P, Picconi O, Boyle P, Melchi CF. Meta-analysis of risk factors for cutaneous melanoma: II. Sun exposure. Eur J Cancer. 2005;41:45–60.
6. Gilchrest BA, Eller MS, Geller AC, Yaar M. The pathogenesis of melanoma induced by ultraviolet radiation. N Engl J Med. 1999;340:1341–8.
7. Jhappan C, Noonan FP, Merlino G. Ultraviolet radiation and cutaneous malignant melanoma. Oncogene. 2003;22:3099–112.
8. Eide MJ, Weinstock MA. Association of UV index, latitude, and melanoma incidence in non-White populations – US surveillance, epidemiology, and end results (SEER) program, 1992 to 2001. Arch Dermatol. 2005;141:477–81.
9. De Fabo EC, Noonan FP, Fears T, Merlino G. Ultraviolet B but not ultraviolet A radiation initiates melanoma. Cancer Res. 2004;64:6372–6.
10. Wang SQ, Setlow R, Berwick M, Polsky D, Marghoob AA, Kopf AW, Bart RS. Ultraviolet A and melanoma: a review. J Am Acad Dermatol. 2001;44:837–46.
11. Moan J, Dahlback A, Setlow RB. Epidemiological support for an hypothesis for melanoma induction indicating a role for UVA radiation. Photochem Photobiol. 1999;70:243–7.
12. Oliveria S, Dusza S, Berwick M. Issues in the epidemiology of melanoma. Expert Rev Anticancer Ther. 2001;1:453–9.
13. Garland C, Garland F, Gorham E. Epidemiologic evidence for different roles of ultraviolet A and B radiation in melanoma mortality rates. Ann Epidemiol. 2003;13:395–404.
14. Curtin JA, Fridlyand J, Kageshita T, Patel HN, Busam KJ, Kutzner H, Cho KH, Aiba S, Brocker EB, LeBoit PE, Pinkel D, Bastian BC. Distinct sets of genetic alterations in melanoma. N Engl J Med. 2005;353:2135–47.
15. Giehl K. Oncogenic Ras in tumor progression and metastasis. Biol Chem. 2005;386:193–205.
16. Campbell PM, Der CJ. Oncogenic Ras and its role in tumor cell invasion and metastasis. Semin Cancer Biol. 2004;14:105–14.
17. Davies H, Bignell GR, Cox C, et al. Mutations of the BRAF gene in human cancer. Nature. 2002;417:949–54.
18. Goodall J, Wellbrock C, Dexter TJ, Roberts K, Marais R, Goding CR. The Brn-2 transcription factor links activated BRAF to melanoma proliferation. Mol Cell Biol. 2004;24:2923–31.
19. Sharma A, Trivedi NR, Zimmerman MA, Tuveson DA, Smith CD, Robertson GP. Mutant V599EB-Raf regulates growth and vascular development of malignant melanoma tumors. Cancer Res. 2005;65:2412–21.
20. Hemesath TJ, Price ER, Takemoto C, Badalian T, Fisher DE. MAP kinase links the transcription factor Microphthalmia to c-Kit signalling in melanocytes. Nature. 1998;391:298–301.
21. Bhatt KV, Spofford LS, Aram G, McMullen M, Pumiglia K, Aplin AE. Adhesion control of cyclin D1 and $p27^{Kip1}$ levels is deregulated in melanoma cells through BRAF–MEK–ERK signaling. Oncogene. 2005;24:3459–71.
22. Gray-Schopfer VC, Cheong SC, Chong H, et al. Cellular senescence in naevi and immortalisation in melanoma: a role for p16? Br J Cancer. 2006;95:496–505.
23. Michaloglou C, Vredeveld LC, Soengas MS, et al. $BRAF^{E600}$-associated senescence-like cell cycle arrest of human naevi. Nature. 2005;436:720–4.
24. Huntington JT, Shields JM, Der CJ, et al. Overexpression of collagenase 1 (MMP-1) is mediated by the ERK pathway in invasive melanoma cells: role of BRAF mutation and fibroblast growth factor signaling. J Biol Chem. 2004;279:33168–76.
25. Ellerhorst JA, Ekmekcioglu S, Johnson MK, Cooke CP, Johnson MM, Grimm EA. Regulation of iNOS by the p44/42 mitogen-activated protein kinase pathway in human melanoma. Oncogene. 2006;25:3956–62.
26. Patton EE, Widlund HR, Kutok JL, et al. BRAF mutations are sufficient to promote nevi formation and cooperate with p53 in the genesis of melanoma. Curr Biol. 2005;15:249–54.
27. Wajapeyee N, Serra RW, Zhu X, Mahalingam M, Green MR. Oncogenic BRAF induces senescence and apoptosis through pathways mediated by the secreted protein IGFBP7. Cell. 2008;132:363–74.
28. Michaloglou C, Vredeveld LC, Mooi WJ, Peeper DS. BRAF(E600) in benign and malignant human tumours. Oncogene. 2008;27:877–95.
29. Dhomen N, Reis-Filho JS, da Rocha Dias S, et al. Oncogenic Braf induces melanocyte senescence and melanoma in mice. Cancer Cell. 2009;15:294–303.
30. Strumberg D, Richly H, Hilger RA, et al. Phase I clinical and pharmacokinetic study of the novel Raf kinase and vascular endothelial growth factor receptor inhibitor BAY 43–9006 in patients with advanced refractory solid tumors. J Clin Oncol. 2005;23:965–72.
31. Eisen T, Ahmad T, Flaherty KT, et al. Sorafenib in advanced melanoma: a phase II randomised discontinuation trial analysis. Br J Cancer. 2006;95:581–6.

32. Rao RD, Holtan SG, Ingle JN, et al. Combination of paclitaxel and carboplatin as second-line therapy for patients with metastatic melanoma. Cancer. 2006; 106: 375–82.
33. Wee S, Jagani Z, Xiang KX, Loo A, Dorsch M, Yao YM, Sellers WR, Lengauer C, Stegmeier F. PI3K pathway activation mediates resistance to MEK inhibitors in KRAS mutant cancers. Cancer Res. 2009;69:4286–93.
34. Ciuffreda L, Del Bufalo D, Desideri M, et al. Growth-inhibitory and antiangiogenic activity of the MEK inhibitor PD0325901 in malignant melanoma with or without BRAF mutations. Neoplasia. 2009;11:720–31.
35. Banerji U, Camidge DR, Verheul HM, et al. The first-in-human study of the hydrogen sulfate (Hydsulfate) capsule of the MEK1/2 inhibitor AZD6244 (ARRY-142886): a phase I open-label multicenter trial in patients with advanced cancer. Clin Cancer Res. 2010;16:1613–23.
36. Stone S, Ping J, Dayananth P, Tavtigian SV, Katcher H, Parry D, Gordon P, Kamb A. Complex structure and regulation of the P16 (MTS1) locus. Cancer Res. 1995;55:2988–94.
37. Haber DA. Splicing into senescence: the curious case of p16 and p19ARF. Cell. 1997;28(91):555–8.
38. Zhang Y, Xiong Y, Yarbrough WG. ARF promotes MDM2 degradation and stabilizes p53: ARF-INK4a locus deletion impairs both the Rb and p53 tumor suppression pathways. Cell. 1998;92:725–34.
39. Levine AJ. p53, the cellular gatekeeper for growth and division. Cell. 1997;88:323–31.
40. Box NF, Terzian T. The role of p53 in pigmentation, tanning and melanoma. Pigment Cell Melanoma Res. 2008;21:525–33.
41. Goldstein AM, Landi MT, Tsang S, Fraser MC, Munroe DJ, Tucker MA. Association of MC1R variants and risk of melanoma in melanoma-prone families with CDKN2A mutations. Cancer Epidemiol Biomarkers Prev. 2005;14:2208–12.
42. Bishop DT, Demenais F, Goldstein AM, et al. Melanoma genetics consortium: geographical variation in the penetrance of CDKN2A mutations for melanoma. J Natl Cancer Inst. 2002;94:894–903.
43. Demenais F. Influence of genes, nevi, and sun sensitivity on melanoma risk in a family sample unselected by family history and in melanoma-prone families. J Natl Cancer Inst. 2004;96:785–95.
44. Puig S, Malvehy J, Badenas C, Ruiz A, et al. Role of the CDKN2A Locus in patients with multiple primary melanomas. J Clin Oncol. 2005;23:3043–51.
45. Goldstein AM, Struewing JP, Chidambaram A, Fraser MC, Tucker MA. Genotype-phenotype relationships in U.S. melanoma-prone families with CDKN2A and CDK4 mutations. J Natl Cancer Inst. 2000;92:1006–10.
46. Chaudru V, Chompret A, Bressac-de Paillerets B, Spatz A, Avril MF, Demenais F. Influence of genes, nevi, and sun sensitivity on melanoma risk in a family sample unselected by family history and in melanoma-prone families. J Natl Cancer Inst. 2004;96:785–95.
47. Eliason MJ, Hansen CB, Hart M, et al. Multiple primary melanomas in a CDKN2A mutation carrier exposed to ionizing radiation. Arch Dermatol. 2007;143:1409–12.
48. Pho L, Grossman D, Leachman SA. Melanoma genetics: a review of genetic factors and clinical phenotypes in familial melanoma. Curr Opin Oncol. 2006;18:173–9.
49. Fargnoli MC, Gandini S, Peris K, Maisonneuve P, Raimondi S. MC1R variants increase melanoma risk in families with CDKN2A mutations: a meta-analysis. Eur J Cancer. 2010;46:1413–20.
50. Box NF, Duffy DL, Chen W, Stark M, Martin NG, Sturm RA, Hayward NK. MC1R genotype modifies risk of melanoma in families segregating CDKN2A mutations. Am J Hum Genet. 2001;69:765–73.
51. van der Velden PA, Sandkuijl LA, Bergman W, Pavel S, van Mourik L, Frants RR, Gruis NA. Melanocortin-1 receptor variant R151C modifies melanoma risk in Dutch families with melanoma. Am J Hum Genet. 2001;69:774–9.
52. Chaudru V, Laud K, Avril MF, Minière A, Chompret A, Bressac-de Paillerets B, Demenais F. Melanocortin-1 receptor (MC1R) gene variants and dysplastic nevi modify penetrance of CDKN2A mutations in French melanoma-prone pedigrees. Cancer Epidemiol Biomarkers Prev. 2005;14:2384–90.
53. Goldstein AM, Chaudru V, Ghiorzo P, et al. Cutaneous phenotype and MC1R variants as modifying factors for the development of melanoma in CDKN2A G101W mutation carriers from 4 countries. Int J Cancer. 2007;121:825–31.
54. Meyle KD, Guldberg P. Genetic risk factors for melanoma. Hum Genet. 2009;126:499–510.
55. Goldstein AM, Chan M, Harland M, et al. Melanoma Genetics Consortium (GenoMEL). High-risk melanoma susceptibility genes and pancreatic cancer, neural system tumors, and uveal melanoma across GenoMEL. Cancer Res. 2006;66:9818–28.
56. Haluska FG, Tsao H, Wu H, Haluska FS, Lazar A, Goel V. Genetic alterations in signaling pathways in melanoma. Clin Cancer Res. 2006;12:2301s–7s.
57. Stokoe D. PTEN. Curr Biol. 2001;11:R502.
58. Dahia PL. PTEN, a unique tumor suppressor gene. Endocr Relat Cancer. 2000;7:115–29.
59. Kandel ES, Hay N. The regulation and activities of the multifunctional serine/threonine kinase Akt/PKB. Exp Cell Res. 1999;253:210–29.
60. Downward J. PI 3-kinase, Akt and cell survival. Semin Cell Dev Biol. 2004;15:177–82.
61. Vivanco I, Sawyers CL. The phosphatidylinositol 3-kinase AKT pathway in human cancer. Nat Rev Cancer. 2002;2:489–501.
62. Datta SR, Brunet A, Greenberg ME. Cellular survival: a play in three Akts. Genes Dev. 1999;13:2905–27.
63. Blume-Jensen P, Hunter T. Oncogenic kinase signalling. Nature. 2001;411:355–65.

64. Plas DR, Thompson CB. Akt-dependent transformation: there is more to growth than just surviving. Oncogene. 2005;24:7435–42.
65. Stiles B, Groszer M, Wang S, Jiao J, Wu H. PTEN less means more. Dev Biol. 2004;273:175–84.
66. Datta SR, Dudek H, Tao X, Masters S, Fu H, Gotoh Y, Greenberg ME. Akt phosphorylation of BAD couples survival signals to the cell-intrinsic death machinery. Cell. 1997;91:231–41.
67. Cardone MH, Roy N, Stennicke HR, Salvesen GS, Franke TF, Stanbridge E, Frisch S, Reed JC. Regulation of cell death protease caspase-9 by phosphorylation. Science. 1998;282:1318–21.
68. Mayo LD, Donner DB. A phosphatidylinositol 3-kinase/Akt pathway promotes translocation of Mdm2 from the cytoplasm to the nucleus. Proc Natl Acad Sci USA. 2001;98:11598–603.
69. Gottlieb TM, Leal JF, Seger R, Taya Y, Oren M. Cross-talk between Akt, p53 and Mdm2: possible implications for the regulation of apoptosis. Oncogene. 2002;21:1299–303.
70. Oren M, Damalas A, Gottlieb T, et al. Regulation of p53: intricate loops and delicate balances. Biochem Pharmacol. 2002;64:865–71.
71. Brunet A, Bonni A, Zigmond MJ, et al. Akt promotes cell survival by phosphorylating and inhibiting a Forkhead transcription factor. Cell. 1999;96:857–68.
72. Romashkova JA, Makarov SS. NF-κB is a target of AKT in anti-apoptotic PDGF signalling. Nature. 1999;401:86–90.
73. Wan YS, Wang ZQ, Shao Y, Voorhees JJ, Fisher GJ. Ultraviolet irradiation activates PI 3-kinase/AKT survival pathway via EGF receptors in human skin in vivo. Int J Oncol. 2001;18:461–6.
74. Waldmann V, Wacker J, Deichmann M. Mutations of the activation-associated phosphorylation sites at codons 308 and 473 of protein kinase B are absent in human melanoma. Arch Dermatol Res. 2001;293:368–72.
75. Waldmann V, Wacker J, Deichmann M. Absence of mutations in the pleckstrin homology (PH) domain of protein kinase B (PKB/Akt) in malignant melanoma. Melanoma Res. 2002;12:45–50.
76. Davies MA, Stemke-Hale K, Tellez C, et al. A novel AKT3 mutation in melanoma tumours and cell lines. Br J Cancer. 2008;99:1265–8.
77. Krasilnikov M, Adler V, Fuchs SY, Dong Z, Haimovitz-Friedman A, Herlyn M, Ronai Z. Contribution of phosphatidylinositol 3-kinase to radiation resistance in human melanoma cells. Mol Carcinog. 1999;24:64–9.
78. Simpson L, Parsons R. PTEN: life as a tumor suppressor. Exp Cell Res. 2001;264:29–41.
79. Maehama T, Dixon JE. The tumor suppressor, PTEN/MMAC1, dephosphorylates the lipid second messenger, phosphatidylinositol 3,4,5-trisphosphate. J Biol Chem. 1998;273:13375–8.
80. Vazquez F, Sellers WR. The PTEN tumor suppressor protein: an antagonist of phosphoinositide 3-kinase signaling. Biochim Biophys Acta. 2000;1470:M21–35.
81. Bonneau D, Longy M. Mutations of the human PTEN gene. Hum Mutat. 2000;16:109–22.
82. Maehama T, Taylor GS, Dixon JE. PTEN and myotubularin: novel phosphoinositide phosphatases. Annu Rev Biochem. 2001;70:247–79.
83. Ali IU, Schriml LM, Dean M. Mutational spectra of PTEN/MMAC1 gene: a tumor suppressor with lipid phosphatase activity. J Natl Cancer Inst. 1999;91:1922–32.
84. Tsao H, Zhang X, Benoit E, Haluska FG. Identification of PTEN/MMAC1 alterations in uncultured melanomas and melanoma cell lines. Oncogene. 1998;16:3397–402.
85. Egger G, Liang G, Aparicio A, Jones PA. Epigenetics in human disease and prospects for epigenetic therapy. Nature. 2004;429:457–63.
86. Mirmohammadsadegh A, Marini A, Nambiar S, Hassan M, Tannapfel A, Ruzicka T, Hengge UR. Epigenetic silencing of the PTEN gene in melanoma. Cancer Res. 2006;66:6546–52.
87. Tsao H, Goel V, Wu H, Yang G, Haluska FG. Genetic interaction between NRAS and BRAF mutations and PTEN/MMAC1 inactivation in melanoma. J Invest Dermatol. 2004;122:337–41.
88. Wu H, Goel V, Haluska FG. PTEN signaling pathways in melanoma. Oncogene. 2003;22:3113–22.
89. Dahia PL, Aguiar RC, Alberta J, et al. PTEN is inversely correlated with the cell survival factor Akt/PKB and is inactivated via multiple mechanisms in haematological malignancies. Hum Mol Genet. 1999;8:185–93.
90. Levy C, Khaled M, Fisher DE. MITF: master regulator of melanocyte development and melanoma oncogene. Trends Mol Med. 2006;12:406–14.
91. Denat L, Larue L. Malignant melanoma and the role of the paradoxal protein microphthalmia transcription factor. Bull Cancer. 2007;94:81–92.
92. Loercher AE, Tank EM, Delston RB, Harbour JW. MITF links differentiation with cell cycle arrest in melanocytes by transcriptional activation of INK4A. J Cell Biol. 2005;168:35–40.
93. Carreira S, Goodall J, Aksan I, et al. Mitf cooperates with Rb1 and activates p21Cip1 expression to regulate cell cycle progression. Nature. 2005;433:764–9.
94. Wellbrock C, Marais R. Elevated expression of MITF counteracts B-RAF stimulated melanocyte and melanoma cell proliferation. J Cell Biol. 2005;170:703–8.
95. Du J, Widlund HR, Horstmann MA, et al. Critical role of CDK2 for melanoma growth linked to its melanocyte-specific transcriptional regulation by MITF. Cancer Cell. 2004;6:565–76.
96. McGill GG, Horstmann M, Widlund HR, et al. Bcl2 regulation by the melanocyte master regulator Mitf modulates lineage survival and melanoma cell viability. Cell. 2002;109:707–18.
97. Garraway LA, Widlund HR, Rubin MA, et al. Integrative genomic analyses identify MITF as a lineage survival oncogene amplified in malignant melanoma. Nature. 2005;436:117–22.

98. Polakis P. Wnt signaling and cancer. Genes Dev. 2000;14:1837–51.
99. Dorsky RI, Moon RT, Raible DW. Control of neural crest cell fate by the Wnt signalling pathway. Nature. 1998;396:370–3.
100. Dorsky RI, Moon RT, Raible DW. Environmental signals and cell fate specification in premigratory neural crest. Bioessays. 2000;22:708–16.
101. Peifer M, Polakis P. Wnt signaling in oncogenesis and embryogenesis – a look outside the nucleus. Science. 2000;287:1606–9.
102. You L, He B, Xu Z, et al. An anti-Wnt-2 monoclonal antibody induces apoptosis in malignant melanoma cells and inhibits tumor growth. Cancer Res. 2004;64:5385–9.
103. Kashani-Sabet M, Range J, Torabian S, et al. A multimarker assay to distinguish malignant melanomas from benign nevi. Proc Natl Acad Sci USA. 2009;106:6268–72.
104. Rubinfeld B, Robbins P, El-Gamil M, Albert I, Porfiri E, Polakis P. Stabilization of β-catenin by genetic defects in melanoma cell lines. Science. 1997;275:1790–2.
105. Rimm DL, Caca K, Hu G, Harrison FB, Fearon ER. Frequent nuclear/cytoplasmic localization of β-catenin without exon 3 mutations in malignant melanoma. Am J Pathol. 1999;154:325–9.
106. Wellbrock C, Rana S, Paterson H, Pickersgill H, Brummelkamp T, Marais R. Oncogenic BRAF regulates melanoma proliferation through the lineage specific factor MITF. PLoS One. 2008;3:2734.
107. Morgan T. The theory of the gene. Am Nat. 1917;51:513–44.
108. Artavanis-Tsakonas S, Rand MD, Lake RJ. Notch signaling: cell fate control and signal integration in development. Science. 1999;284:770–6.
109. Jeffries S, Capobianco AJ. Neoplastic transformation by Notch requires nuclear localization. Mol Cell Biol. 2000;20:3928–41.
110. Allman D, Punt JA, Izon DJ, Aster JC, Pear WS. An invitation to T and more: notch signaling in lymphopoiesis. Cell. 2002;109:S1–11.
111. Ellisen LW, Bird J, West DC, Soreng AL, Reynolds TC, Smith SD, Sklar J. TAN-1, the human homolog of the Drosophila notch gene, is broken by chromosomal translocations in T lymphoblastic neoplasms. Cell. 1991;66:649–61.
112. Sriuranpong V, Borges MW, Ravi RK, Arnold DR, Nelkin BD, Baylin SB, Ball DW. Notch signaling induces cell cycle arrest in small cell lung cancer cells. Cancer Res. 2001;61:3200–5.
113. Gestblom C, Grynfeld A, Ora I, et al. The basic helix-loop-helix transcription factor dHAND, a marker gene for the developing human sympathetic nervous system, is expressed in both high- and low-stage neuroblastomas. Lab Invest. 1999;79:67–79.
114. Grynfeld A, Påhlman S, Axelson H. Induced neuroblastoma cell differentiation, associated with transient HES-1 activity and reduced HASH-1 expression, is inhibited by Notch1. Int J Cancer. 2000;88:401–10.
115. Zagouras P, Stifani S, Blaumueller CM, Carcangiu ML, Artavanis-Tsakonas S. Alterations in Notch signaling in neoplastic lesions of the human cervix. Proc Natl Acad Sci USA. 1995;92:6414–8.
116. Talora C, Sgroi DC, Crum CP, Dotto GP. Specific down-modulation of Notch1 signaling in cervical cancer cells is required for sustained HPV-E6/E7 expression and late steps of malignant transformation. Genes Dev. 2002;16:2252–63.
117. Shou J, Ross S, Koeppen H, de Sauvage FJ, Gao WQ. Dynamics of notch expression during murine prostate development and tumorigenesis. Cancer Res. 2001;61:7291–7.
118. Nicolas M, Wolfer A, Raj K, et al. Notch1 functions as a tumor suppressor in mouse skin. Nat Genet. 2003;33:416–21.
119. Rangarajan A, Talora C, Okuyama R, et al. Notch signaling is a direct determinant of keratinocyte growth arrest and entry into differentiation. EMBO J. 2001;20:3427–36.
120. Lowell S, Jones P, Le Roux I, Dunne J, Watt FM. Stimulation of human epidermal differentiation by δ-notch signalling at the boundaries of stem-cell clusters. Curr Biol. 2000;10:491–500.
121. Hoek K, Rimm DL, Williams KR, et al. Expression profiling reveals novel pathways in the transformation of melanocytes to melanomas. Cancer Res. 2004;64:5270–82.
122. Massi D, Tarantini F, Franchi A, et al. Evidence for differential expression of Notch receptors and their ligands in melanocytic nevi and cutaneous malignant melanoma. Mod Pathol. 2006;19:246–59.
123. Pinnix CC, Lee JT, Liu ZJ, et al. Active Notch1 confers a transformed phenotype to primary human melanocytes. Cancer Res. 2009;69:5312–20.
124. Kang DE, Soriano S, Xia X, Eberhart CG, De Strooper B, Zheng H, Koo EH. Presenilin couples the paired phosphorylation of beta-catenin independent of axin: implications for beta-catenin activation in tumorigenesis. Cell. 2002;110:751–62.
125. Li G, Satyamoorthy K, Herlyn M. N-cadherin-mediated intercellular interactions promote survival and migration of melanoma cells. Cancer Res. 2001;61:3819–25.
126. Liu ZJ, Xiao M, Balint K, et al. Notch1 signaling promotes primary melanoma progression by activating mitogen-activated protein kinase/phosphatidylinositol 3-kinase-Akt pathways and up-regulating N-cadherin expression. Cancer Res. 2006;66:4182–90.
127. Cheng P, Zlobin A, Volgina V, et al. Notch-1 regulates NF-kB activity in hemopoietic progenitor cells. J Immunol. 2001;167:4458–67.
128. Shin HM, Minter LM, Cho OH, et al. Notch1 augments Nf-kB activity by facilitating its nuclear retention. EMBO J. 2006;25:129–38.
129. Weijzen S, Rizzo P, Braid M, et al. Activation of Notch1 signaling maintains the neoplastic phenotype in human Ras-transformed cells. Nat Med. 2002;8:979–86.

130. Kiaris H, Politi K, Grimm LM, et al. Modulation of Notch signaling elicits signature tumors and inhibits hras1-induced oncogenesis in the mouse mammary epithelium. Am J Pathol. 2004;165:695–705.
131. Karin M, Cao Y, Greten FR, Li ZW. NF-kappaB in cancer: from innocent bystander to major culprit. Nat Rev Cancer. 2002;2:301–10.
132. Bonizzi G, Karin M. The two NF-kappaB activation pathways and their role in innate and adaptive immunity. Trends Immunol. 2004;25:280–8.
133. Yamamoto M, Yamazaki S, Uematsu S, et al. Regulation of Toll/IL-1-receptor-mediated gene expression by the inducible nuclear protein IkappaBzeta. Nature. 2004;430:218–22.
134. Kuwata H, Matsumoto M, Atarashi K, Morishita H, Hirotani T, Koga R, Takeda K. IkappaBNS inhibits induction of a subset of Toll-like receptor-dependent genes and limits inflammation. Immunity. 2006;24: 41–51.
135. Bours V, Franzoso G, Azarenko V, Park S, Kanno T, Brown K, Siebenlist U. The oncoprotein Bcl-3 directly transactivates through kappa B motifs via association with DNA-binding p50B homodimers. Cell. 1993;72:729–39.
136. Xiao G, Harhaj EW, Sun SC. NF-kappaB-inducing kinase regulates the processing of NF-kappaB2 p100. Mol Cell. 2001;7:401–9.
137. Basseres DS, Baldwin AS. Nuclear factor-kappaB and inhibitor of kappaB kinase pathways in oncogenic initiation and progression. Oncogene. 2006;25:6817–30.
138. Jost PJ, Ruland J. Aberrant NF-kappaB signaling in lymphoma: mechanisms, consequences, and therapeutic implications. Blood. 2007;109:2700–7.
139. Cilloni D, Martinelli G, Messa F, Baccarani M, Saglio G. Nuclear factor kB as a target for new drug development in myeloid malignancies. Haematologica. 2007;92:1224–9.
140. Dutta J, Fan Y, Gupta N, Fan G, Gélinas C. Current insights into the regulation of programmed cell death by NF-kappaB. Oncogene. 2006;25:6800–16.
141. Luo JL, Kamata H, Karin M. The anti-death machinery in IKK/NF-kappaB signaling. J Clin Immunol. 2005;25:541–50.
142. Burstein E, Duckett CS. Dying for NF-kappaB? Control of cell death by transcriptional regulation of the apoptotic machinery. Curr Opin Cell Biol. 2003;15:732–7.
143. Hayakawa Y, Maeda S, Nakagawa H, et al. Effectiveness of IkappaB kinase inhibitors in murine colitis-associated tumorigenesis. J Gastroenterol. 2009;44:935–43.
144. Demchenko YN, Glebov OK, Zingone A, Keats JJ, Bergsagel PL, Kuehl WM. Classical and/or alternative NF-kappaB pathway activation in multiple myeloma. Blood. 2010;115:3541–52.
145. Siwak DR, Shishodia S, Aggarwal BB, Kurzrock R. Curcumin-induced antiproliferative and proapoptotic effects in melanoma cells are associated with suppression of IkappaB kinase and nuclear factor kappaB activity and are independent of the B-Raf/mitogen-activated/extracellular signal-regulated protein kinase pathway and the Akt pathway. Cancer. 2005;15(04):879–90.
146. Ianaro A, Tersigni M, Belardo G, et al. NEMO-binding domain peptide inhibits proliferation of human melanoma cells. Cancer Lett. 2009;18(274): 331–6.
147. Amiri KI, Richmond A. Role of nuclear factor-κB in melanoma. Cancer Metast Rev. 2005;24:301–31.
148. Meyskens Jr FL, Buckmeier JA, McNulty SE, Tohidian NB. Activation of nuclear factor-kappa B in human metastatic melanoma cells and the effect of oxidative stress. Clin Cancer Res. 1999;5: 1197–202.
149. McNulty SE, Tohidian NB, Meyskens Jr FL. RelA, p50 and inhibitor of kappa B alpha are elevated in human metastatic melanoma cells and respond aberrantly to ultraviolet light B. Pigment Cell Res. 2001;14:456–65.
150. McNulty SE, del Rosario R, Cen D, Meyskens Jr FL, Yang S. Comparative expression of NFkappaB proteins in melanocytes of normal skin vs. benign intradermal naevus and human metastatic melanoma biopsies. Pigment Cell Res. 2004;17:173–80.
151. Yang J, Amiri KI, Burke JR, Schmid JA, Richmond A. BMS-345541 targets inhibitor of kappaB kinase and induces apoptosis in melanoma: involvement of nuclear factor kappaB and mitochondria pathways. Clin Cancer Res. 2006;12:950–60.
152. Dhawan P, Singh AB, Ellis DL, Richmond A. Constitutive activation of Akt/protein kinase B in melanoma leads to up-regulation of nuclear factor-kappaB and tumor progression. Cancer Res. 2002;62: 7335–42.
153. Troppmair J, Hartkamp J, Rapp UR. Activation of NF-kappa B by oncogenic Raf in HEK 293 cells occurs through autocrine recruitment of the stress kinase cascade. Oncogene. 1998;17:685–90.
154. Jo H, Zhang R, Zhang H, et al. NF-kappa B is required for H-ras oncogene induced abnormal cell proliferation and tumorigenesis. Oncogene. 2000;19: 841–9.
155. Richardson PG, Hideshima T, Anderson KC. Bortezomib (PS-341): a novel, first-in-class proteasome inhibitor for the treatment of multiple myeloma and other cancers. Cancer Control. 2003;10:361–9.
156. Markovic SN, Geyer SM, Dawkins F, et al. A phase II study of bortezomib in the treatment of metastatic malignant melanoma. Cancer. 2005;103:2584–9.
157. Kamijo R, Harada H, Matsuyama T, et al. Requirement for transcription factor IRF-1 in NO synthase induction in macrophages. Science. 1994; 263:1612–5.
158. Fukumura D, Kashiwagi S, Jain RK. The role of nitric oxide in tumour progression. Nat Rev Cancer. 2006;6:521–34.
159. Grimm EA, Ellerhorst J, Tang CH, Ekmekcioglu S. Constitutive intracellular production of iNOS and NO in human melanoma: possible role in regulation

159. of growth and resistance to apoptosis. Nitric Oxide. 2008;19:133–7.
160. Russo PA, Halliday GM. Inhibition of nitric oxide and reactive oxygen species production improves the ability of a sunscreen to protect from sunburn, immunosuppression and photocarcinogenesis. Br J Dermatol. 2006;155:408–15.
161. Palmieri G, Capone ME, Ascierto ML, et al. Main roads to melanoma. J Transl Med. 2009;7:86.
162. Martin E, Nathan C, Xie QW. Role of interferon regulatory factor 1 in induction of nitric oxide synthase. J Exp Med. 1994;180:977–84.
163. Xie QW, Kashiwabara Y, Nathan C. Role of transcription factor NF-kappa B/Rel in induction of nitric oxide synthase. J Biol Chem. 1994;269:4705–8.
164. Adcock IM, Brown CR, Kwon O, Barnes PJ. Oxidative stress induces NF kappa B DNA binding and inducible NOS mRNA in human epithelial cells. Biochem Biophys Res Commun. 1994;199:1518–24.
165. Meyskens Jr FL, McNulty SE, Buckmeier JA, et al. Aberrant redox regulation in human metastatic melanoma cells compared to normal melanocytes. Free Radic Biol Med. 2001;31:799–808.
166. Zhang J, Peng B, Chen X. Expression of nuclear factor kappaB, inducible nitric oxide synthesis, and vascular endothelial growth factor in adenoid cystic carcinoma of salivary glands: correlations with the angiogenesis and clinical outcome. Clin Cancer Res. 2005;11:7334–43.
167. MacMicking J, Xie QW, Nathan C. Nitric oxide and macrophage function. Rev Immunol. 1997;15:323–50.
168. Bredt DS. Endogenous nitric oxide synthesis: biological functions and pathophysiology. Free Radic Res. 1999;31:577–96.
169. Geller DA, Billiar TR. Molecular biology of nitric oxide synthases. Cancer Metastasis Rev. 1998;17:7–23.
170. Massi D, Franchi A, Sardi I, et al. Inducible nitric oxide synthase expression in benign and malignant cutaneous melanocytic lesions. J Pathol. 2001;194:194–200.
171. Xie K, Huang S, Dong Z, Juang SH, Gutman M, Xie QW, Nathan C, Fidler IJ. Transfection with the inducible nitric oxide syntheses gene suppresses tumorigenicity and abrogates metastasis by K-1735 murine melanoma cells. J Exp Med. 1995;181:1333–43.
172. Xie K, Wang Y, Huang S, et al. Nitric oxide-mediated apoptosis of K-1735 melanoma cells is associated with downregulation of Bcl-2. Oncogene. 1997;15:771–9.
173. Messmer UK, Ankarcrona M, Nicotera P, Brüne B. p53 expression in nitric oxide induced apoptosis. FEBS Lett. 1994;355:23–6.
174. Rudin CM, Thompson CB. Apoptosis and disease: regulation and clinical relevance of programmed cell death. Annu Rev Med. 1997;48:267–81.
175. Williams GT, Smith CA. Molecular regulation of apoptosis: genetic controls on cell death. Cell. 1993;74:777–9.
176. Krammer PH. The CD95(APO-1/Fas)/CD95L system. Toxicol Lett. 1998;102–103:131–7.
177. Reed JC. Dysregulation of apoptosis in cancer. J Clin Oncol. 1999;17:2941–53.
178. Frisch SM, Screaton RA. Anoikis mechanisms. Curr Opin Cell Biol. 2001;13:555–62.
179. Brune B, Mohr S, Messmer UK. Protein thiol modification and apoptotic cell death as cGMP-independent nitric oxide (NO) signaling pathways. Rev Physiol Biochem Pharmacol. 1996;127:1–30.
180. Tschugguel W, Pustelnik T, Lass H, et al. Inducible nitric oxide synthase (iNOS) expression may predict distant metastasis in human melanoma. Br J Cancer. 1999;79:1609–12.
181. Ahmed B, Van den Oord JJ. Expression of the inducible isoform of nitric oxide synthase in pigment cell lesions of the skin. Br J Dermatol. 2000;142:432–40.
182. Ekmekcioglu S, Ellerhorst J, Smid CM, et al. Inducible nitric oxide synthase and nitrotyrosine in human metastatic melanoma tumors correlate with poor survival. Clin Cancer Res. 2000;6:4768–75.
183. Jemal A, Siegel R, Ward E, Hao Y, Xu J, Murray T, Thun MJ. Cancer statistics, 2008. CA Cancer J Clin. 2008;58:71–96.
184. Chin L, Garraway LA, Fisher DE. Malignant melanoma: genetics and therapeutics in the genomic era. Genes Dev. 2006;20:2149–82.
185. Soengas MS, Lowe SW. Apoptosis and melanoma chemoresistance. Oncogene. 2003;22:3138–51.
186. Miller AJ, Mihm MC. Melanoma. N Engl J Med. 2006;355:51–65.
187. Bevona C, Goggins W, Quinn T. Cutaneous melanomas associated with nevi. Arch Dermatol. 2003;139:1620–4.
188. Rasheed S, Mao Z, Chan JMC, Chan LS. Is melanoma a stem cell tumor? Identification of neurogenic proteins in trans-differentiated cells. J Transl Med. 2005;3:14.
189. Zabierowski SE, Herlyn M. Melanoma stem cells: the dark seed of melanoma. J Clin Oncol. 2008;26:2890–4.

Staging of Melanoma

Zendee Elaba, Michael J. Murphy, Philip Kerr, and Jane M. Grant-Kels

The Melanoma Staging Committee of the American Joint Committee on Cancer (AJCC) was formed in 1998 and is comprised of experts from all relevant medical specialties, including many of the major melanoma centers in North America, Europe, and Australia [1]. This committee set up the AJCC Melanoma Staging Database for the collection of prospective outcome data on melanoma patients from 13 cancer centers and cooperative groups in order to establish and subsequently revise a melanoma staging system [2]. The staging system for melanoma has undergone multiple revisions in the last decade, reflecting the rapid and continuous acquisition of new information and advances in this field [3]. The most recent 7th edition AJCC melanoma staging recommendations are based on multivariate analysis of 30,946 patients with Stages I, II, and III melanoma and 7,972 patients with Stage IV melanoma [4]. The 7th edition AJCC cancer staging system was formally implemented in January 2010.

Z. Elaba, M.D. (✉)
Department of Pathology, Hartford Hospital,
Hartford, CT, USA
e-mail: zendee.elaba@gmail.com

M.J. Murphy, M.D. • P. Kerr, M.D. • J.M. Grant-Kels, M.D.
Department of Dermatology, University
of Connecticut Health Center, Farmington, CT, USA

TNM Classification

The TNM classification system is widely used to characterize cancers, based on the extent of the primary tumor (T), involvement of regional lymph nodes (N), and distant metastasis (M) [5]. The TNM categories for melanoma used in the 7th edition AJCC Staging Manual are outlined in Table 4.1.

T – Primary Tumor

Primary Tumor Thickness

Melanoma thickness (Breslow depth) principally defines the T category, while ulceration and mitotic rate are used as secondary criteria to characterize the primary tumor. Breslow depth is a measurement in millimeters of the thickness of the tumor from the top of the granular layer of the epidermis to the deepest point of invasion [6]. To obtain accurate thickness measurements, the biopsy sample must include the deepest portion of the tumor [7]. The T category thresholds of melanoma thickness are defined as: T1: less than or equal to 1.0 mm, T2: 1.01–2.0 mm, T3: 2.01–4.0 mm, and T4: greater than 4.0 mm [5].

Ulceration

Ulceration, the second determinant of the T category, is regarded as the absence of a completely

Table 4.1 TNM staging categories for cutaneous melanoma

T	Thickness (mm)	Ulceration status/mitoses
Tis	NA	NA
T1	≤1.00	a: Without ulceration and mitosis <1/mm^2 b: With ulceration or mitoses ≥1/mm^2
T2	1.01–2.00	a: Without ulceration b: With ulceration
T3	2.01–4.00	a: Without ulceration b: With ulceration
T4	>4.00	a: Without ulceration b: With ulceration
N	**No. of Metastatic Nodes**	**Nodal Metastatic Burden**
N0	0	NA
N1	1	a: Micrometastasis* b: Macrometastasis†
N2	2–3	a: Micrometastasis* b: Macrometastasis† c: In-transit metastases/satellites without metastatic nodes
N3	≥4 metastatic nodes, or matted nodes, or in-transit metastases/satellites with metastatic nodes	
M	**Site**	**Serum LDH**
M0	No distant metastases	NA
M1a	Distant skin, subcutaneous, or nodal metastases	Normal
M1b	Lung metastases	Normal
M1c	All other visceral metastases	Normal
	Any distant metastasis	Elevated

Tis melanoma in situ, *NA* not applicable, *LDH* lactate dehydrogenase
*Micrometastases are diagnosed after sentinel lymph node biopsy and completion lymphadenectomy
†Macrometastases are defined as clinically detectable nodal metastases confirmed histopathologically

intact epidermis above the primary melanoma on microscopic evaluation [8–10]. Specifically, ulceration is defined as the combination of the following histopathologic features: full-thickness epidermal defect to include absence of stratum corneum and basement membrane, evidence of reactive changes (i.e., fibrin deposition and neutrophils), and thinning, effacement, or reactive hyperplasia of the surrounding epidermis without a history of trauma or recent surgical procedure [5]. A primary melanoma without ulceration is classified under T subcategory "a"; an ulcerated melanoma is grouped under subcategory "b". Ulceration signifies a greater risk for metastases, such that the survival rates for patients of a given T category with ulceration are almost equivalent to patients of the next highest T category without ulceration [7]. To illustrate, the 5-year survival for a T2 ulcerated melanoma (T2b) is ~82%, similar to ~79% for a T3 non-ulcerated melanoma (T3a). Both are categorized as Stage IIA [4]. When multiple primaries are present, the T category is determined by the melanoma with the poorest histopathologic features [7].

Mitotic Rate

In the most recently revised 7th edition AJCC melanoma staging system, the mitotic rate is introduced as a T1 category modifier. Data from the AJCC Melanoma Staging Database and multiple publications have shown that increasing mitotic rate is associated with declining survival rates, particularly within thin melanoma subgroups (Stages I and II) [4, 11–14]. Multiple thresholds of mitotic rate were examined statistically, and the most significant correlation with survival was identified at a threshold of at least 1 mitosis/mm^2 [4]. For T1 melanomas (≤1 mm), a mitotic rate of at least 1 mitosis/mm^2 now replaces Clark level of invasion (used in the 6th edition) as a primary criterion for upgrading the tumor from T1a to T1b [5]. According to the current definition, T1b melanomas are those having a tumor thickness of ≤1.0 mm with the presence of at least 1 mitosis/mm^2 and/or tumor ulceration. The incorporation of mitotic rate to subclassify thin melanomas as T1b in the 7th edition of the AJCC staging system was based on survival studies showing that melanomas with <1 mitosis/mm^2 or <0.5 mm in thickness have a very low risk of nodal micrometastases [5].

With its inclusion in the AJCC staging system, mitotic rate should be assessed in all primary melanomas. The recommended approach is to first identify the area in the dermis showing the most mitotic figures, the so-called "hot spot" [5]. The mitoses in the hot spot are enumerated and the count is then extended to adjacent fields until an area corresponding to 1 mm^2 is evaluated. As a guide, 1 mm^2 corresponds to an area equivalent to approximately four high power fields at ×400 magnification in most, but not all, microscopes. For accuracy, calibration of individual microscopes is recommended [14]. The count is expressed as the number of mitoses/mm^2. If mitoses are sparse and no hot spot can be found, a representative mitosis is chosen from which the count is started and extended to adjacent fields until an area corresponding to 1 mm^2 is again assessed [5, 15]. When the area of the invasive tumor component is less than 1 mm^2, the number of mitoses present in 1 mm^2 of dermal tissue that includes the tumor should be counted and recorded as a number per square millimeter. As an alternative, in tumors with an invasive component less than 1 mm^2 in area, the presence or absence of a mitosis can be designated as at least 1/mm^2 (i.e., "mitogenic") or 0/mm^2 (i.e., "non-mitogenic"), respectively. Some institutions use the designation <1/mm^2 when mitotic figures are not found after examining multiple fields. Most tumor registries interpret this designation "<1/mm^2" as equivalent to zero [4, 5, 15].

N – Regional Lymph Nodes

The N category is based on the status of regional lymph nodes. The number of metastatic nodes is the primary criterion for defining the N category. It has been shown to correlate most strongly with 10-year survival rates compared to other prognostic factors in melanoma patients with regional lymph node metastases [4]. The tumor is classified as N0 when no regional metastasis is detected. N1 is defined as a single nodal metastasis. N2 indicates that two or three nodes are involved, or that in-transit metastases or satellite lesions, including microsatellites (see below) are present in the absence of regional nodal involvement. Those with ≥4 metastatic nodes, matted nodes or in-transit metastases/satellites with metastatic nodes are classified as N3 [5, 7].

Micrometastases Versus Macrometastases

Tumor burden is another important prognostic feature for patients with lymph node metastases, as survival rates differ significantly between patients with micrometastatic versus macrometastatic disease [8, 16, 17]. In a multivariate analysis of prognostic factors among patients with Stage III melanoma, the 5-year overall survival was 67% for patients with nodal micrometastases and 43% for those with nodal macrometastases [18]. Patients who have histopathologically documented nodal metastases [after sentinel lymph node biopsy (SLNB) or elective lymphadenectomy], but with no clinical or radiologic evidence of lymph node metastases, are defined as having micrometastases (subcategory "a") [3, 5]. In the updated AJCC Melanoma Staging Database used for the 7th edition of the AJCC staging manual, more than 90% of micrometastases were detected by SLNB [18]. Patients who have clinical evidence of nodal metastases that are subsequently confirmed by microscopic evaluation, or nodal metastases that show gross extracapsular extension, are defined as having macrometastases (subcategory "b") [5].

Regardless of micrometastatic or macrometastatic status, the number of involved lymph nodes remains the most significant prognostic factor, correlating inversely with survival rates. In multivariate analysis of Stage III patients, the 5-year survival rates for patients with one, two, and three micrometastatic nodes were 71%, 65%, and 61%, respectively. The survival rates for those with similarly stratified macrometastatic nodes were 50%, 43%, and 40%, respectively. When four or more nodes are involved, the 5-year survival rates are ~36% for both groups [18].

Intralymphatic Metastases

The third criterion for defining the N category (subcategory "c") is the presence or absence of satellites or in-transit metastases. Satellite lesions are discontinuous foci of tumor that reside within 5 cm from the primary tumor. In-transit metastases are lesions of discontinuous foci that reside more than 5 cm from the primary tumor. Both tumor foci represent intralymphatic metastases and signify a poorer prognosis [19]. Available data show that there is no significant difference in outcome between these two anatomically defined entities [20]. The presence of in-transit metastases or satellites without metastatic nodes is classified as N2c, while in-transit metastases or satellite lesions associated with regional nodal involvement is categorized as N3 [5]. Microsatellites are defined as any discontinuous nests of metastatic cells that are >0.05 mm in diameter and clearly separated by normal dermis (not fibrosis or inflammation) from the main invasive component of melanoma by a distance of at least 0.3 mm [5]. As in the 6th AJCC edition, the presence of microsatellites is classified in the N2c category.

Immunohistochemical (IHC) Detection of Micrometastases

In the 6th edition of the Cancer Staging Manual, histopathologic confirmation by hematoxylin and eosin (H&E) staining was mandatory to define micrometastasis [15]. With the current availability and use of immunohistochemical (IHC) stains, the AJCC Melanoma Staging Committee now considers it acceptable to classify nodal metastases based solely on IHC staining with at least one melanoma-specific marker (i.e., HMB-45, MelanA/MART-1). In addition, the cells should have malignant morphologic features that are discernible in the IHC-stained tissue [21].

M – Distant Metastasis

The M category is divided into 3 site-based groups that differ significantly with respect to survival: M1a, M1b, and M1c. Both the site(s) of metastases and serum levels of lactate dehydrogenase (LDH) are used to subclassify the M category.

Studies have repeatedly shown that the greatest difference in survival exists between patients with melanoma metastases in visceral sites compared to those with metastases in non-visceral sites [8]. M1a designates patients who have distant metastases in the skin, subcutaneous tissue, or distant lymph nodes, and normal LDH levels. These patients have a relatively better prognosis compared to those with metastases in any other anatomic site(s) [8, 22–24]. M1b defines patients with metastases to the lung and normal LDH levels. They have a slightly better prognosis compared to those individuals with metastases to other visceral sites [22, 25, 26]. Patients with metastases to any other visceral site(s), or any site(s) associated with an elevated LDH level, are classified as M1c. These patients show the worst survival curves [23, 27].

The serum factor LDH is included as a second qualifier of M staging. It has been demonstrated by multiple studies, as well as the updated Melanoma Staging Database, to be an independent and highly significant predictor of survival in Stage IV melanoma patients [5, 8, 23, 28, 29]. An elevated LDH is among the most predictive independent factors of diminished survival upon multivariate analysis, even after accounting for site and number of visceral metastases [24]. In the 2008 AJCC Melanoma Staging Database, the

1- and 2-year overall survival rates for Stage IV patients with normal serum LDH levels were 65% and 40%, respectively. For those with elevated LDH levels, the survival rates were reduced to 32% and 18%, respectively [4]. Hence, when the LDH level is elevated at the time of staging, patients are classified as M1c, regardless of the site of metastasis. For staging purposes, it is recommended that two or more serum LDH determinations are obtained and taken more than 24 h apart [5]. A single determination can yield a false-positive result, as a function of hemolysis or other factors that are not related to melanoma metastases.

The number of metastases at distant sites, previously documented as an important prognostic factor [22, 23, 25, 28–30], is not included in the current staging system. This is due to the lack of standardization of diagnostic tests employed to search for metastases among the published studies. Until better test standardization, the number of metastases cannot be reliably utilized for staging [5].

Metastatic Melanoma of Unknown Primary Site

Metastatic melanoma of unknown primary site is defined as histopathologically confirmed subcutaneous, lymph nodal or visceral metastatic melanoma with no evidence of concomitant cutaneous, mucosal or ocular primary lesion or a previous skin tumor excised without microscopic examination [31]. An accepted theory for possible origin of such a metastatic tumor is an undetected primary melanoma that has undergone spontaneous regression [32]. Patients with metastatic melanoma of unknown primary site have been shown to have a natural history and prognosis that is similar to, or even better than, those with known primary tumors [33, 34]. This suggests that the endogenous immune response which led to the regression of the primary melanoma may somehow contribute to a more favorable outcome [34].

In general, metastatic melanomas of both known and unknown primary sites should be staged with the same criteria. When patients present with lymph node metastases and staging work-up does not reveal any other sites of disease, these metastases should be presumed to be regional (i.e., Stage III, instead of Stage IV). Careful examination of the entire cutaneous surface with special attention to the areas of skin containing lymphatics which drain to that nodal basin should be performed with and without a Wood's lamp in order to look for scars from previous procedures or areas of depigmentation. Pathology from any previous biopsy should be reviewed to check for the possibility of a primary melanoma. Localized metastases to the skin or subcutaneous tissues with no other sites of metastases should also be considered regional disease (Stage III). All other circumstances, including metastases to a visceral site by melanoma of unknown primary site, should be classified as Stage IV disease [5].

Clinical Versus Histopathologic Staging

The definitions of clinical versus histopathologic grouping depend on whether lymph nodes are staged clinically/radiographically or by light microscopic evaluation (Table 4.2).

Clinical Staging

Clinical Stages I and II include patients who have no evidence of regional or distant metastases based on clinical, radiologic, and/or laboratory evaluation. Clinical Stage III includes patients with clinical or radiologic evidence of regional metastases involving either the regional lymph node basin or intralymphatic metastases (satellite or in-transit disease). No subgrouping with respect to the number of metastatic nodes is necessary, and all patients with nodal or intralymphatic regional metastases are classified as clinical Stage III. Clinical Stage IV includes patients with metastases at a distant site(s) and is not further substaged.

Table 4.2 Anatomic stage groupings for cutaneous melanoma

Clinical staging*				Pathologic staging†			
0	Tis	N0	M0	0	Tis	N0	M0
IA	T1a	N0	M0	IA	T1a	N0	M0
IB	T1b	N0	M0	IB	T1b	N0	M0
	T2a	N0	M0		T2a	N0	M0
IIA	T2b	N0	M0	IIA	T2b	N0	M0
	T3a	N0	M0		T3a	N0	M0
IIB	T3b	N0	M0	IIB	T3b	N0	M0
	T4a	N0	M0		T4a	N0	M0
IIC	T4b	N0	M0	IIC	T4b	N0	M0
III	Any T	N > N0	M0	IIIA	T1–4a	N1a	M0
					T1–4a	N2a	M0
				IIIB	T1–4b	N1a	M0
					T1–4b	N2a	M0
					T1–4a	N1b	M0
					T1–4a	N2b	M0
					T1–4a	N2c	M0
				IIIC	T1–4b	N1b	M0
					T1–4b	N2b	M0
					T1–4b	N2c	M0
					Any T	N3	M0
IV	Any T	Any N	M1	IV	Any T	Any N	M1

*Clinical staging includes microstaging of the primary melanoma and clinical/radiologic evaluation for metastases. By convention, it should be used after complete excision of the primary melanoma with clinical assessment for regional and distant metastases

†Pathologic staging includes microstaging of the primary melanoma and pathologic information about the regional lymph nodes after partial (i.e., sentinel node biopsy) or complete lymphadenectomy. Pathologic stage 0 or stage IA patients are the exception; they do not require pathologic evaluation of their lymph nodes

Histopathologic Staging

Histopathologic Stages I and II include patients with no evidence of regional or distant metastases after careful microscopic examination of the regional lymph nodes, in addition to an absence of distant metastases on clinical and radiologic examination. Histopathologic Stage III includes patients showing microscopic evidence of regional metastasis, either in the regional lymph nodes or at intralymphatic sites. For quantitative classification of histopathologic nodal status, careful microscopic evaluation of the resected nodal basin with documentation of the number of lymph nodes examined and the number of those containing metastases should be performed. Histopathologic Stage IV includes patients with microscopic documentation of metastases at one or more distant sites.

Stage Groups

Localized Melanoma (Stages I and II)

Patients with primary melanoma, in the absence of clinical or histopathologic evidence of regional or distant metastases, are categorized into Stages I and II.

Stage I includes patients with low-risk primary melanomas, and is further divided into subgroups "A" and "B" on the basis of ulceration and presence of mitoses. Stage IA includes primary lesions ≤1 mm in thickness and a mitotic rate of <1 mitosis/mm^2, but without ulceration of the overlying epithelium (T1aN0M0). Stage IB includes primary lesions that are either (1) ≤1 mm in thickness with epithelial ulceration or a mitotic rate of at least 1 mitosis/mm^2 (T1bN0M0) or (2) between

1.01 and 2 mm in thickness without ulceration and regardless of mitotic rate (T2N0M0).

Stage II patients with high-risk primary tumors are divided into three subcategories: (1) Stage IIA includes lesions between 1.01 and 2 mm in thickness with ulceration of the overlying epithelium (T2bN0M0), and those >2 mm and ≤4 mm in thickness without epithelial ulceration (T3aN0M0); (2) Stage IIB lesions are >2 mm to 4 mm in thickness with epithelial ulceration (T3bN0M0), or >4 mm in thickness without ulceration (T4aN0M0); and (3) Stage IIC consists of primary lesions >4 mm with overlying ulceration (T4bN0M0).

Regional Metastases (Stage III)

Stage III includes lesions with histopathologically documented involvement of regional lymph nodes or the presence of in-transit or satellite metastases. No substaging is required for clinical Stage III melanoma. For histopathologic stage, the major determinants of outcome are: (1) the number of metastatic lymph nodes; (2) tumor burden (microscopic – detected histopathologically versus macroscopic – detected by physical or radiographic examination and verified microscopically); (3) features of the primary melanoma, including ulceration, mitotic rate and/or Breslow thickness, in the presence of nodal micrometastasis; and (4) presence of satellite or in-transit metastases [20, 35–40]. Of note, tumor features are significant predictors of adverse outcome in patients with nodal micrometastases, but not in those with nodal macrometastases [5].

Using the above prognostic parameters, Stage III is divided into three subgroups with statistically significant differences in survival: (1) Stage IIIA includes patients with 1–3 microscopically involved lymph nodes and without ulceration in the primary tumor (T1-4aN1aM0 or T1-4aN2aM0); (2) Stage IIIB includes: (a) patients with 1–3 microscopically involved lymph nodes and an ulcerated primary tumor (T1-4bN1aM0 or T1-4bN2aM0); (b) those with 1–3 macroscopically involved lymph nodes and a non-ulcerated primary tumor (T1-4aN1bM0 or T1-4aN2bM0); or (c) patients with intralymphatic regional metastases, but without nodal disease (T1-4aN2cM0); and (3) Stage IIIC defines: (a) patients with 1–3 macroscopic lymph node metastases and ulceration in the primary melanoma (T1-4bN1bM0 or T1-4bN2bM0); (b) patients with satellite(s)/in-transit metastases from an ulcerated primary melanoma (T1-4bN2cM0); or (c) any patient with N3 disease, regardless of T status.

Distant Metastases (Stage IV)

Stage IV melanoma is defined by the presence of distant metastases (any M1). Survival differences between the M categories are not statistically significant, and patients are not further substaged [5].

Updates and Changes in the 7th Edition AJCC Melanoma Staging System

Changes in the current edition result from the analysis of an expanded sample size in the melanoma staging database (~17,600 patients in the 6th edition versus ~39,000 patients in the 7th edition), through the collaboration of 17 major cancer centers and organizations [3]. The key features and revisions of the current 2010 AJCC staging system are highlighted as follows:

1. Primary tumor mitotic rate (defined as mitoses/mm^2, not mitoses/10 high power fields) replaces Clark level of invasion in defining the subcategory of T1b. Currently, a mitotic rate of ≥1 mitosis/mm^2 defines T1b; whereas in the 2002 AJCC staging system, T1b melanomas were defined as either ulcerated or with a Clark level IV or V.
2. Either H&E or IHC staining can now be used to define the presence of microscopic nodal metastases. Previously, only H&E staining could be used for staging purposes.
3. The threshold previously used for defining nodal metastasis in the AJCC 6th edition was a metastasis measuring ≥0.2 mm. As a result

of the recent consensus that regional nodal metastatic melanoma of <0.2 mm in diameter is clinically important, nodal tumor deposits of any size are now included in the staging of nodal disease [14]. There is no lower threshold of tumor burden used to define the presence of regional nodal metastasis, and isolated melanoma cells or tumor deposits of <0.1 mm in diameter that are histopathologically or immunohistochemically detected should be considered N+ [4]. As yet, an evidence-based lower threshold of clinically insignificant nodal metastases has not been identified [15].

4. The M category continues to be primarily defined by the site(s) of distant metastases: non-visceral (i.e., skin/soft tissue/distant nodal) (M1a); lung (M1b); and all other visceral metastatic sites (M1c).

5. An increased serum LDH remains a powerful adverse predictor of survival. Regardless of the site of distant disease, patients with elevated LDH are all categorized as M1c.

6. While survival estimates for patients with intralymphatic regional metastases (i.e., satellite and in-transit disease) are somewhat better than for the remaining cohort of patients with Stage IIIB disease, Stage IIIB represents the closest statistical fit for this former group. The definition of intralymphatic regional metastasis has been retained in the current staging system.

7. As recommended by the Melanoma Staging Committee, microsatellites are to be retained in the N2c category. The prognostic significance of this uncommon feature has not been clearly established, but limited evidence shows survival outcome to be similar to patients with satellite metastases [5]. Current published data are insufficient to substantiate a revision of the definitions used in the 6th edition of the staging manual.

8. Metastatic melanoma identified in lymph nodes, skin, or subcutaneous tissues, without a known associated primary melanoma (metastatic melanoma of unknown primary site), is to be classified as Stage III rather than Stage IV disease.

9. Lymphatic mapping and SLNB continue to be important staging tools in melanoma [41], and should be used to identify occult Stage III regional nodal disease among patients who present with clinical Stage IB or Stage II melanoma.

Final Comments and Future Applications

The AJCC Melanoma Staging System recommends that SLNB be accomplished as a staging procedure in melanoma patients for whom results will be used in the subsequent treatment and follow-up decision-making process. In this regard, SLNB is recommended for patients with T2, T3 or T4 melanomas and clinically uninvolved regional lymph nodes (clinical Stage IB and Stage II), in addition to those individuals with T1 melanomas associated with adverse prognostic characteristics: ulceration, mitotic rate ≥1 mitosis/mm^2, and/or Clark level IV.

Melanoma staging critically depends on the identification of the most relevant predictive factors of survival outcome. The need to further subclassify melanomas, particularly those that have already metastasized, and the continuous evolution of our understanding of cancer biology have led to advances beyond purely anatomical staging. Relevant biologic markers that impact disease (i.e., serum LDH) have now been included in the groupings and influence therapeutic selection. In the future, staging and outcome prediction in melanoma patients will be enhanced by the availability of tools that facilitate subcategorization beyond the conventional TNM staging system [42]. Efforts are now geared towards defining genetic markers that may bear predictive prognostic potential in metastatic melanoma [43]. For example, gene expression profiling has been used to establish molecular signatures of disease progression in melanoma and define different subsets of melanoma with varying survival potential. Of note, immune profiling studies have yielded sets of genes that are significantly associated with survival in patients with metastatic melanoma [44].

References

1. Balch CM, Buzaid AC, Atkins MB, et al. A new American Joint Committee on Cancer staging system for cutaneous melanoma. Cancer. 2000;88:1484–91.
2. Balch CM, Soong SJ, Atkins MB, et al. An evidence-based staging system for cutaneous melanoma. CA Cancer J Clin. 2004;54:131–49.
3. Petro A, Schwartz J, Johnson T. Current melanoma staging. Clin Dermatol. 2004;22:223–7.
4. Balch CM, Gershenwald JE, Soong SJ, et al. Final version of 2009 AJCC melanoma staging and classification. J Clin Oncol. 2009;27:6199–206.
5. Edge SE, Byrd DR, Compton CC, et al. AJCC cancer staging manual. New York: Springer; 2009. p. 325–40.
6. Breslow A. Thickness, cross-sectional areas and depth of invasion in the prognosis of cutaneous melanoma. Ann Surg. 1970;172:902–8.
7. Cho YR, Chiang MP. Epidemiology, staging (new system), and prognosis of cutaneous melanoma. Clin Plast Surg. 2010;37:47–53.
8. Balch CM, Soong SJ, Gershenwald JE, et al. Prognostic factors analysis of 17,600 melanoma patients: validation of the American Joint Committee on Cancer melanoma staging system. J Clin Oncol. 2001;19:3622–34.
9. Balch CM, Murad TM, Soong SJ, Ingalls AL, Halpern NB, Maddox WA. A multifactorial analysis of melanoma: prognostic histopathological features comparing Clark's and Breslow's staging methods. Ann Surg. 1978;188:732–42.
10. Balch CM, Wilkerson JA, Murad TM, Soong SJ, Ingalls AL, Maddox WA. The prognostic significance of ulceration of cutaneous melanoma. Cancer. 1980;45:3012–7.
11. Francken AB, Shaw HM, Thompson JF, et al. The prognostic importance of tumor mitotic rate confirmed in 1317 patients with primary cutaneous melanoma and long follow-up. Ann Surg Oncol. 2004;11: 426–33.
12. Barnhill RL, Katzen J, Spatz A, Fine J, Berwick M. The importance of mitotic rate as a prognostic factor for localized cutaneous melanoma. J Cutan Pathol. 2005;32:268–73.
13. Retsas S, Henry K, Mohammed MQ, MacRae K. Prognostic factors of cutaneous melanoma and a new staging system proposed by the American Joint Committee on Cancer (AJCC): validation in a cohort of 1284 patients. Eur J Cancer. 2002;38:511–6.
14. Scolyer RA, Thompson JF, Shaw HM, McCarthy SW. The importance of mitotic rate as a prognostic factor for localized primary cutaneous melanoma. J Cutan Pathol. 2006;33:395–6; author reply 397–399.
15. Gershenwald JE, Soong SJ, Balch CM, American Joint Committee on Cancer (AJCC) Melanoma Staging Committee. 2010 TNM staging system for cutaneous melanoma…and beyond. Ann Surg Oncol. 2010;17:1475–7.
16. Balch CM, Soong S, Ross MI, et al. Long-term results of a multi-institutional randomized trial comparing prognostic factors and surgical results for intermediate thickness melanomas (1.0–4.0 mm). Intergroup Melanoma Surgical Trial. Ann Surg Oncol. 2000;7: 87–97.
17. Cascinelli N, Belli F, Santinami M, Fait V, et al. Sentinel lymph node biopsy in cutaneous melanoma: the WHO Melanoma Program experience. Ann Surg Oncol. 2000;7:469–74.
18. Balch CM, Gershenwald JE, Soong SJ, et al. Multivariate analysis of prognostic factors among 2,313 patients with stage III melanoma: comparison of nodal micrometastases versus macrometastases. J Clin Oncol. 2010;28:2452–9.
19. Rao UN, Ibrahim J, Flaherty LE, Richards J, Kirkwood JM. Implications of microscopic satellites of the primary and extracapsular lymph node spread in patients with high-risk melanoma: pathologic corollary of Eastern Cooperative Oncology Group Trial E1690. J Clin Oncol. 2002;20:2053–7.
20. Buzaid R. Critical analysis of the current AJCC staging system for cutaneous melanoma and proposal of a new staging system. J Clin Oncol. 1997;15:1039–51.
21. Ohsie SJ, Sarantopoulos GP, Cochran AJ, Binder SW. Immunohistochemical characteristics of melanoma. J Cutan Pathol. 2008;35:433–44.
22. Manola J, Atkins M, Ibrahim J, Kirkwood J. Prognostic factors in metastatic melanoma: a pooled analysis of Eastern Cooperative Oncology Group trials. J Clin Oncol. 2000;18:3782–93.
23. Eton O, Legha SS, Moon TE, et al. Prognostic factors for survival of patients treated systemically for disseminated melanoma. J Clin Oncol. 1998;16: 1103–11.
24. Bedikian AY, Johnson MM, Warneke CL, et al. Prognostic factors that determine the long-term survival of patients with unresectable metastatic melanoma. Cancer Invest. 2008;26:624–33.
25. Barth A, Wanek LA, Morton DL. Prognostic factors in 1,521 melanoma patients with distant metastases. J Am Coll Surg. 1995;181:193–201.
26. Balch CM, Soong SJ, Murad TM, Smith JW, Maddox WA, Durant JR. A multifactorial analysis of melanoma. IV. Prognostic factors in 200 melanoma patients with distant metastases (stage III). J Clin Oncol. 1983;1:126–34.
27. Keilholz U, Martus P, Punt CJ, et al. Prognostic factors for survival and factors associated with long-term remission in patients with advanced melanoma receiving cytokine-based treatments: second analysis of a randomised EORTC Melanoma Group trial comparing interferon-alpha2a (IFNalpha) and interleukin 2 (IL-2) with or without cisplatin. Eur J Cancer. 2002;38:1501–11.
28. Franzke A, Probst-Kepper M, Buer J, et al. Elevated pretreatment serum levels of soluble vascular cell adhesion molecule 1 and lactate dehydrogenase as predictors of survival in cutaneous metastatic malignant melanoma. Br J Cancer. 1998;78:40–5.

29. Deichmann M, Benner A, Bock M, et al. S100-Beta, melanoma-inhibiting activity, and lactate dehydrogenase discriminate progressive from nonprogressive American Joint Committee on Cancer stage IV melanoma. J Clin Oncol. 1999;17:1891–6.
30. Brand CU, Ellwanger U, Stroebel W, et al. Prolonged survival of 2 years or longer for patients with disseminated melanoma. An analysis of related prognostic factors. Cancer. 1997;79:2345–53.
31. Das Gupta T, Bowden L, Berg JW. Malignant melanoma of unknown primary origin. Surg Gynecol Obstet. 1963;117:341–5.
32. Giuliano AE, Moseley HS, Morton DL. Clinical aspects of unknown primary melanoma. Ann Surg. 1980;191:98–104.
33. Cormier JN, Xing Y, Feng L, et al. Metastatic melanoma to lymph nodes in patients with unknown primary sites. Cancer. 2006;106:2012–20.
34. Lee CC, Faries MB, Wanek LA, Morton DL. Improved survival after lymphadenectomy for nodal metastasis from an unknown primary melanoma. J Clin Oncol. 2008;26:535–41.
35. Balch CM. Cutaneous melanoma: prognosis and treatment results worldwide. Semin Surg Oncol. 1992;8:400–14.
36. Gershenwald JE, Mansfield PF, Lee JE, Ross MI. Role for lymphatic mapping and sentinel lymph node biopsy in patients with thick (> or = 4 mm) primary melanoma. Ann Surg Oncol. 2000;7:160–5.
37. Bevilacqua RG, Coit DG, Rogatko A, Younes RN, Brennan MF. Axillary dissection in melanoma. Prognostic variables in node-positive patients. Ann Surg. 1990;212:125–31.
38. Morton DL, Wanek L, Nizze JA, Elashoff RM, Wong JH. Improved long-term survival after lymphadenectomy of melanoma metastatic to regional nodes. Analysis of prognostic factors in 1134 patients from the John Wayne Cancer Clinic. Ann Surg. 1991;214:491–9. discussion 499–501.
39. Gershenwald JE, Thompson W, Mansfield PF, et al. Multi-institutional melanoma lymphatic mapping experience: the prognostic value of sentinel lymph node status in 612 stage I or II melanoma patients. J Clin Oncol. 1999;17:976–83.
40. Day CL, Day Jr CL, Harrist TJ, Gorstein F, et al. Malignant melanoma. Prognostic significance of "microscopic satellites" in the reticular dermis and subcutaneous fat. Ann Surg. 1981;194:108–12.
41. Mohr P, Eggermont AM, Hauschild A, Buzaid A. Staging of cutaneous melanoma. Ann Oncol. 2009;20(Suppl 6):vi14–21.
42. Balch CM, Soong SJ. Predicting outcomes in metastatic melanoma. J Clin Oncol. 2008;26:168–9.
43. Haass NK, Smalley KS. Melanoma biomarkers: current status and utility in diagnosis, prognosis, and response to therapy. Mol Diagn Ther. 2009;13:283–96.
44. Bogunovic D, O'Neill DW, Belitskaya-Levy I, et al. Immune profile and mitotic index of metastatic melanoma lesions enhance clinical staging in predicting patient survival. Proc Natl Acad Sci USA. 2009;106:20429–34.

Clinical and Histopathological Parameters in Melanoma

Cheryl Bilinski, Avery LaChance, and Michael J. Murphy

Introduction

A preliminary diagnosis of suspected cutaneous melanoma can be made by a well-trained medical professional in the clinical setting; yet, a definitive diagnosis requires clinicopathological correlation. In addition to diagnostic features, the histopathology of these lesions contains a multitude of clues that can be useful in predicting clinical course and outcome. Found within a thorough dermatopathology report, factors such as (1) age; (2) anatomic location; (3) gender; (4) Breslow thickness; (5) Clark anatomic level; (6) tumor volume; (7) cross-sectional profile; (8) ulceration; (9) mitotic rate; (10) growth phase; (11) regression; (12) host inflammatory response; (13) tumor vascularity; (14) vascular invasion; (15) angiotropism; (16) histologic tumor type; (17) cytologic variation; (18) desmoplasia; (19) neurotropic factors; (20) cytologic atypia; (21) borderline melanocytic lesions; (22) association with a benign melanocytic nevus; (23) paratumoral epidermal hyperplasia; and (24) satellite and/or in-transit metastasis can provide further insight into prognosis for patients with melanoma. This chapter will provide a thorough review of the significance of each of the predictive factors listed above, as well as how they may be interpreted and used by the clinician to guide appropriate therapy and patient education.

Age

Several of studies examining disease-free survival among melanoma patients have found statistically significant differences in outcome amongst individuals in different age brackets. In these studies, increased patient age at diagnosis was found to correlate with a worse prognosis [1–3]. This relationship may be explained by the finding that certain features associated with poor prognosis, including increased tumor thickness, ulceration, regression, and male gender, have a higher prevalence in older patients with melanoma [4]. This correlation is not mirrored in the pediatric population. Although younger children (ages 3–9 years) generally present with thicker lesions that have achieved more advanced stages, these patients tend to have a better 5-year disease-free survival than older children (ages 10–14 years) presenting with melanoma [5].

C. Bilinski, B.A. • A. LaChance, B.A.
University of Connecticut Medical School,
Farmington, CT, USA

M.J. Murphy, M.D. (✉)
Department of Dermatology, University of Connecticut Health Center, Farmington, CT, USA
e-mail: drmichaelmurphy@netscape.net

Anatomic Location

Many studies show that lesions located on an extremity carry a better prognosis than those located on the trunk [6–10]. The prognostic significance of melanoma location with regard to those on extremities has been further evaluated. Interestingly, not all extremity lesions share similar prognoses [11–13]. Of note, survival rates tend to be better in patients with melanomas on the proximal compared to the distal extremity. One study demonstrated increasingly dismal outcomes for leg melanomas located further from the trunk; 10-year survival rates for the thigh, calf, and foot were 94%, 84%, and 66%, respectively, with 5-year survival rates following the same trend [11]. For foot lesions, survival rates are higher for dorsal compared with plantar melanomas [13]. Head and neck melanomas have a poorer prognosis than both truncal and extremity lesions, with lower survival rates for scalp and ear melanomas than for those on the face and neck [14–17]. While there is substantial evidence that melanoma site is an important predictor of survival, some studies have failed to show such a relationship, especially when controlled for other prognostic factors such as Breslow thickness, Clark level, number of positive lymph nodes and gender [1, 18, 19]. Another study showed a disease-free survival advantage for extremity lesions over melanomas of the head and neck and trunk, but failed to demonstrate an improved overall survival rate [20]. Thus, a correlation between anatomic location and prognosis is supported by a number of studies [6–17]. However, the nature of this relationship with other prognostic factors deserves further study.

Gender

For patients younger than 75 years of age, female sex has been found to be a protective factor in melanoma prognosis [2, 9, 21]. Of note, one study involving 5,903 patients showed it to be a highly significant predictor of prolonged survival [7]. The reason for the seemingly protective effect of female sex is currently unknown. However, it may be due, in part, to the fact that women tend to present with thinner lesions [22–25] and at an earlier age than men [2, 5]. In addition, women are more likely to have extremity lesions (excluding those of the hand and foot), while men have a higher incidence of truncal tumors [2]. While these associations are potential confounders, studies that have controlled for lesional thickness between male and female patients suggest that female sex is, in itself, an independent predictor of positive prognosis [22, 23].

Breslow Thickness

Of all histopathological parameters, tumor thickness shows the strongest correlation with survival rates and is considered the most important factor in determining melanoma prognosis [26–30]. The Breslow method is considered the "gold standard" for measurement of tumor thickness. A calibrated ocular micrometer is placed perpendicular to the epidermal surface and the distance from the top of the granular layer to the point of deepest tumor invasion is measured. The latter may be the deep edge of the main tumor mass or of an isolated nest. If ulceration is present, measurement should begin at the ulcer base [26, 31–34]. If the deep aspect of the tumor cannot be evaluated (i.e., following a superficial shave biopsy which transects the tumor), thickness can be defined as "at least ____ mm," with a comment in the dermatopathology report explaining the specimen's limitation [34]. Tumor cells associated with adnexal structures are not taken into account when measuring Breslow thickness, unless the adnexal site is the tumor's sole area of dermal invasion. In the future, this practice may be reevaluated, as recent evidence suggests that there is a significant association between T1 tumors with adnexal involvement beyond 1 mm and positive sentinel lymph node status [32].

Table 5.1 Correlation between Breslow thickness and AJCC Tumor (T) category [26, 31–33]

Breslow thickness	T stage
1 mm or less	T1
>1–2 mm	T2
>2–4 mm	T3
>4 mm	T4

AJCC American Joint Committee on Cancer, *T* tumor

Table 5.2 Relationship between Breslow thickness and Survival [33]

Breslow thickness (mm)	10-year survival rate (%)
0.01–0.5	96
0.51–1.00	89
1.01–2.00	80
2.01–3.00	65
3.01–4.00	57
4.01–6.00	54
>6.00	42

The seventh edition of the American Joint Committee on Cancer (AJCC) Staging Handbook (2009) continues to use Breslow thickness as the primary determinant of the T staging category in melanoma and defines discrete "cutoff groups," as shown in Table 5.1 [26, 31–33]. The appropriateness of these "cutoff groups" is highly debated. Recent studies indicate that tumor thickness is most appropriately considered as a continuous variable [28, 33]. The AJCC notes that the current distinct categories are arbitrary and exist primarily for the purpose of discrete staging. Nonetheless, the current cutoffs are also consistent with "best fit" statistical analysis of the correlation between survival rates and tumor thickness for patients with localized melanoma. Analysis of clinical data from the AJCC Melanoma Staging Database on 27,000 patients with Stage I and Stage II disease is shown in Table 5.2 [33].

While Breslow thickness is the best microscopic indicator of prognosis, it is not a perfect marker and must be considered in combination with other factors. Prolonged survival times have been documented for certain patients with thick melanomas [26]. Likewise, although prognosis for thin melanomas is generally excellent, lesions less than 1 mm in thickness are known to metastasize at a rate of approximately 4.8% [30, 31]. According to one study, features that add to this risk include increased Clark level, presence of ulceration and features of regression. Recently, mitotic rate was also determined to be an important predictor of sentinel lymph node positivity in thin melanomas [30, 33].

Clark Anatomic Level

In 1969, Clark reported five levels of cutaneous melanoma invasion, as outlined in Table 5.3 [32, 35]. These levels describe the depth of tumor invasion in relation to anatomic landmarks [32]. Anatomic depth of invasion reflects tumor biology: the interaction between malignant cells and skin stroma is a crucial determinant of tumor invasion. Consequently, Clark level is used to study the role of biological markers, such as adhesion molecules and matrix metalloproteinases, in melanoma development and progression [32]. Numerous studies demonstrate a significant relationship between prognosis and anatomic depth of invasion, particularly for melanomas that measure 1 mm or less in Breslow thickness [30, 32, 33]. Nevertheless, Clark level has long been considered inferior to Breslow thickness in predicting patient outcome [26, 33, 36–38]. Correlation with patient survival rates is weaker, and assessment of Clark level is inconsistent among pathologists [33]. There are two likely reasons for this. First, there is no defined boundary between the papillary and reticular dermis, which obscures the distinction between level III and level IV lesions. Second, Clark levels are discrete, whereas Breslow thickness can be considered as a continuous variable [39]. Recent evidence shows the prognostic significance of factors such as mitotic rate and ulceration to be superior to that of Clark level, even for thin melanomas [32, 33]. Furthermore, when mitotic rate and ulceration are considered in concert with Breslow thickness, Clark level does not have a significant effect on prognosis [33].

Table 5.3 Clark anatomic level [32, 35]

I	Intraepidermal melanoma/melanoma in situ
II	Invasion of the papillary dermis by single or nested melanoma cells
III	The papillary dermis is filled and widened by melanoma cells, which impinge on the reticular dermis
IV	Invasion of the reticular dermis by melanoma cells
V	Subcutaneous tissue involvement

The sixth edition of the AJCC Cancer Staging Handbook used Clark level to stratify T1 melanomas according to metastatic potential. T1 lesions with Clark level I or II were designated T1a. Clark level III and IV lesions were defined as T1b, and considered to carry a worse prognosis [32, 33]. In the seventh edition of this handbook, the AJCC has replaced anatomic level by mitotic rate as a means of subclassifying T1 lesions [33, 34]. Only when mitotic rate cannot be determined and ulceration is absent should Clark level be used as a tertiary factor to upstage a T1a lesion to a T1b lesion. In such cases, anatomic depth of invasion remains an essential component of the dermatopathology report [33, 34].

Tumor Volume

Tumor volume is quantified by the three-dimensional space occupied by a melanoma lesion, and can be approximated by calculating maximal cross-sectional area (CSA). Breslow's 1970 estimations of CSA proved to hold less prognostic relevance than tumor thickness or anatomic depth of invasion [26]. Recent studies using technologically advanced methods to calculate tumor volume and CSA have found statistically significant relationships between overall survival and these parameters. However, CSA and tumor volume appear to offer no prognostic value over Breslow thickness. Furthermore, measurement is cumbersome. In one study, tumors were sectioned into 2 mm slices. CSA was estimated for each slice, and values were plugged into an algorithm to calculate total tumor volume. CSA has also been measured using digital photography [40]. While these parameters may be closely correlated with prognosis, their measurement is impractical compared to that of Breslow thickness [30].

Cross-Sectional Profile

Melanomas display a range of growth patterns that can be identified by histopathological examination of the cross-sectional profile [30]. Polypoid and verrucous variants are commonly reported [41].

Polypoid, or pedunculated, melanomas display an exophytic growth pattern. A nodule of neoplastic cells, which is often ulcerated and friable, is attached to the skin by a stalk (the latter often composed of benign cells) [42]. Polypoid melanomas carry a poor prognosis with an average 10-year survival rate of less than 40% [43–45]. Depth of invasion has been shown to be an inaccurate predictor of prognosis for pedunculated lesions [39].

Verrucous melanomas display prominent papillomatous epidermal hyperplasia with varying degrees of hyperkeratosis, parakeratosis, and acanthosis [42]. Studies controlling for patient gender, anatomic site and tumor thickness show similar prognoses for verrucous and non-verrucous lesions [46]. However, thickness of these tumors may be overestimated due to the epidermal hyperplasia and papillomatous architecture. Thus, verrucous melanomas may actually carry a worse prognosis than their non-verrucous counterparts [42].

Additional variants have been described, but are rarely reported [41]. These include hemispherical, dome-shaped and plaque-shaped subtypes [30]. Current evidence shows a decrease in 5-year survival rate as the complexity of cross-sectional profile increases. Flat lesions generally have the best prognosis, followed by convex or plateau-like lesions, with the worse prognosis for nodular and polypoid tumors. However, with the exception of polypoid melanomas, survival rates differ minimally between groups [47]. It appears that little additional prognostic information is likely obtained by assessing cross-sectional tumor profile [30].

Ulceration

After Breslow thickness, the AJCC considers ulceration to be the most important parameter in staging localized melanoma. Ulceration is characterized by: (1) full-thickness absence of the epidermis, including stratum corneum and basement membrane; (2) evidence of reactive changes, namely fibrin deposition and neutrophil infiltration; and (3) atrophy or reactive hyperplasia of the epidermis, not explained by trauma or a recent surgical procedure [33, 34].

Ulceration may be an indication of tumor aggressiveness [30, 32]. It is postulated that a lesion ulcerates when angiogenesis cannot keep up with rapid tumor growth; the latter leading to tissue ischemia [28]. Ulcerated melanomas tend to invade through the epidermis, while non-ulcerated tumors lift the overlying skin [34]. Pathologists usually report the presence or absence of ulceration, although there may be additional value in quantifying this parameter (i.e., diameter of ulceration) [30].

Ulceration is positively correlated with tumor thickness. Median thickness at diagnosis is 3.0 mm for ulcerated melanomas and 1.3 mm for non-ulcerated lesions [34]. There is evidence that ulceration is also an independent predictor of survival, especially in melanomas of thickness greater than 1 mm [30, 34]. For patients with Stage I and Stage II melanomas, the presence of ulceration decreases the overall survival rate from 78% to 50% [34]. However, recent data suggest that ulceration may lose independent prognostic significance when considered in conjunction with mitotic rate [34].

While the prognostic significance of ulceration in thin melanomas has been debated, the AJCC continues to use this feature to differentiate between T1a and T1b tumors [30, 32–34]. T1a lesions measure less than or equal to 1 mm in thickness, lack ulceration, and exhibit a mitotic rate of less than 1 mitosis/mm^2. Melanomas of similar thickness, but with ulceration or mitotic count greater than 1 mitosis/mm^2 are classified as T1b [31–34]. The latter group of patients should be considered for sentinel lymph node staging procedures [33, 34]. This difference in clinical management is reasonable in light of the AJCC statistical analysis of survival rates for patients with tumor ulceration. Patients with ulcerated melanomas have survival rates similar to those of patients in the next highest T category with non-ulcerated tumors. For example, a patient with an ulcerated T1 tumor will have an expected survival rate similar to that for a patient with a non-ulcerated T2 tumor, but significantly lower than that for a patient with a non-ulcerated T1 lesion [34]. It is for this reason that evaluation for sentinel lymph node disease is extended to T1b category patients, in addition to those who present with lesions that are T2 or higher [34].

Mitotic Rate

Similar to ulceration, mitotic rate, also called mitotic index [48], is considered a key prognostic factor, particularly for thin melanomas [31–34]. Mitotic rate should be calculated from an area of maximal proliferation [28, 33], and the pathologist must scan the specimen to identify a "mitotic hot spot" in the lesion's dermal component that can be used as a starting point [28, 32–34]. If mitoses are rare or fairly evenly dispersed, and no distinctive "hot spot" can be found, the AJCC recommends that the count begin at a "representative mitosis" [33]. Counting should continue in adjacent fields until an area of 1 mm^2 has been examined [28, 32–34], usually corresponding to about 4 high-power fields using a x40 objective [33]. However, standard light microscopes vary significantly in this respect and should be calibrated to ensure accurate assessment [30, 33, 34].

For melanomas with an invasive component measuring at least 1 mm^2, mitotic index can be reported in mitoses/mm^2 [30, 33, 34]. For lesions with a smaller dermal component, the AJCC recommends dichotomous classification: a melanoma is "mitogenic" if it displays at least 1 mitosis/mm^2, and "nonmitogenic" if it demonstrates less than 1 mitosis/mm^2 [33]. Alternatively, the College of American Pathologists advises extrapolation of mitotic index in such lesions [34].

Some studies have determined mitotic index to be the second most important prognostic factor for melanoma after tumor thickness [33, 49]. As mitotic rate increases, prognosis worsens [30–34, 50]. This relationship is particularly significant for thin melanomas [22, 31, 33, 51]. Recent evidence shows mitotic index to be an independent predictor of lymph node metastases in T1 lesions [50]. As a result, mitotic rate has been introduced as a prognostic factor in the seventh edition of the AJCC Cancer Staging Handbook. Similar to the presence of ulceration, mitotic rate greater than or equal to 1 mitosis/mm^2 upstages a T1 melanoma from T1a to T1b [33].

Opposing studies suggest that there is no relationship between mitotic rate and prognosis [52]. Others indicate that mitotic index is significantly correlated with prognosis, but only because of its association with ulceration and tumor thickness [52]. These authors maintain that mitotic rate is not, in itself, an independent predictor of prognosis and is inextricably intertwined with tumor thickness. If this is true, a "prognostic index", which considers mitotic rate in the context of tumor thickness, may prove to be more appropriate than disparate evaluation of these factors [30, 53, 54].

An alternative method of determining tumor cell proliferation involves the use of immunohistochemistry with MIB-1 antibody (direct against the Ki-67 protein). Ki-67 is expressed in cells during the G_1, S, and G_2, but not G_0 phases of the cell cycle. Therefore, antibodies to this protein function as good markers of proliferative activity. The Ki-67 proliferation index is estimated by the percentage of tumor cell nuclei that stain positively with MIB-1, and can be used as a prognostic indicator in melanoma patients. MIB-1 may also be used to assess the biological potential of borderline melanocytic lesions; however, it is not well-established as a means of differentiating between benign and malignant lesions [32].

Radial and Vertical Growth Phases

Growth pattern is correlated with melanoma stage [3] and subtype [3, 5]; lesions that exhibit a predominantly vertical pattern of growth carry a poorer prognosis than those with a primarily radial pattern [22, 27, 30, 32, 34, 55].

The radial growth phase (RGF) is largely limited to the epidermis, and contributes to increased tumor width, rather than depth [30–34]. Typically, cytology is uniform [34] and dermal mitoses are absent [30]. A microinvasive component may be present [30–34]. However, intradermal nests do not exceed the size of intraepidermal clusters [30] and are cytologically and architecturally similar to the superficial component [32]. If dermal invasion is present, the tumor's intraepidermal portion extends at least three rete ridges beyond the invasive area [31, 34]. RGP lesions are always Clark level I (in-situ) or II (microinvasive) [32].

The presence of vertical growth phase (VGF) correlates with tumor aggressiveness and implies increased likelihood of metastasis [32]. VGF can be defined in two ways: (1) by intradermal nests, at least one of which displays a greater diameter than the largest intraepidermal aggregate, or (2) by the presence of dermal mitoses [30, 34]. Dermal melanoma cells often display different morphology than those of the epidermal component [32]. Architectural distortion of the papillary dermis may be present [32]. VGF lesions are commonly at least Clark Level III or more [32]. A comparison between RGF and VGF is provided in Table 5.4 [22, 27, 30–34, 55].

Melanomas that demonstrate only RGF generally carry an excellent prognosis, and surgical excision is usually curative [32]. However, these lesions do have the potential to metastasize [30, 32, 56]. The presence of an "early vertical growth phase" is associated with a 10% risk of metastasis in the 8 years following diagnosis [32]. Early VGF lesions exhibit primarily a radial growth pattern, but also features indicative of imminent progression to a true vertical pattern. Namely, at least one intradermal nest with divergent cytology exceeds the size of intraepidermal aggregates, cellularity is increased, and dermal mitotic activity may or may not be present [32]. These lesions are regarded as Clark level II, sometimes bordering on level III [32].

Some studies have failed to show a correlation between VGF and poor prognosis, especially for thin melanomas [57, 58]. Varying classification of early VGF lesions may have contributed to

Table 5.4 Comparison between radial growth phase and vertical growth phase

Factor	Radial growth phase	Vertical growth phase
Location	Epidermis	Dermis
Intraepidermal component	Dominant component; uniform cytology; extends at least 3 rete ridges beyond any intradermal nests	Often cytologically and architecturally distinct from intradermal component
Intradermal component	Rare; cytological and architectural uniformity that is similar to superficial component	Present; often morphologically varied
Dermal mitoses	Absent	Usually present
Clark level	I or II	III+
Architectural distortion of papillary dermis	Absent	May be present

this discrepancy. In addition, there is evidence that invasive growth is significantly correlated with other histopathological parameters, such as ulceration and mitotic rate, and may not be independently predictive of prognosis [30].

Regression

Regression is defined as a focal absence of tumor in the epidermis and dermis, bordered on one or both sides by malignant cells in the epidermis, dermis or both [30, 32]. The associated epidermis is atrophied, and the tumor cells are typically replaced by disorganized dermal fibroplasia, melanophages, telangiectasias, and inflammatory cells, most often lymphocytes [28, 30, 32, 34, 59]. Vessels are prominent and oriented perpendicular to the epidermis [32], consistent with scar tissue morphology. The extent of this process can vary from tumor to tumor [30]. In complete regression, melanoma cells are completely absent from both dermis and epidermis. "Severe" regression describes the near or complete replacement of neoplastic cells by dense fibrosis [28].

Regression represents the interaction between melanoma cells and the host immune system [32]. Its prognostic implications are controversial [30, 32, 34]. The majority of studies indicate that the presence of regression is a negative prognostic factor [30, 32, 34, 60–64]. Depending on the criteria used, overall rates of regression in thin melanomas range from 7% to 61%. Additionally, 40–100% of metastatic thin melanomas display regression [63]. This is counterintuitive given that increased host immune response in regressive melanomas negatively correlated with patient outcome [32].

One possible contributor to the discordance between regression and its observed impact is inter-study variation in its definition. Some researchers take into account only complete tumor regression, while others also consider evidence of a partial process. Some studies include the active phase of host immune response, which eventually leads to the microscopic appearance of regression, in their definition. Furthermore, there are no standard criteria to differentiate between true tumor regression and other stromal reactions [59]. As a result, the College of American Pathologists deems tumor regression a significant predictor of poor prognosis only in invasive melanomas with complete regression or regression involving more than 75% of the lesion [34].

Tumor regression is positively correlated with lymph node metastasis and increased tumor vascularity; thus, these factors may be confounders for its negative impact on prognosis [30, 65, 66]. It has been suggested that the interaction between metastatic melanoma cells with host immune cells in lymph nodes could promote regression of the primary tumor [37].

Host Inflammatory Response

The key indicator of the host immune response to melanoma cells is the presence and distribution of tumor-infiltrating lymphocytes (TILs) [30, 32, 34, 67]. To be considered TILs, lymphocytes must surround, directly contact and disrupt VGF tumor cells [32, 34]. Degree of TIL infiltration is stratified into inherently subjective categories: absent, nonbrisk and brisk infiltrates. These are outlined in Table 5.5 [28, 32, 34, 68].

Increasing TIL presence is associated with positive prognosis [30, 34, 67–76]. This is not surprising, as TILs are believed to be cytotoxic and target malignant cells for destruction [32]. Immunohistochemistry can confirm the degree of TIL infiltration observed on hematoxylin and eosin (H&E) staining, and is used experimentally to assess the nature and activity of TILs [32, 67, 73–76]. Markers for T-cell activation, such as CD25 and OX40, can be used to assess prognosis [76]. Large numbers of marker-positive TILs are associated with increased survival rates and negative sentinel lymph node status [32, 74]. Regulatory T-cell (Treg) markers include TIA-1, granzyme B and perforin [32]. Peritumoral positivity for DC-lamp (dendritic cell maturation factor) or CD1a (a marker expressed on Langerhans cells) are also associated with positive prognosis [76]. The relationship between immune cell marker positivity and prognosis indicates the potential for immunotherapy in patients with melanoma [32].

Some studies have failed to show a correlation between TIL infiltration and prognosis [27, 77, 78]. There are several possible explanations. First, some researchers include both RGF and VGF lesions, while others evaluate only invasive tumors [27]. TIL distribution in VGF lesions correlates more strongly with prognosis. Also, there is evidence that TILs may be anergic or functionally deficient, and may not represent a true immune response. When determining prognosis, the TIL activation state may be more important than degree of infiltration [74, 76, 79, 80].

Tumor Vascularity

Tumor vascularity can be evaluated quantitatively (number of vessels) and qualitatively (vessel diameter) on routine H&E sections [30]. Color Doppler sonography has also been used to assess melanoma vascularity in a research setting [81]. Vascular endothelial growth factor (VEGF) and other growth factors, produced by tumor and stromal cells, promote angiogenesis at the base of the invasive vertical phase [59, 82]. Elevated levels of VEGF are associated with increased angiogenesis, lymphangiogenesis and metastasis. VEGF is also increased during the transition from RGF to VGF [83].

Numerous studies have shown a correlation between tumor vascularity and poor prognosis [84–86]. Increased vessel density and vascular cross-sectional area are associated with (1) increased rates of metastasis and (2) decreased overall and relapse-free survival [84, 87–89]. However, some research groups report no relationship between tumor vascularity and prognosis [90–92]. Others report prognostic significance only for thin melanomas, which would imply that vascularity is important only in early stages of lesion development [93]. There is evidence that

Table 5.5 Quantification of host inflammatory response [28, 32, 34, 68]

TILs absent	No lymphocytes, or lymphocytes present do not qualify as TILs; perivascular lymphocytes may be present, within or outside the lesion
TILs nonbrisk	Focal or multifocal lymphocytic infiltration
TILs brisk	Diffuse lymphocytes throughout the entire invasive component of the lesion or across the entire base of the vertical growth phase; some authors maintain that 90% infiltration of the lesion base is sufficient to declare a brisk response

tumor vascularity is a precursor to ulceration and vascular invasion, and that it is correlated with tumor thickness. Thus, vascularity may be a marker for other poor prognostic factors, rather than an independent predictor of survival and metastasis [30].

Vascular Invasion

Vascular invasion is defined as the presence of tumor cells within a vessel lumen [30, 94–96]. Three types of vascular invasion have been identified in melanomas:
1. "Classic," or certain, invasion is defined by the presence of viable neoplastic cells in the vessel lumen.
2. "Uncertain vascular invasion" is said to exist when tumor cells are observed within a vessel wall, but not in the lumen.
3. Perivascular cuffing by melanoma cells is termed "angiotropism" or "extravascular migratory metastasis" [32].

True vascular invasion reflects aggressive tumor biology [32], and is classified by most studies as a negative prognostic factor. It is associated with regional lymph node and distant metastasis, in addition to reduced overall and disease-free survival [94, 97]. The prognostic significance of vascular invasion is particularly strong in T4 melanomas and in patients with lymph node metastases [59, 98]. Classic vascular invasion can be difficult to assess microscopically, as artifact from tissue shrinkage or from the folding of tortuous vessels can create the false impression of lumina [99].

Angiotropism

Angiotropism is defined as the presence of melanoma cells directly opposed to the external surface of lymphatic or microvascular structures. These cells may be arranged in a linear array, an aggregate or both. If only aggregates are present, there must be at least two or more nests at or near the advancing tumor front. No aggregates should be visible in vascular or lymphatic lumina, as this would characterize frank invasion [99, 100].

The few studies that have examined the relationship between angiotropism and metastasis have shown a strong link between the two [100–104]. Melanoma cells are hypothesized to travel along the external surface of vessels; this is one mechanism by which the tumor spreads to near and/or distant sites [99, 105, 106]. Supportive evidence comes from immunopathologic studies showing melanoma cells abutting on, but not invading, external vessel surfaces. Ultrastructural studies have demonstrated an "amorphous matrix," called the angiotumoral complex, which binds neoplastic cells to vascular structures [99, 107–110].

Histological Tumor Type

In 1970, Clark identified three histologic subtypes of melanoma: superficial spreading, nodular, and lentigo maligna [30, 32]. A fourth subtype, acral lentiginous, was added in 1977 [32, 111]. Growth patterns and depth of invasion exhibited by these variants have shown greater prognostic significance than the subtypes themselves [34].

Superficial spreading melanoma (SSM) is by far the most common architectural subtype, comprising 70–80% of all melanomas. SSMs usually arise on skin of the trunk or extremities that has received little or intermittent sun exposure [32, 39]. Clinically, lesions may display a combination of colors, including tan, brown, gray, black, violaceous, and pink. Rarely, they may be blue or white [32]. SSM usually appears as a sharply marginated, palpable papule or nodule of several millimeters in height, often with one or more "peninsula-like" projections [32]. Microscopically, SSMs are likely to be poorly circumscribed [112]. They are primarily composed of atypical epithelioid melanocytes with eosinophilic, amphophilic, or finely pigmented cytoplasm and large nuclei with prominent nucleoli. The migration of single neoplastic cells (pagetoid spread) into a normal or hyperplastic epidermis is common [32, 39, 112]. Dermal nests may vary substantially with regard to size and cytologic features [32]. Given anatomic locations, solar elastosis may be absent [39].

Nodular melanomas (NMs) are also fairly common, comprising 15–30% of melanomas [113]. NMs have a similar anatomic distribution to SSMs, appearing primarily on areas of the trunk and extremities that receive sporadic sun exposure [32]. NM appears as a smooth nodule, ulcerated polyp or elevated plaque without a surrounding flat, pigmented lesion. NMs do not display the range of colors seen in SSMs, and are usually brown, black or blue-black [32]. NMs are defined by a primarily vertical growth pattern. Intraepidermal spread, or RGF, is absent or limited to less than three rete ridges beyond the invasive component. In the dermis, NMs form nests of neoplastic cells that coalesce into an expansile nodule [32, 39, 112].

Approximately 4–15% of melanomas are classified as lentigo maligna melanomas (LMMs) [112]. In contrast to SSMs and NMs, LMMs occur in areas of chronic sun exposure and, by definition, display solar elastosis [32, 112]. LMMs usually appear as irregular, flat, sometimes slightly raised lesions on the face or neck [32]. They range in color from tan to brown to black, and may display dark flecks of pigment on a paler background [32]. Microscopically, LMMs are poorly circumscribed with epidermal atrophy [112]. Spindled melanocytes may predominate [32, 39, 112], and often exhibit large, hyperchromatic nuclei with multinucleation [32]. Neoplastic cells are concentrated in the basal layers of the epidermis [32, 39, 112]. Extension down adnexal structures is often found, but pagetoid spread is uncommon [32, 39].

Acral lentiginous melanomas (ALMs) are rare in white populations (2–8% of all melanomas), but account for 29–72% of melanomas in Asians, African-Americans and Hispanics [113]. These lesions appear on the acral skin of the hands and feet [32, 112]. Neoplastic cells are commonly spindled or banal-appearing [39, 112], and tend to be dispersed as single cells, rather than nests, in the epidermis [112]. Lentiginous elongation of rete ridges may be observed [39].

A 1982 international committee in Sydney, Australia determined that melanoma subtype has no bearing on clinical course or prognosis, and that outcome is most closely associated with tumor thickness [32]. Indeed, most studies have shown minimal prognostic significance of subtype when Breslow thickness is controlled for as a possible confounder [28, 112]. Additionally, the association between NM and ALM with high-risk factors such as vertical growth phase and hand/foot distribution, respectively, may play a role in determining the relationship between histologic tumor type and prognosis. Nevertheless, different studies have used varying criteria to classify melanoma subtype, and LMM and SSM are often found to have a better prognosis than ALM and NM [114–117]. However, not all melanomas fit neatly into these discrete categories [28, 118]. In light of this, recent evidence suggests that melanoma subtypes may be appropriately considered as a spectrum, rather than discrete categories [112].

Importantly, the AJCC TNM staging criteria are derived primarily from data on the most common melanoma subtypes: SSM and NM [33]. The AJCC acknowledges that other types of lesions, namely LMM, ALM and desmoplastic melanoma (DM), may have divergent natural histories. However, no separate staging criteria currently exist to more accurately classify these latter tumors [33].

Cytologic Variants

Melanoma cells exhibit a broad spectrum of cytologic features. Limited available evidence suggests that prognosis may be worsened for certain cytologic variants of melanoma, namely amelanotic, signet-ring, or small cell lesions [30].

Amelanotic cells are characterized by their lack of pigment on H&E staining [6]. Accurate identification of amelanotic lesions may require immunohistochemical studies for evidence of melanocytic differentiation (i.e., S-100, HMB-45, or MART-1). Electron microscopy may be used to identify melanosomes within the tumor cells [39, 42].

Signet-ring cell melanomas are defined by cytoplasmic vacuoles containing vimentin and other intermediate filaments. Nuclei are pushed to the periphery, resulting in the characteristic "signet-ring" morphology [119, 120]. These cytologic variants of melanoma are rare, and found more often in metastatic or recurrent tumors than in primary lesions.

Small cell melanomas are composed of uniform cells and may resemble other small cell neoplasms [39]. It is the only cytologic variant significantly associated with sentinel lymph node metastasis. This risk is further increased by the presence of ulceration in these tumors [56].

Spindle cell melanomas are composed of a prominent fusiform cellular component and scant stroma [42], and may show better survival rates than epithelioid tumors [121].

Spitzoid melanomas exhibit enlarged epithelioid and spindle cells similar to those seen in benign Spitz nevi [40]. While one study showed improved prognosis for children with spitzoid melanomas compared to other variants [122], other case studies demonstrate equivalent survival rates with prolonged follow-up [123].

Nevoid or minimal deviation melanomas resemble benign compound or intradermal nevi when viewed at low power [39, 42]. These lesions display uniform cytology in the VGF with mitotic activity, but may be prognostically favorable [42].

Desmoplasia

The desmoplastic melanoma (DM), a rare histologic variant, is composed of fusiform to spindle-shaped melanocytes within a prominent collagenous stroma [124]. These lesions are usually amelanotic and fibrosing [124, 125]. Diagnostic difficulty is not uncommon, as predominantly fibrous lesions may resemble dermal scars, dermatofibromas or fibrosarcomas [124, 125]. Criteria used to differentiate DMs from benign lesions are the presence of atypical cells, a host inflammatory response and/or overlying lentigo maligna changes. S-100 positivity can be used to confirm melanocytic differentiation [39]; although, MART-1 and HMB-45 are less sensitive in this setting.

DMs tend to occur on sun-damaged skin of the head and neck. Average age of incidence is 10 years older than for other melanoma subtypes [126–132]. Multiple studies have shown patients with DMs to be at lower risk for lymph node metastasis than other melanoma variants of similar thickness [125–127, 133–136]. However, risk of local recurrence may be increased in DMs [127, 129–131, 133, 137]. Some researchers have compared pure DMs, usually defined as tumors that are 80–90% fibrotic, with mixed or combined DMs, which contain more cellular areas. These studies indicate that prognosis may be better for pure DMs [125, 133].

Neurotropic Melanoma

Neurotropism, also called perineural invasion [34], is defined by melanoma infiltration into and extension along nerve fibers [138–140]. Pure neurotropic lesions comprise less than 1% of all melanomas [141]. More commonly, neurotropism is observed in conjunction with desmoplasia in the context of desmoplastic neurotropic melanoma (DNM) [34, 129, 130, 140, 142]. In either case, neurotropism is likely to be an adverse prognostic indicator worthy of mention in the dermatopathology report [30, 34].

Although not as rare as pure neurotropic tumors, DNMs are uncommon. They generally display Schwann-like differentiation and perineural invasion, and may resemble neural sheath tumors [129, 130, 140, 142]. DNMs do not tend to metastasize, but have high local recurrence rates [34, 129, 140, 142–147]. DNMs are generally deeply infiltrative and poorly circumscribed. These features, combined with extension along nerve sheaths, may complicate surgical excision. DNMs may be amelanotic, a feature which is reported to indicate a poorer prognosis [141, 142].

Cytologic Atypia

Limited studies have assessed the correlation between degree of cytologic atypia and melanoma prognosis. Current evidence indicates that this parameter is not as significant as tumor thickness or mitotic activity, and may only be relevant in cases of severe atypia. The latter has been found to correlate with increased rates of metastasis [30].

Borderline Melanocytic Lesions

Borderline lesions, also referred to as melanocytic tumors of uncertain malignant potential (MELTUMP), pose an important diagnostic challenge. These lesions are often composed of epithelioid and/or spindle cells with spitzoid morphology. In such cases, a definitive distinction between a Spitz nevus and malignant spitzoid lesion may be challenging [32]. Key differences are as follows:

Spitz nevi are symmetrical and sharply demarcated [32, 39], with an epidermal component that generally does not extend beyond the dermal constituent. They tend to measure 6 mm or less in greatest diameter [32]. Noticeable epidermal hyperplasia is observed [32, 39], and aggregates of melanocytic cells are often nestled between rete ridges [39]. Melanocytic distribution may be junctional, dermal, or compound [39], and nests are generally uniform, ovoid, and perpendicular to the skin surface [32]. Cells are spindle-shaped, epithelioid, or both. Highly atypical or multinucleated cells and scant mitoses may be present superficially [39]. Melanocytes "mature," by decreasing in size and degree of atypia, in the deep aspect of the lesion [32, 39]. Prominent eosinophilic, hyaline Kamino bodies may be observed at the dermal-epidermal junction [32, 39]. Lymphocytic infiltration tends to be patchy, rather than lichenoid [39]. Melanin may be absent, scarce or abundant [39].

In contrast, malignant spitzoid lesions are asymmetric [32, 39], and may measure greater than 6 mm [32]. Melanocyte maturation is decreased [32, 39], while cytologic atypia is increased [39]. Pagetoid spread (of single cells into the epidermis) is prominent and extends into poorly defined epidermal "shoulders" [32]. Size, shape and orientation of melanocytic nests are variable, and melanin pigment is prominent and irregularly distributed [32]. Epidermal reaction is usually minimal [32, 39]. Mitoses are often atypical and distributed throughout the lesion, including at the base [32, 39]. Mitoses within 0.25 mm of the deep edge signal a particularly poor prognosis [32]. It is reported that malignant lesions do not contain Kamino bodies. Lymphocytic infiltration is more lichenoid than patchy [39].

Borderline lesions display a combination of benign and malignant features. Borderline spitzoid lesions may also be called "borderline spitzoid melanocytic proliferations," "Spitz tumors with severe atypia" or "atypical Spitz tumors." While prognosis is usually favorable, metastasis can occur. These lesions are highly controversial and are often treated like melanomas, including sentinel lymph node biopsy and lymphadenectomy (when the former indicates "metastatic" disease) [32].

Association with a Benign Melanocytic Nevus

Approximately one-quarter to one-third of melanomas are associated with a preexisting benign melanocytic nevus [39, 148]. An estimated 0.00005–0.003% of nevi undergo malignant transformation to become melanoma, and the likelihood of this increases with patient age [148]. The remaining tumors are assumed to have arisen *de novo* [39]. Overall, the literature shows that this distinction has minimal bearing on prognosis [30].

Paratumoral Epidermal Hyperplasia

Melanoma-induced changes in local tissue architecture may play a role in prognosis. Paratumoral epidermal hyperplasia (PTEH) is characterized by epithelial proliferation that directly envelopes a melanoma. One study, which described PTEH as the difference between the deepest paratumoral epidermal penetration and thickness of the adjacent normal epidermis, found PTEH of at least 1 mm to be strongly associated with decreased rates of metastasis [149]. While further research is warranted, it is likely that PTEH is a positive prognostic factor [149].

PTEH should not be confused with pseudoepitheliomatous hyperplasia, which is a nonspecific reactive response that results in overall epithelial, rather than simply paratumoral, proliferation. Unlike PTEH, pseudoepitheliomatous hyperplasia can occur in response to infection, inflammation and trauma, in addition to neoplasia [149–151]. Pseudoepitheliomatous hyperplasia is not uncommon in melanocytic nevi, but is rare in melanomas [150, 152, 153].

Satellite and In-Transit Metastasis

A satellite metastasis, also called microsatellitosis or a microscopic satellite, is a discontinuous tumor cell aggregate measuring 0.05 mm or more in diameter and separated from the primary invasive tumor mass by 0.3–2.0 cm of normal dermis [32–34, 154, 155]. Microsatellites are located deep to the principal tumor mass in the reticular dermis or subcutaneous tissue [32, 34]. The intervening cutaneous tissue should not be fibrotic or inflamed [33]. In-transit metastases are identical to microsatellites, except that they are located, by definition, more than 2 cm from the primary melanoma [154, 155].

Satellite and in-transit metastases are indicative of intralymphatic tumor cell migration from the main mass to regional lymph nodes, and form when melanoma cells become trapped en route between the tumor and those nodes [33, 34, 154, 155]. Their identification is sufficient to declare the presence of intralymphatic metastasis, a defining criterion for AJCC Stage III melanoma [32, 33]. Current evidence does not support microsatellitosis and/or in-transit metastases as independent prognostic factors, likely because the definitions of these entities have fluctuated over time. However, their identification, in the presence of thicker tumors (>1.5 mm), is associated with a higher risk of local recurrence and an increased frequency of regional lymph node disease (12–53%) [33].

Sentinel Lymph Nodes

While sentinel lymph node status is not included in a basic histopathology report for a cutaneous lesion, certain prognostic clues suggestive of an aggressive tumor can be used to indicate the need for its evaluation. The first node draining a cutaneous lesion is considered the sentinel lymph node. Its status is regarded as a good predictor of additional lymphatic metastasis for a number of neoplasms. Patients with cutaneous melanomas staged as 1B or greater may be candidates for sentinel lymph node biopsy. Results of this procedure can be used to detect lymphatic metastasis, correctly stage aggressive cutaneous tumors, and determine appropriate therapy [156]. Of note, sentinel lymph node status has been considered the most important prognostic criterion in predicting survival in melanoma patients [156]. Although an extremely important measure for prognosis and therapy, sentinel lymph node biopsy is a more invasive surgical procedure than cutaneous biopsy or excision. Therefore, clinicopathological correlation and preliminary staging should be used to determine the appropriate patient population requiring sentinel lymph node biopsy.

Conclusion

Accurate reporting is essential for diagnosis, staging and clinical management of patients with melanoma. Table 5.6 provides a summary of prognostic information relating to clinical and histopathological parameters for melanoma contained in the dermatopathology report.

Table 5.6 Summary of prognostic information relating to clinical and histopathological parameters for melanoma contained in the dermatopathology report[a]

Parameter	Prognostic significance	Comment
Age	Increasing age worsens prognosis	
Anatomic location	Acral and head and neck melanoma worse than trunk which is worse than proximal extremity lesions	Value of extremity vs. trunk lesions is controversial
Gender	Female sex improves prognosis	
Breslow thickness[b]	Increasing thickness worsens prognosis	Strongest prognostic factor; should be considered as a continuous variable
Clark anatomic level[b]	Increasing level worsens prognosis	Prognostic value may be increased for thin melanomas
Tumor volume	Increasing tumor volume worsens prognosis	Difficult to calculate
Cross-sectional profile	Polypoid lesions carry worse prognosis	Little additive value beyond other histopathological factors
Ulceration[b]	Ulceration worsens prognosis	Significance in thin lesions is controversial
Mitotic index[b]	Increasing number of mitoses worsens prognosis	Prognostic value may be increased for thin melanomas
Radial and vertical growth phase	VGP carries worse prognosis than RGP	Significance in thin lesions is controversial
Regression	Regression may worsen prognosis	Lack of agreed-on definitions; may only be significant when >75% of lesion is involved
Host inflammatory response	Brisk inflammatory response may improve prognosis	Degree of immune system activation likely more valuable than mere presence of TILs
Tumor vascularity	Increased vascularity may worsen prognosis	May be correlated with other poor prognostic factors, rather than a prognostic factor itself
Angiotropism	Angiotropism worsens prognosis	Limited studies in the literature
Vascular invasion	Vascular invasion worsens prognosis	Potential artifacts can create false vascular spaces
Histologic tumor type	Controversial	Lack of agreed-on definitions; may represent a continuous spectrum, rather than discrete categories
Cell type	Amelanotic, signet-ring cell, and small cell phenotype may worsen prognosis; nevoid and spindle-cell phenotype may improve prognosis	Limited studies in the literature
Desmoplasia	Desmoplasia appears to improve prognosis	Increased local recurrence despite decreased SLN metastases; prognostic value may be increased for thick melanomas
Neurotropism	Neurotropism may worsen prognosis	Increased local recurrence despite decreased SLN metastases; difficult to excise
Cellular atypia	Marked atypia worsens prognosis	Little additive value over other histopathological factors; limited studies in the literature
Association with nevus	Controversial	Little additive value over other histopathological factors
PTEH	PTEH may improve prognosis	Limited studies in the literature
Satellite and in-transit metastasis	Either metastasis worsens prognosis	No prognostic difference between type of metastasis

RGP radial growth phase, *VGP* vertical growth phase, *TILs* tumor-infiltrating lymphocytes, *SLN* sentinel lymph node, *PTEH* paratumoral epidermal hyperplasia
[a]Adapted from Payette et al. [52]
[b]Part of American Joint Committee on Cancer (AJCC) melanoma staging system

References

1. Balzi D, Carli P, Giannotti B, et al. Skin melanoma in Italy: a population-based study on survival and prognostic factors. Eur J Cancer. 1998;34:699–704.
2. Lindholm C, Anderson R, Dufmats M, et al. Invasive cutaneous malignant melanoma in Sweden, 1990–1999. A prospective, population-based study of survival and prognostic factors. Cancer. 2004;101:2067–78.
3. Austin PF, Cruse CW, Lyman G, et al. Age as a prognostic factor in the malignant melanoma population. Ann Surg Oncol. 1994;1:487–94.
4. Chao C, Martin RC, Ross MI, et al. Correlation between prognostic factors and increasing age in melanoma. Ann Surg Oncol. 2004;11:259–64.
5. Ferrari A, Bono A, Baldi M, et al. Does melanoma behave differently in younger children than in adults? A retrospective study of 33 cases of childhood melanoma from a single institution. Pediatrics. 2005;115:649–54.
6. Cochran AJ, Elashoff D, Morton DL, et al. Individualized prognosis for melanoma patients. Hum Pathol. 2000;31:327–31.
7. Garbe C, Buttner P, Bertz J, et al. Primary cutaneous melanoma. Identification of prognostic groups and estimation of individual prognosis for 5093 patients. Cancer. 1995;75:2484–91.
8. Karakousis CP, Driscoll DL. Prognostic parameters in localised melanoma: gender versus anatomical location. Eur J Cancer. 1995;31A:320–4.
9. Levi F, Randimbison L, La Vecchia C, et al. Prognostic factors for cutaneous malignant melanoma in Vaud, Switzerland. Int J Cancer. 1998;78:315–9.
10. Francken AB, Shaw HM, Thompson JF, et al. The prognostic importance of tumor mitotic rate confirmed in 1317 patients with primary cutaneous melanoma and long follow-up. Ann Surg Oncol. 2004;11:426–33.
11. Hsueh EC, Lucci A, Qi K, et al. Survival of patients with melanoma of the lower extremity decreases with distance from the trunk. Cancer. 1999;85:383–8.
12. Talley LI, Soong S, Harrison RA, et al. Clinical outcomes of localized melanoma of the foot: a case-control study. J Clin Epidemiol. 1998;51:853–7.
13. Barnes BC, Seigler HF, Saxby TS, et al. Melanoma of the foot. J Bone Joint Surg Am. 1994;76:892–8.
14. Gillgren P, Mansson-Brahme E, Frisell J, et al. A prospective population-based study of cutaneous malignant melanoma of the head and neck. Laryngoscope. 2000;110:1498–504.
15. Wanebo HJ, Cooper PH, Young DV, et al. Prognostic factors in head and neck melanoma. Effect of lesion location. Cancer. 1988;62:831–7.
16. Leong SP, Accortt NA, Essner R, et al. Impact of sentinel node status and other risk factors on the clinical outcome of head and neck melanoma patients. Arch Otolaryngol Head Neck Surg. 2006;132:370–3.
17. Shumate CR, Carlson GW, Giacco GG, et al. The prognostic implications of location for scalp melanoma. Am J Surg. 1991;162:315–9.
18. Law MM, Wong JH. Evaluation of the prognostic significance of the site of origin of cutaneous melanoma. Am Surg. 1994;60:362–6.
19. Hoersch B, Leiter U, Garbe C. Is head and neck melanoma a distinct entity? A clinical registry-based comparative study in 5702 patients with melanoma. Br J Dermatol. 2006;155:771–7.
20. Nagore E, Oliver V, Botella-Estrada R, et al. Prognostic factors in localized invasive cutaneous melanoma: high value of mitotic rate, vascular invasion and microscopic satellitosis. Melanoma Res. 2005;15:169–77.
21. MacKie RM, Hole D, Hunter JA, et al. Cutaneous malignant melanoma in Scotland: incidence, survival, and mortality, 1979–94. The Scottish Melanoma Group. Br Med J. 1997;315:1117–21.
22. Gimotty PA, Guerry D, Ming ME, et al. Thin primary cutaneous malignant melanoma: a prognostic tree for 10-year metastasis is more accurate than American Joint Committee on Cancer staging. J Clin Oncol. 2004;22:3668–76.
23. Leiter U, Buettner PG, Eigentler TK, et al. Prognostic factors of thin cutaneous melanoma: an analysis of the central malignant melanoma registry of the German Dermatological Society. J Clin Oncol. 2004;22:3660–7.
24. McKinnon JG, Yu XQ, McCarthy WH, et al. Prognosis for patients with thin cutaneous melanoma: long-term survival data from New South Wales Central Cancer Registry and the Sydney Melanoma Unit. Cancer. 2003;98:1223–31.
25. Zalaudek I, Horn M, Richtig E, et al. Local recurrence in melanoma in situ: influence of sex, age, site of involvement and therapeutic modalities. Br J Dermatol. 2003;148:703–8.
26. Breslow A. Thickness, cross-sectional areas and depth of invasion in the prognosis of cutaneous melanoma. Ann Surg. 1970;172:902–8.
27. Barnhill RJ, Fine JA, Roush GC, et al. Predicting five-year outcome for patients with cutaneous melanoma in a population-based study. Cancer. 1996;78:427–32.
28. Crowson AN, Magro CM, Mihm MC. Prognosticators of melanoma, the melanoma report, and the sentinel lymph node. Mod Pathol. 2006;19(suppl 2):S71–87.
29. Breslow A. Tumor thickness, level of invasion and node dissection in stage I cutaneous melanoma. Ann Surg. 1975;182:572–5.
30. Rousseau Jr DL, Ross MI, Johnson MM, et al. Revised American Joint Committee on Cancer staging criteria accurately predict sentinel lymph node positivity in clinically node-negative melanoma patients. Ann Surg Oncol. 2003;10:569–74.

31. Duncan LM. The classification of cutaneous melanoma. Hematol Oncol Clin North Am. 2009;23: 501–13.
32. Piris A, Mihm Jr MC. Progress in melanoma histopathology and diagnosis. Hematol Oncol Clin North Am. 2009;23:467–80.
33. Greene FL, Trotti III A, Fritz AG, Compton CC, Byrd DR, editors. Melanoma of the Skin. In: AJCC Cancer Staging. From the AJCC Cancer Staging Manual, 7th ed. (2010). Springer: Chicago; 2009.
34. Frischberg DP, et al. Protocol for the examination of specimens from patients with melanoma of the skin. College of American Pathology Website. 2009. Available at: http://www.cap.org/apps/cap.portal. Accessed 3 Mar 2011.
35. Clark Jr WH, From L, Bernardino EA, et al. The histogenesis and biologic behavior of primary human malignant melanomas of the skin. Cancer Res. 1969;29:705–27.
36. Balch CM, Murad TM, Soong SJ, et al. A multifactorial analysis of melanoma: prognostic histopathological features comparing Clark's and Breslow's staging methods. Ann Surg. 1978;188:732–42.
37. Buttner P, Garbe C, Bertz J, et al. Primary cutaneous melanoma. Optimized cutoff points of tumor thickness and importance of Clark's level for prognostic classification. Cancer. 1995;75:2499–506.
38. Buzaid AC, Ross MI, Balch CM, et al. Critical analysis of the current American Joint Committee on Cancer staging system for cutaneous melanoma and proposal of a new staging system. J Clin Oncol. 1997;15:1039–51.
39. Rapini RP. Practical dermatopathology. Philadelphia: Elsevier; 2005.
40. Friedman RJ, Rigel DS, Kopf AW, et al. Volume of malignant melanoma is superior to thickness as a prognostic indicator. Preliminary observation. Dermatol Clin. 1991;9:643–8.
41. Beardmore GL, Quinn RL, Little JH. Malignant melanoma in Queensland: pathology of 105 fatal cutaneous melanomas. Pathology. 1970;2:277–86.
42. Rongioletti F, Smoller BR. Unusual histological variants of cutaneous malignant melanoma with some clinical and possible prognostic correlations. J Cutan Pathol. 2005;32:589–603.
43. Larsen TE, Grude TH. A retrospective histological study of 669 cases of primary cutaneous malignant melanoma in clinical stage I. 4. The relation of cross-sectional profile, level of invasion, ulceration and vascular invasion to tumour type and prognosis. Acta Pathol Microbiol Scand A. 1979;87A:131–8.
44. Siminovitch JM, Bergfeld W, Dinner M. Exophytic (pedunculated) malignant melanoma – Cleveland Clinic experience. Ann Plast Surg. 1980;5:432–5.
45. Manci EA, Balch CM, Murad TM, et al. Polypoid melanoma, a virulent variant of the nodular growth pattern. Am J Clin Pathol. 1981;75:810–5.
46. Kuehnl-Petzoldt C, Berger H, Wiebelt H. Verrucouskeratotic variations of malignant melanoma: a clinicopathological study. Am J Dermatopathol. 1982;4: 403–10.
47. Corona R, Scio M, Mele A, et al. Survival and prognostic factors in patients with localised cutaneous melanoma observed between 1980 and 1991 at the Istituto Dermopatico dell'Immacolata in Rome, Italy. Eur J Cancer. 1994;30A:333–8.
48. Schmid-Wendtner MH, Baumert J, Schmidt M, et al. Prognostic index for cutaneous melanoma: an analysis after follow-up of 2715 patients. Melanoma Res. 2001;11:619–26.
49. Azzola MF, Shaw HM, Thompson JF, et al. Tumor mitotic rate is a more powerful prognostic indicator than ulceration in patients with primary cutaneous melanoma: an analysis of 3661 patients from a single center. Cancer. 2003;97:1488–98.
50. Santillan AA, Messina JL, Marzban SS, et al. Pathology review of thin melanoma and melanoma in situ in a multidisciplinary melanoma clinic: impact on treatment decisions. J Clin Oncol. 2010;28: 481–6.
51. Oliveira Filho RS, Ferreira LM, Biasi LJ, et al. Vertical growth phase and positive sentinel node in thin melanoma. Braz J Med Biol Res. 2003;36: 347–50.
52. Payette MJ, Katz M, Grant-Kels JM. Melanoma prognostic factors found in the dermatopathology report. Clin Dermatol. 2009;27:53–74.
53. Schmoeckel C, Braun-Falco O. Prognostic index in malignant melanoma. Arch Dermatol. 1978;114: 871–3.
54. Kopf AW, Gross DF, Rogers GS, et al. Prognostic index for malignant melanoma. Cancer. 1987;59: 1236–41.
55. Lefevre M, Vergier B, Balme B, et al. Relevance of vertical growth pattern in thin level II cutaneous superficial spreading melanomas. Am J Surg Pathol. 2003;27:717–24.
56. Cuellar FA, Vilalta A, Rull R, et al. Small cell melanoma and ulceration as predictors of positive sentinel lymph node in malignant melanoma patients. Melanoma Res. 2004;14:277–82.
57. Glass LF, Guffey JM, Schroer KR, et al. Histopathologic study of recurrent Clark level II melanomas. Semin Surg Oncol. 1993;9:202–7.
58. Mansson-Brahme E, Carstensen J, Erhardt K, et al. Prognostic factors in thin cutaneous malignant melanoma. Cancer. 1994;73:2324–32.
59. Zettersten E, Shaikh L, Ramirez R, et al. Prognostic factors in primary cutaneous melanoma. Surg Clin North Am. 2003;83:61–75.
60. Paladugu RR, Yonemoto RH. Biologic behavior of thin malignant melanomas with regressive changes. Arch Surg. 1983;118:41–4.
61. Sondergaard K, Hou-Jensen K. Partial regression in thin primary cutaneous malignant melanomas clinical stage I. A study of 486 cases. Virchows Arch A Pathol Anat Histopathol. 1985;408:241–7.
62. Shaw HM, Rivers JK, McCarthy SW, et al. Cutaneous melanomas exhibiting unusual biologic behavior. World J Surg. 1992;16:196–202.
63. Guitart J, Lowe L, Piepkorn M, et al. Histological characteristics of metastasizing thin melanomas: a

63. case-control study of 43 cases. Arch Dermatol. 2002; 138:603–8.
64. Slingluff Jr CL, Vollmer RT, Reintgen DT, et al. Lethal "thin" malignant melanoma. Identifying patients at risk. Ann Surg. 1988;208:150–61.
65. Shaw HM, McCarthy SW, McCarthy WH, et al. Thin regressing malignant melanoma: significance of concurrent regional lymph node metastases. Histopathology. 1989;15:257–65.
66. Barnhill RL, Levy MA. Regressing thin cutaneous malignant melanomas (< or =1.0 mm) are associated with angiogenesis. Am J Pathol. 1993;143:99–104.
67. Taylor RC, Patel A, Panageas KS, et al. Tumor-infiltrating lymphocytes predict sentinel lymph node positivity in patients with cutaneous melanoma. J Clin Oncol. 2007;25:869–75.
68. Clark Jr WH, Elder DE, Guerry 4th D, et al. Model predicting survival in stage I melanoma based on tumor progression. J Natl Cancer Inst. 1989;81: 1893–904.
69. Clemente CG, Mihm Jr MC, Bufalino R, et al. Prognostic value of tumor infiltrating lymphocytes in the vertical growth phase of primary cutaneous melanoma. Cancer. 1996;77:1303–10.
70. Day Jr CL, Lew RA, Mihm Jr MC, et al. A multivariate analysis of prognostic factors for melanoma patients with lesions greater than or equal to 3.65 mm in thickness. The importance of revealing alternative Cox models. Ann Surg. 1982;195:44–9.
71. Elder DE, Guerry 4th D, VanHorn M, et al. The role of lymph node dissection for clinical stage I malignant melanoma of intermediate thickness (1.51-3.99 mm). Cancer. 1985;56:413–8.
72. Tuthill RJ, Unger JM, Liu PY, et al. Risk assessment in localized primary cutaneous melanoma: a Southwest Oncology Group study evaluating nine factors and a test of the Clark logistic regression prediction model. Am J Clin Pathol. 2002;118:504–11.
73. Hakansson A, Gustafsson B, Krysander L, et al. Biochemotherapy of metastatic malignant melanoma. Predictive value of tumour-infiltrating lymphocytes. Br J Cancer. 2001;85:1871–7.
74. Ladanyi A, Somlai B, Gilde K, et al. T-cell activation marker expression on tumor-infiltrating lymphocytes as prognostic factor in cutaneous malignant melanoma. Clin Cancer Res. 2004;10:521–30.
75. Movassagh M, Spatz A, Davoust J, et al. Selective accumulation of mature DC Lamp+dendritic cells in tumor sites is associated with efficient T-cell-mediated antitumor response and control of metastatic dissemination in melanoma. Cancer Res. 2004; 64:2192–8.
76. Ladanyi A, Kiss J, Somlai B, et al. Density of DC-LAMP(+) mature dendritic cells in combination with activated T lymphocytes infiltrating primary cutaneous melanoma is a strong independent prognostic factor. Cancer Immunol Immunother. 2007; 56:1459–69.
77. Day Jr CL, Sober AJ, Kopf AW, et al. A prognostic model for clinical stage I melanoma of the lower extremity. Location on foot as independent risk factor for recurrent disease. Surgery. 1981;89:599–603.
78. Spatz A, Shaw HM, Crotty KA, et al. Analysis of histopathological factors associated with prolonged survival of 10 years or more for patients with thick melanomas (>5 mm). Histopathology. 1998;33:406–13.
79. Anichini A, Vegetti C, Mortarini R. The paradox of T-cell-mediated antitumor immunity in spite of poor clinical outcome in human melanoma. Cancer Immunol Immunother. 2004;53:855–64.
80. Marincola FM, Wang E, Herlyn M, et al. Tumors as elusive targets of T-cell-based active immunotherapy. Trends Immunol. 2003;24:335–42.
81. Lassau N, Lamuraglia M, Koscielny S, et al. Prognostic value of angiogenesis evaluated with high-frequency and colour Doppler sonography for preoperative assessment of primary cutaneous melanomas: correlation with recurrence after a 5 year follow-up period. Cancer Imaging. 2006;6:24–9.
82. Vlaykova T, Laurila P, Muhonen T, et al. Prognostic value of tumour vascularity in metastatic melanoma and association of blood vessel density with vascular endothelial growth factor expression. Melanoma Res. 1999;9:59–68.
83. Carlson JA, Ross JS, Slominski A, et al. Molecular diagnostics in melanoma. J Am Acad Dermatol. 2005;52:743–75, quiz 75–8.
84. Kashani-Sabet M, Sagebiel RW, Ferreira CM, et al. Tumor vascularity in the prognostic assessment of primary cutaneous melanoma. J Clin Oncol. 2002;20:1826–31.
85. Barnhill RL, Fandrey K, Levy MA, et al. Angiogenesis and tumor progression of melanoma. Quantification of vascularity in melanocytic nevi and cutaneous malignant melanoma. Lab Invest. 1992;67:331–7.
86. Vlaykova T, Muhonen T, Hahka-Kemppinen M, et al. Vascularity and prognosis of metastatic melanoma. Int J Cancer. 1997;74:326–9.
87. Srivastava A, Laidler P, Davies RP, et al. The prognostic significance of tumor vascularity in intermediate-thickness (0.76–4.0 mm thick) skin melanoma. A quantitative histologic study. Am J Pathol. 1988;133:419–23.
88. Rongioletti F, Miracco C, Gambini C, et al. Tumor vascularity as a prognostic indicator in intermediate-thickness (0.76–4 mm) cutaneous melanoma. A quantitative assay. Am J Dermatopathol. 1996;18: 474–7.
89. Neitzel LT, Neitzel CD, Magee KL, et al. Angiogenesis correlates with metastasis in melanoma. Ann Surg Oncol. 1999;6:70–4.
90. Carnochan P, Briggs JC, Westbury G, et al. The vascularity of cutaneous melanoma: a quantitative histological study of lesions 0.85–1.25 mm in thickness. Br J Cancer. 1991;64:102–7.
91. Graham CH, Rivers J, Kerbel RS, et al. Extent of vascularization as a prognostic indicator in thin (<0.76 mm) malignant melanomas. Am J Pathol. 1994;145:510–4.

92. Busam KJ, Berwick M, Blessing K, et al. Tumor vascularity is not a prognostic factor for malignant melanoma of the skin. Am J Pathol. 1995;147:1049–56.
93. Ilmonen S, Kariniemi AL, Vlaykova T, et al. Prognostic value of tumour vascularity in primary melanoma. Melanoma Res. 1999;9:273–8.
94. Kashani-Sabet M, Sagebiel RW, Ferreira CM, et al. Vascular involvement in the prognosis of primary cutaneous melanoma. Arch Dermatol. 2001;137:1169–73.
95. Setala LP, Kosma VM, Marin S, et al. Prognostic factors in gastric cancer: the value of vascular invasion, mitotic rate and lymphoplasmacytic infiltration. Br J Cancer. 1996;74:766–72.
96. Pinder SE, Ellis IO, Galea M, et al. Pathological prognostic factors in breast cancer. III. Vascular invasion: relationship with recurrence and survival in a large study with long-term follow-up. Histopathology. 1994;24:41–7.
97. Thorn M, Ponten F, Bergstrom R, et al. Clinical and histopathologic predictors of survival in patients with malignant melanoma: a population-based study in Sweden. J Natl Cancer Inst. 1994;86:761–9.
98. Zettersten E, Sagebiel RW, Miller 3rd JR, et al. Prognostic factors in patients with thick cutaneous melanoma (>4 mm). Cancer. 2002;94:1049–56.
99. Lugassy C, Barnhill RL. Angiotropic melanoma and extravascular migratory metastasis: a review. Adv Anat Pathol. 2007;14:195–201.
100. Barnhill RL, Lugassy C. Angiotropic malignant melanoma and extravascular migratory metastasis: description of 36 cases with emphasis on a new mechanism of tumour spread. Pathology. 2004;36:485–90.
101. Gerami P, Shea C, Stone MS. Angiotropism in epidermotropic metastatic melanoma: another clue to the diagnosis. Am J Dermatopathol. 2006;28:429–33.
102. Johnson CS, Ramos-Caro FA, Hassanein AM. Ultralate erysipeloid angiotropic metastatic malignant melanoma. Int J Dermatol. 2001;40:446–7.
103. Shea CR, Kline MA, Lugo J, et al. Angiotropic metastatic malignant melanoma. Am J Dermatopathol. 1995;17:58–62.
104. Moreno A, Espanol I, Romagosa V. Angiotropic malignant melanoma. Report of two cases. J Cutan Pathol. 1992;19:325–9.
105. Barnhill RL. The biology of melanoma micrometastases. Recent Results Cancer Res. 2001;158:3–13.
106. Lugassy C, Barnhill RL, Christensen L. Melanoma and extravascular migratory metastasis. J Cutan Pathol. 2000;27:481.
107. Lugassy C, Dickersin GR, Christensen L, et al. Ultrastructural and immunohistochemical studies of the periendothelial matrix in human melanoma: evidence for an amorphous matrix containing laminin. J Cutan Pathol. 1999;26:78–83.
108. Lugassy C, Eyden BP, Christensen L, et al. Angiotumoral complex in human malignant melanoma characterised by free laminin: ultrastructural and immunohistochemical observations. J Submicrosc Cytol Pathol. 1997;29:19–28.
109. Lugassy C, Shahsafaei A, Bonitz P, et al. Tumor microvessels in melanoma express the beta-2 chain of laminin. Implications for melanoma metastasis. J Cutan Pathol. 1999;26:222–6.
110. Lugassy C, Kleinman HK, Fernandez PM, et al. Human melanoma cell migration along capillary-like structures in vitro: a new dynamic model for studying extravascular migratory metastasis. J Invest Dermatol. 2002;119:703–4.
111. Arrington 3rd JH, Reed RJ, Ichinose H, et al. Plantar lentiginous melanoma: a distinctive variant of human cutaneous malignant melanoma. Am J Surg Pathol. 1977;1:131–43.
112. Weyers W, Euler M, Diaz-Cascajo C, et al. Classification of cutaneous malignant melanoma: a reassessment of histopathologic criteria for the distinction of different types. Cancer. 1999;86:288–99.
113. Swetter SM. Dermatological perspectives of malignant melanoma. Surg Clin North Am. 2003;83:77–95, vi.
114. Hacene K, Le Doussal V, Brunet M, et al. Prognostic index for clinical Stage I cutaneous malignant melanoma. Cancer Res. 1983;43:2991–6.
115. Ringborg U, Afzelius LE, Lagerlof B, et al. Cutaneous malignant melanoma of the head and neck. Analysis of treatment results and prognostic factors in 581 patients: a report from the Swedish Melanoma Study Group. Cancer. 1993;71:751–8.
116. Crocetti E, Mangone L, Lo Scocco G, et al. Prognostic variables and prognostic groups for malignant melanoma. The information from Cox and Classification and Regression Trees analysis: an Italian population-based study. Melanoma Res. 2006;16:429–33.
117. Golger A, Young DS, Ghazarian D, et al. Epidemiological features and prognostic factors of cutaneous head and neck melanoma: a population-based study. Arch Otolaryngol Head Neck Surg. 2007;133:442–7.
118. MacKie RM. Malignant melanoma: clinical variants and prognostic indicators. Clin Exp Dermatol. 2000;25:471–5.
119. Balch CM, Soong SJ, Milton GW, et al. A comparison of prognostic factors and surgical results in 1,786 patients with localized (stage I) melanoma treated in Alabama, USA, and New South Wales, Australia. Ann Surg. 1982;196:677–84.
120. Magro CM, Crowson AM, Mihm MC. Unusual variants of malignant melanoma. Mod Pathol. 2006;19(S2):S41–70.
121. Podnos YD, Jimenez JC, Zainabadi K, et al. Minimal deviation melanoma. Cancer Treat Rev. 2002;28:219–21.
122. Pol-Rodriquez M, Lee S, Silvers DN, et al. Influence of age on survival in childhood spitzoid melanomas. Cancer. 2007;109:1579–83.
123. Fabrizi G, Massi G. Spitzoid malignant melanoma in teenagers: an entity with no better prognosis than

that of other forms of melanoma. Histopathology. 2001;38:448–53.
124. Busam KJ, Mujumdar U, Hummer AJ, et al. Cutaneous desmoplastic melanoma: reappraisal of morphologic heterogeneity and prognostic factors. Am J Surg Pathol. 2004;28:1518–25.
125. Busam KJ. Cutaneous desmoplastic melanoma. Adv Anat Pathol. 2005;12:92–102.
126. Gyorki DE, Busam K, Panageas K, et al. Sentinel lymph node biopsy for patients with cutaneous desmoplastic melanoma. Ann Surg Oncol. 2003;10:403–7.
127. Payne WG, Kearney R, Wells K, et al. Desmoplastic melanoma. Am Surg. 2001;67:1004–6.
128. Jaroszewski DE, Pockaj BA, DiCaudo DJ, et al. The clinical behavior of desmoplastic melanoma. Am J Surg. 2001;182:590–5.
129. Quinn MJ, Crotty KA, Thompson JF, et al. Desmoplastic and desmoplastic neurotropic melanoma: experience with 280 patients. Cancer. 1998;83:1128–35.
130. Carlson JA, Dickersin GR, Sober AJ, et al. Desmoplastic neurotropic melanoma. A clinicopathologic analysis of 28 cases. Cancer. 1995;75:478–94.
131. Skelton HG, Smith KJ, Laskin WB, et al. Desmoplastic malignant melanoma. J Am Acad Dermatol. 1995;32:717–25.
132. Conley J, Lattes R, Orr W. Desmoplastic malignant melanoma (a rare variant of spindle cell melanoma). Cancer. 1971;28:914–36.
133. Hawkins WG, Busam KJ, Ben-Porat L, et al. Desmoplastic melanoma: a pathologically and clinically distinct form of cutaneous melanoma. Ann Surg Oncol. 2005;12:207–13.
134. Thelmo MC, Sagebiel RW, Treseler PA, et al. Evaluation of sentinel lymph node status in spindle cell melanomas. J Am Acad Dermatol. 2001;44:451–5.
135. Cummins DL, Esche C, Barrett TL, et al. Lymph node biopsy results for desmoplastic malignant melanoma. Cutis. 2007;79:390–4.
136. Reed RJ. Minimal deviation melanoma. In: Mihm MC, Murphy GF, Kaufman N, editors. Pathobiology and recognition of malignant melanoma. Baltimore: Williams and Wilkins; 1998. p. 110–52.
137. Egbert B, Kempson R, Sagebiel R. Desmoplastic malignant melanoma. A clinicohistopathologic study of 25 cases. Cancer. 1988;62:2033–41.
138. Su LD, Fullen DR, Lowe L, et al. Desmoplastic and neurotropic melanoma. Cancer. 2004;100:598–604.
139. Reed RJ, Leonard DD. Neurotropic melanoma. A variant of desmoplastic melanoma. Am J Surg Pathol. 1979;3:301–11.
140. Baer SC, Schultz D, Zynnestvedt M, et al. Desmoplasia and neurotropism. Prognostic variables in patients with stage I melanoma. Cancer. 1995;76:2242–7.

141. Newlin HE, Morris CG, Amdur RJ, et al. Neurotropic melanoma of the head and neck with clinical perineural invasion. Am J Clin Oncol. 2005;28:399–402.
142. Anderson TD, Weber RS, Guerry D, et al. Desmoplastic neurotropic melanoma of the head and neck: the role of radiation therapy. Head Neck. 2002;34:1068–71.
143. Madrigal B, Fresno MF, Junquera L, et al. De novo desmoplastic neurotropic melanoma of the lower lip: a neoplasm with ominous behavior. Oral Surg Oral Med Oral Pathol Oral Radiol Endod. 1998;86:452–6.
144. Lin D, Kashani-Sabet M, McCalmont T, et al. Neurotropic melanoma invading the inferior alveolar nerve. J Am Acad Dermatol. 2005;53:S120–2.
145. Fabre B, Gigaud M, Lamant L, et al. [Trigeminal neuralgia presenting as a deep recurrent desmoplastic neurotropic melanoma of a lentigo maligna]. French. Ann Dermatol Venereol. 2003;130:1044–6.
146. Byrne PR, Maiman M, Mikhail A, et al. Neurotropic desmoplastic melanoma: a rare vulvar malignancy. Gynecol Oncol. 1995;56:289–93.
147. Barnhill RL, Bolognia JL. Neurotropic melanoma with prominent melanization. J Cutan Pathol. 1995;22:450–9.
148. Weatherhead SC, Haniffa M, Lawrence CM. Melanomas arising from naevi and de novo melanomas – does origin matter? Br J Dermatol. 2007;156:72–6.
149. Drunkenmolle E, Marsch W, Lubbe D, et al. Paratumoral epidermal hyperplasia: a novel prognostic factor in thick primary melanoma of the skin? Am J Dermatopathol. 2005;27:482–8.
150. Mott RT, Rosenberg A, Livingston S, et al. Melanoma associated with pseudoepitheliomatous hyperplasia: a case series and investigation into the role of epidermal growth factor receptor. J Cutan Pathol. 2002;29:490–7.
151. Hanly AJ, Jorda M, Elgart GW. Cutaneous malignant melanoma associated with extensive pseudoepitheliomatous hyperplasia. Report of a case and discussion of the origin of pseudoepitheliomatous hyperplasia. J Cutan Pathol. 2000;27:153–6.
152. Reis-Filho JS, Gasparetto EL, Schmitt FC, et al. Pseudoepitheliomatous hyperplasia in cutaneous malignant melanoma: a rare and misleading feature. J Cutan Pathol. 2001;28:496–7.
153. Kaddu S, Smolle J, Zenahlik P, et al. Melanoma with benign melanocytic naevus components: reappraisal of clinicopathological features and prognosis. Melanoma Res. 2002;12:271–8.
154. Nakayama T, Taback B, Turner R, et al. Molecular clonality of in-transit melanoma metastasis. Am J Pathol. 2001;158:1371–8.
155. Leon P, Daly JM, Synnestvedt M, et al. The prognostic implications of microscopic satellites in patients with clinical stage I melanoma. Arch Surg. 1991;126:1461–8.
156. Silverio A, McRae M, Ariyan S, et al. Management of the difficult sentinel lymph node in patients with primary cutaneous melanoma. Ann Plast Surg. 2010;65:418–24.

Genetic/Epigenetic Biomarkers: Distinction of Melanoma from Other Melanocytic Neoplasms

Minoru Takata

Introduction

Although it is considered the "gold standard" for classification of cutaneous melanocytic tumors, light microscopic analysis is often equivocal [1]. In some cases, there is considerable disagreement, even among expert pathologists [2–6]. The most frequent diagnostic problem is the distinction of a Spitz nevus from a spitzoid melanoma. One large study, retrospectively reviewing the histopathology of cases presented to a multidisciplinary panel, found a significant change from the original diagnosis in 559 (11%) of 5,136 specimens. In this study, the microscopic interpretation was changed from nevus to melanoma, or vice versa, in 120 (2.3%) of the cases [5]. A misdiagnosis or the incorrect interpretation of a melanocytic lesion can result in unnecessary psychological stress to the patient, under-treatment or over-treatment, and improper follow-up. Thus, diagnostically applicable parameters other than routine histopathology are needed.

Recent investigations have revealed significant differences in genetic alterations between melanomas and benign melanocytic proliferations (reviewed in reference [7]). The distinct patterns of somatic genetic alterations between melanoma and benign melanocytic tumors offer an opportunity to develop diagnostic strategies based on molecular genetic methods. This chapter discusses several molecular genetic analyses, which could be used as additional diagnostic tools, to distinguish melanoma from other melanocytic neoplasms.

Allelic Imbalance (AI) Analysis

Analyses of allelic imbalance (AI) or loss of heterozygosity (LOH) reveal the presence of deletions or gains of specific alleles. PCR amplification of microsatellite polymorphic markers followed by gel electrophoresis is used for this analysis, and can be easily performed on DNA obtained from formalin-fixed paraffin-embedded (FFPE) tissues. If one finds two alleles in the normal tissue of a patient, this marker is regarded as informative. An imbalance is assumed if only one allele is detected in the tumor tissue. It should be noted that contamination of tumor samples by normal cells can produce false-negative results; although, laser capture microdissection may enhance the sensitivity of detection. As some markers will be homozygous at a particular locus and thus uninformative, a combination of markers is normally employed.

Healy et al. [8] allelotyped 41 primary cutaneous melanomas and 32 benign melanocytic nevi,

M. Takata, M.D., Ph.D. (✉)
Department of Dermatology, Okayama University
Postgraduate School of Medical, Dentistry
and Pharmaceutical Sciences, Okayama, Japan
e-mail: mtakata@onyx.ocn.ne.jp

using 45 microsatellite markers that spanned all autosomal arms. They found frequent AI on several arms, including 9p, 10q, 6q, and 18q in primary melanomas. In contrast, 30 of 32 nevi showed no AI. Two nevi demonstrated AI, including a loss of 9p in one case. These latter nevi were described as showing atypical histopathological features that suggested dysplastic nevi. The authors also examined 27 Spitz nevi with markers that showed frequent loss in melanomas, and found that two cases had interstitial deletions of 9p. Thus, AI of 9p may not be confined to melanoma, and other genetic lesions, such as loss of 10q, 6q, and 18q, could be markers of a malignant phenotype [8].

Van Dijk et al. [9] tested the diagnostic utility of AI analysis in a series of 55 tumors that included benign Spitz nevi, Spitz tumors of unclear malignant potential (atypical Spitz tumors), and spitzoid melanomas. Twelve microsatellite markers that mapped to chromosomal arms 1p, 3p, 6q, 8q, 9p, 10q, and 11q were selected for analysis. AI was found in 2 of 12 (17%) typical Spitz nevi, 3 of 9 (33%) atypical Spitz tumors, 12 of 17 (65%) atypical Spitz tumors suspected of being melanomas, and 15 of 17 (88%) spitzoid melanomas. The authors concluded that this approach had no direct applicability for distinguishing between benign and malignant spitzoid tumors [9].

Comparative Genomic Hybridization (CGH)

CGH is a method to detect and map DNA copy number changes throughout the entire genome, using a cytogenetic map supplied by metaphase chromosomes. It involves the simultaneous hybridization of two differentially labeled DNA populations; one from a tumor sample and the other from a healthy donor serving as a reference. Recently, a new variation of the CGH methodology was reported, in which metaphase chromosomes are replaced by arrays of genomic bacterial artificial chromosome clones (array CGH). This allows for accurate quantification of DNA copy number variations over a wide dynamic range and significantly improves the resolution of measurements. Importantly, CGH can be performed on archival FFPE samples, although a relatively large amount of tissue is needed to obtain sufficient DNA [10].

A number of CGH-based studies have found that the majority of melanomas show chromosomal aberrations, whereas benign melanocytic nevi do not [11, 12]. Spitz nevi may demonstrate isolated gain of the short arm of chromosome 11 (11p), a finding that is not observed in melanoma [13]. The clear differences in patterns of aberrations between benign and malignant melanocytic tumors suggest that they could be of diagnostic use. Several cases have been reported in which CGH provided additional information for diagnosis of histopathologically ambiguous spitzoid tumors [10, 14, 15]. Raskin et al. [16] examined copy number variations in 16 atypical Spitz tumors by array CGH, and found chromosomal aberrations in seven cases. However, the vast majority of chromosomal abnormalities observed in these cases are not commonly found in melanomas, suggesting that the atypical Spitz tumor may, in fact, be a distinct entity different from conventional Spitz nevus and melanoma.

CGH may also be useful in solving other diagnostic problems relating to melanocytic tumors, such as distinguishing between a benign proliferative nodule and a melanoma arising within a congenital melanocytic nevus (CMN), and the distinction of malignant blue nevi from benign dermal-based melanocytic proliferations. A recent CGH-based analysis examining neoplasms arising in CMN revealed that proliferative nodules showed numerical aberrations of whole chromosomes. This pattern differed significantly from the findings for melanoma that arose within CMN [17]. In the case of dermal-based melanocytic proliferations, unequivocally benign and malignant lesions show non-overlapping patterns of chromosomal aberration; however, ambiguous tumors can be separated into lesions with and without genomic changes [18]. The differences in CGH patterns may be of diagnostic value in ambiguous cases of these rather rare, but sometimes diagnostically challenging, melanocytic neoplasms.

Multiplex Ligation-Dependent Probe Amplification (MLPA)

MLPA is a novel technique to measure the copy number of up to 45 nucleic acid sequences in one single reaction [19]. This method relies on sequence-specific probe hybridization to genomic DNA, followed by multiplex-PCR amplification of the hybridized probe, and semi-quantitative analysis of the resulting PCR products. The assay is easily performed; requiring only 50 ng of DNA extracted from routinely processed FFPE sections, and thus, may be a superior adjunctive diagnostic tool to CGH. Another advantage of this technique is that it is fast, and multiple samples can be tested in one reaction.

Van Dijk et al. [20] evaluated the reliability of MLPA on DNA isolated from archival melanocytic tumors. They compared MLPA results with those simultaneously determined by CGH, and found 86% concordance of results by both methods. Discordance commonly involved alterations that were detected by MLPA and not by CGH, probably due to a combination of the lower resolution of CGH and occasional false-positive MLPA results. The authors concluded that MLPA is a feasible method to screen large numbers of archival tissues for DNA gains and losses.

Takata et al. [21] examined copy number alterations of 55 melanocytic tumors (24 primary melanomas, 14 Spitz nevi and 17 banal nevi) using commercially available MLPA kits, SALSA P005 and P006. These kits include 76 target genes spanning almost all chromosomal arms. DNA was extracted from archival FFPE tissues. The authors found multiple (≥3) copy number gains and losses in all but two primary melanomas. In contrast, all of the examined Spitz nevi and banal melanocytic nevi showed copy number changes at <2 loci. Receiver operator characteristic curve analysis showed that the threshold value of copy number aberrations corresponding to 98% specificity for melanoma was 2.42, with a sensitivity using this threshold value of 92.5%. This preliminary study indicates that MLPA could be used as an adjunctive diagnostic tool for melanocytic tumors [21].

Fluorescence In Situ Hybridization (FISH)

FISH uses fluorescently labeled probes that are complementary to stretches of genomic DNA. The analysis may be performed on FFPE sections, and can detect cells with aberrations in the presence of significant numbers of adjacent normal cells. However, while gene amplification is rather easy to detect by FISH analysis of FFPE sections, the detection of heterozygous deletion is more difficult (i.e., the detection of a single copy of a gene in a nucleus may be an artifact of tissue-sectioning procedures). Thus, analysis of large numbers of both tumor and normal cells is required to determine a potential decrease in average copy number of a test probe relative to a reference probe. Furthermore, FISH is time-consuming, and can only investigate a few loci at a time.

To overcome the disadvantages of FISH, Gerami et al. [22] used existing data on DNA copy number alterations in melanoma to assemble panels of FISH probes suitable for distinction of melanoma from melanocytic nevi, and tested their validity in large cohorts of melanocytic tumors. The authors found that a four-probe combination targeting 6p25 (RREB1), centromere 6, 6q23 (MYB), and 11q13 (cyclin D1) provided the highest diagnostic discrimination, correctly classifying melanomas with 86.7% sensitivity and 95.4% specificity. As the four probes were labeled with four different colors, one hybridization reaction was sufficient. For the enumeration of FISH signals, ten random nuclei were counted in three selected areas. The same authors further evaluated the diagnostic sensitivity of FISH targeting these four loci in larger numbers of melanocytic nevi and melanomas of different histological subtypes, and confirmed the high performance of this probe set in distinguishing melanoma from nevi. They additionally found that clonal abnormalities in chromosome 6 with increased copies of short arm relative to long arm are common in all melanoma subtypes, and that copy number increase of 11q13 is most common in lentigo maligna melanomas [23]. This probe set has also assisted with the diagnostic classification of melanocytic tumors with ambiguous pathology [22], distinguishing blue nevus-like cutaneous melanoma metastasis from epithelioid blue nevus [24], nevoid melanoma from mitotically active nevus [25], and lentigo maligna from benign junctional nevus [26]. This four-probe FISH assay appears to be a useful diagnostic aid to traditional histopathologic evaluation.

FISH is also helpful in the diagnosis of early acral melanoma in situ. Although early forms of acral melanoma in situ may show clinical features suggestive of malignancy, including large size, variegated color, and/or irregular shape, the light microscopic diagnosis of these tumors may be difficult or even impossible. Often, such lesions show only a slight increase in melanocytes with absent or minimal cytologic atypia [27]. Yamaura et al. [28] performed FISH analysis on clinically atypical, but histopathologically near-normal pigmented lesions on the sole of the foot, and demonstrated cyclin D1 amplifications in normal-appearing intraepidermal melanocytes in some cases. Such lesions show a parallel ridge pattern on dermoscopy, a characteristic finding of acral melanoma in situ [29]. Amplification of the cyclin D1 gene is a genetic hallmark of acral melanoma, detected in atypical melanocytes in the macular portion of overt tumor, as well as in non-atypical melanocytes in the epidermis beyond the histopathologically recognizable border [30, 31]. Thus, lesions containing melanocytes with cyclin D1 amplification appear to represent a latent progression phase of acral melanoma that precedes the atypical melanocytic proliferation in the epidermis [28]. Although cyclin D1 amplification is found in only ~40% of acral melanoma [32], the addition of probes that target other chromosomal regions amplified in this tumor, such as 5p12 [30, 31], could facilitate the detection of early in situ lesions.

Analysis of BRAF, NRAS, and HRAS Gene Mutation

BRAF and NRAS oncogene mutations have been described in melanoma and melanocytic nevi, but are not detected in Spitz nevi (reviewed in references [7, 33]). In contrast, HRAS mutations are found in a subset of Spitz nevi, but not in melanoma [34]. Thus, testing for mutations in these oncogenes may contribute to a more accurate diagnosis of histopathologically ambiguous spitzoid melanocytic lesions. As these mutations are limited to several known hotspots (i.e., codon 600 of the BRAF gene, and codons 12, 13, and 61 of the NRAS and HRAS genes), they are relatively easy to analyze in routinely processed specimens by PCR amplification of a few target exons, followed by sequencing of amplicons.

The results of mutational analyses in published studies [35–42] are summarized in Tables 6.1 and 6.2. Although two studies identified BRAF or NRAS mutations in Spitz nevi and atypical Spitz nevi [35, 37], these mutations are rare in these categories of melanocytic tumors. In contrast, BRAF or NRAS mutations have been detected in 37% of primary spitzoid melanomas.

Table 6.1 Frequency of BRAF and NRAS mutations in published studies

Study	Spitz nevus	Atypical Spitz nevus	Suspected melanoma/ STUMP	Primary spitzoid melanoma	Spitzoid melanoma metastasis	Common primary melanoma
Palmedo [40]	0/21	–	–	2/6	–	–
Gill [38]	0/10	–	–	–	–	–
Lee [39]	–	–	–	1/33	0/2	8/12
van Dijk [42]	0/14	0/16	8/23	30/36	6/7	–
Fullen [37]	5/23	5/25	0/7	2/13	–	–
Takata [41]	0/12	0/11	1/2	1/2	–	15/24
Da Forno [35]	1/16	1/9	3/9	4/27	–	13/25
Emley [36]	0/6	1/13	–	–	–	–
Total	6/102 (6%)	7/74 (9%)	12/41 (29%)	40/107 (37%)	6/9 (67%)	36/61 (59%)

Table 6.2 Frequency of HRAS mutations in published studies

Study	Spitz nevus	Atypical Spitz nevus	Suspected melanoma/ STUMP	Primary spitzoid melanoma	Spitzoid melanoma metastasis	Common primary melanoma
Gill [38]	0/10	–	–	0/9	–	–
van Dijk [42]	4/14	2/16	1/23	0/36	0/7	–
Takata [41]	0/12	0/11	0/2	0/2	–	0/24
Da Forno [35]	0/16	1/9	1/9	0/27	–	0/25
Total	4/52 (8%)	3/36 (8%)	2/34 (6%)	0/74 (0%)	0/7 (0%)	0/49 (0%)

Interestingly, up to 29% of suspected melanoma/spitzoid tumors of uncertain malignant potential (STUMP) showed BRAF or NRAS mutations, suggesting that a substantial number of these tumors were actually melanomas. While HRAS mutations were identified in a few Spitz nevi, atypical Spitz nevi and STUMP, none of the melanomas analyzed showed this aberration. Thus, the presence of a HRAS mutation would favor the diagnosis of a benign melanocytic tumor.

One concerning issue with these analyses is that the grouping of lesions was based on light microscopic examination. The histopathologic diagnosis of spitzoid tumors is notoriously difficult, even for expert pathologists [3, 4]. Thus, a long-term follow-up of patients is imperative to establish the diagnostic value of molecular testing. At the present time, mutational analysis cannot replace conventional light microscopic examination; however, it may provide important additional diagnostic information.

Gene Expression Analysis Using DNA Microarrays

High-density microarrays have been used to monitor the expression of thousands of genes in tissue samples. Recent studies have resulted in the identification of genes that are differentially expressed in benign and malignant melanocytic lesions [43–45]. In one study, Talantov et al. [45] compared the gene expression profiles of primary melanomas and benign melanocytic nevi, identifying two melanoma-specific genes, PLAB and L1CAM. The authors demonstrated the feasibility of using this two-gene combination in a reverse transcription-polymerase chain reaction (RT-PCR) assay to distinguish benign from malignant melanocytic tumors [45]. Alexandrescu et al. [46], who used the same gene expression profile dataset, selected SILV as the most useful marker. They tested SILV expression levels by quantitative RT-PCR in a total of 193 specimens including 98 atypical cases, and showed clear discrimination between melanoma and nevi as well as between different atypia subgroups in the group of atypical samples. Koh et al. [44] successfully employed archival FFPE tissues for microarray gene expression profiling, and also reported genes that showed differential expression between melanomas and melanocytic nevi. However, unlike the Talantov study [45], expression of L1CAM was found to be decreased in melanomas [44]. Kashani-Sabet et al. [43] selected five transcripts (ARPC2, FN1, RGS1, SPP1 and WNT2), which were found to be overexpressed in melanomas compared with melanocytic nevi by gene expression profiling [47], and showed that immunohistochemistry for corresponding proteins can be useful in the distinction of melanocytic tumors. Importantly, this multimarker assay correctly identified ~75% of the cases in which incorrect histopathological diagnoses had been made, including melanomas initially diagnosed as melanocytic nevi. These candidate melanoma-specific markers should be validated in larger cohorts.

Epigenetic Biomarkers

Aberrations in DNA methylation, post-translational modifications of histones, chromatin remodeling, and microRNA expression patterns are epigenetic alterations associated with the development of various human cancers, including melanoma (reviewed in reference [48]). Hypermethylation of CpG islands is one of the most prevalent molecular markers for melanoma. Although the list of methylated genes identified in melanoma continues to grow [48], there have been few attempts to use these genes as diagnostic markers of melanocytic tumors. Takata et al. [41] employed methylation-specific MLPA, a novel method to detect CpG methylation of 25 tumor suppressor genes commonly found in human cancers [49], to examine a series of melanomas and spitzoid tumors. They found CpG methylation in 10 of 24 primary melanomas, but in no Spitz nevi or atypical Spitz tumors. Because CpG methylation can be detected in archival FFPE tissue with rapid and sensitive methylation-specific PCR, this approach may be a promising adjunctive diagnostic tool for melanocytic tumors.

Combination of Mutational Analysis and Methylation-Specific MLPA

While none of the methods discussed above is sufficient as an applicable diagnostic parameter beyond routine histopathology, a combination of molecular assays may be more useful in the distinction of melanoma from benign melanocytic tumors. Takata et al. [41] combined mutational analysis of the BRAF, NRAS and HRAS genes with methylation-specific MLPA (which simultaneously detected CpG methylation and copy number changes of 40 chromosomal sequences in a simple reaction [49]) to examine conventional melanomas and Spitz nevi, as well as atypical spitzoid lesions that had posed diagnostic difficulties. They found at least one genetic and/or epigenetic alteration in almost all melanomas, whereas none of the Spitz nevi with unambiguous histopathology showed such aberrations. Although most of the ambiguous spitzoid lesions, designated as atypical spitzoid tumors, showed no genomic changes, a subset of cases had chromosomal aberrations that included copy number loss of the CDKN2A gene. The authors concluded that this combined analysis may be useful in distinguishing between melanoma and Spitz nevi, and could help to define subgroups of atypical Spitz tumors. The following two cases demonstrate how this combined genetic and epigenetic analysis provides additional information in histopathologically ambiguous cases.

Case 1

A 70-year-old male presented with a pigmented lesion on the sole of his foot (Fig. 6.1). Light microscopic examination showed a well-circumscribed proliferation of spindle cells. The histopathologic diagnoses of two expert dermatopathologists were "Spitz nevus" and "atypical acral nevus, melanoma not ruled out". Combined genetic and epigenetic analysis showed few DNA copy number changes and no mutations in hot spots of the BRAF, NRAS and HRAS genes. However, methylation-specific MLPA revealed CpG methylation of the CDKN2B gene. This finding strongly suggested a melanoma in this case. The patient developed inguinal lymph node metastasis two and a half years after excision of the primary tumor, and died of the disease.

Case 2

A 27-year-old female presented with a pigmented lesion on the groin, clinically diagnosed as a Spitz nevus (Fig. 6.2). Light microscopic examination showed a nodular proliferation of spindled and epithelioid cells in the dermis. Small nests of epithelioid cells with clefting artifacts were also noted in the epidermis. Two pathologists diagnosed this lesion as a melanoma, while the diagnosis of a third pathologist was "atypical Spitz tumor". Methylation-specific MLPA showed neither DNA copy number changes nor CpG methylation. The BRAF, NRAS and HRAS genes were all wild-type. These findings were interpreted as incompatible with a malignant tumor. Because of the histopathologic diagnosis of a melanoma by two pathologists, a sentinel lymph node biopsy was performed with negative results. The patient has been free of disease for 5 years.

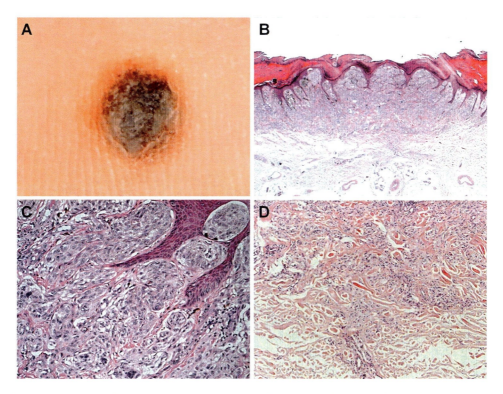

Fig. 6.1 (a) A brownish, slightly keratotic tumor, 6 mm in diameter, on the sole of the foot of a 70-year-old male. (b) Scanning magnification showing a compound proliferation of tumor cells that is laterally well-demarcated. (c) Nests of epithelioid cells in the epidermis and upper dermis. (d) Clear maturation of tumor cells in the deep dermis

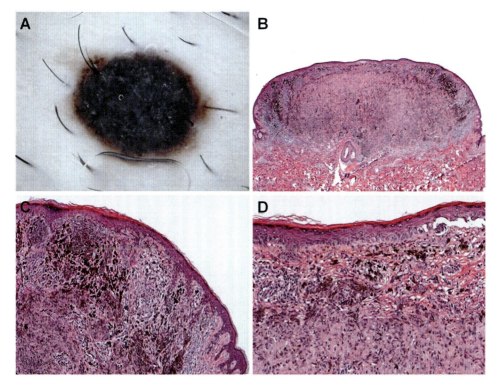

Fig. 6.2 (a) A dermoscopic image of a pigmented tumor on the groin of a 27-year-old female. (b) Scanning magnification shows a nodular proliferation in the dermis with sharp lateral demarcation. (c) The lesion is composed of spindled and epithelioid melanocytes. (d) Proliferation of epithelioid melanocytes within the epidermis and dermis

Conclusion

It is now clear that there are significant differences in genetic and epigenetic alterations among different types of melanocytic tumors. These aberrations can be analyzed in FFPE tissues for diagnostic purposes. Genetic and epigenetic analysis can be of particular diagnostic use in histopathologically ambiguous melanocytic tumors.

References

1. Ruiter DJ, van Dijk MC, Ferrier CM. Current diagnostic problems in melanoma pathology. Semin Cutan Med Surg. 2003;22:33–41.
2. Barnhill RL, Argenyi ZB, From L, et al. Atypical Spitz nevi/tumors: lack of consensus for diagnosis, discrimination from melanoma, and prediction of outcome. Hum Pathol. 1999;30:513–20.
3. Corona R, Mele A, Amini M, et al. Interobserver variability on the histopathologic diagnosis of cutaneous melanoma and other pigmented skin lesions. J Clin Oncol. 1996;14:1218–23.
4. Farmer ER, Gonin R, Hanna MP. Discordance in the histopathologic diagnosis of melanoma and melanocytic nevi between expert pathologists. Hum Pathol. 1996;27:528–31.
5. McGinnis KS, Lessin SR, Elder DE, et al. Pathology review of cases presenting to a multidisciplinary pigmented lesion clinic. Arch Dermatol. 2002;138:617–21.
6. Veenhuizen KC, De Wit PE, Mooi WJ, et al. Quality assessment by expert opinion in melanoma pathology: experience of the pathology panel of the Dutch Melanoma Working Party. J Pathol. 1997;182:266–72.
7. Takata M, Saida T. Genetic alterations in melanocytic tumors. J Dermatol Sci. 2006;43:1–10.
8. Healy E, Belgaid CE, Takata M, et al. Allelotypes of primary cutaneous melanoma and benign melanocytic nevi. Cancer Res. 1996;56:589–93.
9. van Dijk MC, Rombout PD, Mooi WJ, et al. Allelic imbalance in the diagnosis of benign, atypical and malignant Spitz tumours. J Pathol. 2002;197:170–8.
10. Bauer J, Bastian BC. Distinguishing melanocytic nevi from melanoma by DNA copy number changes: comparative genomic hybridization as a research and diagnostic tool. Dermatol Ther. 2006;19:40–9.
11. Bastian BC, Olshen AB, LeBoit PE, Pinkel D. Classifying melanocytic tumors based on DNA copy number changes. Am J Pathol. 2003;163:1765–70.
12. Harvell JD, Kohler S, Zhu S, et al. High-resolution array-based comparative genomic hybridization for distinguishing paraffin-embedded Spitz nevi and melanomas. Diagn Mol Pathol. 2004;13:22–5.
13. Bastian BC, Wesselmann U, Pinkel D, Leboit PE. Molecular cytogenetic analysis of Spitz nevi shows clear differences to melanoma. J Invest Dermatol. 1999;113:1065–9.
14. Bauer J, Bastian B. Genomic analysis of melanocytic neoplasia. Adv Dermatol. 2005;21:81–99.
15. Takata M, Maruo K, Kageshita T, et al. Two cases of unusual acral melanocytic tumors: illustration of molecular cytogenetics as a diagnostic tool. Hum Pathol. 2003;34:89–92.
16. Raskin L, Ludgate M, Iyer RK, et al. Copy number variations and clinical outcome in atypical spitz tumors. Am J Surg Pathol. 2011;35:243–52.
17. Bastian BC, Xiong J, Frieden IJ, et al. Genetic changes in neoplasms arising in congenital melanocytic nevi: differences between nodular proliferations and melanomas. Am J Pathol. 2002;161:1163–9.
18. Maize Jr JC, McCalmont TH, Carlson JA, et al. Genomic analysis of blue nevi and related dermal melanocytic proliferations. Am J Surg Pathol. 2005;29:1214–20.
19. Schouten JP, McElgunn CJ, Waaijer R, et al. Relative quantification of 40 nucleic acid sequences by multiplex ligation-dependent probe amplification. Nucleic Acids Res. 2002;30:e57.
20. van Dijk MC, Rombout PD, Boots-Sprenger SH, et al. Multiplex ligation-dependent probe amplification for the detection of chromosomal gains and losses in formalin-fixed tissue. Diagn Mol Pathol. 2005;14:9–16.
21. Takata M, Suzuki T, Ansai S, et al. Genome profiling of melanocytic tumors using multiplex ligation-dependent probe amplification (MLPA): its usefulness as an adjunctive diagnostic tool for melanocytic tumors. J Dermatol Sci. 2005;40:51–7.
22. Gerami P, Jewell SS, Morrison LE, et al. Fluorescence in situ hybridization (FISH) as an ancillary diagnostic tool in the diagnosis of melanoma. Am J Surg Pathol. 2009;33:1146–56.
23. Gerami P, Mafee M, Lurtsbarapa T, et al. Sensitivity of fluorescence in situ hybridization for melanoma diagnosis using RREB1, MYB, Cep6, and 11q13 probes in melanoma subtypes. Arch Dermatol. 2010;146:273–8.
24. Pouryazdanparast P, Newman M, Mafee M, et al. Distinguishing epithelioid blue nevus from blue nevus-like cutaneous melanoma metastasis using fluorescence in situ hybridization. Am J Surg Pathol. 2009;33:1396–400.
25. Gerami P, Wass A, Mafee M, et al. Fluorescence in situ hybridization for distinguishing nevoid melanomas from mitotically active nevi. Am J Surg Pathol. 2009;33:1783–8.
26. Newman MD, Mirzabeigi M, Gerami P. Chromosomal copy number changes supporting the classification of lentiginous junctional melanoma of the elderly as a subtype of melanoma. Mod Pathol. 2009;22:1258–62.
27. Ishihara Y, Saida T, Miyazaki A, et al. Early acral melanoma in situ: correlation between the parallel ridge pattern on dermoscopy and microscopic features. Am J Dermatopathol. 2006;28:21–7.

28. Yamaura M, Takata M, Miyazaki A, Saida T. Specific dermoscopy patterns and amplifications of the cyclin D1 gene to define histopathologically unrecognizable early lesions of acral melanoma in situ. Arch Dermatol. 2005;141:1413–8.
29. Oguchi S, Saida T, Koganehira Y, et al. Characteristic epiluminescent microscopic features of early malignant melanoma on glabrous skin. A videomicroscopic analysis. Arch Dermatol. 1998;134:563–8.
30. Bastian BC, Kashani-Sabet M, Hamm H, et al. Gene amplifications characterize acral melanoma and permit the detection of occult tumor cells in the surrounding skin. Cancer Res. 2000;60:1968–73.
31. North JP, Kageshita T, Pinkel D, et al. Distribution and significance of occult intraepidermal tumor cells surrounding primary melanoma. J Invest Dermatol. 2008;128:2024–30.
32. Sauter ER, Yeo UC, von Stemm A, et al. Cyclin D1 is a candidate oncogene in cutaneous melanoma. Cancer Res. 2002;62:3200–6.
33. Da Forno PD, Fletcher A, Pringle JH, Saldanha GS. Understanding spitzoid tumours: new insights from molecular pathology. Br J Dermatol. 2008;158:4–14.
34. Bastian BC, LeBoit PE, Pinkel D. Mutations and copy number increase of HRAS in Spitz nevi with distinctive histopathological features. Am J Pathol. 2000;157:967–72.
35. Da Forno PD, Pringle JH, Fletcher A, et al. BRAF, NRAS and HRAS mutations in spitzoid tumours and their possible pathogenetic significance. Br J Dermatol. 2009;161:364–72.
36. Emley A, Yang S, Wajapeyee N, et al. Oncogenic BRAF and the tumor suppressor IGFBP7 in the genesis of atypical spitzoid nevomelanocytic proliferations. J Cutan Pathol. 2010;37:344–9.
37. Fullen DR, Poynter JN, Lowe L, et al. BRAF and NRAS mutations in spitzoid melanocytic lesions. Mod Pathol. 2006;19:1324–32.
38. Gill M, Cohen J, Renwick N, et al. Genetic similarities between Spitz nevus and Spitzoid melanoma in children. Cancer. 2004;101:2636–40.
39. Lee DA, Cohen JA, Twaddell WS, et al. Are all melanomas the same? Spitzoid melanoma is a distinct subtype of melanoma. Cancer. 2006;106:907–13.
40. Palmedo G, Hantschke M, Rutten A, et al. The T1796A mutation of the BRAF gene is absent in Spitz nevi. J Cutan Pathol. 2004;31:266–70.
41. Takata M, Lin J, Takayanagi S, et al. Genetic and epigenetic alterations in the differential diagnosis of malignant melanoma and spitzoid lesion. Br J Dermatol. 2007;156:1287–94.
42. van Dijk MC, Bernsen MR, Ruiter DJ. Analysis of mutations in B-RAF, N-RAS, and H-RAS genes in the differential diagnosis of Spitz nevus and spitzoid melanoma. Am J Surg Pathol. 2005;29:1145–51.
43. Kashani-Sabet M, Rangel J, Torabian S, et al. A multimarker assay to distinguish malignant melanomas from benign nevi. Proc Natl Acad Sci USA. 2009;106:6268–72.
44. Koh SS, Opel ML, Wei JP, et al. Molecular classification of melanomas and nevi using gene expression microarray signatures and formalin-fixed and paraffin-embedded tissue. Mod Pathol. 2009;22:538–46.
45. Talantov D, Mazumder A, Yu JX, et al. Novel genes associated with malignant melanoma but not benign melanocytic lesions. Clin Cancer Res. 2005;11:7234–42.
46. Alexandrescu DT, Kauffman CL, Jatkoe TA, et al. Melanoma-specific marker expression in skin biopsy tissues as a tool to facilitate melanoma diagnosis. J Invest Dermatol. 2010;130:1887–92.
47. Haqq C, Nosrati M, Sudilovsky D, et al. The gene expression signatures of melanoma progression. Proc Natl Acad Sci USA. 2005;102:6092–7.
48. Richards HW, Medrano EE. Epigenetic marks in melanoma. Pigment Cell Melanoma Res. 2009;22:14–29.
49. Nygren AO, Ameziane N, Duarte HM, et al. Methylation-specific MLPA (MS-MLPA): simultaneous detection of CpG methylation and copy number changes of up to 40 sequences. Nucleic Acids Res. 2005;33:e128.

mRNA Biomarkers in Melanoma

Giovanna Chiorino and Maria Scatolini

Introduction

Over the past decade, microarray-based high-throughput gene expression analysis has been employed in an effort to understand the molecular alterations involved in tumorigenesis and disease progression in melanoma. A gene expression array is a small glass-platform containing tens of thousands of sequences corresponding to specific mRNA transcripts. The most recent generation of microarray platforms are able to probe gene expression across the whole genome (Figs. 7.1 and 7.2). These are generally applied to either (1) distinct classes of samples (i.e., primary melanoma and melanoma metastasis) in order to identify genes with class-specific expression patterns or (2) apparently unrelated samples to discover previously unknown classes that are characterized by similar expression profiles. If clinical follow-up is available, gene expression signatures may provide new prognostic markers.

To date, molecular profiling studies of melanoma samples have resulted in interesting, although sometimes inconsistent data. The lack of concordance between studies may be due to different parameters employed with regard to sample selection and experimental design. Many studies have used a small number of samples and arrays with different probe types/densities, making validation across different cohorts difficult. Furthermore, most investigations of transcriptional changes that occur during melanoma progression have been carried out on melanoma cell lines. Cell cultures derived from melanocytes have several limitations. For example, cultured cells are grown outside their natural environment, which may be crucial for maintaining a specific gene expression pattern. Moreover, studies conducted on tissue (and biological fluid) samples are necessary to study the interplay between the tumor and host inflammatory response, in addition to the identification of prognostic markers and therapeutic targets. However, gene expression profiling data derived from primary and/or metastatic melanocytic lesions are scarce. A lack of large collections of banked frozen tumor samples is a contributing factor [1, 2]. However, two recent studies have analyzed the gene expression profiles of large cohorts of formalin-fixed paraffin-embedded (FFPE) tumors [3, 4]. The first study compared the transcriptomes of melanocytic nevi and melanomas, using the Combimatrix 12000 feature CustomArray platform, while the second study used the Illumina DASL Array Human Cancer Panel (502 genes) to investigate the association between gene expression profiles of primary melanoma and patient outcome.

Microarrays can be used to test hundreds-to-thousand of genes in a single experiment and facilitate the performance of data-driven, rather

G. Chiorino, Ph.D. (✉) • M. Scatolini, Ph.D.
Cancer Genomics Laboratory, "Edo ed Elvo Tempia" Foundation, Biella, Italy
e-mail: giovanna.chiorino@fondoedotempia.it

Experimental workflow

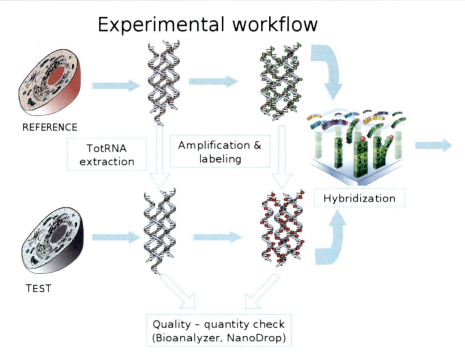

Fig. 7.1 Comparative hybridization involves total RNA isolation from test and reference tissues, mRNA amplification, and labeling with different fluorochromes. RNA quality and quantity are checked. During the hybridization step, labeled samples are applied to a microarray that contains thousands of probes specific for different transcripts

Analytical workflow

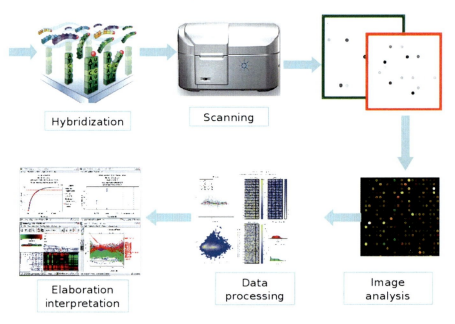

Fig. 7.2 After hybridization, the microarray is scanned and an image is generated for each sample. Results are combined, processed and normalized, and statistical analysis is applied for the selection of differentially expressed transcripts between test and reference samples. When results from many samples are available, class discovery, comparison or prediction tools may be applied to the matrix of differentially expressed genes

than hypothesis-driven, analyses. Moreover, many of the putative biomarkers detected by microarray-based experiments have been subsequently validated using other techniques, such as real-time quantitative polymerase chain reaction (qPCR) and immunohistochemistry [5, 6]. Although gene lists from different studies do not always show significant overlap, enrichment of specific biological processes is a common feature.

In this chapter, we will review the diagnostic and prognostic biomarkers and therapeutic targets in melanoma that have been determined by microarray-based gene expression profiling experiments.

Melanomagenesis

Only a few studies have investigated genes that are differentially expressed in benign and malignant lesions. Among the *in vitro* studies, Hoek et al. [7] compared the expression profiles of a number of melanoma and normal melanocyte cell lines. Genes and pathways modulated in melanoma were identified, including activation of the NOTCH signaling pathway and cancer testis antigens, in addition to downregulation of several genes implicated in immune response, membrane trafficking and growth suppression. In another study, Ryu and colleagues [8] compared melanoma cell lines with primary human melanocyte cultures and reported that normal melanocytes were more similar to aggressive melanomas than their less aggressive counterparts with respect to gene expression. The authors hypothesized that this similarity was due to their proliferative potential.

The first important *in vivo* investigation was conducted by Haqq et al [9]. In this study, the gene expression profiles of a series of normal skin samples, melanocytic nevi, primary melanomas and metastatic melanomas were compared. A number of transcripts useful in discriminating between these lesions were identified. In a follow-up study, Kashani-Sabet et al. [10] described an immunohistochemistry-based diagnostic assay for melanocytic tumors, using five markers [ARPC2, FN1, RGS1, WNT2, and SPP1 (osteopontin)] whose transcripts were found to be overexpressed in melanomas by prior gene expression profiling [9]. Both the intensity and pattern of expression of each marker were noted to be significantly different between melanomas and melanocytic nevi [10]. Based on comparison with the actual histopathological diagnoses, this commercially available multimarker assay is reported to show 95% specificity and 97% sensitivity for diagnosing melanomas arising in melanocytic nevi, 95% accuracy in identifying both Spitz nevi and dysplastic nevi, and 75% accuracy in correctly diagnosing previously misinterpreted melanocytic lesions [9, 10].

Talantov et al. [11] also performed gene expression profiling of normal skin samples, melanocytic nevi and primary melanomas. Similar to Ryu et al. [8], Talantov and colleagues [11] showed that, for a cluster of genes, the expression profiles of benign nevi and melanomas were very similar. In particular, conventional markers of melanocytic differentiation, such as tyrosinase (TYR) and MART-1, were equally overexpressed in both melanoma and nevus tissue specimens. However, Talantov et al. [11] did identify novel genes specifically overexpressed in melanoma. Importantly, the studies by Talantov et al. [11] and Haqq et al. [9] reported a set of common transcripts that could be employed to distinguish melanoma from benign nevi. These included kinesin-like 5 (KNSL5), prostate differentiation factor (PLAB), Cbp/p300-interacting transactivator 1 (CITED1), osteopontin (SPP1), cathepsin B (CSTB), cadherin 3 (CDH3), and presenilin 2 (PSEN2). Interestingly, two of these transcripts, CITED1 and CDH3, were also determined by these and other groups to be differentially expressed in the early stages of melanoma progression [5, 7–9, 11, 12]. Noteworthy is the fact that these two genes were identified in studies using both cell cultures and tissue biopsies. Talantov et al. [11] confirmed the utility of a two-gene (PLAB and L1CAM) reverse transcription (RT)-PCR assay to distinguish between benign and malignant melanocytes in skin and lymph node samples. Importantly, these two markers showed superior performance compared with those commonly employed to determine melanocytic differentiation, such as TYR, gp100/HMB-45, and MART-1 [11].

Koh et al. [3] successfully used archival FFPE tissues for microarray analysis, and also identified genes that were differentially expressed in melanomas and melanocytic nevi. However, in contrast to the study by Talantov et al. [11], expression of L1CAM was found to be decreased in melanomas [3].

Recently, Scatolini et al. [6] performed whole genome expression profiling on a wide variety of melanocytic tumors, including common melanocytic nevi (CMN), dysplastic nevi (DN), radial growth phase (RGP) melanoma, vertical growth phase (VGP) melanoma and metastatic tumors. For each progression step, they found genes that had been previously described in association with (melanoma) tumorigenesis, in addition to novel transcripts. A small number of differentially expressed genes were found between CMN and RGF melanoma; these were largely involved in the deregulation of intra/intercellular adhesion. Among them, three transcripts were common to previous studies: Hairy/enhancer-of-split related with YRPW motif 1 (HEY1) [5, 7, 11, 12], homo sapiens growth differentiation factor 15 (GDF15) [11, 12], and homo sapiens glycoprotein M6A, transcript variant 1, GPM6A [7].

A patented combined noninvasive/tape-stripping and gene-based assay (MelDTect™) is also available for the detection of melanoma [13]. RNA is harvested from the surface layer of the skin, without the need for biopsy, and analyzed using a 19-gene classifier. This test is purported to demonstrate a sensitivity of 100% and a specificity of 88% in discriminating melanomas from melanocytic nevi (Sherman Chang, Ph.D., personal communication, 2010) [13].

Dysplastic Nevi and Melanoma Progression

Direct comparison of CMN and DN samples has revealed a small number of differentially expressed genes associated with cellular adhesion and neurogenesis (n=24) [6]. A potent neurite outgrowth inhibitor (RTN4) was found to be expressed at lower levels in DN compared with CMN. In contrast, CD44 was found to be differentially upregulated in DN. CD44 is a cell-surface glycoprotein involved in cell-cell interactions, cell adhesion, migration and possibly metastasis (in the setting of malignant tumors). Comparing DN with RGP melanoma, a large number of deregulated transcripts were found (n=100); most of which are involved in transcriptional regulation (i.e., EP300, BHLHB2, FBXO18, CNBP, and POLR2B) [6]. However, multiclass comparison identified a group of genes expressed by both DN and VGP melanoma at higher levels than in CMN, but downregulated in RGP melanoma. These included a set of mismatch repair system transcripts (PMS2, PMS2L2, PMS2L3, and PMS2L5). DN show variable risk to develop into melanoma, as evidenced by the heterogeneity of their global transcriptional changes [6]. To date, DN have been categorized according to morphological criteria, without any molecular characterization. In the study by Scatolini et al. [6], the expression pattern of a group of genes enriched in cellular detoxification, RNA processing and antigen presentation separated DN into two subclasses: (1) one similar to RGP melanoma, with expression levels higher than in CMN and (2) one similar to VGP melanoma, with expression levels lower than in CMN [6].

From RGP Melanoma to VGP Melanoma: The Big Step

Numerous studies suggest that the transition from RGP melanoma to VGP melanoma in primary lesions is the most critical step in melanoma progression.

Haqq et al. [9] were the first group to apply high-throughput gene expression analysis to the RGF and VGF components of a single melanoma lesion. They found that a number of genes were downregulated in VGP. Reduced expression of corresponding proteins for two transcripts (MMP10 and CDH3) was subsequently validated by immunohistochemistry in a cohort of VGP melanoma samples [9].

Using whole genome expression profiling of tissue specimens representing normal skin, benign and atypical nevi, and early- and advanced-stage melanoma, Smith et al. [5] determined that significant molecular changes occur with the transition from RGP to VGP disease. The principal enriched biological processes included mitotic cell cycle, cell proliferation, and immune response. Moreover, Smith et al. [5] selected the top 50 genes that were either upregulated or downregulated in the advanced-stage melanomas. Upregulated genes with the greatest fold-change included osteopontin 1 (SPP1) and Cbp/p300-interacting transactivator 1 (CITED1). Dermicidin (DCD) was found to be the most downregulated gene [5]. From the results of their *in vitro* study, Ryu et al. [8] identified two distinct groups of melanoma cell lines ("less aggressive" and "more aggressive"), based on differences in their gene expression patterns. The less aggressive group comprised RGP melanoma and some VGP melanoma cell lines. The more aggressive group was characterized by some VGP melanoma and all the metastatic melanoma cell lines. Genes with altered expression in the latter group were involved in cell cycle control, cell proliferation, DNA repair and replication (i.e., CDCA2, NCAPH, NCAPG, NCAPG2, PBK, NUSAP1, BIRC5, ESCO2, HELLS, MELK, GINS1, GINS4, RAD54L, TYMS, and DHFR), and negative regulation of apoptosis (BIRC5/survivin). The less aggressive group of melanomas expressed higher levels of genes associated with cellular adhesion and melanocytic differentiation (i.e., CDH3, CDH1, c-KIT, PAX3, CITED1/MSG-1, TYR, MELANA, MC1R, and OCA2).

Scatolini et al. [6] also analyzed transcriptional changes associated with the transition from RGP to VGP melanoma, identifying 540 differentially expressed genes. Results indicated that this process is characterized by a general decrease in the ability of melanoma cells to undergo apoptosis, supported by altered regulation of DAPL1, TP63, SMAD3, and TNFRSF25. Another important feature was synergy between the Wnt and mitogen-activated protein kinase (MAPK) pathways in both melanoma growth phases, which may represent an important mechanism underpinning the pathogenesis and progression of this tumor [6]. In addition, five of the modulated transcripts identified (AP1S2, PLP1, BCL2A1, KRT77, and STARD3NL) were previously reported by Smith et al. [5] to be differentially expressed between nevi/melanoma in situ and advanced-stage melanomas. However, unlike the study by Smith et al. [5], Scatolini and colleagues [6] did not find mitotic cell cycle regulation and cell proliferation to be the predominant overrepresented biological processes. This may be due to the fact that Smith et al. [5] did not separate common nevi, atypical lesions and in situ melanomas into unique classes.

From Primary Melanoma to Metastatic Disease

In order to identify a metastatic phenotype for melanoma, Bittner et al. [14] used cDNA microarrays to analyze the gene expression profiles of biopsies and cell cultures of primary tumors. They identified the downregulation of genes involved in cell spreading, migration and focal adhesion (integrin-beta 1, integrin-beta 3, integrin-alpha 1, sindecan 4, and vinculin), that may be associated with less aggressive tumor behavior.

To investigate the invasive capacity of melanoma, Roesch et al. [15] combined laser capture microdissection with cDNA microarray technology and compared the gene expression profiles of the invasive margin and tumor core in nine cases of VGP melanoma. Genes encoding PEPCK, TEB4, the ribosomal protein L19, the interleukin-3 receptor alpha subunit, the inositol 1,4,5-triphosphate 3-kinase isoenzyme, and three anonymous expressed sequence tags (ESTs) were capable of separating the two classes of melanoma tissue.

Haqq et al. [9] reported that melanoma metastases could be divided in two distinct groups. Moreover, a correlation between the RGP melanoma signature and one of the metastatic classes was identified, suggesting that a small, but clinically significant proportion of metastases may arise from this growth phase of primary melanoma.

Hoek et al. [16] carried out three separate DNA microarray analyses on a total of 86 melanoma cultures. The authors identified three different sample cohorts representing melanoma groups with different metastatic potential. A model for the transition from weakly to strongly metastatic melanoma was proposed, in which TGF-beta signaling upregulates genes for vasculogenic/extracellular matrix remodeling factors and Wnt signal inhibitors. Interestingly, the expression pattern of one of the Hoek subgroups [16] strongly correlated with the weakly metastatic signature identified by Bittner et al. [14].

A study by Jaeger et al. [17] analyzed the gene expression signature of microdissected melanoma cells, derived from primary melanoma and melanoma metastasis. More than 300 genes were identified to be differentially expressed between both groups, with the overrepresented gene ontology categories including cell cycle regulation, mitosis, cell communication, and cell adhesion.

Riker et al. [12] compared the transcriptomic profiles of primary melanomas and melanoma metastases (lymph node, subcutaneous and distant metastases). Metastatic tumors expressed higher levels of MAGE, GPR19, BCL2A1, MMP14, SOX5, BUB1, and RGS20, but showed relative underexpression of SPRR1A/B, KRT16/17, CD24, LOR, GATA3, MUC15, and TMPRSS4. The transition from non-metastatic expression levels to metastatic expression levels occurred as primary melanomas increased in thickness. Riker et al. [12] identified several putative genes associated with tumor progression and metastasis, including SPP1, MITF, CITED1, GDF-15, c-Met, and several of the HOX loci, some of which were reported by other studies [7, 11]. A number of genes believed to be important for suppression of tumor growth (PITX-1, CST-6, PDGFRL, DSC-3, POU2F3, and CLCA2) were also identified [12]. Only two genes (LGALS7 and SFN), both of which were underexpressed in the metastasis signature, were common to the studies by Riker et al. [12] and Jaeger et al. [17].

In a study comparing metastatic melanoma cell lines, Jeffs et al. [18] identified an invasion signature that was characterized by decreased expression of developmental and lineage specification genes (MITF, EDNRB, DCT, and TYR) and increased expression of genes involved in extracellular environment interaction (PLAUR, VCAN, and HIF1a). Interestingly, a 24-gene overlap between the 96-gene signature of Jeffs et al. [18] and that reported by Hoek et al. [16] was found. Overlapping genes were involved in melanin biosynthesis, pigmentation, development and lineage specification, and included MITF. Moreover, the 96-gene signature was capable of classifying normal skin, benign nevi and primary melanomas in the Talantov et al. [11] dataset. Similar to the Riker et al. [12] and Haqq et al. [9] data, melanocytic nevi with molecular profiles similar to malignant tumors were identified [18].

Scatolini et al. [6] determined genes that were differentially expressed between VGP melanoma and metastatic tumors. Although only a small cohort of metastasis from different sites were analyzed (n=5), their expression profiles were rather homogeneous and showed high concordance with the results of studies by Jaeger et al. [17] and Riker et al. [12]. In metastatic melanoma, there is alteration of pathways involved in cell cycle and DNA repair. As shown in Table 7.1, most of the modulated transcripts are underexpressed in metastatic tumors and can be classified into a small number of families: laminins, collagens, kallikreins, keratins, cadherins, desmocollins, etc.

More recently, Eichhoff et al. [19] have suggested that melanoma cells are capable of cycling between proliferative and invasive phases (phenotype-switching model). Based on their microarray data, they analyzed protein expression in a matched primary/metastasis pair from a melanoma patient [19]. The expression of the proliferative phenotype markers Melan-A and Mitf inversely correlated with the expression of both the invasive phenotype marker Wnt5A and the hypoxia marker Glut-1. Protein expression patterns were similar in the primary and metastasis samples. Eichhoff et al. [19] hypothesized that disease progression involves melanoma cells retaining the capacity to regulate the expression of metastasis-promoting factors according to changing microenvironmental conditions.

Table 7.1 Families of transcripts underexpressed in the transition from primary to metastatic melanoma

Gene Family	Gene symbol	Gene Family	Gene symbol
Laminins	LAMC2[a]	Cadherins	CDH1[a]
	LAMA3[a]		CDH13
	LAMB3[a]		CELSR1
Collagens	COL13A1	Cystatins	CSTA[a]
	COL17A1[a]		CST6[a,b]
	COL4A6[a]		CSTB
Kallikreins	KLK5	Serpins	SERPINEB3[a,b]
	KLK7[a]		SERPINE2B
	KLK8[a,b]		SERPINEB5[a,b]
	KLK10[a,b]		SERPINEB13
	KLK11[a,b]		SERPINEB7[b]
Keratins	KRT6B[a]	Calcium-binding proteins	S100A8[a]
	KRT10[a]		S100A14[a,b]
	KRT14[a]		S100A7[a,b]
	KRT23[a]		S100A9[a]
	KRT80		S100A10
	KRT17[a,b]		S100P[a]
	KRT33A		S100A2[a]
	KRT6A[a]	Small proline-rich proteins	SPRR1B[a]
	KRT5[a,b]		SPRR1A[a]
	KRT2A		SPRR2D
	KRT16[a,b]		SPRR2E
	KRT15[a]	Desmocollins	DSC3[a,b]
	KRT6E		DSC1[a,b]

Adapted from Scatolini et al. [6]
[a]Indicate results in agreement with Jaeger et al. [17]
[b]Indicate results in agreement with Riker et al. [12]

Gene Expression Profiling and Outcome

DNA microarray technology has also been used to identify supplemental prognostic indicators to the Breslow thickness, as well as biomarkers of patient survival and treatment response. The most extensive study of this type was conducted on behalf of the Melanoma Group of the European Organization for the Research and Treatment of Cancer (EORTC) [20]. Winnepennickx et al. [20] collected 83 primary melanomas from 58 patients, and used an oligonucleotide-based microarray to identify 254 genes that were associated with distant metastasis-free survival. Twenty-three of these genes were studied at the protein level by immunohistochemistry, with the expression of five markers (MCM4, MCM3, MCM6, KPNA2, and geminin) found to be statistically associated with overall survival [20]. In multivariate regression analysis adjusted for tumor thickness, ulceration, age and gender, the expression of MCM4 and MCM6 were still significantly associated with overall survival in these patients [20].

A follow-up investigation by Kauffmann et al. [21] on 60 fresh/frozen primary melanomas (with and without metastases) determined that differential expression of 48 genes (predominantly overexpression of DNA repair genes) was associated with metastatic progression and poor prognosis.

Gene expression profiling studies by Conway et al. [4] and Jewell et al. [22], on FFPE primary melanomas, confirmed that upregulation of SPP1 (osteopontin) and DNA repair genes (predominantly those involved in double-strand break repair, RAD51, RAD52, and TOP2A) were associated with poor prognostic histopathological features and predicted reduced relapse-free survival. These data support the hypothesis that maintenance of genomic stability (via intact DNA repair pathways) is required for melanoma progression, and influences response to chemotherapeutic agents and radiotherapy [21, 22]. Interestingly, the prognostic role of SPP1 had been previously reported by other microarray studies on frozen tissue samples [17, 23] and immunohistochemical assays for SPP1 protein expression [24]. Of note, Conway et al. [4] applied the Illumina DASL assay to RNA extracted from FFPE tissue. With the most recent version of this technology, large cohorts of archival samples can now be analyzed on a whole genome scale (~24,000 genes).

Based on their prior cDNA microarray studies [9], Kashani-Sabet et al. [25] described a three-marker (NCOA3, SPP1, and RGS1) immunohistochemistry-based assay with independent prognostic significance vis-à-vis sentinel lymph node status and disease-specific survival in patients with primary melanoma.

In another study, Mandruzzato et al. [26] correlated gene expression to survival in a cohort of 38 melanoma patients with metastatic disease (stages III and IV). A 30-probe-set survival prediction model was generated. Transcripts overexpressed in patients with longer survival included those associated with innate and acquired immunity (i.e., IL-4R, TNFAIP3, and CD2), confirming the interplay between immunological mechanisms and the biological behavior of melanoma. In contrast, the poor-survival group was characterized by the expression of genes related to cellular proliferation and tissue invasion (i.e., GJB2, CSPG4, and MCM3) [26].

Investigations by John et al. [27], Bogunovic et al. [28], and Jönsson et al. [29] have also determined that transcriptomic profiles are capable of distinguishing clinical outcomes in patients with metastatic melanoma. These studies included both treated (i.e., radiotherapy, immunotherapy, and/or chemotherapy) and untreated patients with metastatic disease [27–29]. John et al. [27] developed a 21-gene prognostic predictor and identified a list of differentially expressed transcripts between good and poor prognosis classes of patients, including molecules involved in Wnt signaling, nuclear factor kappa B and apoptosis pathways, and immune response. The study by Bogunovic et al. [28] underlined the prognostic role of immune response and cell proliferation-related genes, which are positively and negatively associated with survival, respectively. The authors reported that gene expression signatures, as well as quantification of tumor-infiltrating leukocytes, CD3+ cells and the mitotic index, improved upon the ability of TNM staging to predict post-recurrence survival in patients with melanoma [28]. Jönsson et al. [29] used global gene expression profiles to stratify stage IV melanoma patients who had received standard treatment with dacarbazine (DTIC). Using hierarchical clustering, they identified four distinct tumor subtypes characterized by gene signatures representing diverse biological mechanisms. These subtypes were named proliferative, high-immune response, pigmentation and normal-like, reflecting the pattern of genes representative for each subtype. Importantly, they observed a significant difference in clinical outcome between the four tumor classes, with the proliferative subtype having the worst prognosis. Results suggested a predictive role of the pigmentation subtype with respect to DTIC treatment. The authors also investigated the prognostic impact of *a priori*-defined genes related to immune response signaling, using their own and other publicly available melanoma datasets. Significantly poor overall survival was observed in tumors with low expression of immune response genes. Moreover, their findings suggested that expression of T-cell-related genes should be explored as a potential predictive factor for response to immunotherapy in melanomas.

In an interesting study designed to evaluate survival, antiapoptotic, antioxidant and proapoptotic genes and their signaling pathways in melanoma cells, Su et al. [30] developed a third-generation human mitochondria-focused cDNA microarray and profiled 21 melanoma cell lines and three normal melanocyte controls. Two distinct types of melanoma cells were identified, each with a specific set of deregulated survival-apoptosis genes. The presence of two different survival pathways in melanoma indicates that drugs targeting both pathways need to be designed and developed. Above all, these results highlight the necessity to "genetically pre-select" appropriate patient populations before clinical trials with proapoptotic agents, such as oblimersen, are undertaken.

Finally, Augustine et al. [31] reported that gene expression signatures can be used to predict response to chemotherapy in patients with in-transit metastatic melanoma.

Conclusion

The studies described in this chapter report several potential diagnostic and prognostic markers for melanoma, as well as gene expression signatures associated with different clinical and histopathological classes of melanocytic tumors. A number of genes, such as CDH3 and SPP1, have been identified in more than one study and validated in large cohorts both at the mRNA and protein level. For an in-depth comparative analysis of human melanoma gene expression, we suggest an interesting review on the impact of genomics in our understanding of melanoma progression and metastasis [32]. With regard to gene expression signatures, many studies show little or no overlap in identified transcripts. However, most studies are in agreement concerning which biological processes are (1) altered during melanoma progression and (2) present among different prognostic classes of patients. In addition, histopathological parameters are not sufficient to definitively classify melanocytic lesions in some instances. Molecular testing could be used to identify subgroups of tumors characterized by similar biological process alterations and behavior, supplementing microscopic analysis. A clear example is the molecular characterization of dysplastic nevi, which is not in line with their current histopathological classification. Furthermore, the molecular analysis of metastatic lesions could be tailored to select biological processes, such as apoptosis, immune system response, DNA repair, pigmentation and cell proliferation, since their alteration has been associated with differential clinical outcome. Results of microarray-based studies indicate that metastatic melanoma is biologically diverse, and reiterate the importance of tailoring clinical trials to the molecular and cellular profiles of tumors in individual patients. In the near future, the availability of novel profiling methodologies applicable to large cohorts of archival FFPE tissue will facilitate the identification of robust biomarkers that are translatable to clinical practice.

References

1. Hoek KS. DNA microarray analyses of melanoma gene expression: a decade in the mines. Pigment Cell Res. 2007;20:466–84.
2. Hoek KS. Melanoma progression, gene expression and DNA microarrays. G Ital Dermatol Venereol. 2009;144:39–49.
3. Koh SS, Opel ML, Wei JP, et al. Molecular classification of melanomas and nevi using gene expression microarray signatures and formalin-fixed and paraffin-embedded tissue. Mod Pathol. 2009;22: 538–46.
4. Conway C, Mitra A, Jewell R, et al. Gene expression profiling of paraffin-embedded primary melanoma using the DASL assay identifies increased osteopontin expression as predictive of reduced relapse-free survival. Clin Cancer Res. 2009;15: 6939–46.
5. Smith AP, Hoek K, Becker D. Whole-genome expression profiling of the melanoma progression pathway reveals marked molecular differences between nevi/melanoma in situ and advanced-stage melanomas. Cancer Biol Ther. 2005;4:1018–29.
6. Scatolini M, Mello-Grand M, Grosso E, et al. Altered molecular pathways in melanocytic lesions. Int J Cancer. 2010;126:1869–81.
7. Hoek KS, Rimm DL, Williams KR, et al. Expression profiling reveals novel pathways in the transformation of melanocytes to melanomas. Cancer Res. 2004;64: 5270–82.
8. Ryu B, Kim DS, Deluca AM, et al. Comprehensive expression profiling of tumor cell lines identifies molecular signatures of melanoma progression. PLoS One. 2007;2:e594.
9. Haqq C, Nosrati M, Sudilovsky D, et al. The gene expression signatures of melanoma progression. Proc Natl Acad Sci USA. 2005;102:6092–7.
10. Kashani-Sabet M, Rangel J, Torabian S, et al. A multimarker assay to distinguish malignant melanomas from benign nevi. Proc Natl Acad Sci USA. 2009;106: 6268–72.
11. Talantov D, Mazumder A, Yu JX, et al. Novel genes associated with malignant melanoma but not benign melanocytic lesions. Clin Cancer Res. 2005;11: 7234–42.
12. Riker AI, Enkemann SA, Fodstad O, et al. The gene expression profiles of primary and metastatic melanoma yields a transition point of tumor progression and metastasis. BMC Med Genomics. 2008;1:13.
13. DermTech International. Available at http://dermtech.com/technology/melanoma-detection/index.php. Accessed 2 Sept 2010.
14. Bittner M, Meltzer P, Chen Y, et al. Molecular classification of cutaneous malignant melanoma by gene expression profiling. Nature. 2000;406:536–40.

15. Roesch A, Vogt T, Stolz W, et al. Discrimination between gene expression patterns in the invasive margin and the tumour core of malignant melanomas. Melanoma Res. 2003;13:503–9.
16. Hoek KS, Schlegel NC, Brafford P, et al. Metastatic potential of melanomas defined by specific gene expression profiles with no BRAF signature. Pigment Cell Res. 2006;19:290–302.
17. Jaeger J, Koczan D, Thiesen HJ, et al. Gene expression signatures for tumor progression, tumor subtype, and tumor thickness in laser-microdissected melanoma tissues. Clin Cancer Res. 2007;13:806–15.
18. Jeffs AR, Glover AC, Slobbe LJ, et al. A gene expression signature of invasive potential in metastatic melanoma cells. PLoS One. 2009;4:e8461.
19. Eichhoff OM, Zipser MC, Xu M, et al. The immunohistochemistry of invasive and proliferative phenotype switching in melanoma: a case report. Melanoma Res. 2010;20:349–55.
20. Winnepenninckx V, Lazar V, Michiels S, et al. Gene expression profiling of primary cutaneous melanoma and clinical outcome. J Natl Cancer Inst. 2006;98:472–82.
21. Kauffmann A, Rosselli F, Lazar V, et al. High expression of DNA repair pathways is associated with metastasis in melanoma patients. Oncogene. 2008;27:565–73.
22. Jewell R, Conway C, Mitra A, et al. Patterns of expression of DNA repair genes and relapse from melanoma. Clin Cancer Res. 2010;16:5211–21.
23. Zhou Y, Dai DL, Martinka M, et al. Osteopontin expression correlates with melanoma invasion. J Invest Dermatol. 2005;124:1044–52.
24. Rangel J, Nosrati M, Torabian S, et al. Osteopontin as a molecular prognostic biomarker for melanoma. Cancer. 2008;112:144–50.
25. Kashani-Sabet M, Venna S, Nosrati M, et al. A multimarker prognostic assay for primary cutaneous melanoma. Clin Cancer Res. 2009;15:6987–92.
26. Mandruzzato S, Callegaro A, Turcatel G, et al. A gene expression signature associated with survival in metastatic melanoma. J Transl Med. 2006;4:50.
27. John T, Black MA, Toro TT, et al. Predicting clinical outcome through molecular profiling in stage III melanoma. Clin Cancer Res. 2008;14:5173–80.
28. Bogunovic D, O'Neill DW, Belitskaya-Levy I, et al. Immune profile and mitotic index of metastatic melanoma lesions enhance clinical staging in predicting patient survival. Proc Natl Acad Sci USA. 2009;106:20429–34.
29. Jönsson G, Busch C, Knappskog S, et al. Gene expression profiling-based identification of molecular subtypes in stage IV melanomas with different clinical outcome. Clin Cancer Res. 2010;16:3356–67.
30. Su DM, Zhang Q, Wang X, et al. Two types of human malignant melanoma cell lines revealed by expression patterns of mitochondrial and survival-apoptosis genes: implications for malignant melanoma therapy. Mol Cancer Ther. 2009;8:1292–304.
31. Augustine CK, Jung SH, Sohn I, et al. Gene expression signatures as a guide to treatment strategies for in-transit metastatic melanoma. Mol Cancer Ther. 2010;9:779–90.
32. Ren S, Liu S, Howell Jr P, et al. The impact of genomics in understanding human melanoma progression and metastasis. Cancer Control. 2008;15:202–15.

Epigenetic Biomarkers in Melanoma

Suhu Liu, Suping Ren, Paul M. Howell Jr., and Adam I. Riker

Epigenetics, defined in its most basic sense as a stable heritable change in gene function that is not a result of changes in the actual DNA sequence, has been one of the fastest growing fields of cancer research over the past decade. DNA promoter methylation is known to directly inhibit gene expression and is a common occurrence during tumor formation and progression. This action may lead to the formation of a heterochromatic environment at the promoter or other sites by histone deacetylases to further suppress target genes. MicroRNAs are short, ~22 nucleotides in length, fragments of single-stranded RNA that bind the 3′-untranslated region (3′-UTR) of complementary mRNA sequences, inhibiting their translation and signaling them for destruction, in many cases. These processes are highly interactive and, when their expression, activity or safe-guards are deregulated, they serve to propagate aberrant gene expression toward uncontrolled cellular proliferation, evasion of apoptosis, and an increased invasive potential. Development of therapies targeting the actions of some important epigenetic modulators have proven somewhat successful and with good tolerance in the clinic for patients with melanoma and other cancers. Currently, the only epigenetic drugs approved by the FDA for the treatment of cancer are Vidaza® (azacytidine) and Dacogen® (decitabine), two DNA hypomethylating agents, and Zolinza® (vorinostat), a histone deacetylase inhibitor; although, these are only approved for blood-based malignancies, as these tumors have been the most responsive to date. To this point, the effective treatment of solid tumors, including melanoma, has proven more difficult. Despite different drug targets, an up-regulation of silenced tumor suppressor genes is a common effect. Given the vast potential of epigenetic-based therapies for cancer, it is important to establish a panel of epigenetic biomarkers in order to better tailor treatment and uncover epigenetic modes which regulate normal and tumor cell processes.

S. Liu, M.D., Ph.D.
Harvard University, Dana-Farber Cancer Institute, Boston, MA, USA

S. Ren, M.D., Ph.D. • P.M. Howell Jr., B.S.
Mitchell Cancer Institute, University of South Alabama, Mobile, AL, USA

A.I. Riker, M.D. (✉)
Department of Surgery, Ochsner Medical Center, Ochsner Cancer Institute, Ochsner Health System, New Orleans, LA, USA
e-mail: ariker1234@gmail.com

Introduction

The transformation and malignant progression of human cells is a complex process, involving the initiation of uncontrolled proliferation, unlimited replicative potential, resistance to apoptosis, invasion of tissue and tumor cell angiogenesis, with final implantation and subsequent growth within secondary sites. Over the last decade, cancer researchers worldwide have found that epigenetic processes appear to be intimately involved at each of these steps along the metastatic process, thereby allowing for the discovery of numerous potential therapeutic targets and tumor markers in a multitude of cancers. Epigenetics can be simply defined as stable heritable changes in gene function that are not a result of changes in the actual DNA sequence.

Heritable epigenetically silenced regions of DNA are generally characterized by specific identifying markers, such as the methylation of DNA itself, or methylation and loss of acetylation associated with the histones that regulate DNA transcription. This results in a heterochromatic-like cellular environment that may involve either one or several genes. Hypermethylated gene promoter regions comprised of CpG dinucleotides with global hypomethylation, di- or trimethylation of histone 3 lysine 9 (H3K9me2 or H3K9me3), H3K27me3, and loss of both H4K16 acetylation and trimethylation of H4K20 are all hallmarks of cancer [1–4]. DNA methyltransferases (DNMTs) and methyl-CpG-binding domain (MBD) proteins maintain silencing of DNA regions via covalent modification of CpG dinucleotide cytosines. In a similar fashion, histone deacetylases (HDACs) maintain silencing of a region of chromatin by removing transcriptionally-activating acetyl groups from histones marked by histone acetyltransferases (HATs). Histone methyltransferases (HMTs) and the heterochromatin protein 1 (HP1) gene act to further silence chromatin and counter the actions of histone demethylases (HDMs). Most recently, microRNAs (miRNAs) have been described for their capacity to regulate the cellular landscape by binding target mRNAs (up to hundreds per single miRNA) and preventing their translation.

Deregulation of epigenetic states has been implicated in the formation and progression of multiple cancers, including melanoma. DNMTs and HDACs are commonly over-expressed in cancer and have the capacity to down-regulate the expression of several known tumor suppressor genes (TSGs). As such, drugs targeting these enzymes have an inherent tumor-specificity, with inhibitors of the transcriptionally-repressive HDAC and DNMT complexes currently being studied for their therapeutic effects [5]. Both have produced a wealth of basic and translational knowledge as well as data lending to their efficacies, low side-effect profile and tolerability, and specificity for various tumor types. The complexity in the sheer number and interaction of proteins and small RNAs involved in epigenetic regulation has spurred great interest for identifying therapeutic targets and effective diagnostic and prognostic tumor biomarkers.

Notable melanoma diagnostic biomarkers have included S-100, MART-1, gp100, and Ki-67, which, when utilized as a combined panel of markers, are sufficient for distinguishing melanoma from non-melanocytic tumors. Ki-67 is currently the most efficient marker at separating benign from malignant melanocytic lesions [6]. Some of the most common and effective prognostic indicators are S100β, MIA (melanoma inhibitory activity) and LDH (lactate dehydrogenase). S100β and MIA are markers routinely used in Europe for early detection of melanoma tumor relapse or metastasis during patient follow-up. The American Joint Committee on Cancer (AJCC) notes serum LDH levels as a significant predictor of survival in stage IV metastatic melanoma, incorporating LDH levels into the most recent version of the AJCC staging system [7]. LDH, a non-specific marker that indicates high tumor load, is the strongest independent prognostic factor in stage IV metastatic melanoma [6].

Serological screening is an important method for biomarker identification in cancer patients. Circulating DNA, miRNA and histones in peripheral blood allow for a minimally invasive means of identification and measurement of epigenetic markers. Serum mass spectrometry-based proteomic profiling and immunological assays can also provide valuable methods for both diagnostic and prognostic determinations of disease. For example, stage I primary melanoma and stage IV metastatic melanoma can be effectively differentiated by examining their respective serum proteomic profiles [8], with serum amyloid A (SAA) found to be a significant individual discriminator [9]. Employing immunoassays, Findeisen et al. [9] further described the superior capacity of combined SAA and C-reactive protein (CRP) over S100β analysis for predicting progression-free and overall survival in a cohort of 399 stage I-III melanoma patients. Qiu and Wang [10] presented a method for plasma membrane protein detection utilizing stable isotope labeling by amino acids in cell culture (SILAC), liquid chromatography-mass spectrometry, and cell surface biotinylation and affinity peptide purification with patient-paired primary and metastatic melanoma cell lines. Use of biotinylation and peptide purification in turn resulted in reduced cytoplasmic and non-membrane protein contamination.

It is important to bear in mind a few points when seeking to characterize the utility of a biomarker: (1) redundancy: does the marker display unique qualities in normal and tumor cells, capable of differentiating between the two, or is it capable of differentiating between tumor type or stage?; (2) reliability: how strongly or often does the marker correlate with diagnostic, prognostic, or chemoresistance measurements?; (3) specificity: how specific is the marker for its indication(s) class(es); (4) therapeutic potential: how may the presence or therapeutic manipulation of this marker benefit the ultimate goal of developing personalized treatment strategies?; are therapies targeting the marker or its pathologic indication available or reasonably possible?; and is the drug specificity such that inhibition or activation of the target likely to result in too many unknown/non-specific cellular events?; and (5) detection: is there a reliable and reasonable procedure available for detection of the marker and all pertinent data regarding its indication(s) in the patient? We thus seek to effectively examine the current field of epigenetic biomarkers in melanoma.

DNA Methylation

DNA methylation refers to the methylation of C-5 of cytosines, which occur as part of a CpG dinucleotide; the only clearly identified epigenetic modification of DNA in mammalian cells [11]. The mammalian DNA methylation machinery is made up of two components: DNMTs, which establish and maintain genome-wide DNA methylation patterns, and the MBD proteins, which are involved in 'reading' and interpreting the methylation patterns. Properly established and maintained DNA methylation patterns are essential for mammalian development and normal functioning in humans, with changes in DNA methylation patterns being important characteristics of most human cancers. In general, cancer cells have reduced levels of genomic DNA methylation and contain aberrantly hypermethylated CpG islands, both of which contribute to malignant transformation and progression. The full extent and sequence context of DNA hypermethylation and hypomethylation is still relatively unknown.

Aberrant DNA Hypermethylation

The molecular and cellular processes associated with promoter region CpG hypermethylation act as an alternate and/or complementary mechanism to gene deletion or mutation, resulting in the inactivation of specific gene expression and function. DNA hypermethylation contributes to gene silencing by preventing the binding of activating transcription factors and by attracting repressor complexes that induce the formation of inactive chromatin structures. Numerous TSGs and miRNAs have been shown to be regulated by DNA hypermethylation in different types of cancer. To date, more than 50 protein-encoding genes have been identified to be aberrantly hypermethylated during some phase of melanoma progression and metastasis (Table 8.1) [12]. However, there are only two miRNAs, miR-34a [13] and miR-9 [14], shown to be methylated in melanoma. Although the exact function of most of these aberrantly silenced genes and miRNAs is still unknown, most data would support the notion that they possess a wide range of alternative gene functions, such as cell cycle control, apoptosis, cell signaling, tumor cell invasion and metastasis, angiogenesis, and immune recognition [15].

The 14-3-3σ gene, also known as stratifin, was first identified as an epithelial cell antigen (HME-1), exclusively expressed in human epithelia. It has been implicated in p53-mediated

Table 8.1 Genes with an altered DNA methylation status in melanoma (modified from Sigalotti et al. [196])

Pathway	Gene	Methylation status in melanoma[a]	%
Apoptosis	DAPKβ	Methylated	19
	HSPB6	Methylated	100
	HSPB8	Methylated	69
	RASSF1A	Methylated	19–69
	TMS1	Methylated	8–50
	TNFRSF10C	Methylated	57
	TNFRSF10D	Methylated	80
	TP53INP1	Methylated	19
	TRAILR1	Methylated	13–80
	XAF1	Methylated	–
Anchorage-independent growth	TPM1	Methylated	8
Cell cycle	CDKN1B	Methylated	0–9
	CDKN1C	Methylated	35
	CDKN2A	Methylated	10–76
	TSPY	Methylated	100
Cell fate determination	MIB2	Methylated	19
	APC	Methylated	15–17
	WIF1	Methylated	–
Chromatin remodeling	NPM2	Methylated	50
Degradation of misfolded proteins	DERL3	Methylated	23
Differentiation	ENC1	Methylated	6
	GDF15	Methylated	75
	HOXB13	Methylated	20
DNA repair	MGMT	Methylated	0–63
Drug metabolism	CYP1B1	Methylated	100
	DNAJC15	Methylated	50
Extracellular matrix	COL1A2	Methylated	63–80
	MFAP2	Methylated	30
Immune recognition	BAGE	Demethylated	83
	HLA class I	Methylated	–
	HMW-MAA	Methylated	–
	MAGE-A1, -A2, -A3, -A4	Demethylated	–
Inflammation	PTGS2	Methylated	20
Invasion/metastasis	CCR7	No CpG island	–
	CDH1	Methylated	88
	CDH8	Methylated	10
	CDH13	Methylated	44
	CXCR4	Methylated	–
	DPPIV	Methylated	80
	EPB41L3	Methylated	5
	SERPINB5	Methylated	13–100
	LOX	Methylated	45
	SYK	Methylated	3–30
	TFPI-2	Methylated	13–29
	THBD	Methylated	20–60
	TIMP3	Methylated	13
Proliferation	MT1G	Methylated	21
	WFDC1	Methylated	20–25

(continued)

Table 8.1 (continued)

Pathway	Gene	Methylation status in melanoma[a]	%
Signaling	DDIT4L	Methylated	29
	ERα	Methylated	17–51
	PGRβ	Methylated	56
	PRDX2	Methylated	8
	PTEN	Methylated	0–62
	3-OST-2	Methylated	15–56
	RARRES1	Methylated	13
	RARβ2	Methylated	13–70
	RIL	Methylated	88
	SOCS1	Methylated	75–76
	SOCS2	Methylated	44–75
	SOCS3	Methylated	60
	UNC5C	Methylated	23
Vesicle transport	Rab33A	Methylated	100
Transcription	HAND1	Methylated	15–63
	OLIG2	Methylated	63
	NKX2-3	Methylated	63
	PAX2	Methylated	38
	PAX7	Methylated	31
	RUNX3	Methylated	4–29
Unknown[b]	BST2	Methylated	50
	FAM78A	Methylated	8
	HS3ST2	Methylated	56
	LRRC2	Methylated	5
	LXN	Methylated	95
	PCSK1	Methylated	60
	PPP1R3C	Methylated	25
	PTPRG	Methylated	8
	QPCT	Methylated	100
	SLC27A3	Methylated	46

APAF-1 Apoptotic Protease Activating Factor 1, *APC* adenomatous polyposis coli, *BAGE* B melanoma antigen, *BST2* bone marrow stromal cell antigen 2, *CCR7* chemokine (C-C motif) receptor 7, *CDH1* cadherin 1, *CDH8* cadherin 8, *CDH13* cadherin 13, *CDKN1B* cyclin-dependent kinase inhibitor 1B, *CDKN1C* cyclin-dependent kinase inhibitor 1C, *CDKN2A* cyclin-dependent kinase inhibitor 2A, *COL1A2* alpha 2 type I collagen, *CXCR4* chemokine (C-X-C motif) receptor 4, *CYP1B1* cytochrome P450, family 1, subfamily B, polypeptide 1, *DAPK* death-associated protein kinase, *DDIT4L* DNA-damage-inducible transcript 4-like, *DERL3* Der1-like domain family, member 3, *DNAJC15* DnaJ homolog, subfamily C, member 15, *DPPIV* dipeptidyl peptidase IV, *ENC1* ectodermal-neural cortex-1, *EPB41L3* erythrocyte membrane protein band 4.1-like 3, *ERα* estrogen receptor alpha, *FAM78A* family with sequence similarity 78, member A, *GDF15* growth differentiation factor 15, *HAND1* heart and neural crest derivatives expressed 1, *HLA class I* human leukocyte class I antigen, *HMW-MAA* high molecular weight melanoma associated antigen, *HOXB13* homeobox B13, *HS3ST2* heparan sulfate (glucosamine) 3-O-sulfotransferase 2, *HSPB6* heat shock protein, alpha-crystallin-related, B6, *HSPB8* heat shock 22 kDa protein 8, *LRRC2* leucine rich repeat containing 2, *LOX* lysyl oxidase, *LXN* latexin, *MAGE* melanoma-associated antigen, *MFAP2* microfibrillar-associated protein 2, *MGMT* O-6-methylguanine-DNA methyltransferase, *MIB2* mindbomb homolog 2, *MT1G* metallothionein 1G, *NKX2-3* NK2 transcription factor related, locus 3, *NPM2* nucleophosmin/nucleoplasmin 2, *OLIG2* oligodendrocyte lineage transcription factor 2, *PAX2* paired box 2, *PAX7* paired box 7, *PCSK1* proprotein convertase subtilisin/kexin type 1, *PGRβ* progesterone receptor β, *PPP1R3C* protein phosphatase 1, regulatory (inhibitor) subunit 3C, *PRDX2* peroxiredoxin, *PTEN* phosphatase and tensin homologue, *PTGS2* prostaglandin-endoperoxide synthase 2, *PTPRG*, protein tyrosine phosphatase, receptor type, G, *QPCT* glutaminyl-peptide cyclotransferase, *RARB* retinoid acid receptor β2, *RASSF1A* RAS association domain family 1, *RIL* reversion-induced LIM, *RUNX3* runt-related transcription factor 3, *SERPINB5* serpin peptidase inhibitor, clade B, member 5, *SLC27A3* solute carrier family 27, *SOCS* suppressor of cytokine signaling, *SYK* spleen tyrosine kinase, *TFPI-2* tissue factor pathway inhibitor-1, *THBD* thrombomodulin, *TIMP3* tissue inhibitor of metalloproteinase 3, *TMS1* target of methylation silencing 1, *TNFRSF10C* tumor necrosis factor receptor superfamily, member 10C, *TNFRSF10D* tumor necrosis factor receptor superfamily, member 10D, *TP53INP1* tumor protein p53 inducible nuclear protein 1, *TPM1* tropomyosin 1 (alpha), *TRAILR1* TNF-related apoptosis inducing ligand receptor 1, *TSPY* testis specific protein, Y-linked, *UNC5C* Unc-5 homologue C, *WFDC1* WAP four-disulfide core domain 1, *WIF1* Wnt inhibitory factor 1, *XAF1* XIAP associated factor 1

[a]Methylation status of the gene found in melanoma as compared to that found in normal tissue
[b]To be determined

G2/M cell cycle arrest and acts as a TSG in colorectal cancer [16]. Gene silencing of 14-3-3σ by CpG hypermethylation has been found to occur in many human epithelial cancers, including breast cancer [17], hepatocellular carcinoma [18], vulval squamous neoplasia [19], gastric carcinoma [20], oral carcinoma [21], and epithelial ovarian cancer [22, 23], as well as prostate and endometrial carcinoma [23]. Most recently, 14-3-3σ gene expression and regulation was investigated in melanoma, with the 14-3-3σ gene found to be highly expressed in human skin, but undetectable in either normal human melanocytes or melanoma cells [24]. Unlike epithelial cancers, the promoter CpG islands in the 14-3-3σ gene are heavily methylated in both normal melanocytes and most melanoma cells in a cell-lineage specific manner [24]. Spontaneous demethylation of 14-3-3σ CpG islands was not observed in clinical melanoma tissue samples or in short-passaged melanoma cell lines. These results indicate that 14-3-3σ might have a tentative negative effect on melanoma progression, as recently demonstrated by Schultz et al. [25]. On the other hand, since 14-3-3σ is methylated in melanoma in a cell-lineage specific manner, the methylation status of 14-3-3σ is not suitable as a marker for evaluating disease progression in melanoma patients.

Aberrant DNA Hypomethylation

Epigenetic silencing of TSGs is a well-documented and important cellular phenomenon; although, there is relatively little research into the role of hypomethylation in the initiation and transformation events of melanoma. It was recently demonstrated that hypomethylation in cancers may contribute to tumor progression by inducing genomic instability via the demethylation of transposons and peri-centromeric repeats [26]. For instance, genome-wide hypomethylation was observed in mice that carried a hypomorphic DNMT1 and developed aggressive T-cell lymphomas [27]. This demonstrated the potential consequences of tumor development as a result of spontaneously-occurring or chemically-induced DNA hypomethylation. The molecular basis for hypomethylation-induced tumors in this model involves chromosomal instability events accompanied by the activation of endogenous retroviral elements. Further evidence has shown that extensive DNA hypomethylation in lung cancer occurs specifically at repetitive sequences, through the analysis of the hypermethylation patterns of promoter regions in squamous cell carcinoma of the lung and matched normal lung tissue [28]. These findings validate the role of DNA methylation in maintaining the stability of the human genome and the suppression of transposable elements in mammalian cells.

DNA hypomethylation not only exists at repetitive sequences of the genome in tumors, but also at specific promoter regions, possibly resulting in the activation of genes with suspected oncogenic activities [26]. A few such genes have been reported in several types of cancer, including: cyclin D2, maspin [29, 30], and R-RAS [26] promoter CpG hypomethylation and over-expression in gastric cancer; MN/CA9 in renal cancer [31]; SNCG/BC SG1 in breast and ovarian cancer [32]; BORIS/CTCFL in ovarian cancer [33]; heparinase in bladder cancer [34]; WNT5A, CRIP1, and S100P in prostate cancer [35]; and c-ROS in malignant gliomas [36]. Importantly, cancer-testis antigens (CTAs) and several other related genes have been shown to be aberrantly hypomethylated in melanomas, such as PRAME (preferentially expressed antigen of melanoma), SSX 1-5 (sarcoma, synovial, breakpoint 1-5), GAGE 1-6 (G antigen 1-6), MAGE-A2, -A3 and -A4 (melanoma antigen) [37], HMW-MAA (high molecular weight melanoma-associated antigen) [38], NY-ESO-1 (New York esophageal squamous cell carcinoma 1) [39], and PI5 (protease inhibitor 5/maspin) [40].

Expression of these genes appears to be suppressed in normal human skin melanocytes, primarily due to presumably heavily methylated promoter regions in a cell lineage-specific manner. However, these same genes can exist in a demethylated state and are aberrantly re-expressed in subsets of melanoma cells. The biological significance of gene re-expression continues to be poorly understood, with current evidence suggesting that their reactivation may contribute to overall tumorigenesis. It is clear that the expression of these tumor antigens can result in their recognition and possible destruction by the host immune system. There is also evidence showing that CTA gene products can influence a range of cellular processes, including cell signaling, transcription, translation, and chromosomal recombination [41]. For instance, recent data suggested that NY-ESO-1 promotes growth in normal and human non-small cell lung cancer cell lines [42]. Additionally, there are data suggesting that expression of MAGE genes in cancer cells contributes directly to the malignant phenotype and response to therapy [41].

Clinical Applications

It appears that epigenetic alterations in cancer cells affect virtually every cellular pathway involved in cell cycle progression, apoptosis, cell survival, angiogenesis, and immunogenicity. Therefore, it is not surprising that 'epigenetic drugs' display pleiotropic activities. The use of demethylating agents in clinical practice for the treatment of patients with cancer has increased in recent years. The therapeutic goal is to reverse such hypermethylated regions in order to 'reactivate' those genes involved in either tumor suppression or some other related function, possibly contributing to the regression of established tumors. There are several agents that are capable of inhibiting DNMTs and associated with the capacity to reactivate silenced genes and induce differentiation or apoptosis of malignant cells. The most intensively studied class of such agents are the DNMT inhibitors, which include 5-azacytidine (5-aza, azacytidine) and 5-aza-2'-deoxycytidine (decitabine), currently approved in the United States for the treatment of patients with myelodysplastic syndromes (MDS) [43].

Combinations of demethylation drugs with chemotherapy, interferon, and tumor vaccines have been proposed as a means to increase their clinical efficacy; since genes involved in chemotherapy and/or interferon resistance and CTAs are all at least partially modulated by promoter gene methylation. In pre-clinical murine experiments, such combination therapies have shown some impressive results, with evidence of tumor regression [44, 45]. Clinical trials have also shown limited, but promising results [46]. These clinical trials demonstrated that demethylation agents (decitabine) can be combined safely with carboplatin, causing epigenetic changes in patients with solid tumors. Decitabine can also be safely administered with, and may enhance the activity of, high-dose interleukin-2 (IL-2), with responses occurring in 31% of melanoma patients [47].

Although reactivation of TSGs and inhibition of tumor growth through the use of demethylating agents has been well documented, there is concern that the lack of specificity of current demethylating agents often produces global hypomethylation of the genome, resulting in not only re-expression of previously silenced TSGs, but also activation of 'tumor-promoting genes'. Further research is needed to determine appropriate patient selection and dosing schedules. As we identify new genes and improve our current understanding of the epigenetic mechanisms involved in melanoma, we foresee the development of an array-based DNA methylation assay capable of identifying a panel of methylated genes within a freshly procured melanoma sample. By doing so, we can selectively modulate these promoter regions utilizing demethylating agents or HDAC inhibitors, thereby resulting in the re-activation of methylation-suppressed gene function.

DNA Methylation as Biomarkers in Melanoma

Due to the extensive differential methylation patterns between malignant cells and normal cells, aberrantly hypermethylated or hypomethylated genes or genetic loci may serve as clinically useful biomarkers for early detection of disease, tumor classification, and response to treatment with classical chemotherapeutic agents, target compounds, and epigenetic drugs. Numerous studies have shown the promise of DNA methylation as potential biomarkers with clinical applications. Furthermore, the demonstration of identical patterns of DNA methylation in cancer cells and in circulating DNA in bodily fluids of the same patient has opened the possibility for the development of non-invasive or minimally invasive diagnostic tests [48]. Although cancer cells show both aberrant regional hypermethylation and global as well as regional hypomethylation, most work on biomarker identification is still limited to aberrantly hypermethylated genes or genomic loci. Indeed, there are several potential advantages for utilizing DNA methylation as biomarkers [49]. First, changes in the status of DNA methylation are characteristic of neoplastic cells. Different patterns can be useful in diagnosing and classifying tumors of different histology. Second, techniques for methylation detection, such as methylation-specific polymerase chain reaction (MS-PCR), are both quick and sensitive. Third, compared to protein or RNA biomarkers, DNA is very stable and can be obtained from a wide variety of sources.

Several studies have demonstrated the clinical utility of detecting circulating methylated tumor-related genes in the peripheral blood of cancer patients, employing quantitative methylation-specific PCR (Q-MS-PCR) for gene methylation analysis of clinical samples [50]. For instance, significantly less frequent circulating methylated RASSF1A was reported for biochemotherapy responders compared with non-responders, with methylation of RASSF1A significantly correlated with overall survival and biochemotherapy response [51]. Furthermore, Mori et al. [52] reported that estrogen receptor alpha (ER-A) methylation is predictive of melanoma progression. Although the role of ER-A in melanoma is unknown, it was found to be methylated more frequently in metastatic than primary melanomas. In addition, serum methylated ER-A was detected more frequently in advanced compared to localized melanomas and was the only factor predictive of both progression-free and overall survival in patients treated with biochemotherapy [52]. Such data suggest that this biomarker may indeed be considered an unfavorable prognostic factor when discussing treatment options with patients.

The true source of tumor-related methylated DNA in serum is unknown. Circulating tumor cells (CTCs) in the peripheral blood may be one potential source of serum methylated DNA. To test this hypothesis, Koyanagi et al. [53] obtained matched pairs of peripheral blood lymphocytes and serum specimens simultaneously from 50 stage IV melanoma patients before the administration of biochemotherapy. Peripheral blood leukocytes were analyzed for three mRNA markers of CTCs: MART-1, GalNAc-T, and MAGE-A3; with sera analyzed for two methylated DNA markers: RASSF1A and RAR-β2. The number of detected CTC markers was found to correlate with the overall percentage of methylated DNA in the peripheral blood [53]. A significant difference in overall survival in this group of patients treated with biochemotherapy was also noted [53].

There are still many lingering questions concerning specific methylation phenotypes, such as a CpG island methylator phenotype (CIMP) in melanoma. It is often perceived that cancer cells can be classified according to their degree of DNA methylation, with those cancers with higher levels of promoter region methylation representing a clinically and etiologically distinct group that is best characterized by what is described as 'epigenetic instability' [54]. The CIMP is marked by methylation of both tumor-related genes and multiple non-coding methylated-in-tumor (MINT) loci. In gastric and colorectal cancer, the existence of such CIMPs have been described and found to be associated with tumor development. The CIMP has also been shown to be a predictive marker of survival benefit from adjuvant 5-fluorouracil-based chemotherapy in patients with colorectal carcinoma that is metastatic to regional lymph nodes [55].

The question of whether there are also CIMPs that exist for melanoma was recently pursued by Tanemura et al. [56]. They investigated the methylation status of promoter CpG islands of six tumor-related genes (WIF1, TFPI2, RASSF1A, RARh2, SOCS1, and GATA4) and a panel of MINT loci (MINT1, MINT2, MINT3, MINT12, MINT17, MINT25, and MINT31) in primary and metastatic tumors of different clinical stages ($n = 122$). They found that an increase in hypermethylation of four tumor-related genes, that included WIF1, TFPI2, RASSF1A, and SOCS1, was associated with advancing clinical tumor stage. This finding indicates that a CIMP pattern is associated with advancing clinical stage of melanoma. Interestingly, the methylation status of MINT31 was associated with disease outcome in stage III melanoma patients, with its methylation found to be a significant predictor of improved overall survival. Future prospective large-scale studies will be necessary in order to validate CIMP-positive primary melanomas as being of high risk of metastasis or recurrence.

Thus, the detection of hypermethylated DNA may contribute to a more sensitive classification system for melanoma, with the further identification of prognostic markers as predictors of outcome to treatment. It is also possible that a panel of methylation markers, rather than a single marker, may be more valuable in predicting the overall prognosis of melanoma patients. As more prognostic markers are identified, it will be important to validate their utility by examining their gene expression related to clinical outcome in a series of properly staged patients with melanoma.

Histone Modifications

Epigenetic modifications of histones are vital for normal human development and the maintenance of cellular homeostasis. Such modifications may include acetylation, methylation, ubiquitination, phosphorylation, sumoylation, proline isomerization, and ADP ribosylation [1]. While DNA methylation represses target gene expression, the marking of histone tails by alternative means can result in repressive or activating potential. As these modifications directly and indirectly affect gene expression, they also hold an important role in the development and progression of cancer. Many hallmarks of cancer, such as insensitivity to growth inhibitory and apoptotic signals, increased potential for proliferation, capacity for invasion and metastasis, and maintenance of angiogenesis, are indeed induced and/or maintained by certain epigenetic states [57, 58]. Several authors have reported on the utilization of certain modified histone states, particularly involving acetylation and methylation, as biomarkers for numerous cancers, including those of the breast [59], prostate [4, 60], lung [61, 62], and esophagus [63]. The characterization of those involved in melanoma may help to identify biomarkers for developmental risk, diagnosis, prognosis, metastatic propensity, and chemoresistance [3, 64, 65].

Eukaryotic DNA is found in the nucleus packaged into dense chromatin, a tightly twisted compaction of DNA, histones (H1, H2A, H2B, H3, and H4; each with their own specialized variants) and non-histone proteins. The functional unit of chromatin is the nucleosome, which consists of a histone octamer of two H2A-H2B dimers and an H3-H4 tetramer around which ~147 bp of core DNA is wound ~1.7 times. Histone H1 acts to link nucleosomes together for a higher order compaction of chromatin. Between each nucleosome lies a stretch of ~50 bp, which gives the overall appearance of 'beads on a string' in actively transcribed euchromatin. The NH_2-terminal histone domain extends from the core as a charged histone 'tail'. Amino acid residues such as lysine and arginine contribute to the overall basic properties of the histone tail and to the binding of the negatively charged DNA phosphate backbone.

Post-translational modification of these and other residues on the nucleosomal tails primes the sites for unique interaction with chromatin remodeling complexes and transcription factors, thus providing a myriad of ways to affect chromatin assembly and gene expression. Specific combinations of histone modifications determine the overall expression status of a region of chromatin, the proposed 'histone code'. This code may be useful as a marker for predicting past and future gene expression trends and targeting unique cell characteristics based on a current and fluid epigenetic 'fingerprint' [66–69]. While numerous covalent modifications of histones are known, two have been identified as effective cancer biomarkers, acetylation and methylation [3, 4, 59–63].

Histone Acetylation and Methylation

DNA-binding histones are directly targeted by the lysine-modifying proteins, HATs and HDACs, affecting the strength with which they bind and segregate DNA from the transcriptional machinery. Specifically, reversible acetylation of the ε-amino group on N-terminal tail lysine residues reduces the positive charge of the histone and alleviates the charge-attraction between it and DNA, relaxing chromatin and making DNA more accessible to DNA transcription factors.

Lysine acetylation is associated with open, transcriptionally active euchromatin. Furthermore, lysine acetylation can regulate protein stability through either directly or indirectly affecting protein interaction with the cell ubiquitination machinery [70], regulating gene expression through the modification of higher-order chromatin folding [71], and recruiting transcriptional activators such as the SWI/SNF adenosine triphosphatase (ATP)-dependent chromatin remodeling complex [72, 73]. Notably, loss of the tumor suppressor SNF5, the core subunit of this complex, is associated with increased chemoresistance and poor patient survival in melanoma [74], which in many instances requires the presence of the ATPase subunit, BRG1 [75]. Lysine deacetylation is thus associated with tightly bound, inactive heterochromatin and is important for its repression of tumor suppressor genes during cancer progression.

Methylation and demethylation of histones is mediated by HMTs and HDMs, respectively. While lysine acetylation is transcriptionally activating, lysine methylation can be either repressive (H3K9, H3K27) or activating (H3K4), depending on the location of the methylated residues and the degree of methylation in the region. Furthermore, acetylation and methylation of histones may in turn lead to the epigenetic modification of DNA, and vice versa. For instance, Fuks et al. [76] show that the methyl-CpG-binding protein, MeCP2, binds methylated CpG (met-CpG) sites and recruits both HDAC and H3K9-specific HMT activity. HDACs and HMTs work together at this met-CpG site by removal of the acetyl group from H3K9 in order to allow room for methyl group addition, an initiation factor for the formation of heterochromatin [77, 78]. Additionally, a complex of the HMTs, G9a and GLP independently regulates both H3K9 and DNA methylation in murine and human embryonic stem cell populations [78, 79]. Histone methylation may also regulate gene transcription independent of promoter DNA methylation [80]. These types of interactions are vital for establishing a more complete and coherent description of the current cellular environment by which to define important markers.

Clinical Applications

Regulation of histone modifications has shown to be a valuable approach for halting and reversing tumor development, either directly or through the enhancement of chemosensitivity to certain drug classes. In cancer, many TSGs are found to be down-regulated jointly through promoter hypermethylation and the reversible deacetylation of lysine residues of local histones by HDACs [81]. Furthermore, HDACs are known to act on proteins that regulate cellular differentiation, proliferation, gene expression, and death [82, 83]. Reversible epigenetic mechanisms allow for the manipulation of tumor cell activity at a level that can produce widespread, immediate and inheritable change. Therefore, HDAC inhibitors are currently being studied as treatment for patients with multiple cancers, including melanoma.

The cell type-specific anti-tumor effects of HDAC inhibitors are generally thought to result in large part from the re-expression of TSGs and increased acetylation of non-histone proteins, including p53, Hsp90, NF-κB, and tubulin, which are active in multiple cellular processes [84]. Notably, protein acetylation may either stabilize the protein or promote its degradation; for example, HDAC2 and p300 are rapidly degraded upon treatment with the HDAC inhibitors valproic acid (valproate, VPA) or butyrate [85, 86]. Targeting HDACs is also somewhat tumor-specific as they are known to be over-expressed in many cancers. Multiple HDAC inhibitors have been shown to inhibit angiogenesis through attenuation of vascular endothelial growth factor (VEGF) [87] and also to induce generation of reactive oxygen species (ROS) [88], premature chromatid separation [89], autophagic cell death [90], and cell senescence [91] in transformed cells. More general effects of treatment with HDAC inhibitors are the induction of intrinsic (mitochondrial) and extrinsic (death receptor-mediated) apoptotic pathways [92], growth arrest, and differentiation *in vitro* and *in vivo* [93, 94]; albeit only about 2–20% of genes show a change in expression after HDAC inhibitor treatment in tumor cells, most of those genes being involved in cell growth and survival [95]. Boyle et al. [96] described an equal number of genes repressed or reactivated in melanoma cell lines treated with either butyrate or suberic bishydroxamate (SBHA), consistent with findings in other tumor cell types.

The importance of chemoresistance and the current lack of effective treatment strategies for advanced stage melanoma cannot be overstated. To this end, HDAC inhibitors have been used to identify and modulate the expression of notable chemoresistance markers. Class III β-tubulin (TUBB3) over-expression promotes resistance to taxane derivative chemotherapies and demonstrates up-regulation in normal melanocytes and a majority of primary melanoma tumors, albeit gradually lost in a subset of melanomas with increasing stage of disease [97]. Recently, Akasaka et al. [97] described the correlation of TUBB3 protein expression with chemosensitivity to paclitaxel-induced apoptosis in melanoma cells. Upon treatment of the human melanoma cell line HMV-I with an HDAC inhibitor, TUBB3 expression was induced, correlating with increased TUBB3 promoter region H3/4 acetylation. HDAC inhibitor-promotion of retinoic acid (RA)-signaling was also recently shown to be counteracted to a great degree by the retinoic acid receptor (RAR) and PRAME [98]. Suppression of these proteins resulted in the sensitization of cells to HDAC inhibitors both *in vitro* and in mouse xenografts.

Combination decitabine and the HDAC inhibitor belinostat (PXD101) markedly increased the expression of methylation-silenced MLH1 and MAGE-A1 *in vitro* and *in vivo* over decitabine alone and enhanced cisplatin sensitivity of previously resistant ovarian cancer xenografts [99]. Combination therapies, particularly using HDAC and DNMT inhibitors, have produced clinically relevant data and are currently being employed as effective treatment strategies. The joint action of 'opening up' chromatin and releasing repressive CpG methylation allows for the re-expression of silenced TSGs.

Similar patient data from combinations of HDAC inhibitors with other drug classes have also been achieved. In a recent case presented by Daud et al. [100], VPA potentiated the cytotoxicity and DNA strand cleavage induced by a novel topoisomerase I inhibitor, karenitecin (KTN), in melanoma cell lines and a metastatic melanoma xenograft. Furthermore, inclusion of this combination therapy in a small phase I/II trial for patients with stage IV melanoma was associated with disease stabilization in 47% (7 of 15) of patients. Exhibition of hyperacetylation of histones in peripheral blood mononuclear cells and CTCs indicates an important ability to serologically verify HDAC inhibitor activity. Munster et al. [101] reported on combination vorinostat and another notable topoisomerase inhibitor, doxorubicin, and described HDAC2 pre-treatment expression correlating with post-treatment hyperacetylation, indicating the potential for HDAC2 expression to act as a marker predictive of HDAC inhibition. Vo et al. [102] recently described an up-regulation in tumor expression of MHC and tumor-associated antigens and an increase in proliferation and activity of adoptively transferred gp100 melanoma antigen-specific pmel-1 T-cells after treatment of B16 murine melanoma cells with combination HDAC inhibitor (LAQ824) and adoptive transfer lymphocytes, validating these findings with combination LAQ824 and the melanoma antigen tyrosinase-related protein 2 (TRP2). Histone acetylation mechanisms thus play a major role in multiple cellular processes and are proving a viable field for tumor marker discovery.

With the advent of epigenetic therapy for cancer and the presence of a myriad of interactions between various epigenetic effectors, interest in development and use of HMT inhibitors for deciphering the least well understood of these effectors has recently been growing. It was not until 2005 that chaetocin, a fungal metabolite, became the first lysine-specific HMT inhibitor to be described [103]. G9a, an H3K9 HMT, was screened against for inhibitors using a panel of 125,000 compounds [104]. One inhibitor was identified to selectively target G9a and reduce H3K9me2 formation, without competing with the S-adenosyl methionine cofactor. Transient demethylation was evident upon removing the inhibitor from the cells, an important note for therapeutic development. RNA interference knockdown of G9a and SUV39H1, another H3K9 HMT, in PC3 prostate cancer cells resulted in marked reduction of cell growth including telomeric shortening [80]. Independently, SUV39H1 knockdown resulted in G2/M arrest, while G9a knockdown resulted in a 1.7-fold increase in total DNA, associated with a near doubling of chromosome number, in addition to abnormal centrosome number and morphology in 25% of cells. Of note, gene up-regulation was not seen after knockdown of either HMT for the vast majority of 39,000 genes included in an mRNA microarray, indicating a possible non-gene-based mechanism by which HMTs propagate malignancy.

Combination HMT and HDAC inhibitor treatment has been shown to reduce levels of the HMT enhancer of zeste homolog 2 (EZH2) and induce apoptosis in acute myeloid leukemia cells above independent treatment levels [105]. DZNep (3-deazaneplanocin A) is one of a few new HMT-inhibiting compounds currently being studied. It is found to inhibit global histone methylation (including that of H3K27 and H4K20), significantly reduce PRC2 levels, and induce re-expression of some TSGs in a reversible manner, inducing apoptosis of breast cancer cells [106, 107].

Histone Modifications as Biomarkers in Melanoma

Some members of the three main HAT families, GNAT [general control non-depressible 5 (Gcn5)-related N-acetyltransferase], MYST [named for family members MOZ, Ybf2-Sas3, Sas2, and Tip60, and which also includes HBO1, MOF, GCN5, PCAF (p300/CBP-binding associated factor) and MORF (MOZ-related factor)], and p300/CBP (adenoviral E1A-associated protein, 300 kDa; CREB-binding protein), have been described in melanoma-associated systems. Tip60 and HBO1 present in a complex with the putative melanoma tumor suppressors ING3 and ING4, respectively [108–111]. Notably, down-regulation of nuclear ING3 or cytosolic accumulation in primary melanomas of 2 mm or greater Breslow thickness is correlated with a reduced 5-year survival rate, while its phosphorylation inhibits melanoma growth through down-regulation of cyclin B1 and reduction of downstream cyclin-dependent kinase (CDK) 1 activity [111].

Both Tip60 and HBO1 also functionally link NF-κB [112–114], while acetylation by Tip60, GCN5, and PCAF can stabilize the transcription factor c-Myc [115, 116], all of which are putative melanoma oncoproteins [117–122]. Bhoumik et al. [123] described the promotion of Tip60 degradation through the interaction of activating transcription factor-2 (ATF2), which recruits Tip60 to acetylate histones H2B and H4, and Cul3 ubiquitin ligase. Inhibition of ATF2 expression was further shown to induce Tip60 protein expression in a panel of melanoma and prostate cancer cell lines, while down-regulation of ATF2 inhibits melanoma proliferation *in vitro* and tumor growth *in vivo* [124]. Increased ATF2 localization to the nucleus is a marker of poorer melanoma prognosis; while its cytoplasmic sequestration has been shown to inhibit mouse xenograft tumor growth [125]. Sakuraba et al. [126] recently provided clinical data correlating Tip60 down-regulation in 5 of 38 (13%) primary colorectal cancer specimens with increased tumor size, poor differentiation, peritoneal dissemination, distant metastasis and higher TNM classification stage.

CBP and p300 have been shown to associate with microphthalmia-associated transcription factor (MITF), a melanocyte lineage survival oncogene [127–129], that transcriptionally regulates melanoma invasiveness, proliferation, and apoptosis [130], and which is mostly up-regulated in metastatic melanomas [131], and associated with decreased survival in metastatic melanoma patients [132]. Reduced expression or activity of p300/CBP has also been shown to inhibit growth and induce senescence in melanocytes and melanoma cells via the down-regulation of cyclin E due to deacetylation at its promoter [133].

The DEK proto-oncogene, noted for its involvement in leukemogenesis and interaction with histones, has been described as a potent inhibitor of both p300 and PCAF expression and activity [134]. DEK is amplified in melanoma (chromosome 6p, a commonly amplified melanoma locus) and is expressed in metastatic lesions. Long- and short-term knockdown of DEK has been found to result in premature melanoma senescence and reduced chemoresistance to DNA-damaging agents [135]. Its anti-apoptotic role may be due to p53 inhibition in some systems. However, short hairpin RNA directed against DEK produced no change in p53 or p53-dependent apoptosis in a melanoma model; although up-regulation of anti-apoptotic MCL-1 was noted [135].

HDACs generally act as part of transcriptionally repressive complexes and can reverse the actions of HATs, inducing growth arrest, differentiation, and apoptosis [136]. Importantly, HDACs may have either tumor suppressing or oncogenic effects depending on their targets; for example, HDACs reactivate the expression of proteins such as CDK inhibitor-1 (CDKN1/p21) [137] and urokinase plasminogen activator (uPA), a tissue degrading protein implicated in tumor cell invasion and metastasis, potentially resulting in the induction of cellular senescence/apoptosis or promotion of tumor cell invasion [138], respectively. Currently, 18 known human HDACs have been described [139, 140]; separated into four classes based on structural homology to yeast HDACs, mechanism of enzyme activity, and cellular localization.

Histone deacetylase 1 (HDAC1) is a potent inhibitor of H3 and H4 acetylation and involved in the mediation of human melanocyte senescence, likely a result of increased association of HDAC1 and the retinoblastoma (RB) protein [133, 141]. HDAC1 histone deacetylation is also an important prerequisite for H3K9 di- and trimethylation; its trimethylation being a marker of senescence in melanocytes and melanocytic nevi [141]. Notably, Schultz et al. [25] described the induction of melanoma cell senescence by 14-3-3σ, evident in part by increased H3K9 methylation levels following over-expression of 14-3-3σ [25]. The metastasis suppressor BRMS1, a noted HDAC1 co-repressor, has recently been shown to suppress expression of uPA via recruitment of HDAC1 to the NF-κB binding site of the uPA promoter and reducing acetylation of p65 in the metastatic melanoma cell line C8161.9 [142].

Oncostatin M (OSM), an IL-6 type cytokine and STAT3 activator, is a noted suppressor of melanoma cell proliferation that is highly regulated via histone acetylation near its promoter [143]. Lacreusette et al. [144] describe an immunotherapeutic approach, utilizing tumor-infiltrating lymphocytes (TILs) in stage III melanoma patients, whereby there was a relationship between responsiveness of cancer cells to Oncostatin M and/or IL-6 and survival. Such resistance may be due to the inhibition of OSM gene expression by HDACs during melanoma cell proliferation. Other tumor types may also display promoter region hypermethylation by DNMTs, particularly colorectal cancer [145].

Histone methylation plays a key role in establishing and maintaining stable gene expression patterns during cellular differentiation and embryonic development. Methylation of H3K4, K36, and K79 are generally associated with gene activation, while gene silencing generally results from methylation of H3K9, K20, or K27 [57]. Lysine-dependent kinase 1 (LSD1), an HDM, specifically demethylates di- and monomethylated H3K4 and K9; for example, H3K4me2 may become H3K4me1 and finally H3K4me0. In this manner, LSD1 may activate or silence gene expression depending on its target. Recently, recruitment of LSD1 by the melanoma oncogene Myc and transient LSD1-mediated demethylation of H3K4 at the Myc E-box DNA binding site has been shown to induce local DNA oxidation, promoting Myc target gene mRNA transcription [146].

Polycomb group (PcG) proteins, which commonly harbor HMT domains, remodel chromatin such that transcription factors cannot bind promoters. PcG proteins in complex are termed polycomb repressive complexes (PRCs), and their repressive function is stable over multiple generations, only overcome by germline differentiation processes. Over-expression of PcGs is correlated with severity and invasiveness of some cancers [147]. One of the best described oncogenic PcGs is EZH2. Expression of EZH2 as a member of PRC 2/3 allows activity of its SET (suppressor of variegation-enhancer of zeste-trithorax) HMT domain to methylate H3K27 and purportedly H3K9 [148]. EZH2 is significantly up-regulated in melanoma and associated with poor prognosis in prostate, breast and other cancers [149–151].

Two identified polymorphisms of EZH2 have also recently been associated with reduced lung cancer risk [152]. The co-expression of the EZH2 and Ras genes is required for the epigenetic silencing of the Fas gene, also responsible for anchorage-independent growth and tumorigenicity [153]. It may also act as a platform for DNMT function by facilitating DNA methylation and repressing E-cadherin gene expression, thought to be important during epithelial-mesenchymal cell-type transition (EMT) involved in tumor cell invasion and metastasis. Furthermore, EZH2 represses the expression of RUNX3, an important tumor suppressor gene that up-regulates the cell cycle regulators $p21^{WAF1/Cip1}$ and $p57^{KIP2}$ and the pro-apoptotic protein Bim [154, 155].

Wang et al. [156] described the identification of two *Drosophila* polycomb-like (PCL) protein human homologs, hPCL3S and hPCL3L, short and long mRNA, respectively. Northern blot analysis revealed the absence of both in normal melanocytes, while their expressions were dramatically higher in all tested melanoma cell lines, including those derived from radial and vertical growth phase primaries and metastatic tumors. Additionally, a stage IV melanoma tissue sample and all tested stage III skin cancers expressed higher hPCL3 and hPCL3S levels, respectively, than did earlier stage samples.

MicroRNAs

MicroRNAs are endogenous, ~22 nucleotide in length, non-coding RNAs that play a central role in gene regulation and expression through direct interaction with mRNA either by inhibiting mRNA translation [157–160] or promoting mRNA degradation [161–163]. There are currently several hundred confirmed miRNA sequences in humans, with computational predictions suggesting that the total count might be more than 1,000 [164]. The regulatory nature of miRNAs, combined with the large number of presumptive target genes, suggests that they are essential regulators of a wide range of cellular processes. Recent evidence is emerging that particular miRNAs may play an important role in human cancer epigenetic pathogenesis.

It is important to understand the basic molecular mechanisms involved in miRNA-mediated gene silencing. Briefly, miRNA is originally transcribed by RNA polymerase II as a long primary miRNA (pri-miRNA) [165]. It is then processed into a 60–70 nucleotide miRNA precursor (pre-miRNA) by Drosha, a member of the nuclear RNase III family. The pre-miRNA is transported from the nucleus to the cytoplasm by RanGTP/exportin 5, where it is subsequently cleaved by DICER to generate 20–22 nucleotide duplexes. Generally, only one strand of the duplex serves as mature miRNA [166, 167]. Single-stranded miRNA is incorporated into a ribonucleoprotein effector complex known as the RNA-induced silencing complex (RISC). This complex identifies target messages based on complementarities between the 'guide' miRNA and the mRNA, resulting in either endonucleolytic cleavage of targeted mRNA or translational repression [168–170].

Most recently, researchers have shown that miRNAs are not only inactivating factors for translation, but play a more diverse role in the regulation of gene expression [171]. Li et al. [172] identified several double-stranded RNAs (dsRNAs) that activate E-cadherin, $p21^{WAF1/Cip1}$, and VEGF gene expression by targeting non-coding regulatory regions in gene promoters. They revealed synthesized 21-nt dsRNAs targeting selected promoter regions of human genes that, when transfected into human cell lines, resulted in long-lasting and sequence-specific induction of the target genes. Ørom et al. [173] also revealed that the miRNA miR-10a interacts with the 5′-UTR of ribosomal protein mRNAs and enhances their translation.

Since miRNA-mediated regulation can affect the expression of hundreds of genes on several chromosomes, unique patterns of altered miRNA expression provide complex fingerprints that may serve as diagnostic markers for tumorigenesis [171, 172]. A few studies have examined the miRNA profiles within melanoma cell lines [174] or tumor samples [175, 176]. Zhang et al. examined 45 primary cultured melanoma cell lines by array comparative genomic hybridization (aCGH) and observed that many genomic loci that contain miRNA-coding sequences are frequently affected (85.9%) by copy number abnormalities [176]. Among 59 of the NCI-60 cell lines (derived from melanoma, leukemia, and cancers of the gastrointestinal tract, kidney, ovary, breast, prostate, lung, and central nervous system), Gaur et al. [174] identified a set of 15 miRNAs with significant differential expression in the eight melanoma cell lines studied. It appeared that the melanoma cell lines clustered into an independent terminal branch based on miRNA expression.

Increasing evidence shows that expression of miRNA genes is deregulated in human cancer, thus epigenetically adjusting their target gene mRNA expression accordingly [177–185]. Specific miRNA over-expression or under-expression has been shown to correlate with particular tumor histologies, with over-expression resulting in the down-regulation of TSGs, whereas their under-expression could lead to oncogene up-regulation [176]. For example, let-7, down-regulated in lung cancer, suppresses Ras [181]; miR-15 and miR-16, deleted or down-regulated in leukemia, suppress BCL2 [182]; and miR-17-5p and miR-20a control the balance of cell death and proliferation driven by the proto-oncogene c-Myc [183]. Clear evidence indicates that miRNA polycistron miR-17-92 serves as an oncogene in lymphoma [184] and lung cancer [185]. In addition, miR-372 and miR-373 are novel oncogenes in testicular germ cell tumors and act by neutralizing p53-mediated CDK inhibition, possibly through direct inhibition of the expression of the tumor-suppressor LATS2 [186].

Several miRNAs have been identified as playing key roles in human melanoma epigenetic pathogenesis (Table 8.2). The first report linking the deregulated expression of a single miRNA to its function in melanoma tumorigenesis was published by Bemis et al. [50]. They examined the expression of mature miR-137 that was capable of down-regulating MITF expression in melanoma cell lines, with MITF previously shown to be a master regulator of melanocyte development, survival, and function [130, 187, 188]. They further identified a 15-bp variable nucleotide tandem repeat sequence, which alters the processing and function of miR-137 in melanoma cell lines [50]. In another study, Müller et al. [188] determined let-7a to be an important regulator of integrin $\beta(3)$ expression; the latter is known to play an important role in melanoma progression and invasion. Melanoma cells transfected with synthetic let-7a molecules show repressed expression of integrin $\beta(3)$ that is accompanied by reduced invasive potential, as observed in Boyden chamber assays. As a corollary, induction of integrin $\beta(3)$ gene expression with let-7a anti-miR resulted in invasive behavior of transfected melanocytes [188]. It appears that the loss of let-7a expression is involved in the development and progression of melanoma. Schultz et al. [189] found that members of the let-7 family of miRNAs were significantly down-regulated in primary melanomas compared with benign melanocytic nevi. Over-expression of let-7b in melanoma cells *in vitro* resulted in the down-regulation of expression of cyclins D1, D3, and A, as well as CDK4, all of which have been described to play a role in melanoma development. The effect of let-7b on protein expression is due to targeting of the 3′-UTRs of individual mRNAs. In line with its down-modulating effects on cell cycle regulators, let-7b inhibited cell cycle progression and anchorage-independent growth of melanoma cells.

Müller et al. [190] summarized the functional characterization of single miRNA species in melanoma cells in a review published in 2009. They underlined the role of miRNAs in the pathogenesis of melanoma, as well as future prospects in diagnosis and therapy. This group also carried out a detailed comparison of the miRNAomes of normal human melanocytes with well-characterized

Table 8.2 miRNAs altered in melanoma (modified from Sigalotti et al. [196])

Pathway	miRNA	Targeted gene	Expression[a]
Apoptosis	miR-15b	–	Up-regulated
	miR-155	NIK (?), SKI (?)	Down-regulated
Cell cycle	miR-193b	Cyclin D1	Down-regulated
	miR 17–92 cluster	c-MYC	Up-regulated
	miR 106–363 cluster	Rbp1-like (?)	Up-regulated
	miR-137	MITF	Down-regulated
	miR-182	MITF, FOXO3	Up-regulated
	miR-221/-222	c-KIT, p27	Up-regulated
	let-7b	cyclins A, D1, D3, CDK4	Down-regulated
Invasion/metastasis	miR-373	–	Up-regulated
	miR-137	MITF	Down-regulated
	miR-182	MITF, FOXO3	Up-regulated
	let-7a	ITGB3	Down-regulated
	miR-34b	MET	Down-regulated
	miR-34c	MET	Down-regulated
	miR-199a*	MET	Down-regulated
Unknown[b]	miR-17-5p	–	Up-regulated
	miR-146a	–	Down-regulated
	miR-146b	–	Down-regulated
	miR-16	–	Up-regulated
	miR-21	–	Up-regulated
	miR-22	–	Up-regulated
	miR-106b	–	Up-regulated
	miR-125b	–	Down-regulated
	miR-200c	–	Down-regulated
	miR-203	–	Down-regulated
	miR-204	–	Down-regulated
	miR-205	–	Down-regulated
	miR-211	–	Down-regulated
	miR-214	–	Down-regulated
	miR-768-3p	–	Down-regulated

CDK4 cyclin-dependent kinase 4, *FOXO3* forkhead box O3, *ITGB3* integrin beta 3, *MITF* microphthalmia-associated transcription factor, *NIK* nuclear factor-inducing kinase, *Rbp1-like* retinoblastoma binding protein 1-like, *SKI* v-ski sarcoma viral oncogene homolog
[a]Level of expression of miRNAs in melanoma as compared to that found in normal melanocytes
[b]To be determined
*Passenger strand/star arm

melanoma cell lines derived from primary tumors and melanoma metastases [191]. The experimental setup of this study made it possible to identify miRNAs differentially expressed in each step of melanoma tumorigenesis, such as early development and metastasis. The most important findings can be summarized as follows: (1) expression of a high number of miRNAs is deregulated in melanoma cells compared with normal melanocytes, with the bulk of miRNAs up-regulated in melanoma cell lines; (2) the bulk of those miRNAs found to be most strongly deregulated were not previously described to be of importance in tumor development; (3) heterogeneity of melanoma cells causes intrinsic changes in the expression of some miRNAs, which makes it necessary to analyze sets of cell lines/tissue samples in order to minimize the effects of individual alterations. It is interesting to note that several miRNAs, proven to harbor oncogenic or tumor-suppressive potential in other types of tumors, were also found to be deregulated in melanoma. Thus, these miRNAs may also be relevant in melanoma pathobiology; although the mechanisms by which they exert their function in this cancer subtype remain to be elucidated.

The transcriptional regulation of miRNA expression in several tumor types has recently been examined, with epigenetic modification of DNA identified as a key mechanism. Saito et al. [192] demonstrated that the induction of a small subset of miRNAs was followed by the inhibition of DNA methylation and histone deacetylation. One of these miRNAs – miR-127, located within a CpG island – is generally down-regulated in most cancer cells compared with corresponding normal cells. MiR-127 was found to be up-regulated following treatment with chromatin-modifying drugs, while the target gene BCL6 was translationally repressed [192]. Meng et al. [193] reported that another CpG island-embedded miRNA, miR-370, showed IL-6-driven methylation regulation in cholangiocarcinoma cells. The authors demonstrated that IL-6 can enhance the growth of cholangiocarcinoma cells by repressing the expression of miR-370 epigenetically. Interestingly, the demethylation agent 5-aza-2′-deoxycytidine had an opposite effect on the expression of miR-370, but only in malignant cells. Among its predicted targets, the oncogene MAP3K8 was identified, which may explain the altered growth of tumor cells in this context. These data illustrate the complex network involving an inflammation-associated cytokine, DNA methylation, the expression of a miRNA, and its target protein-coding gene [193].

In a study of lung adenocarcinoma, Brueckner et al. [194] reported that the let-7a-3 locus is generally hypomethylated and that its expression can be epigenetically modulated. Another group has identified the promyelocytic leukemia zinc finger (PLZF) transcription factor as a repressor of miR-221 and miR-222 via direct binding to their putative regulatory region(s) in melanoma [195]. Specifically, PLZF silencing in melanomas unblocks miR-221 and miR-222, which in turn controls neoplastic progression through down-modulation of p27$^{Kip1/CDKN1B}$ and c-KIT receptor, leading to enhanced proliferation and differentiation blockade of melanoma cells, respectively. *In vitro* and *in vivo* functional studies confirmed the key role of miR-221/-222 in regulating the progression of human melanoma, thus suggesting that targeted therapies suppressing miR-221/-222 may prove beneficial in advanced tumors [195].

Conclusions

With the realization that epigenetic heterogeneity is a major driving force in cancer development and progression, and known to be further involved in some enigmatic and seemingly indecipherable disease states, an enlightened assessment of the effectiveness of current and future biomarkers is needed. Accordingly, the most effective epigenetic-based therapies for melanoma are likely to come from some combination of DNA-, histone- and miRNA-directed modalities rather than the targeting of a specific pathway or effector molecule. Next generation high-throughput technologies will allow researchers to overcome many of the boundaries that have precluded efficient study of epigenetic influences on cellular events to date, for example: (1) the myriad combinations of post-translational modifications possible; (2) unknown and unanticipated interactions between modifications; (3) antibody specificity for a growing number of markers; and (4) availability of sufficient sample quantity and quality for current measurement systems.

References

1. Ellis L, Atadja PW, Johnstone RW. Epigenetics in cancer: targeting chromatin modifications. Mol Cancer Ther. 2009;8:1409–20.
2. Jenuwein T, Allis CD. Translating the histone code. Science. 2001;293:1074–80.
3. Fraga MF, Ballestar E, Villar-Garea A, et al. Loss of acetylation at Lys16 and trimethylation at Lys20 of histone H4 is a common hallmark of human cancer. Nat Genet. 2005;37:391–400.
4. Seligson DB, Horvath S, Shi T, et al. Global histone modification patterns predict risk of prostate cancer recurrence. Nature. 2005;435:1262–6.
5. Howell Jr PM, Liu S, Ren S, Behlen C, Fodstad O, Riker AI. Epigenetics in human melanoma. Cancer Control. 2009;16:200–18.
6. Ugurel S, Utikal J, Becker JC. Tumor biomarkers in melanoma. Cancer Control. 2009;16:219–24.
7. Balch CM, Gershenwald JE, Soong SJ, et al. Final version of 2009 AJCC melanoma staging and classification. J Clin Oncol. 2009;27:6199–206.
8. Mian S, Ugurel S, Parkinson E, et al. Serum proteomic fingerprinting discriminates between clinical stages and predicts disease progression in melanoma patients. J Clin Oncol. 2005;23:5088–93.

9. Findeisen P, Zapatka M, Peccerella T, et al. Serum amyloid A as a prognostic marker in melanoma identified by proteomic profiling. J Clin Oncol. 2009;27: 2199–208.
10. Qiu H, Wang Y. Quantitative analysis of surface plasma membrane proteins of primary and metastatic melanoma cells. J Proteome Res. 2008;7:1904–15.
11. Bird A. DNA methylation patterns and epigenetic memory. Genes Dev. 2002;16:6–21.
12. Liu S, Ren S, Howell P, Fodstad O, Riker AI. Identification of novel epigenetically modified genes in human melanoma via promoter methylation gene profiling. Pigment Cell Melanoma Res. 2008;21: 545–58.
13. Lodygin D, Tarasov V, Epanchintsev A, et al. Inactivation of miR-34a by aberrant CpG methylation in multiple types of cancer. Cell Cycle. 2008;7:2591–600.
14. Lujambio A, Calin GA, Villanueva A, et al. A microRNA DNA methylation signature for human cancer metastasis. Proc Natl Acad Sci USA. 2008;105:13556–61.
15. Rothhammer T, Bosserhoff AK. Epigenetic events in malignant melanoma. Pigment Cell Res. 2007;20: 92–111.
16. Hermeking H, Lengauer C, Polyak K, et al. 14-3-3 sigma is a p53-regulated inhibitor of G2/M progression. Mol Cell. 1997;1:3–11.
17. Umbricht CB, Evron E, Gabrielson E, Ferguson A, Marks J, Sukumar S. Hypermethylation of 14-3-3 sigma (stratifin) is an early event in breast cancer. Oncogene. 2001;20:3348–53.
18. Iwata N, Yamamoto H, Sasaki S, et al. Frequent hypermethylation of CpG islands and loss of expression of the 14-3-3 sigma gene in human hepatocellular carcinoma. Oncogene. 2000;19:5298–302.
19. Gasco M, Sullivan A, Repellin C, et al. Coincident inactivation of 14-3-3sigma and p16INK4a is an early event in vulval squamous neoplasia. Oncogene. 2002;21:1876–81.
20. Kang YH, Lee HS, Kim WH. Promoter methylation and silencing of PTEN in gastric carcinoma. Lab Invest. 2002;82:285–91.
21. Gasco M, Bell AK, Heath V, et al. Epigenetic inactivation of 14-3-3 sigma in oral carcinoma: association with p16(INK4a) silencing and human papillomavirus negativity. Cancer Res. 2002;62: 2072–6.
22. Akahira JI, Aoki M, Suzuki T, et al. Expression of EBAG9/RCAS1 is associated with advanced disease in human epithelial ovarian cancer. Br J Cancer. 2004;90:2197–202.
23. Mhawech P, Benz A, Cerato C, et al. Downregulation of 14-3-3sigma in ovary, prostate and endometrial carcinomas is associated with CpG island methylation. Mod Pathol. 2005;18:340–8.
24. Liu S, Howell P, Ren S, Fodstad O, Riker AI. The 14-3-3sigma gene promoter is methylated in both human melanocytes and melanoma. BMC Cancer. 2009;9:162.
25. Schultz J, Ibrahim SM, Vera J, Kunz M. 14-3-3sigma gene silencing during melanoma progression and its role in cell cycle control and cellular senescence. Mol Cancer. 2009;8:53.
26. Nishigaki M, Aoyagi K, Danjoh I, et al. Discovery of aberrant expression of R-RAS by cancer-linked DNA hypomethylation in gastric cancer using microarrays. Cancer Res. 2005;65:2115–24.
27. Howard G, Eiges R, Gaudet F, Jaenisch R, Eden A. Activation and transposition of endogenous retroviral elements in hypomethylation induced tumors in mice. Oncogene. 2008;27:404–8.
28. Rauch TA, Zhong X, Wu X, et al. High-resolution mapping of DNA hypermethylation and hypomethylation in lung cancer. Proc Natl Acad Sci USA. 2008;105:252–7.
29. Akiyama Y, Maesawa C, Ogasawara S, Terashima M, Masuda T. Cell-type-specific repression of the maspin gene is disrupted frequently by demethylation at the promoter region in gastric intestinal metaplasia and cancer cells. Am J Pathol. 2003;163: 1911–9.
30. Oshimo Y, Nakayama H, Ito R, et al. Promoter methylation of cyclin D2 gene in gastric carcinoma. Int J Oncol. 2003;23:1663–70.
31. Cho M, Uemura H, Kim SC, et al. Hypomethylation of the MN/CA9 promoter and upregulated MN/CA9 expression in human renal cell carcinoma. Br J Cancer. 2001;85:563–7.
32. Gupta RA, Tejada LV, Tong BJ, et al. Cyclooxygenase-1 is overexpressed and promotes angiogenic growth factor production in ovarian cancer. Cancer Res. 2003;63:906–11.
33. Woloszynska-Read A, James SR, Link PA, Yu J, Odunsi K, Karpf AR. DNA methylation-dependent regulation of BORIS/CTCFL expression in ovarian cancer. Cancer Immun. 2007;7:21.
34. Ogishima T, Shiina H, Breault JE, et al. Promoter CpG hypomethylation and transcription factor EGR1 hyperactivate heparanase expression in bladder cancer. Oncogene. 2005;24:6765–72.
35. Wang Q, Williamson M, Bott S, et al. Hypomethylation of WNT5A, CRIP1 and S100P in prostate cancer. Oncogene. 2007;26:6560–5.
36. Jun HJ, Woolfenden S, Coven S, et al. Epigenetic regulation of c-ROS receptor tyrosine kinase expression in malignant gliomas. Cancer Res. 2009;69: 2180–4.
37. Sigalotti L, Coral S, Nardi G, et al. Promoter methylation controls the expression of MAGE2, 3 and 4 genes in human cutaneous melanoma. J Immunother. 2002;25:16–26.
38. Luo W, Wang X, Kageshita T, Wakasugi S, Karpf AR, Ferrone S. Regulation of high molecular weight-melanoma associated antigen (HMW-MAA) gene expression by promoter DNA methylation in human melanoma cells. Oncogene. 2006;25:2873–84.
39. James SR, Link PA, Karpf AR. Epigenetic regulation of X-linked cancer/germline antigen genes by DNMT1 and DNMT3b. Oncogene. 2006;25:6975–85.

40. Wada K, Maesawa C, Akasaka T, Masuda T. Aberrant expression of the maspin gene associated with epigenetic modification in melanoma cells. J Invest Dermatol. 2004;122:805–11.
41. Simpson AJ, Caballero OL, Jungbluth A, Chen YT, Old LJ. Cancer/testis antigens, gametogenesis and cancer. Nat Rev Cancer. 2005;5:615–25.
42. Glazer CA, Smith IM, Ochs MF, et al. Integrative discovery of epigenetically derepressed cancer testis antigens in NSCLC. PLoS One. 2009;4:e8189.
43. Howell PM, Liu Z, Khong HT. Demethylating agents in the treatment of cancer. Pharmaceuticals. 2010;3: 2022–44.
44. Morita S, Iida S, Kato K, Takagi Y, Uetake H, Sugihara K. The synergistic effect of 5-aza-2′-deoxycytidine and 5-fluorouracil on drug-resistant tumors. Oncology. 2006;71:437–45.
45. Reu FJ, Bae SI, Cherkassky L, et al. Overcoming resistance to interferon-induced apoptosis of renal carcinoma and melanoma cells by DNA demethylation. J Clin Oncol. 2006;24:3771–9.
46. Appleton K, Mackay HJ, Judson I, et al. Phase I and pharmacodynamic trial of the DNA methyltransferase inhibitor decitabine and carboplatin in solid tumors. J Clin Oncol. 2007;25:4603–9.
47. Gollob JA, Sciambi CJ, Peterson BL, et al. Phase I trial of sequential low-dose 5-aza-2′-deoxycytidine plus high-dose intravenous bolus interleukin-2 in patients with melanoma or renal cell carcinoma. Clin Cancer Res. 2006;12:4619–27.
48. Kagan J, Srivastava S, Barker PE, Belinsky SA, Cairns P. Towards clinical application of methylated DNA sequences as cancer biomarkers: a joint NCI's EDRN and NIST workshop on standards, methods, assays, reagents and tools. Cancer Res. 2007;67: 4545–9.
49. Mulero-Navarro S, Esteller M. Epigenetic biomarkers for human cancer: the time is now. Crit Rev Oncol Hematol. 2008;68:1–11.
50. Bemis LT, Chen R, Amato CM, et al. MicroRNA-137 targets microphthalmia-associated transcription factor in melanoma cell lines. Cancer Res. 2008;68:1362–8.
51. Mori T, O'Day SJ, Umetani N, et al. Predictive utility of circulating methylated DNA in serum of melanoma patients receiving biochemotherapy. J Clin Oncol. 2005;23:9351–8.
52. Mori T, Martinez SR, O'Day SJ, et al. Estrogen receptor-alpha methylation predicts melanoma progression. Cancer Res. 2006;66:6692–8.
53. Koyanagi K, Mori T, O'Day SJ, Martinez SR, Wang HJ, Hoon DS. Association of circulating tumor cells with serum tumor-related methylated DNA in peripheral blood of melanoma patients. Cancer Res. 2006;66:6111–7.
54. Issa JP. CpG island methylator phenotype in cancer. Nat Rev Cancer. 2004;4:988–93.
55. Van Rijnsoever M, Elsaleh H, Joseph D, McCaul K, Iacopetta B. CpG island methylator phenotype is an independent predictor of survival benefit from 5-fluorouracil in stage III colorectal cancer. Clin Cancer Res. 2003;9:2898–903.
56. Tanemura A, Terando AM, Sim MS, et al. CpG island methylator phenotype predicts progression of malignant melanoma. Clin Cancer Res. 2009;15: 1801–7.
57. Esteller M. Epigenetics in cancer. N Engl J Med. 2008;358:1148–59.
58. Guil S, Esteller M. DNA methylomes, histone codes and miRNAs: tying it all together. Int J Biochem Cell Biol. 2009;41:87–95.
59. Elsheikh SE, Green AR, Rakha EA, et al. Global histone modifications in breast cancer correlate with tumor phenotypes, prognostic factors, and patient outcome. Cancer Res. 2009;69:3802–9.
60. Isharwal S, Miller MC, Marlow C, Makarov DV, Partin AW, Veltri RW. p300 (histone acetyltransferase) biomarker predicts prostate cancer biochemical recurrence and correlates with changes in epithelia nuclear size and shape. Prostate. 2008;68:1097–104.
61. Barlési F, Giaccone G, Gallegos-Ruiz MI, et al. Global histone modifications predict prognosis of resected non small-cell lung cancer. J Clin Oncol. 2007;25:4358–64.
62. Van Den Broeck A, Brambilla E, Moro-Sibilot D, et al. Loss of histone H4K20 trimethylation occurs in preneoplasia and influences prognosis of non-small cell lung cancer. Clin Cancer Res. 2008;14:7237–45.
63. Tzao C, Tung HJ, Jin JS, Sun GH, Hsu HS, Chen BH, Yu CP, Lee SC. Prognostic significance of global histone modifications in resected squamous cell carcinoma of the esophagus. Mod Pathol. 2009;22:252–60.
64. Fiegl H, Elmasry K. Cancer diagnosis, risk assessment and prediction of therapeutic response by means of DNA methylation markers. Dis Markers. 2007;23:89–96.
65. Seligson DB, Horvath S, McBrian MA, et al. Global levels of histone modifications predict prognosis in different cancers. Am J Pathol. 2009;174:1619–28.
66. Yoo CB, Jones PA. Epigenetic therapy of cancer: past, present and future. Nat Rev Drug Discov. 2006;5:37–50.
67. Ducasse M, Brown M. Epigenetic aberrations and cancer. Mol Cancer. 2006;5:60.
68. Esteller M. Cancer epigenomics: DNA methylomes and histone-modification maps. Nat Rev Genet. 2007;8:286–98.
69. Wang Y, Fischle W, Cheung W, Jacobs S, Khorasanizadeh S, Allis CD. Beyond the double helix: writing and reading the histone code. Novartis Found Symp. 2004;259:3–17; discussion 17–21, 163–169.
70. Sadoul K, Boyault C, Pabion M, Khochbin S. Regulation of protein turnover by acetyltransferases and deacetylases. Biochimie. 2008;90:306–12.
71. Verdone L, Agricola E, Caserta M, Di Mauro E. Histone acetylation in gene regulation. Brief Funct Genomic Proteomic. 2006;5:209–21.
72. Santos-Rosa H, Caldas C. Chromatin modifier enzymes, the histone code and cancer. Eur J Cancer. 2005;41:2381–402.

73. Wang GG, Allis CD, Chi P. Chromatin remodeling and cancer, Part II: ATP-dependent chromatin remodeling. Trends Mol Med. 2007;13:373–80.
74. Lin H, Wong RP, Martinka M, Li G. Loss of SNF5 expression correlates with poor patient survival in melanoma. Clin Cancer Res. 2009;15:6404–11.
75. Wang X, Sansam CG, Thom CS, Metzger D, Evans JA, Nguyen PT, Roberts CW. Oncogenesis caused by loss of the SNF5 tumor suppressor is dependent on activity of BRG1, the ATPase of the SWI/SNF chromatin remodeling complex. Cancer Res. 2009;69:8094–101.
76. Fuks F, Hurd PJ, Wolf D, Nan X, Bird AP, Kouzarides T. The methyl-CpG-binding protein MeCP2 links DNA methylation to histone methylation. J Biol Chem. 2003;278:4035–40.
77. Yamada T, Fischle W, Sugiyama T, Allis CD, Grewal SI. The nucleation and maintenance of heterochromatin by a histone deacetylase in fission yeast. Mol Cell. 2005;20:173–85.
78. Tachibana M, Matsumura Y, Fukuda M, Kimura H, Shinkai Y. G9a/GLP complexes independently mediate H3K9 and DNA methylation to silence transcription. EMBO J. 2008;27:2681–90.
79. Link PA, Gangisetty O, James SR, Woloszynska-Read A, Tachibana M, Shinkai Y, Karpf AR. Distinct roles for histone methyltransferases G9a and GLP in cancer germ-line antigen gene regulation in human cancer cells and murine embryonic stem cells. Mol Cancer Res. 2009;7:851–62.
80. Kondo Y, Shen L, Cheng AS, et al. Gene silencing in cancer by histone H3 lysine 27 trimethylation independent of promoter DNA methylation. Nat Genet. 2008;40:741–50.
81. Bonazzi VF, Irwin D, Hayward NK. Identification of candidate tumor suppressor genes inactivated by promoter methylation in melanoma. Genes Chromosomes Cancer. 2009;48:10–21.
82. Minucci S, Pelicci PG. Histone deacetylase inhibitors and the promise of epigenetic (and more) treatments for cancer. Nat Rev Cancer. 2006;6:38–51.
83. Xu WS, Parmigiani RB, Marks PA. Histone deacetylase inhibitors: molecular mechanisms of action. Oncogene. 2007;26:5541–52.
84. Lin H, Chen C, Shuan L, Weng J, Chen C. Targeting histone deacetylase in cancer therapy. Med Res Rev. 2006;26:397–413.
85. Krämer OH, Zhu P, Ostendorff HP, et al. The histone deacetylase inhibitor valproic acid selectively induces proteasomal degradation of HDAC2. EMBO J. 2003;22:3411–20.
86. Li Q, Su A, Chen J, Lefebvre YA, Haché RJ. Attenuation of glucocorticoid signaling through targeted degradation of p300 via the 26s proteasome pathway. Mol Endocrinol. 2002;16:2819–27.
87. Qian DZ, Kato Y, Shabbeer S, Wei Y, Verheul HM, Salumbides B, Sanni T, Atadja P, Pili R. Targeting tumor angiogenesis with histone deacetylase inhibitors: the hydroxamic acid derivative LBH589. Clin Cancer Res. 2006;12:634–42.
88. Carew JS, Giles FJ, Nawrocki ST. Histone deacetylase inhibitors: mechanisms of cell death and promise in combination cancer therapy. Cancer Lett. 2008;269:7–17.
89. Magnaghi-Jaulin L, Eot-Houllier G, Fulcrand G, Jaulin C. Histone deacetylase inhibitors induce premature sister chromatid separation and override the mitotic spindle assembly checkpoint. Cancer Res. 2007;67:6360–7.
90. Shao Y, Gao Z, Marks PA, Jiang X. Apoptotic and autophagic cell death induced by histone deacetylase inhibitors. Proc Natl Acad Sci USA. 2004;101:18030–5.
91. Xu WS, Perez G, Ngo L, Gui CY, Marks PA. Induction of polyploidy by histone deacetylase inhibitor: a pathway for antitumor effects. Cancer Res. 2005;65:7832–9.
92. Hwang JJ, Kim YS, Kim MJ, Jang S, Lee JH, Choi J, Ro S, Hyun YL, Lee JS, Kim CS. A novel histone deacetylase inhibitor, CG0006, induces cell death through both extrinsic and intrinsic apoptotic pathways. Anticancer Drugs. 2009;20:815–21.
93. Lafon-Hughes L, Di Tomaso MV, Méndez-Acuña L, Martínez-López W. Chromatin-remodelling mechanisms in cancer. Mutat Res. 2008;658:191–214.
94. Rosato RR, Almenara JA, Dai Y, Grant S. Simultaneous activation of the intrinsic and extrinsic pathways by histone deacetylase (HDAC) inhibitors and tumor necrosis factor-related apoptosis-inducing ligand (TRAIL) synergistically induces mitochondrial damage and apoptosis in human leukemia cells. Mol Cancer Ther. 2003;2:1273–84.
95. Yang XJ, Seto E. HATs and HDACs: from structure, function and regulation to novel strategies for therapy and prevention. Oncogene. 2007;26:5310–8.
96. Boyle GM, Martyn AC, Parsons PG. Histone deacetylase inhibitors and malignant melanoma. Pigment Cell Res. 2005;18:160–6.
97. Akasaka K, Maesawa C, Shibazaki M, Maeda F, Takahashi K, Akasaka T, Masuda T. Loss of class III beta-tubulin induced by histone deacetylation is associated with chemosensitivity to paclitaxel in malignant melanoma cells. J Invest Dermatol. 2009;129:1516–26.
98. Epping MT, Wang L, Plumb JA, Lieb M, Gronemeyer H, Brown R, Bernards R. A functional genetic screen identifies retinoic acid signaling as a target of histone deacetylase inhibitors. Proc Natl Acad Sci USA. 2007;104:17777–82.
99. Steele N, Finn P, Brown R, Plumb JA. Combined inhibition of DNA methylation and histone acetylation enhances gene re-expression and drug sensitivity in vivo. Br J Cancer. 2009;100:758–63.
100. Daud AI, Dawson J, DeConti RC, et al. Potentiation of a topoisomerase I inhibitor, karenitecin, by the histone deacetylase inhibitor valproic acid in melanoma: translational and phase I/II clinical trial. Clin Cancer Res. 2009;15:2479–87.
101. Munster PN, Marchion D, Thomas S, et al. Phase I trial of vorinostat and doxorubicin in solid tumours:

histone deacetylase 2 expression as a predictive marker. Br J Cancer. 2009;101:1044–50.
102. Vo DD, Prins RM, Begley JL, et al. Enhanced antitumor activity induced by adoptive T-cell transfer and adjunctive use of the histone deacetylase inhibitor LAQ824. Cancer Res. 2009;69:8693–9.
103. Greiner D, Bonaldi T, Eskeland R, Roemer E, Imhof A. Identification of a specific inhibitor of the histone methyltransferase SU(VAR)3-9. Nat Chem Biol. 2005;1:143–5.
104. Kubicek S, O'Sullivan RJ, August EM, et al. Reversal of H3K9me2 by a small-molecule inhibitor for the G9a histone methyltransferase. Mol Cell. 2007;25:473–81.
105. Fiskus W, Wang Y, Sreekumar A, et al. Combined epigenetic therapy with the histone methyltransferase EZH2 inhibitor 3-deazaneplanocin A and the histone deacetylase inhibitor panobinostat against human AML cells. Blood. 2009;114:2733–43.
106. Tan J, Yang X, Zhuang L, Jiang X, Chen W, Lee PL, Karuturi RK, Tan PB, Liu ET, Yu Q. Pharmacologic disruption of Polycomb-repressive complex 2-mediated gene repression selectively induces apoptosis in cancer cells. Genes Dev. 2007;21:1050–63.
107. Miranda TB, Cortez CC, Yoo CB, Liang G, Abe M, Kelly TK, Marquez VE, Jones PA. DZNep is a global histone methylation inhibitor that reactivates developmental genes not silenced by DNA methylation. Mol Cancer Ther. 2009;8:1579–88.
108. Doyon Y, Selleck W, Lane WS, Tan S, Côté J. Structural and functional conservation of the NuA4 histone acetyltransferase complex from yeast to humans. Mol Cell Biol. 2004;24:1884–96.
109. Doyon Y, Cayrou C, Ullah M, Landry AJ, Côté V, Selleck W, Lane WS, Tan S, Yang XJ, Côté J. ING tumor suppressor proteins are critical regulators of chromatin acetylation required for genome expression and perpetuation. Mol Cell. 2006;21:51–64.
110. Li J, Martinka M, Li G. Role of ING4 in human melanoma cell migration, invasion and patient survival. Carcinogenesis. 2008;29:1373–9.
111. Wang Y, Dai DL, Martinka M, Li G. Prognostic significance of nuclear ING3 expression in human cutaneous melanoma. Clin Cancer Res. 2007;13:4111–6.
112. Baek SH, Ohgi KA, Rose DW, Koo EH, Glass CK, Rosenfeld MG. Exchange of N-CoR corepressor and Tip60 coactivator complexes links gene expression by NF-kappaB and beta-amyloid precursor protein. Cell. 2002;110:55–67.
113. Contzler R, Regamey A, Favre B, Roger T, Hohl D, Huber M. Histone acetyltransferase HBO1 inhibits NF-kappaB activity by coactivator sequestration. Biochem Biophys Res Commun. 2006;350:208–13.
114. Calao M, Burny A, Quivy V, Dekoninck A, Van Lint C. A pervasive role of histone acetyltransferases and deacetylases in an NF-kappaB-signaling code. Trends Biochem Sci. 2008;33:339–49.
115. Frank SR, Parisi T, Taubert S, Fernandez P, Fuchs M, Chan HM, Livingston DM, Amati B. MYC recruits the TIP60 histone acetyltransferase complex to chromatin. EMBO Rep. 2003;4:575–80.
116. Patel JH, Du Y, Ard PG, et al. The c-MYC oncoprotein is a substrate of the acetyltransferases hGCN5/PCAF and TIP60. Mol Cell Biol. 2004;24:10826–34.
117. Hussein MR, Haemel AK, Wood GS. Apoptosis and melanoma: molecular mechanisms. J Pathol. 2003;199:275–88.
118. Ryu B, Kim DS, Deluca AM, Alani RM. Comprehensive expression profiling of tumor cell lines identifies molecular signatures of melanoma progression. PLoS One. 2007;2:e594.
119. Zhuang D, Mannava S, Grachtchouk V, et al. C-MYC overexpression is required for continuous suppression of oncogene-induced senescence in melanoma cells. Oncogene. 2008;27:6623–34.
120. Ueda Y, Richmond A. NF-kappaB activation in melanoma. Pigment Cell Res. 2006;19:112–24.
121. Treszl A, Adány R, Rákosy Z, Kardos L, Bégány A, Gilde K, Balázs M. Extra copies of c-myc are more pronounced in nodular melanomas than in superficial spreading melanomas as revealed by fluorescence in situ hybridisation. Cytometry B Clin Cytom. 2004;60:37–46.
122. Schlagbauer-Wadl H, Griffioen M, van Elsas A, et al. Influence of increased c-Myc expression on the growth characteristics of human melanoma. J Invest Dermatol. 1999;112:332–6.
123. Bhoumik A, Singha N, O'Connell MJ, Ronai ZA. Regulation of TIP60 by ATF2 modulates ATM activation. J Biol Chem. 2008;283:17605–14.
124. Bhoumik A, Ronai Z. ATF2: a transcription factor that elicits oncogenic or tumor suppressor activities. Cell Cycle. 2008;7:2341–5.
125. Bhoumik A, Huang TG, Ivanov V, Gangi L, Qiao RF, Woo SL, Chen SH, Ronai Z. An ATF2-derived peptide sensitizes melanomas to apoptosis and inhibits their growth and metastasis. J Clin Invest. 2002;110:643–50.
126. Sakuraba K, Yasuda T, Sakata M, et al. Down-regulation of Tip60 gene as a potential marker for the malignancy of colorectal cancer. Anticancer Res. 2009;29:3953–5.
127. Garraway LA, Widlund HR, Rubin MA, et al. Integrative genomic analyses identify MITF as a lineage survival oncogene amplified in malignant melanoma. Nature. 2005;436:117–22.
128. Sato S, Roberts K, Gambino G, Cook A, Kouzarides T, Goding CR. CBP/p300 as a co factor for the Microphthalmia transcription factor. Oncogene. 1997;14:3083–92.
129. Price ER, Ding HF, Badalian T, Bhattacharya S, Takemoto C, Yao TP, Hemesath TJ, Fisher DE. Lineage-specific signaling in melanocytes C-kit stimulation recruits p300/CBP to microphthalmia. J Biol Chem. 1998;273:17983–6.
130. Dynek JN, Chan SM, Liu J, Zha J, Fairbrother WJ, Vucic D. Microphthalmia-associated transcription factor is a critical transcriptional regulator of melanoma inhibitor of apoptosis in melanomas. Cancer Res. 2008;68:3124–32.

131. Lomas J, Martin-Duque P, Pons M, Quintanilla M. The genetics of malignant melanoma. Front Biosci. 2008;13:5071–93.
132. Ugurel S, Houben R, Schrama D, Voigt H, Zapatka M, Schadendorf D, Bröcker EB, Becker JC. Microphthalmia-associated transcription factor gene amplification in metastatic melanoma is a prognostic marker for patient survival, but not a predictive marker for chemosensitivity and chemotherapy response. Clin Cancer Res. 2007;13:6344–50.
133. Bandyopadhyay D, Okan NA, Bales E, Nascimento L, Cole PA, Medrano EE. Down-regulation of p300/CBP histone acetyltransferase activates a senescence checkpoint in human melanocytes. Cancer Res. 2002;62:6231–9.
134. Ko SI, Lee IS, Kim JY, Kim SM, Kim DW, Lee KS, Woo KM, Baek JH, Choo JK, Seo SB. Regulation of histone acetyltransferase activity of p300 and PCAF by proto-oncogene protein DEK. FEBS Lett. 2006;580:3217–22.
135. Khodadoust MS, Verhaegen M, Kappes F, et al. Melanoma proliferation and chemoresistance controlled by the DEK oncogene. Cancer Res. 2009;69:6405–13.
136. Shankar S, Srivastava RK. Histone deacetylase inhibitors: mechanisms and clinical significance in cancer. HDAC inhibitor-induced apoptosis. Adv Exp Med Biol. 2008;615:261–98.
137. Ocker M, Schneider-Stock R. Histone deacetylase inhibitors: signalling towards p21cip1/waf1. Int J Biochem Cell Biol. 2007;39:1367–74.
138. Pulukuri SM, Gorantla B, Rao JS. Inhibition of histone deacetylase activity promotes invasion of human cancer cells through activation of urokinase plasminogen activator. J Biol Chem. 2007;282:35594–603.
139. Mottet D, Castronovo V. Histone deacetylases: target enzymes for cancer therapy. Clin Exp Metastasis. 2008;25:183–9.
140. Gallinari P, Di Marco S, Jones P, Pallaoro M, Steinkühler C. HDACs, histone deacetylation and gene transcription: from molecular biology to cancer therapeutics. Cell Res. 2007;17:195–211.
141. Bandyopadhyay D, Curry JL, Lin Q, Richards HW, Chen D, Hornsby PJ, Timchenko NA, Medrano EE. Dynamic assembly of chromatin complexes during cellular senescence: implications for the growth arrest of human melanocytic nevi. Aging Cell. 2007;6:577–91.
142. Cicek M, Fukuyama R, Cicek MS, Sizemore S, Welch DR, Sizemore N, Casey G. BRMS1 contributes to the negative regulation of uPA gene expression through recruitment of HDAC1 to the NF-kappaB binding site of the uPA promoter. Clin Exp Metastasis. 2009;26:229–37.
143. Lacreusette A, Nguyen JM, Pandolfino MC, Khammari A, Dreno B, Jacques Y, Godard A, Blanchard F. Loss of oncostatin M receptor beta in metastatic melanoma cells. Oncogene. 2007;26:881–92.
144. Lacreusette A, Lartigue A, Nguyen JM, et al. Relationship between responsiveness of cancer cells to Oncostatin M and/or IL-6 and survival of stage III melanoma patients treated with tumour-infiltrating lymphocytes. J Pathol. 2008;216:451–9.
145. Deng G, Kakar S, Okudiara K, Choi E, Sleisenger MH, Kim YS. Unique methylation pattern of oncostatin m receptor gene in cancers of colorectum and other digestive organs. Clin Cancer Res. 2009;15:1519–26.
146. Amente S, Bertoni A, Morano A, Lania L, Avvedimento EV, Majello B. LSD1-mediated demethylation of histone H3 lysine 4 triggers Myc-induced transcription. Oncogene. 2010;29:3691–702.
147. Sauvageau M, Sauvageau G. Polycomb group genes: keeping stem cell activity in balance. PLoS Biol. 2008;6:e113.
148. Schwartz YB, Pirrotta V. Polycomb silencing mechanisms and the management of genomic programmes. Nat Rev Genet. 2007;8:9–22.
149. Varambally S, Dhanasekaran SM, Zhou M, et al. The polycomb group protein EZH2 is involved in progression of prostate cancer. Nature. 2002;419:624–9.
150. Simon JA, Lange CA. Roles of the EZH2 histone methyltransferase in cancer epigenetics. Mutat Res. 2008;647:21–9.
151. Zeidler M, Kleer CG. The Polycomb group protein Enhancer of Zeste 2: its links to DNA repair and breast cancer. J Mol Histol. 2006;37:219–23.
152. Yoon KA, Gil HJ, Han J, Park J, Lee JS. Genetic polymorphisms in the polycomb group gene EZH2 and the risk of lung cancer. J Thorac Oncol. 2010;5:10–6.
153. Gazin C, Wajapeyee N, Gobeil S, Virbasius CM, Green MR. An elaborate pathway required for Ras-mediated epigenetic silencing. Nature. 2007;449:1073–7.
154. Fujii S, Ito K, Ito Y, Ochiai A. Enhancer of zeste homologue 2 (EZH2) down-regulates RUNX3 by increasing histone H3 methylation. J Biol Chem. 2008;283:17324–32.
155. Yang X, Karuturi RK, Sun F, Aau M, Yu K, Shao R, Miller LD, Tan PB, Yu Q. CDKN1C (p57) is a direct target of EZH2 and suppressed by multiple epigenetic mechanisms in breast cancer cells. PLoS One. 2009;4:e5011.
156. Wang S, Robertson GP, Zhu J. A novel human homologue of *Drosophila* polycomblike gene is up-regulated in multiple cancers. Gene. 2004;343:69–78.
157. Ambros V. The functions of animal microRNAs. Nature. 2004;431:350–5.
158. Bartel DP. MicroRNAs: genomics, biogenesis, mechanism, and function. Cell. 2004;116:281–97.
159. Lee RC, Feinbaum RL, Ambros V. The C. elegans heterochronic gene lin-4 encodes small RNAs with antisense complementarity to lin-14. Cell. 1993;75:843–54.

160. Reinhart BJ, Slack FJ, Basson M, Pasquinelli AE, Bettinger JC, Rougvie AE, Horvitz HR, Ruvkun G. The 21-nucleotide let-7 RNA regulates developmental timing in Caenorhabditis elegans. Nature. 2000;403:901–6.
161. Krützfeldt J, Rajewsky N, Braich R, Rajeev KG, Tuschl T, Manoharan M, Stoffel M. Silencing of microRNAs in vivo with 'antagomirs'. Nature. 2005;438:685–9.
162. Lim LP, Lau NC, Garrett-Engele P, Grimson A, Schelter JM, Castle J, Bartel DP, Linsley PS, Johnson JM. Microarray analysis shows that some microRNAs downregulate large numbers of target mRNAs. Nature. 2005;433:769–73.
163. Sood P, Krek A, Zavolan M, Macino G, Rajewsky N. Cell-type-specific signatures of microRNAs on target mRNA expression. Proc Natl Acad Sci USA. 2006;103:2746–51.
164. Molnár V, Tamási V, Bakos B, Wiener Z, Falus A. Changes in miRNA expression in solid tumors: an miRNA profiling in melanomas. Semin Cancer Biol. 2008;18:111–22.
165. Kim VN. MicroRNA biogenesis: coordinated cropping and dicing. Nat Rev Mol Cell Biol. 2005;6:376–85.
166. Kosik KS, Krichevsky AM. The elegance of the microRNAs: a neuronal perspective. Neuron. 2005;47:779–82.
167. Lee Y, Ahn C, Han J, Choi H, Kim J, Yim J, Lee J, Provost P, Rådmark O, Kim S, Kim VN. The nuclear RNase III Drosha initiates microRNA processing. Nature. 2003;425:415–9.
168. Denli AM, Tops BB, Plasterk RH, Ketting RF, Hannon GJ. Processing of primary microRNAs by the Microprocessor complex. Nature. 2004;432:231–5.
169. Hammond SM, Bernstein E, Beach D, Hannon GJ. An RNA-directed nuclease mediates post-transcriptional gene silencing in *Drosophila* cells. Nature. 2000;404:293–6.
170. Chen C, Ridzon DA, Broomer AJ, et al. Real-time quantification of microRNAs by stem-loop RT-PCR. Nucleic Acids Res. 2005;33:e179.
171. Takamizawa J, Konishi H, Yanagisawa K, et al. Reduced expression of the let-7 microRNAs in human lung cancers in association with shortened postoperative survival. Cancer Res. 2004;64:3753–6.
172. Li LC, Okino ST, Zhao H, Pookot D, Place RF, Urakami S, Enokida H, Dahiya R. Small dsRNAs induce transcriptional activation in human cells. Proc Natl Acad Sci USA. 2006;103:17337–42.
173. Ørom UA, Nielsen FC, Lund AH. MicroRNA-10a binds the 5'UTR of ribosomal protein mRNAs and enhances their translation. Mol Cell. 2008;30:460–71.
174. Gaur A, Jewell DA, Liang Y, Ridzon D, Moore JH, Chen C, Ambros VR, Israel MA. Characterization of microRNA expression levels and their biological correlates in human cancer cell lines. Cancer Res. 2007;67:2456–68.
175. Lu J, Getz G, Miska EA, et al. MicroRNA expression profiles classify human cancers. Nature. 2007;435:834–8.
176. Zhang L, Huang J, Yang N, et al. MicroRNAs exhibit high frequency genomic alterations in human cancer. Proc Natl Acad Sci USA. 2006;103:9136–41.
177. Croce CM, Calin GA. miRNAs, cancer, and stem cell division. Cell. 2005;122:6–7.
178. Gregory RI, Shiekhattar R. MicroRNA biogenesis and cancer. Cancer Res. 2005;65:3509–12.
179. Calin GA, Sevignani C, Dumitru CD, et al. Human microRNA genes are frequently located at fragile sites and genomic regions involved in cancers. Proc Natl Acad Sci USA. 2004;101:2999–3004.
180. McManus MT. MicroRNAs and cancer. Semin Cancer Biol. 2003;13:253–8.
181. Johnson SM, Grosshans H, Shingara J, et al. RAS is regulated by the let-7 microRNA family. Cell. 2005;120:635–47.
182. Cimmino A, Calin GA, Fabbri M, et al. miR-15 and miR-16 induce apoptosis by targeting BCL2. Proc Natl Acad Sci USA. 2005;102:13944–9.
183. O'Donnell KA, Wentzel EA, Zeller KI, Dang CV, Mendell JT. c-Myc-regulated microRNAs modulate E2F1 expression. Nature. 2005;435:839–43.
184. He L, Thomson JM, Hemann MT, et al. A microRNA polycistron as a potential human oncogene. Nature. 2005;435:828–33.
185. Hayashita Y, Osada H, Tatematsu Y, et al. A polycistronic microRNA cluster, miR-17-92, is overexpressed in human lung cancers and enhances cell proliferation. Cancer Res. 2005;65:9628–32.
186. Voorhoeve PM, le Sage C, Schrier M, et al. A genetic screen implicates miRNA-372 and miRNA-373 as oncogenes in testicular germ cell tumors. Cell. 2006;124:1169–81.
187. Levy C, Khaled M, Fisher DE. MITF: master regulator of melanocyte development and melanoma oncogene. Trends Mol Med. 2006;12:406–14.
188. Müller DW, Bosserhoff AK. Integrin beta 3 expression is regulated by let-7a miRNA in malignant melanoma. Oncogene. 2008;27:6698–706.
189. Schultz J, Lorenz P, Gross G, Ibrahim S, Kunz M. MicroRNA let-7b targets important cell cycle molecules in malignant melanoma cells and interferes with anchorage-independent growth. Cell Res. 2008;18:549–57.
190. Müller DW, Bosserhoff A. Role of miRNAs in the progression of malignant melanoma. Br J Cancer. 2009;101:551–6.
191. Müller DW, Rehli M, Bosserhoff AK. miRNA expression profiling in melanocyte and melanoma cell lines reveals miRNAs associated with formation and progression of malignant melanoma. J Invest Dermatol. 2009;129:1740–51.
192. Saito Y, Liang G, Egger G, Friedman JM, Chuang JC, Coetzee GA, Jones PA. Specific activation of microRNA-127 with downregulation of the proto-oncogene BCL6 by chromatin-modifying drugs in human cancer cells. Cancer Cell. 2006;9:435–43.

193. Meng F, Wehbe-Janek H, Henson R, Smith H, Patel T. Epigenetic regulation of microRNA-370 by interleukin-6 in malignant human cholangiocytes. Oncogene. 2007;27:378–86.
194. Brueckner B, Stresemann C, Kuner R, Mund C, Musch T, Meister M, Sültmann H, Lyko F. The human let-7a-3 locus contains an epigenetically regulated microRNA gene with oncogenic function. Cancer Res. 2007;67:1419–23.
195. Felicetti F, Errico MC, Bottero L, et al. The promyelocytic leukemia zinc finger-microRNA-221/-222 pathway controls melanoma progression through multiple oncogenic mechanisms. Cancer Res. 2008;68:2745–54.
196. Sigalotti L, Covre A, Fratta E, et al. Epigenetics of human cutaneous melanoma: setting the stage for new therapeutic strategies. J Transl Med. 2010;8:56.

MicroRNA Biomarkers in Melanoma

Jim Kozubek, Faseeha Altaf, and Soheil Sam Dadras

Introduction

The frontiers of cell science are a *terra incognita*. At least some of the protein function(s) of cells and the systems biology that are emerging have been traced to single base changes in the genome, single nucleotide polymorphisms, or more rare mutations that help to explain functional alterations in the bustling life of a cancer cell. However, even the most ambitious genome-wide association studies have, in most cases, failed to adequately explain complex traits or the underpinnings of pathology, placing in doubt the dogma of the "common-disease, common-variant" hypothesis – a theory that the commonality of some diseases must imply a common set of identifiable triggers. It has long been presumed that these triggers would be visible at the level of the DNA template. Only recently, a paradigm shift has begun to emerge in genetics. New discoveries are proving that epigenetics and noncoding RNA (ncRNA) account for a level of regulatory control that can evade detection in simple examinations of the DNA template. Such regulatory changes routinely "put the slip" on cancer investigators who are focused exclusively on gene mutations and/or single nucleotide polymorphisms. In fact, exploration of these furtive systems under ncRNA control is revealing new access points into the genome, and may provide a "torch" to reveal the mechanistic changes in some of the darkest pathologies of cancer cells.

Cancers of the skin are the most common of all cancers. Melanoma is a cancer that arises from the melanocytes or the pigment-producing cells of the skin. Trends show the worldwide prevalence of melanoma has risen over the past three decades, dissimilar to other cancer types. In fact, melanoma incidence is increasing faster than any other form of cancer in the United States, and it is now the sixth most common form of cancer diagnosed in this country. Though not the most common form of skin cancer, melanoma is the most serious and, by far, one of the deadliest. The National Cancer Institute estimated 68,120 newly identified melanoma cases and 8,700 deaths from melanoma in 2010 [1].

A number of studies have identified potential risk factors for melanoma development. Risk factors vary by skin type and include patient age, prior personal and family medical histories, and increased frequency or presence of atypical melanocytic nevi. Ultraviolet (UV) radiation exposure is the major environmental factor contributing to melanoma incidence. A higher incidence of

J. Kozubek, M.S.
Department of Genetics and Developmental Biology,
University of Connecticut Health Center,
Farmington, CT, USA

F. Altaf, B.S.
University of Connecticut (Storrs campus),
Storrs, CT, USA

S.S. Dadras, M.D., Ph.D. (✉)
Departments of Dermatology and Genetics and
Developmental Biology, University of Connecticut
Health Center, Farmington, CT, USA
e-mail: dadras@uchc.edu

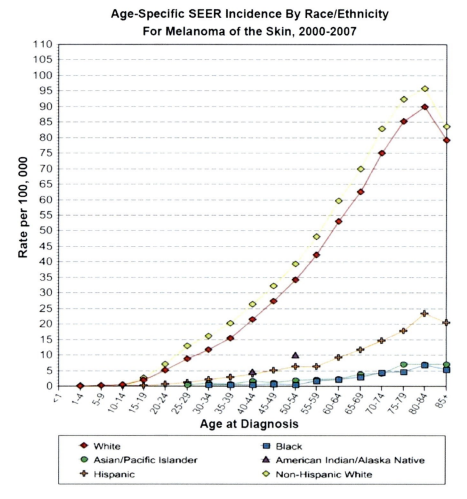

Fig. 9.1 Age-specific incidence of melanoma in the United States distinguished by race. These results show an age-dependent increase in the incidence of melanoma in non-Hispanic white, white and Hispanic individuals of both sexes in the United States from 2000 to 2007. Data source is Surveillance, Epidemiology and End Results (*SEER*, http://seer.cancer.gov/). Cancer sites include invasive cases. Incidence source is SEER 17 areas (San Francisco, Connecticut, Detroit, Hawaii, Iowa, New Mexico, Seattle, Utah, Atlanta, San Jose-Monterey, Los Angeles, Alaska Native Registry, Rural Georgia, Kentucky, Louisiana, New Jersey, and California excluding SF/SJM/LA). Hispanics and non-Hispanics are not mutually exclusive from whites, blacks, Asian/Pacific Islanders, and American Indians/Alaska Natives

melanoma is reported in fair-skinned people. Furthermore, epidemiological analysis suggests gender and genetics also affect melanoma incidence. According to the American Cancer Society, the occurrence of melanoma in whites is more than ten times the incidence in African Americans. These results show an age-dependent increase in the incidence of melanoma in non-Hispanic white, white and even Hispanic individuals of both sexes in the United States from 2000 to 2007 (Fig. 9.1). In fact, recent studies demonstrate an increase in melanoma incidence among Hispanics in California [2] and Florida [3].

Indeed, melanoma results from complex etiologies and deregulation of cell functions with disparate origins (Fig. 9.2). A few of these origins have been well characterized and, for the purposes of discussion, we can consider one of the most well-known causes of initiation: overexposure to ambient sunlight. The sun's warm rays can be inviting, but sunlight also contains UV radiation that can damage DNA, particularly in keratinocytes,

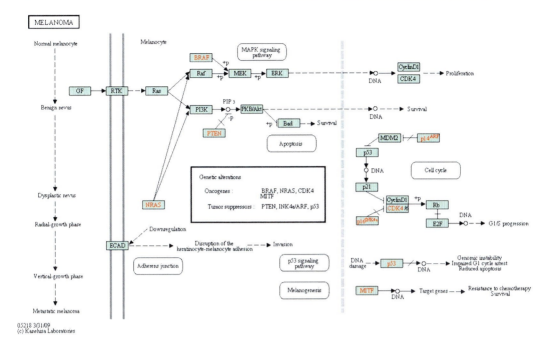

Fig. 9.2 Summary of known molecular pathways in melanoma. This pathway summary is obtained from KEGG pathway program. Melanoma arises from the malignant transformation of pigment-producing cells, melanocytes. The only known environmental risk factor is exposure to ultraviolet (*UV*) radiation. In addition, people with fair skin are at increased risk. Melanoma pathogenesis is also driven by genetic factors. Oncogenic NRAS mutations activate both Raf-MEK-ERK and PI3K-Akt effector pathways. The Raf-MEK-ERK pathway may also be activated via mutations in the BRAF gene. The PI3K-Akt pathway may also be activated through loss or mutation of the inhibitory tumor suppressor gene PTEN. These mutations arise early in melanoma pathogenesis and are preserved throughout tumor progression. Melanoma development has been shown to be strongly associated with inactivation of the p16INK4a/cyclin-dependent kinases 4 and 6/retinoblastoma protein (p16INK4a/CDK4,6/pRb) and p14ARF/human double minute 2/p53 (p14ARF/HDM2/p53) tumor suppressor pathways. MITF and TP53 are further implicated in melanoma progression

through the induction of pyrimidine-pyrimidine dimers. The TP53 gene has many roles, one of which is to activate $p21^{cip/WAF1}$, a cyclin-dependent kinase inhibitor, in response to DNA damage and thereby arrest the cell cycle or trigger cell death by apoptosis (programmed cell death) [2]. The DNA mismatch repair apparatus can help out by self-editing the pyrimidine dimers. However, these governing genes are not impregnable to sun damage. UV-induced mutations that occur in the TP53 or DNA damage repair genes themselves can prevent skin cells from repair or apoptosis. Skin cells exposed to sunlight over a prolonged duration are often more resistant to apoptosis and die at a slower rate due to compromised TP53 or DNA repair genes. More mutations are permitted to accumulate in skin cells (epidermal keratinocytes and melanocytes), as they continue to divide.

Melanoma can present as cutaneous, mucosal, or ocular in origin. In fact, four major types of cutaneous melanoma exist. From most frequent to least common, these four major types are: (1) superficial spreading melanoma, (2) nodular melanoma, (3) lentigo maligna melanoma, and (4) acrolentiginous melanoma. Following diagnosis, the melanoma is staged based on the histopathologic parameters of the primary tumor (i.e., tumor thickness, ulceration and mitotic index) and the status of the sentinel lymph node, as defined by the American Joint Committee on Cancer [3]. Treatment options vary by type, by stage, and by location of the tumor. Recognition of early and localized melanoma allows for cure by surgery. Metastatic melanoma, on the contrary, can be lethal. Regionally and distantly spread melanomas show high resistance to current treatment modalities. Therefore, a capacity to diagnose melanoma before it reaches a metastatic stage and the development of exceptionally potent drugs to combat metastatic disease remain enduring translational goals within melanoma research. To date, physicians make diagnostic and prognostic evaluations that are based on biopsies which provide microscopic evidence of melanoma and its histopathologic prognostic parameters. However, evaluations based on ostensive qualities in biopsied tissues can be an inaccurate science in some cases. In addition, accurate prognostic biomarkers are currently lacking. Only in the past decade have scientists discovered and are now beginning to learn how to exploit a novel intrinsic regulatory mechanism in the genome for the purpose of making diagnoses and combating melanoma.

Overview of microRNAs

RNA interference (RNAi) explains how endogenous ncRNA molecules are processed by a series of enzymes called Drosha, DGCR8 and DICER into final mature forms of just 18–23 nucleotides in length [4]. These small ncRNA molecules, called microRNA (miRNA), can latch onto messenger RNA (mRNA) under the guardianship of a multiprotein complex called the RNA –Induced Silencing Complex (RISC), and degrade or disrupt their translation into protein. This newly discovered mechanism of miRNA regulation is helping to clarify our understanding of a major conundrum in genomics – namely, how an organism can be so complex while relying on so few genes. miRNA regulation also has implications for research into complex disease states, including melanoma.

Recent research efforts show miRNA molecules to be associated with melanoma progression and the development of metastasis. miRNAs spring from introns and intragenic regions, shadowy facets of the genome that were once considered mere scaffolding by some, and even "junk DNA" by others. These molecules are generated in a precursor form as short hairpins, up to 140 nucleotides in length, before undergoing processing into short, single-stranded RNA molecules.

The "loop" and unused arm, or "star" arm, of the precursor molecule are degraded by enzymes that naturally dispose of single-stranded RNA molecules adrift in the cytoplasm. The "mature" arm, averaging 22 nucleotides in length and containing a critical 7 nucleotide "seed" region, is placed under RISC guardianship. The RISC binds the mature arm to a complementary region on a 3′-untranslated region (UTR) of an mRNA transcript, resulting in degradation, or "silencing," of the transcript, and preventing it from ever translating into a protein. Therefore, the complementary binding of miRNAs to UTRs represses translation and inhibits gene expression. In fact, a prevailing theory on their origin suggests that miRNAs emerged as a mechanism to shut down exogenous double-stranded RNA viruses, but later became incorporated as a means to enhance the regulatory complexity of the genome. It should come as no surprise that miRNAs are proving to play critical roles in the homeostasis of cellular life, while the recognition of pervasive deregulation of miRNA in cancers is a rapidly emerging research field. miRNAs have the potential to be clinically relevant biomarkers in both early- and late-stage melanomas. In the future, miRNAs may have important diagnostic [5] and prognostic [6] applications with regard to melanoma, and represent therapeutic targets in this disease.

microRNAs as Novel Therapeutics

Consider that therapeutic drugs are typically classified as one of two types. One type is targeted therapy in which the introduction of a drug, such as the ATP-blocker Gleevec®, can inhibit biosynthesis or "gum up" a pathway. A second type of therapeutic agent summons the power of innate systems within the body, like a leviathan to fight disease. An example of the latter type of strategy would be the employment of an antibody or adjuvant to stimulate the host immune system to use its own organic defense systems to ward off a disease. RNAi, via the triggering of miRNAs, is being actively investigated as an emerging prospect in this second class of therapeutics. It should be noted that many technical limitations are emerging. The first of which is accurate identification of miRNA targets. The short stature of miRNAs is an intrinsic property that enables these molecules to target theoretically hundreds of genes. Web-based algorithms, such as PicTar and TargetScan, identify hundreds of theoretical gene targets based on sequence complementarity between a miRNA and the 3'-UTRs of mRNA transcripts. Therefore, the broad efficacy of miRNAs can enable them to control entire gene networks and other properties, such as "cell-to-cell adherence", if not "invasiveness," making them particularly attractive triggers for evaluating cancer progression. miRNAs can function like a skeleton key, opening an entire isle of prison doors with one turn. However, the ubiquity of their targets also remains a prevailing paradox in this field, since the worm ball of targets and pathways that any given miRNA may influence is difficult to untangle. Furthermore, the use of *in vivo* models to modulate miRNA represents a cautious exercise, since the potential to regulate an entire cell network is a power not to be taken lightly. To date, most research has centered on cell cultures and mouse tumor models. miRNA levels may be artificially induced with viral vectors and silenced with "antagomirs," exogenous single-stranded RNA that can now be procured from a small number of start-up companies. Thus, researchers typically employ quantitative real-time polymerase chain reaction (qRT-PCR) to quantify the expression level(s) of miRNA in cultured primary cells or cell lines, and then use a gene expression profiling method to identify potential targets. Once a researcher narrows hundreds of computational targets down to a few that appear to be under the influence of a deregulated miRNA, the researcher typically mutates or deletes the 3'-UTR of the mRNA transcript and expresses it ectopically in a cell line. Rescuing of the target mRNA usually indicates that a key target gene has been identified. In any case, the quantification of miRNA expression and identification of target genes employs a principle called "consistency," that is used to decipher relationships between molecules.

Questions remain regarding the reliability and accuracy of cultured cell lines to extrapolate diagnostic profiles of miRNA in the context of a given organism. Several studies, including work in our own laboratory, have shown disparities between miRNA expression patterns in established melanoma cell lines and melanoma tissue samples. Recently, some researchers have begun to use archival formalin-fixed, paraffin-embedded (FFPE) tissue samples as RNA sources, replete with a history of clinical information, in an effort to profile miRNA content. Formalin fixation with paraffin embedding is a process of preserving tissue samples in a waxed state and generally breaks up longer RNA molecules, such as mRNA. Seminal work in this area has proven that miRNAs consistently survive this process and the use of FFPE tissue to produce miRNA profiles is now considered a *fait accompli* [7, 8]. Use of FFPE human tissue samples should provide a more relevant biomarker discovery platform to construct miRNA signatures that more closely reflect disease progression. Due to the complexity of the networks that miRNAs influence, initial uses of the now ~2,000 human miRNAs discovered would most likely be diagnostic and/or prognostic in nature.

microRNA Nomenclature

Prior to a review of some recent findings, a short primer on miRNA nomenclature is in order. miRNAs are generally introduced by number, such as hsa-miR-101, where "hsa" refers to the genus and species, *Homo sapiens*. If dropped, in the case of miR-101, it is implied to refer to humans. The number typically indicates the order of discovery, such that miR-101 was identified prior to miR-201. The earliest miRNAs to be discovered are members of the let-7 family and are referred to with a "let" rather than "miR" prefix. Both "let" and "lin" are idiosyncratic prefixes that have been preserved from the earliest days of miRNA taxonomy. As the naming system progressed, miRNAs were named according to both function and location. miR-17-5p, miR-18a and miR-20a are all members of the miR-17-92 cluster and spring from the same genomic region. However, miRNAs often spring from more than one place in the genome, and antecedent numbers such as miR-194-1 and miR-194-2 are used to denote this. In addition, miRNAs with closely related function(s) can be denoted by letters, as is the case with the miR-200a, miR-200b and miR-200c family. Sometimes mature miRNA can spring from opposite ends of the same precursor molecule, thereby gaining a directional distinction, as in miR-142-3p and miR-142-5p. In some cases, the mature arm of the precursor molecule is not always the functional component – sometimes it is degraded, while the star arm is guarded by RISC; for example, miR-123*.

Deregulated microRNAs in Melanoma

Let's now turn to some examples of emerging miRNA profiles in melanoma. The expression of let-7a, a founding member of the let-7 family, has been shown to be down-regulated in melanoma cell lines compared to ordinary, primary melanocyte cell lines [9]. In fact, computational analysis places let-7a in sequence complementarity with the 3'-UTR of integrin β_3 mRNA, a precursor to a protein that is an essential component in the construction of vitronectin receptors. These receptors are built under the command of the Raf-MEK-extracellular signal-regulated kinase (ERK) signaling pathway and have a role in actin fiber organization and anchorage of cells to the extracellular matrix. Transfection of cell lines with exogenous let-7a molecules results in down-regulation of integrin β_3. In contrast, the introduction of a let-7a antagomir leads to up-regulation of the integrin β_3 gene and promotes the invasive capacity of melanocytes. Thus, let-7a represents a "trigger" on a pathway with a confirmed role in anchorage independence and migration. Let-7b, a close family member, plays a role in extracellular matrix integrity, compromising it. The let-7b molecule has been shown to regulate a transcript that encodes Basigin, an inducer of a metalloproteinase which degrades the extracellular matrix [10]. Transfection of murine melanoma cells with let-7b results in reduced cellular migration and metastasis (i.e., more let-7b is associated with less metalloproteinase). The implication is that healthy skin melanocytes require a basal level of let-7a and let-7b to uphold extracellular matrix integrity, and melanomas can reduce the levels of these miRNAs as a mechanism for tissue invasion. Furthermore, let-7b interferes with cellular proliferation and colony formation (anchorage-independent growth) in melanoma cell lines [11]. These data reinforce the tumor suppressive functions of both let-7a and let-7b.

In a few striking instances, miRNAs appear to unilaterally control cellular properties. According to Glud et al. [12], the addition of exogenous miR-125b to human metastatic melanoma cell lines resulted in the induction of cellular senescence. This indicates that miR-125b is apt to be down-regulated in melanoma. Indeed, predicted targets of miR-125b include the E2F family of proteins, which are overexpressed in melanoma and regulate the $p16^{CDKN2A}$ pathway, the latter implicated in cellular senescence and cell cycle arrest (Fig. 9.1). In addition, miR-125b expression levels show an inverse correlation with Akt3/Protein Kinase B, a kinase that is associated with more aggressive melanomas; at high levels promoting cell survival, cell proliferation and anti-apoptosis effects. Follow-up work by Glud et al. [13], using archival FFPE samples, proved that miR-125b expression levels are reduced in metastatic melanomas compared to primary melanomas, suggesting that it could be useful biomarker for metastatic progression. Along a similar line, miR-205 was shown to undergo substantial down-regulation in melanoma tissue samples, archival FFPE samples and cell lines [14, 15]; being connected thus far to E2F1, one of the most well studied and prolific cell cycle transcription factors.

Many other miRNAs are being connected to cell cycle regulation in melanoma. Itself a target of an interferon (IFN)-β-mediated exoribonuclease, miR-221 has been shown to be a regulator of the cyclin-dependent kinase inhibitor $p27^{kip1}$, with down-regulation of miR-221 found to be related to its metastatic effects as a result of this cell cycle connection [16]. One study used qRT-PCR analysis of melanocytes and melanoma cell lines to determine that miR-146a, miR-146b and miR-155 undergo down-regulation in melanoma cell lines, while miR-17-5p, miR-18a and miR-20a (encoded through the miR-17-92 cluster) were up-regulated [17]. Indeed, the up-regulation of miR-17-5p has been demonstrated by other investigators [18, 19], with miR-146a found to have a role in cellular senescence [20]. In addition, Levati et al. [17] showed that ectopic expression of miR-155 reduced cellular proliferation in 12 of 13 melanoma cell lines, indicating its importance as a tumor suppressor. A computationally predicted target of miR-155 is SKI, a gene product that functions as a transcriptional co-repressor and conspires with important cell cycle regulators, including Rb and SMAD family members.

In a similar vein, miR-137 shows sequence complementarity (TargetScan) to the 3'-UTR of the mRNA transcript for carboxyl terminal binding protein I (CtBPI), a transcriptional co-repressor of tumor suppressor genes. Deng et al. [21] used a luciferase reporter assay to show that miR-137 suppresses CtBPI activity. This suppressive function was lost when the 3'-UTR of the target mRNA transcript was deleted [21]. Thus, miR-137 may be down-regulated in melanoma in order to increase CtBPI, thereby dampening tumor suppressor effects. For example, PTEN, a tumor suppressor, is a proven CtBPI target [22]. In addition, CtBPI may modulate the activity of the Ink4 family of tumor suppressors. The Ink4 region encodes for three cell cycle inhibitors – p16Ink4a and p15Ink4b, which function in the Rb pathway by inhibiting CDK4 and CDK6, and Ink4a/Arf, which attains a suppressive function by stabilizing p53 [23]. It is not surprising that miR-137 is located at chromosome site 1p22, a recognized melanoma "hot spot".

Furthermore, it is becoming apparent that miR-137 may have a broader role in melanoma initiation and progression, due to its recent connection with microphthalmia-associated transcription factor (MITF) [24]. This transcription factor is a master regulator of melanocyte development and is thought to be up-regulated in melanocytes as a means to protect the skin against UV radiation-induced DNA damage. Computational algorithms have shown that miR-27a, miR-32, miR-124, miR-137 and miR-148 possess conserved binding sites to the 3'-UTR of MITF. To test their biological function(s), Haflidadottir et al. [25] used a mouse MITF 3'-UTR luciferase reporter construct and showed that addition of miR-137 and miR-148 mimics reduced the signal, while mutations of the MITF 3'-UTR restored the signal. In the same study, western blotting showed down-regulation of MITF protein with the introduction of miR-148 and miR-137 [25]. Therefore, only two of these five computationally relevant miRNAs may actually be triggers on this pathway. Using a green fluorescent protein and MITF 3'-UTR showed down-regulation of the fluorescent tag in cell lines with addition of miR-137, while no such reduction occurred with a GFP empty vector [26]. The conservation rate of the MITF 3'-UTR sequence in 11 vertebrate species is reported to be 36%, a high rate of conservation for a noncoding region [26].

miR-182 is located at chromosomal loci 7q31-34 and flanked by the c-MET and BRAF genes. It has been shown that the expression of miR-182 increases from primary to metastatic melanoma, promoting cell migration and survival through suppression of MITF and FOXO3 [27]. Western blotting has demonstrated near disappearance of an MITF signal and reduction in FOXO3 in response to the addition of exogenous miR-182, while introduction of an antagomir rescued these proteins. Coupling of the target genes in a luciferase construct resulted in attenuation of the signal in response to increasing miR-182 in a dose-dependent relationship. It is perhaps no surprise that miR-182 and flanking partners c-MET and BRAF can jointly up-regulate with unique targets in melanoma.

BRAF is a component of a mitogenic pathway and its constitutive up-regulation typically results in bystander signals that induce cellular senescence in otherwise normal, healthy cells. BRAF proto-oncogene is point-mutated (T1799A) in ~65% of melanoma tumors. BRAF^{T1799A} encodes BRAF^{V600E} [28], a constitutively active protein serine kinase that elicits sustained activation of the mitogen-activated protein kinase (MAPK) pathway (Fig. 9.2). The induction of BRAF in healthy cells has been connected to the up-regulation of miR-34a, which in turn targets and down-regulates the oncogene MYC, thus dampening mitogenic effects [20]. miR-34a has also been shown to target the 3′-UTR of c-MET [29]. According to a number of researchers, miR-34a represents a tumor suppressor [5, 19]. miR-34a undergoes down-regulation in uveal melanoma cells, leading to up-regulation of c-MET and resulting in higher levels of Akt and cell cycle-related proteins [29]. Such instances of oncogenes exerting their regulatory control through miRNA pathways are not uncommon. The entire miR-34 family of genes is a direct transcriptional target of p53, invoking broad communication networks. miR-34b, miR-34c and miR-199a* have also been connected to c-MET [30], a potent oncogene that has proven roles in tumor invasion [31]. Transfection of cancer cell lines with all three of these miRNAs resulted in down-regulation of c-MET, while introduction of antagomirs rescued c-MET expression to normal levels [30]. In this study, a luciferase assay was used to confirm direct binding. Furthermore, miR-34b, miR-34c and miR-199a* were shown to impede the invasive capacity of cancerous cells compared to controls (i.e., arresting their ability to scatter in chamber assays).

miR-210, located on chromosome 11, has been shown to target MNT, a known MYC antagonist. To understand its role, consider that hypoxia-inducible factor (HIF-1α) causes cell cycle arrest by inhibition of c-MYC via binding of its cell cycle partner MAX and abrogation of MYC-MAX heterodimerization; however, in contrast, HIF-2α promotes MYC-MAX stabilization. miR-210 is found to be up-regulated under hypoxic conditions. Research has demonstrated that miR-210 is a direct target of both HIF-1α and HIF-2α, and overrides hypoxia-induced cell cycle arrest [32]. Western blotting has shown that miR-210 over-expression is connected to reduced levels of MNT protein. MNT interacts with MAX and thus antagonizes the MYC-MAX dimer. Thus, HIFs can induce miR-210 in order to reduce MNT and, thereby, promote MYC activation in the process of tumorigenesis.

Recent work in our own laboratory has shown that miR-451 undergoes down-regulation from primary to metastatic melanoma samples (unpublished results). In fact, miR-451 is placed squarely under the control of E2A, a transcription factor that is ubiquitinated and degraded in the Notch signaling pathway. Furthermore, miR-451 has been experimentally proven to repress MYC in mouse models [33]. These findings immediately elevate the status of miR-451 in cancer research, identifying it as a suppressor of one of the most notorious tumor oncogenes. Moreover, cancer stem cells have been found to rely on Notch and Wnt signaling pathways for perpetual renewal [34–36]. Notch is a receptor with an intercellular domain that fragments and translocates to the nucleus, leading to the transcription of MYC, and contributing indirectly to Ras-mediated cell transformation [2]. Thus, Notch not only contributes to down-regulation of miR-451, a suppressor of MYC, but also transcribes MYC as an endpoint. To take these connections to a dynamic new level, consider that Wnt, Notch and the Transforming Growth Factor-β (TGF-β) family of cytokines are known inducers of epithelial-to-mesenchymal transition (EMT) [37–40]. EMT is a process in which cancer cells can change their phenotype, in an effort to invade through the basal lamina and promote widespread metastasis. This process is mediated via the down-regulation of membrane-bound glycoprotein E-cadherin, which results in reduced cell-cell adherence [34]. Of note, E2A is associated with E-cadherin regulation [2] and TGF-β has been shown to up-regulate E2A proteins in epithelial cells [41], reducing the amount of E-cadherin available for cell-cell structural adhesion. Thus, cancers may use E2A in more than one way – its down-regulation connected to the promotion of MYC and its up-regulation associated with reduced E-cadherin expression.

miR-451 is unique in that it is DICER independent [42, 43] and has comparatively few computational gene targets. In fact, just 14 targets were identified in a TargetScan search, compared to most miRNAs that typically have hundreds of algorithmically suitable targets. Even so, miR-451 has previously been connected to glucose metabolism in cancer cells [44, 45]. The kinase LBK1 is phosphorylated by other kinases in a mitogenic pathway, with the addition of a phosphate group to it resulting in activation of AMPK, a kinase that then promotes glucose uptake and energy conservation under stressful or hypoxic conditions. However, tumorigenic cells can use energy perpetually in a state of aerobic glycolysis, the so-called "Warberg Effect," and AMPK activation can be suppressed in melanoma cells [44]. In low-glucose situations, cells normally sit tight and miR-451 is reduced by targeting of its binding partner, enabling LBK1 activation and thereby AMPK elevation. In cancer, miR-451 down-regulation has been associated with cell migration; while its up-regulation is associated with anti-apoptotic cellular proliferation via unrestrained mTOR signaling and poorer rates of patient survival [45].

miR-137, which was previously discussed as targeting CtBPI, also appears to contribute to regulation of the extracellular matrix. As stated, miR-137 undergoes down-regulation in melanoma leading to up-regulation of CtBPI [21]. Furthermore, the CtBPI-interacting E box repressor ZEB is a proven negative regulator of E-cadherin, while the transcription factor E1A may promote E-cadherin expression by disrupting the CtBPI/ZEB partnership.

miR 214 has been shown to be elevated in metastatic melanoma cell lines compared to primary melanoma cell lines [46]. Of note, miR-214 was found to be over-expressed in primary melanoma cell lines using lentiviral vectors, and completely repressed with antisense inhibitors in metastatic melanoma cell lines. Cells that received a boost of miR-214 became invasive and mobile, with improved adhesion of fibrin, laminin and collagen; while those that had miR-214 occluded demonstrated adhesion defects [46]. A luciferase assay connected miR-214 to the 3'-UTR of the mRNA transcript for integrin α3 (ITGA3) and transcription factor AP-2γ (TFAP2C), which have, among other roles, direct regulatory control over E-cadherin, connecting these genes to pro-metastatic behaviors. miR-214 over-expression was also connected to c-MET up-regulation [46].

miR-193b has been shown to undergo significant down-regulation in cutaneous melanoma [18]. In a recent profiling experiment, over-expression of miR-193b was associated with reduced cellular proliferation and down-regulation of hundreds of genes, with 18 of these computationally matched to miR-193b, including the mRNA transcript for Cyclin D1; a luciferase assay confirmed binding of these two molecules. This study also confirmed that miR-200c, miR-203, miR-204, miR-205 and miR-211 undergo down-regulation in the transition from common melanocytic nevus to melanoma. Indeed, miR-205 and miR-200c down-regulation and miR-146 up-regulation in melanoma reaffirm findings by Philippidou et al. [15]. In addition, miR-200c has been shown to regulate E-cadherin by targeting its partnering repressors ZEB1 and ZEB2 [47]. miR-203 is found to undergo tumor-specific methylation in cancer cell lines with a series of putative cell cycle targets [48], providing a striking example of how miRNA and epigenetic effects can conspire in tumor pathology.

miR-196a is reported to be down-regulated in melanoma cell lines and fresh/frozen tissue samples, with proven ties to the transcription factor HOX-C8 [49]. Transfection of cell lines with a miR-196a expression plasmid was correlated with reduced HOX-C8 expression, and a 3'-UTR HOX-C8 luciferase construct confirmed homologous binding to miR-196a. Abrogation of miR-196a resulted in increased HOX-C8 levels, associated with: (1) increases in the downstream target Osteopontin, an integrin binding phosphoprotein that is involved in extracellular matrix adhesion; (2) reduction in the levels of

Cadherin-11, a protein that localizes β-catenin to the cell membrane; and (3) reduction in Calponin-1, a protein that stabilizes the cytoskeleton.

microRNAs and Prognostication in Melanoma Patients

miRNAs are attracting interest not only for their role(s) in cancer-related pathways, but also as potential prognostic markers. For instance, miR-150 was shown by Segura et al. [6] to be a statistically significant prognostic indicator in melanoma, with its down-regulation being correlated with higher disease-free survival. miR-211 has captured attention as a tumor suppressor [50–52], perhaps unsurprising since it is located in intron region 6 of the melastatin gene TRPM1, a known tumor suppressor [53]. Levy et al. [50] made this discovery while surveying miR-211 in HeLa cells and connected it to growth factor targets IGF2R, TGFBR2 and NFAT5. Boyle et al. [51], also working with HeLa cells, demonstrated miR-211 down-regulation with enhancement of the transcription factor BRN2, a downstream target in the MAPK pathway that has been shown to be up-regulated in BRAF-mutant mice. In addition, Mazar et al. [52] reported a connection between miR-211 and the ion channel gene KCNMA1.

In a study by Mueller et al. [54], microarray data showed miR-133a, miR-199b, miR-453, miR-520f, miR-521 and miR-551b to be up-regulated threefold in the transition from melanocytes to primary melanoma cells, and again from primary melanoma cells to metastatic melanoma cells. Of note, miR-141 and miR-145 were associated with early progression of melanoma, undergoing up-regulation in primary melanoma cells lines as compared with normal human epidermal melanocytes [54]. Another in vitro study demonstrated miR-133a up-regulation and miR-145 down-regulation in melanoma, and additionally proved that miR-126 undergoes down-regulation in metastatic melanoma cell lines compared to primary melanoma cell lines [55]. miRNA profiling studies, based on microarray technology and qRT-PCR validation, have shown that miR-17-5p undergoes up-regulation, and miR-181a and miR-194 show down-regulation, in melanoma [54]. miR-373 is strongly induced in primary melanoma and undergoes a twofold up-regulation in invasive melanoma cells [54]; however, the contribution of miR-373 to melanoma pathobiology has been disputed by others [56].

Future of microRNAs in Melanoma Management

The literature is quickly becoming inundated with miRNA profiling studies. However, trends are difficult to sort out since, just like oncogenes and tumor suppressors, miRNAs appear to make modal contributions to cancer progression. In other words, a miRNA can contribute to cancer progression in one particular cancer type or underpin a specific cancerous phenotype, while the same miRNA may behave differently in other cancer types, suggesting that miRNAs are highly cell-type specific in their function. A goal of ongoing and future miRNA research will be to narrow the scope of this field and define a small set of dependable diagnostic and prognostic miRNA biomarkers in melanoma. It is likely that this will happen in three ways: (1) first, through the brute force of profiling studies, either using next generation sequencing (NGS) or microarray platforms, which enable miRNA trends to emerge in melanoma clinical specimens; (2) second, through continued plumbing of networks by evaluating miRNA levels with NGS and qRT-PCR, coupled with experimental testing that compromises the 3′-UTR of theoretical gene targets in order to test connections, and supported by protein profiling to examine the effects of a miRNA on gene networks and pathways; and (3) third, through investigations of the role of DICER and/or other enzymes of the miRNA biogenesis pathway in melanoma progression.

In a recent study, we examined the expression patterns and clinical relevance of DICER in cutaneous melanoma [57]. We showed that a large proportion of cutaneous melanomas exhibited up-regulation of DICER, which was significantly associated with aggressive cancer features. For the first time, we demonstrated definitive evidence that DICER up-regulation is specific to the malignant proliferation of melanocytes (melanoma), but not keratinocytes (carcinoma) or fibroblasts (sarcoma), in a study of 404 human skin tumors. DICER expression was evaluated in various subtypes of primary melanomas (i.e., arising on glabrous (subungual, palm and sole) skin, non-glabrous skin, the eye, and at mucosal sites (oral, urothelial and anal mucosa)), in addition to metastatic tumors (variety of organs), and compared to that of melanocytic nevi. Our immunostaining results clearly showed that DICER up-regulation was specific to cutaneous, acrolentiginous and metastatic melanomas [57]. We then carried out a pooled analysis using two recent large studies that profiled gene expression patterns in cutaneous tumors. This analysis corroborated our immunostaining data and indicated that at least a component of DICER up-regulation in melanoma is due to differences in mRNA accumulation. Deregulation of DICER, or other enzymes in the miRNA biogenesis pathway, may be a common central feature that is shared by several solid cancers and used to globally regulate the biogenesis of oncomirs [58–65]. From our pooled analysis focusing on all known enzymes that participate in the biogenesis and maturation of canonical miRNAs, we also propose the possibility of a more general phenomenon where several deregulated RNAi enzymes, in addition to DICER, may influence the various steps in melanoma progression (Fig. 9.3).

Our results show definitive up-regulation of DICER in cutaneous melanoma compared to other skin cancer types, and correlating with more aggressive tumor behavior. When confirmed by independent studies in larger cohorts, increased DICER expression may serve as a clinically useful prognostic biomarker for individuals with cutaneous melanoma. In addition, an understanding of DICER deregulation and its influence on the expression patterns of mature miRNAs may uncover novel therapeutic targets in melanoma.

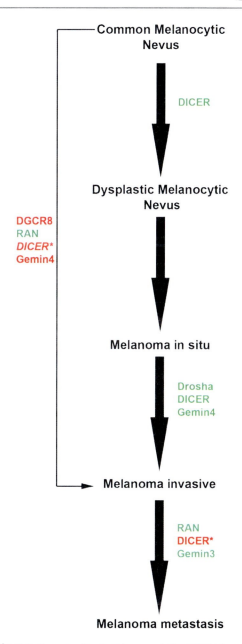

Fig. 9.3 Enzymes involved in canonical miRNA biogenesis are deregulated during melanoma progression. Combined DICER immunoreactivity, presented herein (denoted by *asterisk* '*'), and mRNA transcriptional profiling [66, 67] for DICER and other enzymes in the miRNA biogenesis pathway showed global changes in their expression levels during tumor progression. Enzymes shown in *red* are up-regulated and those in *green* are down-regulated. Up-regulation of DICER* from common melanocytic nevus to invasive melanoma was reported by both our study [57] and those of other investigators [66, 67]. DICER, DGCR8 and Gemin4 ranked among the top 20 percentile of most significantly altered genes

References

1. Institute NC. 51-Year trends in U.S. cancer death rates In: SEER Cancer Statistics Review, 1975–2000: http://seer.cancer.gov/statfacts/html/melan. Accessed 1 June 2011.
2. Weinberg R. The biology of cancer. New York: Garland Science; 2007.
3. Balch CM, Gershenwald JE, Soong SJ, Thompson JF, Atkins MB, et al. Final version of 2009 AJCC melanoma staging and classification. J Clin Oncol. 2009;27:6199–206.
4. Fire A, Xu S, Montgomery MK, Kostas SA, Driver SE, et al. Potent and specific genetic interference by double-stranded RNA in Caenorhabditis elegans. Nature. 1998;391:806–11.
5. Chan E, Patel R, Nallur S, Ratner E, Bacchiocchi A, et al. MicroRNA signatures differentiate melanoma subtypes. Cell Cycle. 2011;10(11):1845–52.
6. Segura MF, Belitskaya-Levy I, Rose AE, Zakrzewski J, Gaziel A, et al. Melanoma MicroRNA signature predicts post-recurrence survival. Clin Cancer Res. 2010;16:1577–86.
7. Ma Z, Lui WO, Fire A, Dadras SS. Profiling and discovery of novel miRNAs from formalin-fixed, paraffin-embedded melanoma and nodal specimens. J Mol Diagn. 2009;11:420–9.
8. Liu A, Xu X. MicroRNA isolation from formalin-fixed, paraffin-embedded tissues. Methods Mol Biol. 2011;724:259–67.
9. Muller DW, Bosserhoff AK. Integrin beta 3 expression is regulated by let-7a miRNA in malignant melanoma. Oncogene. 2008;27:6698–706.
10. Fu TY, Chang CC, Lin CT, Lai CH, Peng SY, et al. Let-7b-mediated suppression of basigin expression and metastasis in mouse melanoma cells. Exp Cell Res. 2011;317:445–51.
11. Schultz J, Lorenz P, Gross G, Ibrahim S, Kunz M. MicroRNA let-7b targets important cell cycle molecules in malignant melanoma cells and interferes with anchorage-independent growth. Cell Res. 2008;18: 549–57.
12. Glud M, Manfe V, Biskup E, Holst L, Dirksen AM, et al. MicroRNA miR-125b induces senescence in human melanoma cells. Melanoma Res. 2011;21: 253–6.
13. Glud M, Rossing M, Hother C, Holst L, Hastrup N, et al. Downregulation of miR-125b in metastatic cutaneous malignant melanoma. Melanoma Res. 2010;20: 479–84.
14. Dar AA, Majid S, de Semir D, Nosrati M, Bezrookove V, et al. miRNA-205 suppresses melanoma cell proliferation and induces senescence via regulation of E2F1 protein. J Biol Chem. 2011;286:16606–14.
15. Philippidou D, Schmitt M, Moser D, Margue C, Nazarov PV, et al. Signatures of microRNAs and selected microRNA target genes in human melanoma. Cancer Res. 2010;70:4163–73.
16. Das SK, Sokhi UK, Bhutia SK, Azab B, Su ZZ, et al. Human polynucleotide phosphorylase selectively and preferentially degrades microRNA-221 in human melanoma cells. Proc Natl Acad Sci USA. 2010;107: 11948–53.
17. Levati L, Pagani E, Romani S, Castiglia D, Piccinni E, et al. MicroRNA-155 targets the SKI gene in human melanoma cell lines. Pigment Cell Melanoma Res. 2011;24:538–50.
18. Chen J, Feilotter HE, Pare GC, Zhang X, Pemberton JG, et al. MicroRNA-193b represses cell proliferation and regulates cyclin D1 in melanoma. Am J Pathol. 2010;176:2520–9.
19. Greenberg E, Hershkovitz L, Itzhaki O, Hajdu S, Nemlich Y, et al. Regulation of cancer aggressive features in melanoma cells by MicroRNAs. PLoS One. 2011;6:e18936.
20. Christoffersen NR, Shalgi R, Frankel LB, Leucci E, Lees M, et al. p53-independent upregulation of miR-34a during oncogene-induced senescence represses MYC. Cell Death Differ. 2010;17:236–45.
21. Deng Y, Deng H, Bi F, Liu J, Bemis LT, et al. MicroRNA-137 targets carboxyl-terminal binding protein 1 in melanoma cell lines. Int J Biol Sci. 2011;7:133–7.
22. Chinnadurai G. The transcriptional corepressor CtBP: a foe of multiple tumor suppressors. Cancer Res. 2009;69:731–4.
23. Mroz EA, Baird AH, Michaud WA, Rocco JW. COOH-terminal binding protein regulates expression of the p16INK4A tumor suppressor and senescence in primary human cells. Cancer Res. 2008;68:6049–53.
24. Bemis LT, Chen R, Amato CM, Classen EH, Robinson SE, et al. MicroRNA-137 targets microphthalmia-associated transcription factor in melanoma cell lines. Cancer Res. 2008;68:1362–8.
25. Haflidadottir BS, Bergsteinsdottir K, Praetorius C, Steingrimsson E. miR-148 regulates Mitf in melanoma cells. PLoS One. 2010;5:e11574.
26. Hallsson JH, Haflidadottir BS, Schepsky A, Arnheiter H, Steingrimsson E. Evolutionary sequence comparison of the Mitf gene reveals novel conserved domains. Pigment Cell Res. 2007;20:185–200.
27. Segura MF, Hanniford D, Menendez S, Reavie L, Zou X, et al. Aberrant miR-182 expression promotes melanoma metastasis by repressing FOXO3 and microphthalmia-associated transcription factor. Proc Natl Acad Sci USA. 2009;106:1814–9.
28. Davies H, Bignell GR, Cox C, Stephens P, Edkins S, et al. Mutations of the BRAF gene in human cancer. Nature. 2002;417:949–54.
29. Yan D, Zhou X, Chen X, Hu DN, Dong XD, et al. MicroRNA-34a inhibits uveal melanoma cell proliferation and migration through downregulation of c-Met. Invest Ophthalmol Vis Sci. 2009;50:1559–65.
30. Migliore C, Petrelli A, Ghiso E, Corso S, Capparuccia L, et al. MicroRNAs impair MET-mediated invasive growth. Cancer Res. 2008;68:10128–36.

31. Comoglio PM, Trusolino L. Invasive growth: from development to metastasis. J Clin Invest. 2002; 109:857–62.
32. Zhang Z, Sun H, Dai H, Walsh RM, Imakura M, et al. MicroRNA miR-210 modulates cellular response to hypoxia through the MYC antagonist MNT. Cell Cycle. 2009;8:2756–68.
33. Li X, Sanda T, Look AT, Novina CD, von Boehmer H. Repression of tumor suppressor miR-451 is essential for NOTCH1-induced oncogenesis in T-ALL. J Exp Med. 2011;208:663–75.
34. Takebe N, Harris PJ, Warren RQ, Ivy SP. Targeting cancer stem cells by inhibiting Wnt, Notch, and Hedgehog pathways. Nat Rev Clin Oncol. 2011;8: 97–106.
35. McGovern M, Voutev R, Maciejowski J, Corsi AK, Hubbard EJ. A "latent niche" mechanism for tumor initiation. Proc Natl Acad Sci USA. 2009;106: 11617–22.
36. Reya T, Clevers H. Wnt signalling in stem cells and cancer. Nature. 2005;434:843–50.
37. Dissanayake SK, Wade M, Johnson CE, O'Connell MP, Leotlela PD, et al. The Wnt5A/protein kinase C pathway mediates motility in melanoma cells via the inhibition of metastasis suppressors and initiation of an epithelial to mesenchymal transition. J Biol Chem. 2007;282:17259–71.
38. Vincan E, Barker N. The upstream components of the Wnt signalling pathway in the dynamic EMT and MET associated with colorectal cancer progression. Clin Exp Metastasis. 2008;25:657–63.
39. Massague J. TGFbeta in cancer. Cell. 2008;134: 215–30.
40. Yang J, Weinberg RA. Epithelial-mesenchymal transition: at the crossroads of development and tumor metastasis. Dev Cell. 2008;14:818–29.
41. Kondo M, Cubillo E, Tobiume K, Shirakihara T, Fukuda N, et al. A role for Id in the regulation of TGF-beta-induced epithelial-mesenchymal transdifferentiation. Cell Death Differ. 2004;11:1092–101.
42. Cifuentes D, Xue H, Taylor DW, Patnode H, Mishima Y, et al. A novel miRNA processing pathway independent of Dicer requires Argonaute2 catalytic activity. Science. 2010;328:1694–8.
43. Cheloufi S, Dos Santos CO, Chong MM, Hannon GJ. A dicer-independent miRNA biogenesis pathway that requires Ago catalysis. Nature. 2010;465:584–9.
44. Zheng B, Jeong JH, Asara JM, Yuan YY, Granter SR, et al. Oncogenic B-RAF negatively regulates the tumor suppressor LKB1 to promote melanoma cell proliferation. Mol Cell. 2009;33:237–47.
45. Godlewski J, Nowicki MO, Bronisz A, Nuovo G, Palatini J, et al. MicroRNA-451 regulates LKB1/AMPK signaling and allows adaptation to metabolic stress in glioma cells. Mol Cell. 2010;37:620–32.
46. Penna E, Orso F, Cimino D, Tenaglia E, Lembo A, et al. microRNA-214 contributes to melanoma tumour progression through suppression of TFAP2C. EMBO J. 2011;30:1990–2007.
47. Korpal M, Lee ES, Hu G, Kang Y. The miR-200 family inhibits epithelial-mesenchymal transition and cancer cell migration by direct targeting of E-cadherin transcriptional repressors ZEB1 and ZEB2. J Biol Chem. 2008;283:14910–4.
48. Furuta M, Kozaki KI, Tanaka S, Arii S, Imoto I, et al. miR-124 and miR-203 are epigenetically silenced tumor-suppressive microRNAs in hepatocellular carcinoma. Carcinogenesis. 2010;31:766–76.
49. Mueller DW, Bosserhoff AK. MicroRNA miR-196a controls melanoma-associated genes by regulating HOX-C8 expression. Int J Cancer. 2010;129(5): 1064–74.
50. Levy C, Khaled M, Iliopoulos D, Janas MM, Schubert S, et al. Intronic miR-211 assumes the tumor suppressive function of its host gene in melanoma. Mol Cell. 2010;40:841–9.
51. Boyle GM, Woods SL, Bonazzi VF, Stark MS, Hacker E, et al. Melanoma cell invasiveness is regulated by miR-211 suppression of the BRN2 transcription factor. Pigment Cell Melanoma Res. 2011;24:525–37.
52. Mazar J, DeYoung K, Khaitan D, Meister E, Almodovar A, et al. The regulation of miRNA-211 expression and its role in melanoma cell invasiveness. PLoS One. 2010;5:e13779.
53. Duncan LM, Deeds J, Hunter J, Shao J, Holmgren LM, et al. Down-regulation of the novel gene melastatin correlates with potential for melanoma metastasis. Cancer Res. 1998;58:1515–20.
54. Mueller DW, Rehli M, Bosserhoff AK. miRNA expression profiling in melanocytes and melanoma cell lines reveals miRNAs associated with formation and progression of malignant melanoma. J Invest Dermatol. 2009;129:1740–51.
55. Molnar V, Tamasi V, Bakos B, Wiener Z, Falus A. Changes in miRNA expression in solid tumors: an miRNA profiling in melanomas. Semin Cancer Biol. 2008;18:111–22.
56. Satzger I, Mattern A, Kuettler U, Weinspach D, Voelker B, et al. MicroRNA-15b represents an independent prognostic parameter and is correlated with tumor cell proliferation and apoptosis in malignant melanoma. Int J Cancer. 2010;126:2553–62.
57. Ma Z, Swede H, Cassarino DC, Fleming E, Fire A, Dadras SS. Up-regulated Dicer expression in patients with cutaneous melanoma. PLoS ONE. 2011;6(6): e20494.
58. Karube Y, Tanaka H, Osada H, Tomida S, Tatematsu Y, et al. Reduced expression of Dicer associated with poor prognosis in lung cancer patients. Cancer Sci. 2005;96:111–5.
59. Sugito N, Ishiguro H, Kuwabara Y, Kimura M, Mitsui A, et al. RNASEN regulates cell proliferation and affects survival in esophageal cancer patients. Clin Cancer Res. 2006;12:7322–8.
60. Chiosea S, Jelezcova E, Chandran U, Acquafondata M, McHale T, et al. Up-regulation of dicer, a component of the MicroRNA machinery, in prostate adenocarcinoma. Am J Pathol. 2006;169:1812–20.

61. Chiosea S, Jelezcova E, Chandran U, Luo J, Mantha G, et al. Overexpression of Dicer in precursor lesions of lung adenocarcinoma. Cancer Res. 2007;67:2345–50.
62. Muralidhar B, Goldstein LD, Ng G, Winder DM, Palmer RD, et al. Global microRNA profiles in cervical squamous cell carcinoma depend on Drosha expression levels. J Pathol. 2007;212:368–77.
63. Chiosea SI, Barnes EL, Lai SY, Egloff AM, Sargent RL, et al. Mucoepidermoid carcinoma of upper aerodigestive tract: clinicopathologic study of 78 cases with immunohistochemical analysis of Dicer expression. Virchows Arch. 2008;452:629–35.
64. Merritt WM, Lin YG, Han LY, Kamat AA, Spannuth WA, et al. Dicer, Drosha, and outcomes in patients with ovarian cancer. N Engl J Med. 2008;359:2641–50.
65. Jakymiw A, Patel RS, Deming N, Bhattacharyya I, Shah P, et al. Overexpression of dicer as a result of reduced let-7 MicroRNA levels contributes to increased cell proliferation of oral cancer cells. Genes Chromosomes Cancer. 2010;49:549–59.
66. Scatolini M, Grand MM, Grosso E, Venesio T, Pisacane A, et al. Altered molecular pathways in melanocytic lesions. Int J Cancer. 2010;126:1869–81.
67. Riker AI, Enkemann SA, Fodstad O, Liu S, Ren S, et al. The gene expression profiles of primary and metastatic melanoma yields a transition point of tumor progression and metastasis. BMC Med Genomics. 2008;1:13.

MicroRNAs as Biomarkers and Therapeutic Targets in Melanoma

Daniel W. Mueller and Anja K. Bosserhoff

MicroRNAs (abbreviated: miRNAs) represent a class of small non-coding RNAs, initially discovered in the nematode *Caenorhabditis elegans*. In 1993, the labs of Victor Ambros [1] and Gary Ruvkun [2] cooperatively characterized the structure and function of lin-4, the founding member of today's rapidly growing molecule class termed microRNAs. However, it was not until the year 2000 that Reinhart and colleagues detected a second miRNA species – let-7 [3]. Given that the sequence of let-7 was actually conserved in a large variety of Metazoens from *Drosophila* to humans (in contrast to lin-4 which is specific to *Caenorhabditis*; [4, 5]), this fueled further miRNA research and eventually revealed that miRNAs are involved in posttranscriptional gene regulation in virtually all multicellular organisms. Today, it is widely accepted that deregulated expression of miRNAs plays a major role in the formation and progression of a wide range of human tumors [6–8], including melanoma [9–11]. Therefore, miRNAs harbor great potential to serve as molecular biomarkers and even therapeutic targets in diverse tumor types [12–14]. With regard to melanoma, where (a) early detection of primary lesions is necessary to ensure optimal outcome and (b) highly efficient therapeutic strategies beneficial for broad cohorts of patients still do not exist, miRNAs could potentially be utilized to improve patient survival in the future [15, 16].

miRNA Biogenesis and Function

Transcription of miRNA Genes and Processing in the Nucleus

MicroRNA genes are embedded in both intergenic and intragenic regions of the human genome, thereby encoding single miRNAs or clusters of multiple miRNAs arranged in a polycistronic manner [17]. As a first step, miRNA genes are transcribed into pri-miRNAs (primary miRNA transcripts; Fig. 10.1). In most cases, transcription is mediated by RNA polymerase II, resulting in 5′-methyl-guanosine capped and polyadenylated pri-miRNAs which are up to several kilo bases in length and contain local stem-loop structures [18, 19]. Specific subsets of miRNAs are initially transcribed by RNA polymerase III [20]. While still present in the nuclear compartment, the pri-miRNA is endonucleolytically cleaved by the so-called microprocessor complex consisting of RNase III enzyme Drosha (RNASEN) and its co-factor DGCR8 (DiGeorge syndrome critical region on chromosome 8; also known as Pasha (Partner of Drosha) in *D. melanogaster* and *C. elegans*) [21, 22]. DGCR8 interacts with the ~33 bp stem-loop as well as the adjacent unpaired flanking regions within the pri-miRNA, supporting Drosha-mediated cleavage

D.W. Mueller, Ph.D. • A.K. Bosserhoff, Ph.D. (✉)
Institute of Pathology, Molecular Pathology,
University of Regensburg, Regensburg, Germany
e-mail: anja.bosserhoff@klinik.uni-regensburg.de

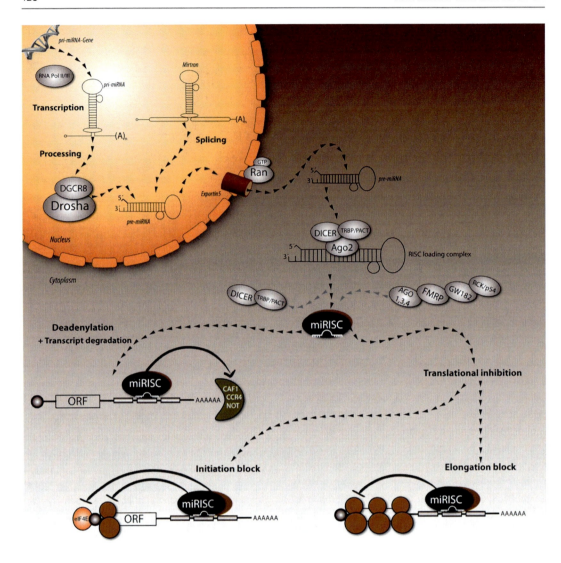

Fig. 10.1 Schematic overview of miRNA biogenesis and function. Please refer to paragraph "miRNA biogenesis and function" for detailed explanations of the molecular mechanisms involved in each step (Reprinted from [11]. With kind permission from Springer publishing)

in the stem region [23, 24]. Rapid translocation of the resulting pre-miRNA to the cytoplasm occurs via the Ran-GTP-dependent nuclear export factor Exportin 5 (EXP5), a member of the nuclear transport receptor family [25]. Thereby, recognition of the >14 bp double-stranded RNA (dsRNA) stem together with a short (one to eight nucleotides) 3′ overhang ensures export of only correctly processed pre-miRNAs [26]. Interestingly, a specific sub-group of pre-miRNAs exists that can be exported from the nucleus circumventing Drosha processing. These so-called mirtrons are located in very short introns and form hairpins resembling pre-miRNA molecules after splicing releases them from their host transcripts [27].

Cytoplasmic Processing and Modes of miRNA-Mediated Gene Silencing

In the cytoplasm, maturation of pre-miRNAs is mediated by a multi-enzyme complex called RISC loading complex (RLC). The main components of the RLC are RNase III enzyme Dicer, the dsRNA-binding domain proteins TRBP (TAR RNA-binding protein) and PACT (protein activator of PKR), as well as Ago2 (Argonaute-2), the latter building the complex's core [28, 29]. TRBP and PACT facilitate Dicer-mediated cleavage of the pre-miRNA, which occurs near the terminal loop and gives rise to an RNA duplex of ~22 nucleotides with two nucleotide overhangs on each 3' terminus [30, 31]. Subsequently, Dicer and its co-factors TRBP and PACT dissociate from the miRNP (micro-ribonucleoprotein complex), and the miRNA duplex is separated into the guide strand (which is functional in gene silencing) and the passenger strand (miRNA*; which usually gets degraded). Currently, it appears that there is no universal helicase responsible for unwinding of the miRNA duplex, but rather specific helicases that may differentially regulate subgroups of miRNAs [32]. In some cases, a helicase is not required for duplex unwinding [33, 34]. Selection of the guide strand is based on the presence of a thermodynamically less stable base pair at the 5' end of the duplex, and is followed by unwinding and loading onto a RISC (RNA-induced silencing complex) [35]. The assembly of this miRISC (miRNA-induced silencing complex) is a dynamic process coupled with the preceding steps of pre-miRNA processing. Key components of the miRISC are proteins of the Argonaute (AGO) family, FMRP (fragile X mental retardation protein), and P-body components including GW182 and RCK/p54 – all of which are essential for miRNA-mediated gene repression [36]. Guided by the mature miRNA, the miRISC subsequently recognizes and binds target sequences in the 3' untranslated regions (3'UTRs) of specific mRNAs, inhibiting their translation into protein. Even today, the general rules for the initial miRNA::mRNA interaction, which are fundamental for target recognition, are only incompletely determined experimentally and bioinformatically [37–41].

The resulting miRNA-induced posttranscriptional silencing can either be mediated by destabilization of the target mRNA [42–45] or by repression of protein translation [46, 47]; both pathways act cooperatively, but yet independently of each other. Destabilization of target mRNAs starts with recruitment of the P-body component GW182 by Argonaute proteins [48]. GW182 then mediates binding of the CAF1:CCR4:NOT1 deadenylase complex to the target mRNA. Deadenylation is followed by removal of the 5'-methyl-guanosine cap via the DCP1:DCP2 decapping complex, ultimately leading to $5' \rightarrow 3'$ exonucleolytic degradation of mRNA by exonuclease XRN1 [49–51]. However, there is still a lack of consensus concerning the mechanism(s) by which miRNAs induce repression of mRNA translation. While many experiments point towards initiation of translation as a target for repression, there is also evidence that diverse post-initiation steps could be affected (reviewed in [52]). It remains to be elucidated whether miRNAs are actually capable of controlling translation by multiple mechanisms or if these discrepancies can be attributed to the different experimental approaches utilized [53, 54]. The mechanisms involved in miRNA biogenesis and function are summarized in Fig. 10.1.

The general pathway of miRNA biogenesis and function is complicated by a large number of regulatory interventions, in which a vast quantity of yet unidentified proteins is likely involved. There may be specific alterations to the pathway for every individual miRNA or at least for distinct subgroups of these molecules. In addition, miRNAs not only repress gene expression, but are also able to induce expression of specific genes under certain cellular conditions (for recent and comprehensive reviews on regulation of miRNA expression and function, see references [32, 52, 55–57]). To date, more than 800 miRNAs have been discovered in the human genome (http://microrna.sanger.ac.uk/; [58]), and are estimated to regulate ~30% of all human transcripts [39]. MiRNAs have been shown to be involved in the normal regulation of a variety of cellular processes, such as proliferation, apoptosis, cell-cycle control, and differentiation [59–64]. As a consequence, abnormalities in miRNA activity may contribute to the pathogenesis and progression of various types of human cancers (reviewed in [65, 66]), including melanoma (reviewed in [9, 11]; see Fig. 10.2 and Table 10.1).

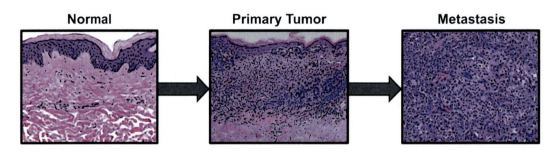

miR-17-92, miR-30b/d, miR-182, miR-210, miR-214, miR-221/222, miR-532-5p

let-7a/b, miR-34a/b/c, miR-193b, miR-196a, miR-205, miR-211

Fig. 10.2 Schematic overview of most prominent validated miRNAs deregulated during melanomagenesis. MiR-17-92, miR-30b/d, miR-182, miR-210, miR-214, miR-221/222, and miR-532-5p have been shown to be upregulated during melanoma progression, potentially acting as oncogenes. In contrast, expression of the miRNAs let-7a/b, miR-34a/b/c, miR-193b, miR-196a, miR-205 and miR-211 is diminished in melanoma cells, assigning them a role as tumor-suppressive microRNAs. For references, please refer to Table 10.1 (Modified and reprinted from [9]. With kind permission from the *British Journal of Cancer*)

Table 10.1 MicroRNAs known to be deregulated in melanomagenesis and considered to be potentially suitable for therapeutic approaches

miRNA	Gain/loss in melanoma cells	Cause of gain/loss	Verified target(s) in melanoma	Reference(s)
let-7a	↓	Not yet determined	N-Ras, integrin beta3	[75, 129, 131, 132, 136]
let-7b	↓	Not yet determined	Cyclin D1, EMMPRIN	[29, 131, 137]
miR-17-92	↑	Not yet determined	BIM (?)	[72, 131, 132, 138]
miR-30b/d	↑	Amplification of 8q24 (?)	GALNT7	[139]
miR-34a	↓	Hypermethylation	None	[140]
miR-34b/c	↓	Hypermethylation	MET (?)	[141, 142]
miR-137	↓ (?)	Amplification of a VNTR in the 5'UTR of the pri-miRNA	MITF, CtBP1	[143, 144]
miR-182	↑	Amplification of 7q31-34	MITF, FOXO3	[145]
miR-193b	↓	Not yet determined	Cyclin D1	[131]
miR-196a	↓	Not yet determined	HOX-B7, HOX-C8	[86, 132, 146, 147]
miR-205	↓	Not yet determined	E2F1, E2F5	[148]
miR-210	↑	Hypoxia or constitutive HIF-1α activity (?)	MNT (?)	[84, 149]
miR-211	↓	Melastatin (TRPM1) down-regulation	KCNMA1, TGFBR2, NFAT5, BRN2, PRAME	[150–153]
miR-214	↑	Copy number gain (?)	TFAP2C, ITGA3	[154]
miR-221/222	↑	Loss of PLZF expression, MITF level, down-regulation of hPNP^{old-35}	c-KIT, p27^{Kip1}	[72, 132, 155–157]
miR-532-5p	↑	Not yet determined	RUNX3 (?)	[158]

(?) Pending confirmation

Studies on Global miRNA Expression and General Potential of miRNAs to Serve as Biomarkers in Melanoma

Initial Studies on Global miRNA Expression, Including Data on Melanoma Cells

As evidence of the participation of deregulated miRNA expression in carcinogenesis accumulated, a plethora of initial studies examining global miRNA expression patterns in various types of cancers were performed. Of note, the first studies published by Lu et al. [67], Zhang et al. [68], Gaur et al. [69], and Blower et al. [70] contained both melanoma tissue samples and melanoma cell lines. A number of general conclusions were reached from these studies. Firstly, miRNA expression profiles reflect the developmental lineage and differentiation state of solid tumors [67, 69]. For example, poorly differentiated tumors can be successfully classified by their miRNA expression profiles, in contrast to their respective mRNA profiles [67, 69]. This allowed Rosenfeld and colleagues to construct a classifier consisting of 48 miRNAs that was capable of determining the origin of metastatic tumors of unknown primary origin with high accuracy [71]. The latter finding could prove relevant for diagnosis of unknown primary melanomas, which represent ~5% of all melanoma cases. Secondly, it was recognized that a large number of miRNAs are subject to DNA copy number abnormalities in cancers, indicating that copy number alterations of miRNA genes may partially account for deregulation of miRNA expression. With regard to melanoma samples, it was shown that 85.9% of genomic loci harboring one or more of 283 examined miRNA genes exhibited DNA copy number alterations and that some of these changes were specific to this form of skin cancer [68]. In addition, 15 miRNAs (4 up- and 11 down-regulated) showed significantly different expression in eight melanoma cell lines (included in the NCI-60 panel), separating them from the other cancer cell lines investigated [69]. Unfortunately, due to the aims and experimental approaches of the studies cited here, no information on specific miRNAs or subsets of miRNAs differentially expressed in melanoma cells compared to their normal biological correlate (i.e., benign melanocytes) could be derived. Nevertheless, the data obtained underlined the potential of miRNA profiling to identify miRNAs with diagnostic, staging and prognostic value in melanoma, as well as targets for novel approaches to therapy of this potentially lethal disease.

miRNA Profiling of Melanocytes and Melanoma Cell Lines and Usefulness of Formalin-Fixed Paraffin-Embedded (FFPE) Tissue Samples for the Discovery of miRNA Biomarkers

Mueller et al. [72] were the first to perform a detailed comparison of miRNA expression between normal human melanocytes and well-characterized melanoma cell lines derived from primary tumors and melanoma metastases. Their most important findings can be summarized as follows: (1) expression of a high number of miRNAs is deregulated in melanoma cell lines compared to normal melanocytes; the majority of miRNAs investigated were up-regulated in melanomas; (2) the majority of miRNAs found to be most strongly deregulated were not previously described to be of importance in tumor development; and (3) heterogeneity of melanoma cells results in intrinsic variability in the expression of some miRNAs, making it necessary to analyze sets of cell lines/tissue samples in order to minimize the effects of individual alterations. The experimental setup of this study aimed to identify miRNAs differentially expressed in different stages of melanoma tumorigenesis (such as early development and metastasis), which could then be analyzed for their cellular function in melanomagenesis and their potential as therapeutic targets in the future [72]. Accordingly, appropriately selected cell lines were used. A miRNA classifier for melanoma staging or general diagnostic purposes was not investigated. Such a classifier can only be created by performing large scale analysis of miRNA expression on a sizeable quantity of melanoma tissue samples derived from primary tumors and metastases (preferably including paired primary tumor/metastases samples from the same patient). Originally, this appeared to be a major challenge in the study of melanoma, as fresh tissue samples from primary tumors are difficult to obtain. This is due to the therapeutic guidelines in most countries, which require microscopic analysis of the whole primary tumor to determine histopathological prognostic parameters, including Breslow thickness. Fortunately, formalin-fixed and paraffin-embedded (FFPE) specimens of melanocytic lesions have been found to be a suitable starting material for miRNA expression profiling [73–75]. Recent studies have demonstrated that: (1) small-RNA fractions of sufficient quality for miRNA expression profiling can be extracted from FFPE melanocytic lesions; and (2) miRNA expression profiles derived from FFPE material closely resemble those derived from fresh/frozen samples. Importantly, miRNA expression profiles are not significantly affected by variations in the duration of formalin fixation or storage in paraffin [76–78]. For a number of reasons, miRNA is a much more vigorous analyte than mRNA in FFPE tissue. Large RNA molecules are chemically modified by addition of hydroxymethyl groups to the nucleic acid backbones during formalin fixation [79]. Additionally, formaldehyde facilitates depurination of nucleic acids as well as the hydrolysis of phosphodiester bonds [80, 81]. Of note, it is difficult to extract mRNAs of >300 bp from FFPE tissue [82]. Therefore, mRNA-based gene expression profiles derived from FFPE tissue show only low correlation to profiles derived from fresh/frozen tissue [74, 77]. In contrast, miRNAs are well preserved in FFPE samples. Due to their small size and their association with protein complexes, they can be easily extracted and are additionally shielded from modification reactions and degradation pathways. Remarkably, it has been shown that miRNAs are stable for up to 10 years (or even longer) in FFPE tissues [75, 79, 83].

Ma et al. [75] provide a simple and efficient protocol for extraction of small RNA fractions from FFPE sections. They noted the importance of performing two cycles of deparaffinization; the use of siliconized tubes throughout the whole procedure (small RNAs were found to otherwise adhere to the walls of regular plastic tubes); and proteinase K digestion is essential to release RNA from the tissue sections. MiRNA fractions in quantities and qualities suitable for miRNA expression profiling can be readily recovered from FFPE tissue samples using either customized protocols or commercial kits, making archival FFPE material a unique basis for the identification of miRNAs with prognostic relevance in melanoma. The possibility of performing miRNA expression profiling on FFPE tissue samples has many important advantages. There is a bulk of archival material available, collected over decades of pathological examination of melanocytic lesions, with every single sample representing a morphologically-defined case accurately staged by trained pathologists. Furthermore, FFPE samples are associated with detailed disease history (including data on clinical outcome and disease-specific survival). Correlating this clinico-pathological data with miRNA expression profiles will potentially help to optimize cancer prognosis and/or treatment response. It is of utmost importance to note that useful miRNA expression profiles can only be obtained if contamination of FFPE melanoma samples by non-tumorous cells is eliminated or minimized (such as by the use of laser capture microdissection).

There is now an obvious need for comparative studies analyzing large sets of FFPE samples of clearly defined melanoma tissues with available clinical data, benign melanocytic lesions and normal human melanocytes from several different donors, using robust and reliable experimental platforms. This will be essential to definitively identify miRNAs associated with disease parameters, and potentially identify diagnostic and/or prognostic biomarkers. Fortunately, during the last 2 years, studies with these aims have started to emerge.

Attempts to Identify miRNAs that Can Serve as Molecular Biomarkers in Melanoma Diagnosis and Prognosis

In 2010, Ralf Gutzmer's group published the first study on a miRNA with the potential to serve as an independent prognostic marker in melanoma [84]. Determining expression levels of a defined set of miRNAs in FFPE tissue samples of primary melanomas derived from 128 patients with available detailed clinical follow-up information, this group demonstrated that high intratumoral levels of miR-15b were significantly associated with poor recurrence-free survival and overall survival. MiR-15b overexpression was found to be a statistically independent parameter of disease-free survival ($p=0.015$) and overall survival ($p=0.013$), in addition to other well-known prognostic factors (i.e., Breslow-index and ulceration of the primary tumor), on multivariate Cox analysis [84].

Furthermore, Eva Hernando's group analyzed the expression of 611 miRNAs in 59 FFPE specimens of melanoma metastases derived from patients with detailed clinical follow-up [85]. By correlating miRNA profiles with post-recurrence survival, they identified a signature composed of 18 up-regulated miRNAs that was significantly associated with longer survival. A miRNA classifier consisting of six of these miRNAs (miR-150, miR-342-3p, miR-455-3p, miR-145, miR-155, and miR-497) was able to predict post-recurrence survival in their sample set with an estimated accuracy of ~80%. Notably, this classifier was able to significantly risk-stratify stage III melanoma patients into "better" and "worse" prognostic categories based on survival probability, in contrast to the AJCC standard classification system (stages IIIB and IIIC). Interestingly, Segura and co-workers also found that nearly all miRNAs included in a prolonged survival miRNA classifier were related to the site of metastasis. These findings suggest that subsets of miRNAs could serve as signatures predictive for which organs will develop metastases in melanoma patients. Additional studies will be necessary to determine if the classifier constructed can predict for the risk of metastases in patients with primary melanoma [85].

Another study by Caramuta and colleagues investigated if miRNA expression profiles could separate melanoma patients into those with shortened versus prolonged survival [86]. They specifically analyzed lymph node metastases and reported that down-regulation of miR-191, combined with up-regulation of miR-193a, miR-193b, miR-365, miR-338, and let-7i, identified melanoma patients with poor outcomes.

In an innovative approach, Jukic and colleagues identified miRNAs differentially expressed between melanomas from individuals at different extremes of age (i.e., young patients <30 years old and older patients >60 years old) [87]. Working with a limited set of tumor samples, they demonstrated that primary melanomas in older patients differ in their miRNA expression profiles from melanomas in younger individuals. These results might potentially reflect differences in the biological processes affected and/or, as remains to be investigated, age-dependent differences in the melanocytes from which these lesions arose.

Interestingly, miRNA classifiers could potentially be used to discriminate between different melanoma subtypes. The first evidence for this hypothesis was reported by Chan and colleagues who profiled the expression of 384 miRNAs in primary melanoma cell cultures derived from 42 patients and a pool of three normal melanocyte samples [88]. They identified a cohort of seven miRNAs that were differentially expressed in acral compared to non-acral melanomas, theoretically serving as a molecular signature that defines the acral lentiginous subtype of this tumor. If validated in larger samples sets (particularly in melanoma tissue samples, and not solely cell lines), such a signature could potentially support not only pathologists' decisions in cases with ambiguous histopathology, but also be used to select for appropriate treatment regimens among different melanoma subtypes.

Potential of Blood-Based miRNA Biomarker Discovery in Clinical Samples

Recently, another promising source for miRNAs of prognostic value has emerged – the blood of melanoma patients. MiRNAs have been found to be surprisingly stable and readily detectable in serum and plasma, in contrast to other circulating nucleic acids, and thus show the potential to serve as diagnostic and/or prognostic markers in human blood samples [89–95]. The use of routinely processed clinical samples in miRNA biomarker discovery is facilitated by the resistance of circulating miRNAs to: (1) incubation at room-temperature for several hours; (2) repeated freeze-thaw cycles; and (3) endogenous RNase activity [91, 93, 94]. Additionally, the expression profile of serum miRNAs appears to be reproducible and consistent in healthy individuals, but shows significant changes in the sera of cancer patients, with miRNA levels either elevated or reduced [93, 94]. Based on these findings, it was speculated that under healthy conditions, most serum miRNAs are derived from circulating blood cells; while during cancer pathogenesis and progression, miRNAs may also be released by the tissues affected [93]. Indeed, Mitchell and colleagues were able to demonstrate that miRNAs derived from human prostate cancer cells and xenografted into mice entered the circulation of these animals [91]. Variations in the abundances of these tumor-derived miRNAs within the serum were at least in part correlated to the tumor burden of the animals [91]. Two basic prerequisites towards a potential miRNA serum biomarker can be concluded from these findings: (1) it must be expressed at moderate-to-high levels by cancer cells; and (2) it should be undetectable or present at only low levels in the serum of normal individuals. This suggests that serum miRNAs are better-suited to studies evaluating an up-regulation of their expression; a fact underlined by the generally low levels of serum miRNAs [89, 91].

A number of different reliable and robust protocols for the extraction of miRNAs from human serum and plasma, as well as for the profiling of serum miRNA expression, have already been developed [89, 94]. Sufficient amounts of serum miRNAs for expression profiling can be extracted from as little as one milliliter (1 ml) of serum. Furthermore, both qRT-PCR-based and microarray-based techniques are suitable for reliable expression profiling of serum miRNAs [89–95]. However, if serum miRNAs are to be routinely used as biomarkers in the future, standardization of the profiling methods employed will be necessary. While the extraction of miRNAs from blood samples using a simple phenol/chloroform extraction protocol seems to be sufficient and can be easily adopted, several issues have to be considered regarding which technique is employed for expression profiling of circulating miRNAs. Firstly, if using the microarray-based technique, it should be noted that different labeling methods may affect the expression pattern found. In general, labeling: (1) by incorporation of modified oligonucleotides; (2) using an extended poly-A tail; or (3) with a modified primer is preferred. Secondly, if amplification steps are performed during the protocol, they can produce different expression patterns as a result of differential efficiencies within the amplification process. Thirdly, if using a qRT-PCR-based setup, a common normalization molecule has to be defined, as 5S rRNA and U6 snRNA (two molecules routinely used as internal controls in miRNA qRT-PCR reactions) are not stable in serum. A miRNA ubiquitously expressed throughout tissues and cell lines – namely miR-16 – appears to be an ideal candidate for this purpose [95, 96].

Although there is currently no assay available to examine miRNA signatures in the serum or plasma of cancer patients for routine diagnostic purposes, some promising results have already been obtained [7, 8, 89–93, 95]. For example, Lawrie et al. [95] reported that miR-21 levels were significantly elevated in the sera of individuals with diffuse large B-cell lymphoma, and that miR-21 serum levels were additionally associated with relapse-free survival in these patients. Mitchell et al. [91] found that serum levels of miR-141 can distinguish patients with prostate cancer from healthy controls; thereby, establishing a blood-based PCR approach for the detection of human prostate cancer. A similar experimental setup was utilized to detect serum miRNAs in ovarian cancer patients [90]. Taylor and Gercel-Taylor [92] showed that the miRNA content of both ovarian tumor cells and circulating exosomes was highly similar, and could be used to distinguish cancer patients from individuals with benign ovarian disease and normal controls. Chen et al. [93] demonstrated that serum expression levels of miR-25 and miR-223 were elevated in patients with non-small cell lung carcinoma (NSCLC), and that these circulating miRNAs could serve as blood-based biomarkers for this tumor. Lodes et al. [89] determined serum miRNA expression patterns for five types of human cancer (prostate, colon, ovarian, breast, and lung) and showed that the resulting patterns can be utilized to correctly discriminate between normal and cancer patient blood samples in most cases.

To date, more than 100 studies have assessed the potential use of serum or plasma miRNAs as tumor biomarkers (reviewed in [97]). These studies underline the important impact serum/plasma miRNAs could have on future diagnostic and prognostic applications in virtually all types of human cancers (i.e., prostate cancer, colorectal cancer, lung cancer, ovarian cancer, breast cancer, and others) [98–102].

The first efforts to identify melanoma-specific blood-based biomarkers were reported by Eckart Meese and his group [103]. Fundamental to their experiments was a commercially available microarray-based platform developed in cooperation with Febit Biomed GmbH (Heidelberg, Germany). This technology was used to identify sets of 24 and 48 miRNAs, respectively, which provided accurate discrimination of patients with NSCLC or multiple sclerosis from healthy individuals with an accuracy of 95% [7, 8]. Screening the expression of 866 miRNAs in the blood of 20 healthy control individuals, a test set of 24 melanoma patients and an independent validation set (comprising 11 additional melanoma patients), they identified a 16 miRNA signature which achieved a classification accuracy of 97.4%, a specificity of 95% and a sensitivity of 98% [103]. Studies involving larger patient cohorts will be necessary to determine if the classifier constructed will actually be able to allow for early melanoma detection, as proposed by the authors. The same is true for the concept of using peripheral blood cells for miRNA biomarker discovery, instead of either circulating protein-bound miRNAs or exosomal miRNAs as performed by most other groups [97]. Nevertheless, it should be highlighted that the commercially available biochip platform on which these experiments were performed could potentially be optimized for routine diagnostic use in near future.

Kanemaru and colleagues found levels of a single circulating miRNA, miR-221, to be significantly elevated in the sera of melanoma patients [104]. Analyzing 94 melanoma patients and 20 healthy controls, they additionally revealed that stage I–IV melanoma patients had even higher miR-221 levels than patients with melanoma in situ. Moreover, miR-221 levels tended to decrease after surgical removal of the primary tumor and to rise again at the time of disease recurrence [104]. On the one hand, miR-221 could be an interesting biomarker due to its well-characterized functional networking in melanoma (reviewed in [11]). However, miR-211 overexpression has also been observed in a variety of other tumors, so that the specificity of this biomarker for melanoma may not be sufficiently pronounced.

In conclusion, serum miRNAs represent a "gold mine" for the identification of biomarkers with the promise of diagnostic, prognostic and therapeutic response prediction [97]. The most obvious advantage of blood-based biomarkers is that sample collection represents a non-invasive procedure, without the requirement for biopsy or other invasive techniques that limit the application of some currently available diagnostic procedures [105, 106]. Unfortunately, the use of only a single serum biomarker molecule might limit the sensitivity, specificity, accuracy, and thus the usefulness of blood-based diagnostic tools currently implemented in the clinic. An approach that employs several different serum miRNAs, serving as a "fingerprint" for a specific type of cancer, may prove to outperform traditional protocols and have a huge impact on diagnosis, including determining cancer classification, estimating prognosis, predicting therapeutic efficacy, maintaining surveillance following surgery, and forecasting disease recurrence.

It is expected that additional retrospective studies on blood samples of melanoma patients will soon be performed as reliable methodologies are now available and a multitude of blood samples from well-documented melanoma cases are stored in clinical archives. Of note, a group from the University of Leicester aims to identify serum miRNA biomarkers which can determine clinical outcome in patients with advanced melanoma [107]. The availability of high-throughput approaches for global miRNA characterization and simple, universally applicable methods for miRNA quantification (i.e., qRT-PCR) suggest that the discovery-validation pipeline for miRNA biomarkers in melanoma has the potential to be highly efficient and to proceed rather quickly.

Future Prospects for miRNAs as Melanoma Biomarkers

As is true for other cancer types where tumor markers for early neoplastic transformation remain to be discovered, melanoma biomarkers that distinguish between benign melanocytic nevi and early melanoma are urgently needed – especially when one considers that the ability to metastasize may be a very early event in the pathogenesis of melanoma. MiRNA biomarkers hopefully harbor the potential to suit not only this purpose, but also to separate primary melanomas with the risk for metastasis from non-metastasizing tumors. Although miRNA analysis is unlikely to replace existing tools for tumor diagnosis and management (such as immunohistochemical staining and detection of serum marker-proteins), miRNA biomarkers offer huge benefits if used to complement such established methodologies.

Identification of miRNAs Deregulated in Melanoma and Their Potential to be Utilized for Future Targeted-Melanoma Therapy

Recent Progress in Exploitation of RNA Interference for Cancer Therapy

Although the discovery of RNA interference (RNAi) can be dated back to barely more than a decade ago, this comparatively short period of time has been sufficient to not only recognize the potential utility of this cellular mechanism for the treatment of human diseases such as cancer, but also to engineer RNAi-based technologies already applicable in the clinical setting.

To date, artificially designed siRNAs (small inhibitory RNA molecules) are almost exclusively used for therapeutic purposes (for recent reviews on clinical trials of siRNA-based therapeutics, see [108–110]). Remarkable advancements in the delivery of siRNAs to target tissues have been made, including the optimization of siRNA molecule stability in the bloodstream, the transduction of siRNAs across biological membranes, and cell type-specific delivery (reviewed in [108, 111–114]). Considering that localized siRNA delivery directly to the tissue affected has several distinct advantages over systemic siRNA administration, it may be of special interest for the treatment of primary melanoma tumors that Inoue and colleagues reported successful transduction of siRNAs into skin cells by intradermal injection of unmodified siRNA molecules followed by *in vivo* electroporation [115]. With regard to the treatment of melanoma metastases, improvements in systemic delivery achieved by the development of modifications stabilizing siRNAs in the bloodstream, as well as the engineering of siRNA carriers (such as liposomes, polymer-based nanoparticles, and siRNA-cholesterol conjugates), thereby optimizing siRNA uptake by tumor cells, could prove beneficial [108, 111–114]. Davis et al. were the first to report efficient and cancer cell-specific RNAi in humans by systemic administration of a targeted nanovesicle siRNA delivery system in three metastatic melanoma patients [116]. In addition, direct intra-tumoral injection of siRNA delivery complexes may be applicable to primary tumors and localized metastases, if this method can be translated from animal xenograft models into the clinical setting [117, 118].

Advantages of Utilizing miRNAs for RNAi-Based Gene Therapy

Due to the fact that both synthetic miRNA mimetics (dsRNA molecules in which one strand closely resembles a major miRNA sequence) and miRNA-antagonizing molecules (anti-miRs; single-stranded RNAs (ssRNAs) which are perfectly complementary to a miRNA, thus preventing binding of this miRNA to its target mRNAs) share high structural similarity to siRNAs, techniques developed for administration of siRNA therapeutics should also be suitable for miRNA-based applications. MiRNAs offer some intriguing advantages over siRNAs when employed in RNAi-based therapeutic approaches. In contrast to an siRNA which only targets one mRNA, a single miRNA is capable of regulating the expression of dozens to hundreds of target genes [59]. As a consequence, modulating the expression level of only one miRNA would have a broad impact on several cellular functions. With regard to cancer treatment, this implies that multiple oncogenic pathways could be manipulated by altering the expression levels of a single miRNA species. On the one hand, considering that tumors are of notably heterogeneous nature, this promiscuity of miRNAs is one of the most obvious advantages when using these molecules for therapeutic gene silencing. On the other hand, it may be difficult to anticipate the entirety of effects triggered by modifying miRNA expression in a particular tissue. Fortunately, the mode of action of miRNA-mediated gene silencing may help to attenuate this latter concern to some degree, as explained by the following. Firstly, it has been suggested that robust silencing of an mRNA is only obtained if several binding sites for a specific miRNA are present in the 3′UTR of the transcript, whereas the presence of only a single target site will result in lower efficiency of silencing [119]. Therefore, as a specific miRNA does not repress all of its target genes with the same efficacy, it is thought that through careful selection of appropriate miRNAs, the effects exerted on intended pathways will be profound whereas effects on unintended pathways can be limited [113]. Secondly, it appears that the deregulation of expression of at least some of the miRNAs involved in cancer formation and progression is very specific and exclusive to malignant cells. This conclusion stems from studies demonstrating that miRNA expression profiles can accurately separate tumor cells from their healthy biological correlates [67, 69, 71, 120]. This indicates that the reconstitution of a miRNA lost during the malignant transformation of tumor cells would potentially not have a strong impact on the surrounding healthy tissue in which the miRNA is already strongly expressed under physiological conditions. Of course, the same would be true when antagonizing an oncogenic miRNA in tumor cells, as miRNA inhibitors would probably produce no effect in those cells which do not express the miRNA at a detectable level. Taking both these arguments into consideration, it has been suggested that miRNAs known to be involved in a particular process could be exploited for therapeutic purposes without the knowledge of all of their target genes [113]. Nevertheless, attention must be drawn to any potential side-effects caused by the possible future use of miRNA therapeutics, as a result of the extensive impact of these molecules on global gene expression.

Another important advantage of utilizing miRNAs, instead of siRNAs, for RNAi-based therapy is that the modulation of gene expression would not be exclusively limited to genes up-regulated during oncogenesis. Although the introduction of miRNA mimetics into tumor cells will lead to down-regulation of their target genes (as well as transfection of a siRNA promotes silencing of its single target gene), antagonizing miRNA function through administration of anti-miR molecules will result in re-expression of the corresponding target genes in transfected tumor cells. The availability of miRNA mimetics for the re-establishment of tumor-suppressive miRNA expression, as well as anti-miRs for blockade of oncogenic miRNA function, strongly broadens the possible applications of miRNA agents in RNAi-based therapy.

Besides the use of miRNA mimetics and anti-miRs, several other potential applications that exploit the principles of miRNA-mediated RNAi for targeted therapy have recently been developed. For example, target protectors (RNA-binding oligonucleotides, which are complementary to miRNA binding sites in the 3′UTR of the corresponding transcript) were reported to successfully prevent miRNA-mediated silencing of specific target genes [121, 122]. This technique could prove beneficial if only specific transcripts are expected to be relieved from miRNA control. Additionally, promising results have been obtained in experiments utilizing differential expression of miRNAs in tumor cells and healthy tissue to improve specificity and efficacy of gene and stem cell therapy, in addition to viral oncolytics in animal models (reviewed in [123]). Basically, the transgene already expressed under a tissue-specific promoter is additionally engineered to harbor several artificial binding sites perfectly complementary to the 3'UTR of a specific miRNA. By selecting a miRNA which is highly abundant in healthy cells but whose expression is lost in tumor cells, the transgenic transcript gets silenced in healthy cells but remains stable in tumor cells, ultimately leading to selective transgene expression only in tumorous cells [124, 125]. Therefore, miRNA-based techniques show considerable potential if used to complement other approaches for targeted gene therapy.

Several recent findings further highlight both the applicability and great potential of miRNA-based therapeutics. Sakari Kauppinen's group was the first to demonstrate successful and well-tolerated LNA-mediated miRNA silencing in non-human primates [126]. This was also the starting point for the first miRNA-targeted drug to enter clinical trials (miravirsen, SPC3649), under the leadership of Santoris Pharma A/S (Hoersholm, Denmark). Most recently, Kauppinen and his co-workers have developed a method to synchronously knock-down all members of a miRNA family that share the same seed sequence, using a single seed-targeting tiny LNA molecule [127]. Interestingly, miRNAs have also recently been found to be implicated in drug resistance mechanisms in tumors [128], indicating that miRNA therapeutics could enhance the efficiency of traditional chemo- or radio-therapeutic applications in otherwise resistant cancers. Furthermore, miRNAs have been identified as potential key targets in the fight against cancer-promoting/sustaining stem cells [13].

miRNAs Suitable for RNAi-Based Therapeutic Approaches in Melanoma

Several miRNAs deregulated during the pathogenesis and progression of melanoma have already been identified (extensively reviewed in [11]; see Fig. 10.2). For some of these miRNAs, the causes for their loss or gain of expression, as well as for one or more of their related target genes, in melanoma cells have been determined (Table 10.1). Although research into the global impact of miRNAs on melanomagenesis is still in its infancy, there are already some promising candidates that could potentially be used for therapeutic RNAi purposes. In the medium term, the rapidly advancing characterization of the melanoma miRNAome (representing the entity that encompasses all miRNAs expressed by melanoma cells) and the concomitant detection of significant changes in the expression levels of specific miRNAs as compared to normal, healthy melanocytes will accelerate the identification of potent miRNA targets for future therapeutic intervention [72, 129–132].

Unfortunately, there is no currently available data on efforts to optimize *in vivo* delivery of miRNA mimetics or anti-miRs into human melanoma cells, nor studies utilizing miRNA-mediated RNAi for the treatment of melanocytic tumors in a clinical setting. Nevertheless, Huynh and colleagues have demonstrated that targeting of miR-182 by intraperitoneal injection of a 2' sugar modified anti-miR containing a phosphorothioate backbone resulted in reduced melanoma metastases to the liver and spleen in a mouse model [133]. Of note, despite the authors detecting some degree of acute hepatitis in anti-miR treated animals, liver toxicity did not reach levels as severe as those previously observed with shRNA-based approaches [134, 135].

Future Prospects for miRNA-Based Therapeutics in the Treatment of Melanoma

The recent progress achieved in siRNA technology builds a stable foundation for the engineering of miRNA-based applications for the treatment of human cancers, including melanoma. However, there are still many obstacles to be negotiated before miRNA therapeutics can be routinely applied in the clinic. As outlined above, the main hurdle is the accurate estimation of unwanted side-effects when therapeutically modulating the expression level of a particular miRNA in its tissue-specific context. It is the responsibility of basic researchers to proceed with the identification and verification of miRNA target genes, so that existing bioinformatical algorithms can be optimized to better suit this purpose. Only a complete understanding of miRNA function and its impact on the global cellular network of pathways will ultimately lead to the development of miRNA-based therapeutics.

Acknowledgements The authors are deeply indebted to Dr. Richard Bauer for the excellent graphical artwork of Fig. 10.1.

References

1. Lee RC, Feinbaum RL, Ambros V. The C. elegans heterochronic gene lin-4 encodes small RNAs with antisense complementarity to lin-14. Cell. 1993; 75(5):843–854.
2. Wightman B, Ha I, Ruvkun G. Posttranscriptional regulation of the heterochronic gene lin-14 by lin-4 mediates temporal pattern formation in C. elegans. Cell. 1993;75(5):855–862.
3. Reinhart BJ, Slack FJ, Basson M, Pasquinelli AE, Bettinger JC, Rougvie AE, et al. The 21-nucleotide let-7 RNA regulates developmental timing in Caenorhabditis elegans. Nature. 2000;403(6772): 901–906.
4. Pasquinelli AE, Reinhart BJ, Slack F, Martindale MQ, Kuroda MI, Maller B, et al. Conservation of the sequence and temporal expression of let-7 heterochronic regulatory RNA. Nature. 2000;408(6808): 86–89.
5. Slack FJ, Basson M, Liu Z, Ambros V, Horvitz HR, Ruvkun G. The lin-41 RBCC gene acts in the C. elegans heterochronic pathway between the let-7 regulatory RNA and the LIN-29 transcription factor. Mol Cell. 2000;5(4):659–669.
6. Negrini M, Nicoloso MS, Calin GA. MicroRNAs and cancer-new paradigms in molecular oncology. Curr Opin Cell Biol. 2009;21(3):470–9.
7. Farazi TA, Spitzer JI, Morozov P, Tuschl T. miRNAs in human cancer. J Pathol. 2011;223(2):102–15.
8. Lee SK, Calin GA. Non-coding RNAs and cancer: new paradigms in oncology. Discov Med. 2011; 11(58):245–54.
9. Mueller DW, Bosserhoff AK. Role of miRNAs in the progression of malignant melanoma. Br J Cancer. 2009;101(4):551–556.
10. Howell Jr PM, Li X, Riker AI, Xi Y. MicroRNA in melanoma. Ochsner J. 2010;10(2):83–92.
11. Mueller DW, Bosserhoff AK. miRNAs in malignant melanoma. In: Bosserhoff A, editor. Melanoma development: molecular biology, genetics and clinical application. Wien: Springer; 2011.
12. Garzon R, Marcucci G, Croce CM. Targeting microRNAs in cancer: rationale, strategies and challenges. Nat Rev Drug Discov. 2010;9(10): 775–89.
13. Leal JA, Feliciano A, Lleonart ME. Stem cell MicroRNAs in senescence and immortalization: novel players in cancer therapy. Med Res Rev. 2011. [Epub Ahead of Print].
14. Cortez MA, Ivan C, Zhou P, Wu X, Ivan M, Calin GA. microRNAs in cancer: from bench to bedside. Adv Cancer Res. 2010;108:113–57.
15. Gremel G, Rafferty M, Lau TY, Gallagher WM. Identification and functional validation of therapeutic targets for malignant melanoma. Crit Rev Oncol Hematol. 2009;72(3):194–214.
16. Sigalotti L, Covre A, Fratta E, Parisi G, Colizzi F, Rizzo A, Danielli R, Nicolay HJ, Coral S, Maio M. Epigenetics of human cutaneous melanoma: setting the stage for new therapeutic strategies. J Transl Med. 2010;8:56.
17. Lee Y, Jeon K, Lee JT, Kim S, Kim VN. MicroRNA maturation: stepwise processing and subcellular localization. EMBO J. 2002;21(17):4663–4670.
18. Lee Y, Kim M, Han J, Yeom KH, Lee S, Baek SH, et al. MicroRNA genes are transcribed by RNA polymerase II. EMBO J. 2004;23(20):4051–4060.
19. Cai X, Hagedorn CH, Cullen BR. Human microRNAs are processed from capped, polyadenylated transcripts that can also function as mRNAs. RNA. 2004;10(12):1957–1966.
20. Borchert GM, Lanier W, Davidson BL. RNA polymerase III transcribes human microRNAs. Nat Struct Mol Biol. 2006;13(12):1097–1101.
21. Lee Y, Ahn C, Han J, Choi H, Kim J, Yim J, et al. The nuclear RNase III Drosha initiates microRNA processing. Nature. 2003;425(6956): 415–419.
22. Landthaler M, Yalcin A, Tuschl T. The human DiGeorge syndrome critical region gene 8 and Its D. melanogaster homolog are required for miRNA biogenesis. Curr Biol. 2004;14(23):2162–2167.
23. Han J, Lee Y, Yeom KH, Nam JW, Heo I, Rhee JK, et al. Molecular basis for the recognition of primary microRNAs by the Drosha-DGCR8 complex. Cell. 2006;125(5):887–901.
24. Zeng Y, Cullen BR. Efficient processing of primary microRNA hairpins by Drosha requires flanking nonstructured RNA sequences. J Biol Chem. 2005; 280(30):27595–27603.
25. Kim VN. MicroRNA precursors in motion: exportin-5 mediates their nuclear export. Trends Cell Biol. 2004;14(4):156–159.
26. Zeng Y, Cullen BR. Sequence requirements for micro RNA processing and function in human cells. RNA. 2003;9(1):112–123.
27. Berezikov E, Chung WJ, Willis J, Cuppen E, Lai EC. Mammalian mirtron genes. Mol Cell. 2007;28(2): 328–336.
28. Gregory RI, Chendrimada TP, Cooch N, Shiekhattar R. Human RISC couples microRNA biogenesis and posttranscriptional gene silencing. Cell. 2005;123(4): 631–640.

29. MacRae IJ, Ma E, Zhou M, Robinson CV, Doudna JA. In vitro reconstitution of the human RISC-loading complex. Proc Natl Acad Sci USA. 2008;105(2):512–517.
30. Hutvagner G, McLachlan J, Pasquinelli AE, Balint E, Tuschl T, Zamore PD. A cellular function for the RNA-interference enzyme Dicer in the maturation of the let-7 small temporal RNA. Science. 2001;293(5531):834–838.
31. Knight SW, Bass BL. A role for the RNase III enzyme DCR-1 in RNA interference and germ line development in Caenorhabditis elegans. Science. 2001;293(5538):2269–2271.
32. Winter J, Jung S, Keller S, Gregory RI, Diederichs S. Many roads to maturity: microRNA biogenesis pathways and their regulation. Nat Cell Biol. 2009;11(3):228–234.
33. Diederichs S, Haber DA. Dual role for argonautes in microRNA processing and posttranscriptional regulation of microRNA expression. Cell. 2007;131(6):1097–1108.
34. Matranga C, Tomari Y, Shin C, Bartel DP, Zamore PD. Passenger-strand cleavage facilitates assembly of siRNA into Ago2-containing RNAi enzyme complexes. Cell. 2005;123(4):607–620.
35. Khvorova A, Reynolds A, Jayasena SD. Functional siRNAs and miRNAs exhibit strand bias. Cell. 2003;115(2):209–216.
36. Filipowicz W, Bhattacharyya SN, Sonenberg N. Mechanisms of post-transcriptional regulation by microRNAs: are the answers in sight? Nat Rev Genet. 2008;9(2):102–114.
37. Nielsen CB, Shomron N, Sandberg R, Hornstein E, Kitzman J, Burge CB. Determinants of targeting by endogenous and exogenous microRNAs and siRNAs. RNA. 2007;13(11):1894–1910.
38. Grimson A, Farh KK, Johnston WK, Garrett-Engele P, Lim LP, Bartel DP. MicroRNA targeting specificity in mammals: determinants beyond seed pairing. Mol Cell. 2007;27(1):91–105.
39. Lewis BP, Burge CB, Bartel DP. Conserved seed pairing, often flanked by adenosines, indicates that thousands of human genes are microRNA targets. Cell. 2005;120(1):15–20.
40. Brennecke J, Stark A, Russell RB, Cohen SM. Principles of microRNA-target recognition. PLoS Biol. 2005;3(3):e85.
41. Doench JG, Sharp PA. Specificity of microRNA target selection in translational repression. Genes Dev. 2004;18(5):504–511.
42. Wu L, Fan J, Belasco JG. MicroRNAs direct rapid deadenylation of mRNA. Proc Natl Acad Sci USA. 2006;103(11):4034–4039.
43. Behm-Ansmant I, Rehwinkel J, Izaurralde E. MicroRNAs silence gene expression by repressing protein expression and/or by promoting mRNA decay. Cold Spring Harb Symp Quant Biol. 2006;71:523–530.
44. Giraldez AJ, Mishima Y, Rihel J, Grocock RJ, Van Dongen S, Inoue K, et al. Zebrafish MiR-430 promotes deadenylation and clearance of maternal mRNAs. Science. 2006;312(5770):75–9.
45. Wu L, Belasco JG. Micro-RNA regulation of the mammalian lin-28 gene during neuronal differentiation of embryonal carcinoma cells. Mol Cell Biol. 2005;25(21):9198–9208.
46. Pillai RS, Bhattacharyya SN, Artus CG, Zoller T, Cougot N, Basyuk E, et al. Inhibition of translational initiation by Let-7 MicroRNA in human cells. Science. 2005;309(5740):1573–1576.
47. Standart N, Jackson RJ. MicroRNAs repress translation of m7G ppp-capped target mRNAs in vitro by inhibiting initiation and promoting deadenylation. Genes Dev. 2007;21(16):1975–1982.
48. Till S, Lejeune E, Thermann R, Bortfeld M, Hothorn M, Enderle D, et al. A conserved motif in Argonaute-interacting proteins mediates functional interactions through the Argonaute PIWI domain. Nat Struct Mol Biol. 2007;14(10):897–903.
49. Behm-Ansmant I, Rehwinkel J, Doerks T, Stark A, Bork P, Izaurralde E. mRNA degradation by miRNAs and GW182 requires both CCR4:NOT deadenylase and DCP1:DCP2 decapping complexes. Genes Dev. 2006;20(14):1885–1898.
50. Eulalio A, Rehwinkel J, Stricker M, Huntzinger E, Yang SF, Doerks T, et al. Target-specific requirements for enhancers of decapping in miRNA-mediated gene silencing. Genes Dev. 2007;21(20):2558–2570.
51. Eulalio A, Huntzinger E, Nishihara T, Rehwinkel J, Fauser M, Izaurralde E. Deadenylation is a widespread effect of miRNA regulation. RNA. 2009;15(1):21–32.
52. Chekulaeva M, Filipowicz W. Mechanisms of miRNA-mediated post-transcriptional regulation in animal cells. Curr Opin Cell Biol. 2009;21(3):452–460.
53. Kong YW, Cannell IG, de Moor CH, Hill K, Garside PG, Hamilton TL, et al. The mechanism of microRNA-mediated translation repression is determined by the promoter of the target gene. Proc Natl Acad Sci USA. 2008;105(26):8866–8871.
54. Cannell IG, Kong YW, Bushell M. How do microRNAs regulate gene expression? Biochem Soc Trans. 2008;36(Pt 6):1224–1231.
55. Kim VN, Han J, Siomi MC. Biogenesis of small RNAs in animals. Nat Rev Mol Cell Biol. 2009;10(2):126–139.
56. Davis BN, Hata A. Regulation of microRNA biogenesis: a miRiad of mechanisms. Cell Commun Signal. 2009;7:18.
57. Krol J, Loedige I, Filipowicz W. The widespread regulation of microRNA biogenesis, function and decay. Nat Rev Genet. 2010;11(9):597–610.
58. Griffiths-Jones S, Saini HK, Van Dongen S, Enright AJ. miRBase: tools for microRNA genomics. Nucleic Acids Res. 2008;36(Database issue):D154–D158.
59. Krek A, Grun D, Poy MN, Wolf R, Rosenberg L, Epstein EJ, et al. Combinatorial microRNA target predictions. Nat Genet. 2005;37(5):495–500.

60. Lee YS, Kim HK, Chung S, Kim KS, Dutta A. Depletion of human micro-RNA miR-125b reveals that it is critical for the proliferation of differentiated cells but not for the down-regulation of putative targets during differentiation. J Biol Chem. 2005;280: 16635–16641.
61. Johnson SM, Grosshans H, Shingara J, Byrom M, Jarvis R, Cheng A, Labourier E, Reinert KL, Brown D, Slack FJ. RAS is regulated by the let-7 microRNA family. Cell. 2005;120:635–647.
62. Lim LP, Lau NC, Garrett-Engele P, Grimson A, Schelter JM, Castle J, Bartel DP, Linsley PS, Johnson JM. Microarray analysis shows that some microRNAs downregulate large numbers of target mRNAs. Nature. 2005;433:769–773.
63. John B, Enright AJ, Aravin A, Tuschl T, Sander C, Marks DS. Human MicroRNA targets. PLoS Biol. 2004;2:e363.
64. Kiriakidou M, Nelson PT, Kouranov A, Fitziev P, Bouyioukos C, Mourelatos Z, Hatzigeorgiou A. A combined computational-experimental approach predicts human microRNA targets. Genes Dev. 2004;18:1165–1178.
65. Mirnezami AH, Pickard K, Zhang L, Primrose JN, Packham G. MicroRNAs: key players in carcinogenesis and novel therapeutic targets. Eur J Surg Oncol. 2009;35(4):339–347.
66. Visone R, Croce CM. MiRNAs and cancer. Am J Pathol. 2009;174(4):1131–1138.
67. Lu J, Getz G, Miska EA, Alvarez-Saavedra E, Lamb J, Peck D, et al. MicroRNA expression profiles classify human cancers. Nature. 2005;435(7043): 834–838.
68. Zhang L, Huang J, Yang N, Greshock J, Megraw MS, Giannakakis A, et al. microRNAs exhibit high frequency genomic alterations in human cancer. Proc Natl Acad Sci U S A. 2006;103(24):9136–9141.
69. Gaur A, Jewell DA, Liang Y, Ridzon D, Moore JH, Chen C, et al. Characterization of microRNA expression levels and their biological correlates in human cancer cell lines. Cancer Res. 2007;67(6):2456–2468.
70. Blower PE, Verducci JS, Lin S, Zhou J, Chung JH, Dai Z, et al. MicroRNA expression profiles for the NCI-60 cancer cell panel. Mol Cancer Ther. 2007;6(5):1483–1491.
71. Rosenfeld N, Aharonov R, Meiri E, Rosenwald S, Spector Y, Zepeniuk M, et al. MicroRNAs accurately identify cancer tissue origin. Nat Biotechnol. 2008;26(4):462–469.
72. Mueller DW, Rehli M, Bosserhoff AK. miRNA expression profiling in melanocytes and melanoma cell lines reveals miRNAs associated with formation and progression of malignant melanoma. J Invest Dermatol. 2009;129(7):1740–1751.
73. Glud M, Klausen M, Gniadecki R, Rossing M, Hastrup N, Nielsen FC, et al. MicroRNA expression in melanocytic nevi: the usefulness of formalin-fixed, paraffin-embedded material for miRNA microarray profiling. J Invest Dermatol. 2009;129(5): 1219–1224.
74. Liu A, Tetzlaff MT, Vanbelle P, Elder D, Feldman M, Tobias JW, et al. MicroRNA expression profiling outperforms mRNA expression profiling in formalin-fixed paraffin-embedded tissues. Int J Clin Exp Pathol. 2009;2(6):519–527.
75. Ma Z, Lui WO, Fire A, Dadras SS. Profiling and discovery of novel miRNAs from formalin-fixed, paraffin-embedded melanoma and nodal specimens. J Mol Diagn. 2009;11(5):420–429.
76. Siebolts U, Varnholt H, Drebber U, Dienes HP, Wickenhauser C, Odenthal M. Tissues from routine pathology archives are suitable for microRNA analyses by quantitative PCR. J Clin Pathol. 2009;62(1): 84–88.
77. Xi Y, Nakajima G, Gavin E, Morris CG, Kudo K, Hayashi K, et al. Systematic analysis of microRNA expression of RNA extracted from fresh frozen and formalin-fixed paraffin-embedded samples. RNA. 2007;13(10):1668–1674.
78. Lawrie CH, Soneji S, Marafioti T, Cooper CD, Palazzo S, Paterson JC, et al. MicroRNA expression distinguishes between germinal center B cell-like and activated B cell-like subtypes of diffuse large B cell lymphoma. Int J Cancer. 2007;121(5):1156–1161.
79. Doleshal M, Magotra AA, Choudhury B, Cannon BD, Labourier E, Szafranska AE. Evaluation and validation of total RNA extraction methods for microRNA expression analyses in formalin-fixed, paraffin-embedded tissues. J Mol Diagn. 2008;10(3):203–211.
80. Masuda N, Ohnishi T, Kawamoto S, Monden M, Okubo K. Analysis of chemical modification of RNA from formalin-fixed samples and optimization of molecular biology applications for such samples. Nucleic Acids Res. 1999;27(22):4436–4443.
81. Srinivasan M, Sedmak D, Jewell S. Effect of fixatives and tissue processing on the content and integrity of nucleic acids. Am J Pathol. 2002;161(6):1961–1971.
82. Cronin M, Pho M, Dutta D, Stephans JC, Shak S, Kiefer MC, et al. Measurement of gene expression in archival paraffin-embedded tissues: development and performance of a 92-gene reverse transcriptase-polymerase chain reaction assay. Am J Pathol. 2004;164(1):35–42.
83. Li J, Smyth P, Flavin R, Cahill S, Denning K, Aherne S, et al. Comparison of miRNA expression patterns using total RNA extracted from matched samples of formalin-fixed paraffin-embedded (FFPE) cells and snap frozen cells. BMC Biotechnol. 2007;7:36.
84. Satzger I, Mattern A, Kuettler U, Weinspach D, Voelker B, Kapp A, et al. MicroRNA-15b represents an independent prognostic parameter and is correlated with tumor cell proliferation and apoptosis in malignant melanoma. Int J Cancer. 2010;126(11): 2553–2562.
85. Segura MF, Belitskaya-Lévy I, Rose AE, Zakrzewski J, Gaziel A, Hanniford D, Darvishian F, Berman RS, Shapiro RL, Pavlick AC, Osman I, Hernando E. Melanoma MicroRNA signature predicts post-recurrence survival. Clin Cancer Res. 2010;16(5): 1577–86.

86. Caramuta S, Egyházi S, Rodolfo M, Witten D, Hansson J, Larsson C, Lui WO. MicroRNA expression profiles associated with mutational status and survival in malignant melanoma. J Invest Dermatol. 2010;130(8):2062–70.
87. Jukic DM, Rao UN, Kelly L, Skaf JS, Drogowski LM, Kirkwood JM, Panelli MC. Microrna profiling analysis of differences between the melanoma of young adults and older adults. J Transl Med. 2010;8:27.
88. Chan E, Patel R, Nallur S, Ratner E, Bacchiocchi A, Hoyt K, Szpakowski S, Godshalk S, Ariyan S, Sznol M, Halaban R, Krauthammer M, Tuck D, Slack FJ, Weidhaas JB. MicroRNA signatures differentiate melanoma subtypes. Cell Cycle. 2011;10(11):1845–52.
89. Lodes MJ, Caraballo M, Suciu D, Munro S, Kumar A, Anderson B. Detection of cancer with serum miRNAs on an oligonucleotide microarray. PLoS One. 2009;4(7):e6229.
90. Resnick KE, Alder H, Hagan JP, Richardson DL, Croce CM, Cohn DE. The detection of differentially expressed microRNAs from the serum of ovarian cancer patients using a novel real-time PCR platform. Gynecol Oncol. 2009;112(1):55–59.
91. Mitchell PS, Parkin RK, Kroh EM, Fritz BR, Wyman SK, Pogosova-Agadjanyan EL, et al. Circulating microRNAs as stable blood-based markers for cancer detection. Proc Natl Acad Sci USA. 2008;105(30):10513–10518.
92. Taylor DD, Gercel-Taylor C. MicroRNA signatures of tumor-derived exosomes as diagnostic biomarkers of ovarian cancer. Gynecol Oncol. 2008;110(1):13–21.
93. Chen X, Ba Y, Ma L, Cai X, Yin Y, Wang K, et al. Characterization of microRNAs in serum: a novel class of biomarkers for diagnosis of cancer and other diseases. Cell Res. 2008;18(10):997–1006.
94. Gilad S, Meiri E, Yogev Y, Benjamin S, Lebanony D, Yerushalmi N, et al. Serum microRNAs are promising novel biomarkers. PLoS One. 2008;3(9):e3148.
95. Lawrie CH, Gal S, Dunlop HM, Pushkaran B, Liggins AP, Pulford K, et al. Detection of elevated levels of tumour-associated microRNAs in serum of patients with diffuse large B-cell lymphoma. Br J Haematol. 2008;141(5):672–675.
96. Levati L, Alvino E, Pagani E, Arcelli D, Caporaso P, Bondanza S, et al. Altered expression of selected microRNAs in melanoma: antiproliferative and proapoptotic activity of miRNA-155. Int J Oncol. 2009;35(2):393–400.
97. Cortez MA, Bueso-Ramos C, Ferdin J, Lopez-Berestein G, Sood AK, Calin GA. Medscape. MicroRNAs in body fluids-the mix of hormones and biomarkers. Nat Rev Clin Oncol. 2011;8(8):467–77.
98. Hu Z, Chen X, Zhao Y, Tian T, Jin G, Shu Y, Chen Y, Xu L, Zen K, Zhang C, Shen H. Serum microRNA signatures identified in a genome-wide serum microRNA expression profiling predict survival of non-small-cell lung cancer. J Clin Oncol. 2010; 28(10):1721–6.
99. Ng EK, Chong WW, Jin H, Lam EK, Shin VY, Yu J, Poon TC, Ng SS, Sung JJ. Differential expression of microRNAs in plasma of patients with colorectal cancer: a potential marker for colorectal cancer screening. Gut. 2009;58(10):1375–81.
100. Heneghan HM, Miller N, Kerin MJ. Circulating miRNA signatures: promising prognostic tools for cancer. J Clin Oncol. 2010;28(29):e573–4. author reply e575–6.
101. Ho AS, Huang X, Cao H, Christman-Skieller C, Bennewith K, Le QT, Koong AC. Circulating miR-210 as a novel hypoxia marker in pancreatic cancer. Transl Oncol. 2010;3(2):109–13.
102. Yamamoto Y, Kosaka N, Tanaka M, Koizumi F, Kanai Y, Mizutani T, Murakami Y, Kuroda M, Miyajima A, Kato T, Ochiya T. MicroRNA-500 as a potential diagnostic marker for hepatocellular carcinoma. Biomarkers. 2009;14(7):529–38.
103. Leidinger P, Keller A, Borries A, Reichrath J, Rass K, Jager SU, Lenhof HP, Meese E. High-throughput miRNA profiling of human melanoma blood samples. BMC Cancer. 2010;10:262.
104. Kanemaru H, Fukushima S, Yamashita J, Honda N, Oyama R, Kakimoto A, Masuguchi S, Ishihara T, Inoue Y, Jinnin M, Ihn H. The circulating microRNA-221 level in patients with malignant melanoma as a new tumor marker. J Dermatol Sci. 2011;61(3):187–93.
105. Duffy MJ. Role of tumor markers in patients with solid cancers: a critical review. Eur J Intern Med. 2007;18(3):175–184.
106. Roulston JE. Limitations of tumour markers in screening. Br J Surg. 1990;77(9):961–962.
107. http://www2.le.ac.uk/ebulletin/news/press-releases/2000-2009/2009/06/nparticle 2009-06-3049 29817456.
108. Whitehead KA, Langer R, Anderson DG. Knocking down barriers: advances in siRNA delivery. Nat Rev Drug Discov. 2009;8(2):129–138.
109. Wang J, Lu Z, Wientjes MG, Au JL. Delivery of siRNA therapeutics: barriers and carriers. AAPS J. 2010;12(4):492–503.
110. Burnett JC, Rossi JJ, Tiemann K. Current progress of siRNA/shRNA therapeutics in clinical trials. Biotechnol J. 2011;6(9):1130–46.
111. Grimm D. Small silencing RNAs: state-of-the-art. Adv Drug Deliv Rev. 2009;61(9):672–703.
112. Gondi CS, Rao JS. Concepts in in vivo siRNA delivery for cancer therapy. J Cell Physiol. 2009;220(2):285–291.
113. Love TM, Moffett HF, Novina CD. Not miR-ly small RNAs: big potential for microRNAs in therapy. J Allergy Clin Immunol. 2008;121(2):309–319.
114. Yuan X, Naguib S, Wu Z. Recent advances of siRNA delivery by nanoparticles. Expert Opin Drug Deliv. 2011;8(4):521–36.
115. Inoue T, Sugimoto M, Sakurai T, Saito R, Futaki N, Hashimoto Y, et al. Modulation of scratching behavior by silencing an endogenous cyclooxygenase-1 gene in the skin through the administration of siRNA. J Gene Med. 2007;9(11):994–1001.

116. Davis ME, Zuckerman JE, Choi CH, Seligson D, Tolcher A, Alabi CA, Yen Y, Heidel JD, Ribas A. Evidence of RNAi in humans from systemically administered siRNA via targeted nanoparticles. Nature. 2010;464(7291):1067–70.
117. Grzelinski M, Urban-Klein B, Martens T, Lamszus K, Bakowsky U, Hobel S, et al. RNA interference-mediated gene silencing of pleiotrophin through polyethylenimine-complexed small interfering RNAs in vivo exerts antitumoral effects in glioblastoma xenografts. Hum Gene Ther. 2006;17(7):751–766.
118. Niu XY, Peng ZL, Duan WQ, Wang H, Wang P. Inhibition of HPV 16 E6 oncogene expression by RNA interference in vitro and in vivo. Int J Gynecol Cancer. 2006;16(2):743–751.
119. Doench JG, Petersen CP, Sharp PA. siRNAs can function as miRNAs. Genes Dev. 2003;17(4): 438–442.
120. Calin GA, Croce CM. MicroRNA signatures in human cancers. Nat Rev Cancer. 2006;6(11):857–866.
121. Choi WY, Giraldez AJ, Schier AF. Target protectors reveal dampening and balancing of Nodal agonist and antagonist by miR-430. Science. 2007;318(5848):271–274.
122. Esau C, Davis S, Murray SF, Yu XX, Pandey SK, Pear M, et al. miR-122 regulation of lipid metabolism revealed by in vivo antisense targeting. Cell Metab. 2006;3(2):87–98.
123. Brown BD, Naldini L. Exploiting and antagonizing microRNA regulation for therapeutic and experimental applications. Nat Rev Genet. 2009;10(8): 578–585.
124. Brown BD, Gentner B, Cantore A, Colleoni S, Amendola M, Zingale A, et al. Endogenous microRNA can be broadly exploited to regulate transgene expression according to tissue, lineage and differentiation state. Nat Biotechnol. 2007;25(12): 1457–1467.
125. Wolff LJ, Wolff JA, Sebestyen MG. Effect of tissue-specific promoters and microRNA recognition elements on stability of transgene expression after hydrodynamic naked plasmid DNA delivery. Hum Gene Ther. 2009;20(4):374–388.
126. Elmén J, Lindow M, Schütz S, Lawrence M, Petri A, Obad S, Lindholm M, Hedtjärn M, Hansen HF, Berger U, Gullans S, Kearney P, Sarnow P, Straarup EM, Kauppinen S. LNA-mediated microRNA silencing in non-human primates. Nature. 2008;452(7189): 896–9.
127. Obad S, dos Santos CO, Petri A, Heidenblad M, Broom O, Ruse C, Fu C, Lindow M, Stenvang J, Straarup EM, Hansen HF, Koch T, Pappin D, Hannon GJ, Kauppinen S. Silencing of microRNA families by seed-targeting tiny LNAs. Nat Genet. 2011;43(4): 371–8.
128. Giovannetti E, Erozenci A, Smit J, Danesi R, Peters GJ. Molecular mechanisms underlying the role of microRNAs (miRNAs) in anticancer drug resistance and implications for clinical practice. Crit Rev Oncol Hematol. 2011. [Epub Ahead of Print].
129. Schultz J, Lorenz P, Gross G, Ibrahim S, Kunz M. MicroRNA let-7b targets important cell cycle molecules in malignant melanoma cells and interferes with anchorage-independent growth. Cell Res. 2008;18(5):549–557.
130. Stark MS, Tyagi S, Nancarrow DJ, Boyle GM, Cook AL, Whiteman DC, Parsons PG, Schmidt C, Sturm RA, Hayward NK. Characterization of the melanoma miRNAome by deep sequencing. PLoS One. 2010;5(3):e9685.
131. Chen J, Feilotter HE, Paré GC, Zhang X, Pemberton JG, Garady C, Lai D, Yang X, Tron VA. MicroRNA-193b represses cell proliferation and regulates cyclin D1 in melanoma. Am J Pathol. 2010;176(5):2520–9.
132. Philippidou D, Schmitt M, Moser D, Margue C, Nazarov PV, Muller A, Vallar L, Nashan D, Behrmann I, Kreis S. Signatures of microRNAs and selected microRNA target genes in human melanoma. Cancer Res. 2010;70(10):4163–73.
133. Huynh C, Segura MF, Gaziel-Sovran A, Menendez S, Darvishian F, Chiriboga L, Levin B, Meruelo D, Osman I, Zavadil J, Marcusson EG, Hernando E. Efficient in vivo microRNA targeting of liver metastasis. Oncogene. 2011;30(12):1481–8.
134. Grimm D, Streetz KL, Jopling CL, Storm TA, Pandey K, Davis CR, Marion P, Salazar F, Kay MA. Fatality in mice due to oversaturation of cellular microRNA/short hairpin RNA pathways. Nature. 2006;441(7092):537–41.
135. Martin JN, Wolken N, Brown T, Dauer WT, Ehrlich ME, Gonzalez-Alegre P. Lethal toxicity caused by expression of shRNA in the mouse striatum: implications for therapeutic design. Gene Ther. 2011;18(7): 666–73.
136. Muller DW, Bosserhoff AK. Integrin beta 3 expression is regulated by let-7a miRNA in malignant melanoma. Oncogene. 2008;27(52):6698–6706.
137. Fu TY, Chang CC, Lin CT, Lai CH, Peng SY, Ko YJ, Tang PC. Let-7b-mediated suppression of basigin expression and metastasis in mouse melanoma cells. Exp Cell Res. 2011;317(4):445–51.
138. Levati L, Alvino E, Pagani E, Arcelli D, Caporaso P, Bondanza S, Di Leva G, Ferracin M, Volinia S, Bonmassar E, Croce CM, D'Atri S. Altered expression of selected microRNAs in melanoma: antiproliferative and proapoptotic activity of miRNA-155. Int J Oncol. 2009;35(2):393–400.
139. Gaziel-Sovran A, Segura MF, Di Micco R, Collins MK, Hanniford D, Vega-Saenz de Miera E, Rakus JF, Dankert JF, Shang S, Kerbel RS, Bhardwaj N, Shao Y, Darvishian F, Zavadil J, Erlebacher A, Mahal LK, Osman I, Hernando E. miR-30b/30d regulation of GalNAc transferases enhances invasion and immunosuppression during metastasis. Cancer Cell. 2011;20(1):104–18.
140. Lodygin D, Tarasov V, Epanchintsev A, Berking C, Knyazeva T, Körner H, Knyazev P, Diebold J, Hermeking H. Inactivation of miR-34a by aberrant CpG methylation in multiple types of cancer. Cell Cycle. 2008;7(16):2591–600.

141. Lujambio A, Esteller M. CpG island hypermethylation of tumor suppressor microRNAs in human cancer. Cell Cycle. 2007;6(12):1455–9.
142. Migliore C, Petrelli A, Ghiso E, Corso S, Capparuccia L, Eramo A, Comoglio PM, Giordano S. MicroRNAs impair MET-mediated invasive growth. Cancer Res. 2008;68(24):10128–36.
143. Bemis LT, Chen R, Amato CM, Classen EH, Robinson SE, Coffey DG, et al. MicroRNA-137 targets microphthalmia-associated transcription factor in melanoma cell lines. Cancer Res. 2008;68(5):1362–1368.
144. Deng Y, Deng H, Bi F, Liu J, Bemis LT, Norris D, Wang XJ, Zhang Q. MicroRNA-137 targets carboxyl-terminal binding protein 1 in melanoma cell lines. Int J Biol Sci. 2011;7(1):133–7.
145. Segura MF, Hanniford D, Menendez S, Reavie L, Zou X, Alvarez-Diaz S, et al. Aberrant miR-182 expression promotes melanoma metastasis by repressing FOXO3 and microphthalmia-associated transcription factor. Proc Natl Acad Sci USA. 2009;106(6):1814–1819.
146. Braig S, Mueller DW, Rothhammer T, Bosserhoff AK. MicroRNA miR-196a is a central regulator of HOX-B7 and BMP4 expression in malignant melanoma. Cell Mol Life Sci. 2010;67(20):3535–48.
147. Mueller DW, Bosserhoff AK. MicroRNA miR-196a controls melanoma-associated genes by regulating HOX-C8 expression. Int J Cancer. 2011;129(5):1064–74.
148. Dar AA, Majid S, de Semir D, Nosrati M, Bezrookove V, Kashani-Sabet M. miRNA-205 suppresses melanoma cell proliferation and induces senescence via regulation of E2F1 protein. J Biol Chem. 2011;286(19):16606–14.
149. Zhang Z, Sun H, Dai H, Walsh RM, Imakura M, Schelter J, Burchard J, Dai X, Chang AN, Diaz RL, Marszalek JR, Bartz SR, Carleton M, Cleary MA, Linsley PS, Grandori C. MicroRNA miR-210 modulates cellular response to hypoxia through the MYC antagonist MNT. Cell Cycle. 2009;8(17):2756–68.
150. Mazar J, DeYoung K, Khaitan D, Meister E, Almodovar A, Goydos J, Ray A, Perera RJ. The regulation of miRNA-211 expression and its role in melanoma cell invasiveness. PLoS One. 2010;5(11):e13779.
151. Levy C, Khaled M, Iliopoulos D, Janas MM, Schubert S, Pinner S, Chen PH, Li S, Fletcher AL, Yokoyama S, Scott KL, Garraway LA, Song JS, Granter SR, Turley SJ, Fisher DE, Novina CD. Intronic miR-211 assumes the tumor suppressive function of its host gene in melanoma. Mol Cell. 2010;40(5):841–9.
152. Boyle GM, Woods SL, Bonazzi VF, Stark MS, Hacker E, Aoude LG, Dutton-Regester K, Cook AL, Sturm RA, Hayward NK. Melanoma cell invasiveness is regulated by miR-211 suppression of the BRN2 transcription factor. Pigment Cell Melanoma Res. 2011;24(3):525–37.
153. Sakurai E, Maesawa C, Shibazaki M, Yasuhira S, Oikawa H, Sato M, Tsunoda K, Ishikawa Y, Watanabe A, Takahashi K, Akasaka T, Masuda T. Downregulation of microRNA-211 is involved in expression of preferentially expressed antigen of melanoma in melanoma cells. Int J Oncol. 2011;39(3):665–72.
154. Penna E, Orso F, Cimino D, Tenaglia E, Lembo A, Quaglino E, Poliseno L, Haimovic A, Osella-Abate S, De Pittà C, Pinatel E, Stadler MB, Provero P, Bernengo MG, Osman I, Taverna D. microRNA-214 contributes to melanoma tumour progression through suppression of TFAP2C. EMBO J. 2011;30(10):1990–2007.
155. Felicetti F, Errico MC, Bottero L, Segnalini P, Stoppacciaro A, Biffoni M, et al. The promyelocytic leukemia zinc finger-microRNA-221/-222 pathway controls melanoma progression through multiple oncogenic mechanisms. Cancer Res. 2008;68(8):2745–2754.
156. Igoucheva O, Alexeev V. MicroRNA-dependent regulation of cKit in cutaneous melanoma. Biochem Biophys Res Commun. 2009;379(3):790–794.
157. Das SK, Sokhi UK, Bhutia SK, Azab B, Su ZZ, Sarkar D, Fisher PB. Human polynucleotide phosphorylase selectively and preferentially degrades microRNA-221 in human melanoma cells. Proc Natl Acad Sci U S A. 2010;107(26):11948–53.
158. Kitago M, Martinez SR, Nakamura T, Sim MS, Hoon DS. Regulation of RUNX3 tumor suppressor gene expression in cutaneous melanoma. Clin Cancer Res. 2009;15(9):2988–2994.

Mitochondrial DNA Biomarkers in Melanoma

Mark L. Steinberg

Mitochondrial DNA Alterations in Metabolic Diseases and Cancer

The mitochondrial genome is a small [16,569 base pair (bp)], maternally-inherited circular DNA, that is present in copy numbers ranging from only a few to several thousand in the cytosol of a mammalian cell. The mitochondrial genome contains 37 genes. Of these, 13 genes encode polypeptides that represent components of the major respiratory chain complexes. Seven of these are components of complex I (NADH dehydrogenase), three are components of complex IV (cytochrome c oxidase), two are components of the ATP synthase complex (complex V), and one is the cytochrome b subunit of complex III. There are also genes for 12S and 16S ribosomal RNAs and 22 mitochondrial tRNAs (Fig. 11.1). The mitochondrial DNA (mtDNA), which is completely sequestered within the mitochondrial compartment, is unbound by protein complexes and subjected to oxidative damage to a much greater extent than nuclear DNA (nDNA). This is attributed to the accumulation of reactive oxygen species (ROS) that are generated within the mitochondrial matrix during electron transport [1, 2]. In addition, DNA repair is much more limited in mitochondria than in the nucleus. In mitochondria, mammalian cell nucleotide excision repair enzymes (glycosylases) have been demonstrated, but mismatch repair and recombinatorial repair mechanisms appear to be lacking [3–5]. Therefore, alterations in mtDNA are relatively stable over time and tend to persist in a cell lineage over many generations.

Mutations in regions of the genome that encode components of the electron transport chain are known to cause respiratory chain malfunction and result in genetic diseases that are transmitted to offspring via the mitochondria. A number of metabolic diseases, mostly myopathies and neuropathies, caused by mutagenic changes in these genes have been described (Table 11.1) [6–9]. Recently, mitochondrial dysfunction has been implicated in the process of carcinogenesis, because of the involvement of mitochondria in apoptotic pathways [10] and the activation of oncogenic signaling pathways by ROS [11]. There have been a number of recent studies linking alterations in mtDNA to cancers of skin [12–14], breast [15], oral epithelium [16], lung [17], bladder [18], gastrointestinal tract [19, 20], and cervix [21].

M.L. Steinberg, Ph.D. (✉)
Department of Chemistry, The City College of New York, New York, NY, USA
e-mail: marste@sci.ccny.cuny.edu

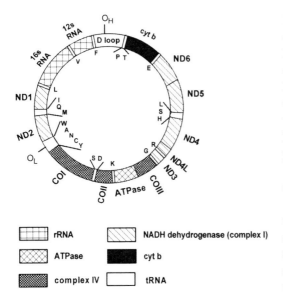

Fig. 11.1 A map of the mitochondrial genome. The genome encodes two ribosomal RNAs and components of complexes I, III, IV and V: seven genes encoding proteins of the NADH dehydrogenase complex (ND1, ND2, ND3, ND4, ND4L, ND5, ND6) in complex I, one gene encoding a cytochrome b polypeptide (cyt b) of complex III, three genes (COI, COII, COIII) that encode polypeptide components of cytochrome oxidase (complex IV), and one gene that encodes a polypeptide in the Fo subunit of the FoF1 ATPase (complex V). There are also genes for 22 tRNAs scattered around the mitochondrial genome. Their approximate locations are indicated along the inner circle by the single letter amino acid codes which denote the amino acid specificity of each tRNA. The locations of the heavy (purine-rich) and light (pyrimidine-rich) strand replication origins are indicated by OH and OL, respectively

Mitochondrial DNA Replication and DNA Instability

The Mitochondrial Genome

The two complementary strands of mtDNA are distinguished on the basis of their G (guanine) or C (cytosine) content, and are designated as either heavy (H-strand; high G content) or light (L-strand; high C content). Each of the two strands has its own replication origin. The two replication origins are separated from one another by a distance representing approximately two thirds of the genome (from the direction of DNA replication).

Replication is initiated asynchronously at the two origins, with the L-strand being replicated first. Initiation of DNA replication from the L-strand origin creates a single-stranded segment of the H-strand, known as the D-loop. The D-loop spans the region between nucleotides (nt) 576–16024, which contains the two mtDNA promoters (an H-strand promoter at nt 545–567 and an L-strand promoter at nt 392–445; summarized in Wallace [2]). A large fraction of the stable alterations that are found in mtDNA occur within the D-loop [22]. This finding has been attributed to the fact that the D-loop is transiently present as a single-stranded segment just after the initiation of DNA synthesis from the L-strand origin. In the single-stranded state, damage to the unpaired strand cannot be repaired by normal template-driven repair mechanisms, particularly excision repair. The single-stranded segment is also much more likely to undergo base mispairing between the single strand and the nascent strands of the replicating DNA; replication of the mispaired duplex can result in the formation of deletions. The clustering of nucleotide changes in the D-loop makes this segment a particularly rich source of potential biomarkers. Two highly polymorphic regions exist within the D-loop, known as hypervariable regions: (HVR1; nt 16024–16365 and HVR2; nt 73–340). HVR2 contains a polycytosine microsatellite segment (nt 303–315) that is particularly mutable. MtDNA alterations in HVR1 and HVR2 are used as markers of genetic lineage, and forensically as biomarkers of different ethnic and racial groupings [23].

Mutations Related to Exposure to Ultraviolet Radiation

There is a strong causal link between exposure to ultraviolet radiation (UVR) from sun exposure and all forms of skin cancer, including melanoma [24]. One particular type of mutagenic DNA damage, which is caused directly by the UVA component of UVR, is covalent bonding between adjacent pyrimidine residues to form cyclobutane dimers (CBD). These lesions are highly mutagenic, as they tend to produce C→T and CC→TT

Table 11.1 Genetic diseases of mitochondrial DNA

Disease[a]	Manifestations	Mitochondrial DNA alteration
DAD (diabetes mellitus and deafness)	Early-onset diabetes and deafness	10,423 bp deletion: nt 14812 → nt 4389
KSS/CEOP (Kearns-Sayre syndrome/chronic external ophthalmoplegia)	Early-onset cerebellar ataxia, paralysis of the extraocular muscles (ophthalmoplegia)	4,977 bp deletion (common deletion): nt 8470 → nt 8482
LHON (Leber's hereditary optic neuropathy)	Degeneration of the optic nerves and retina, Wolff-Parkinson-White syndrome	Multiple SNPs nt 3460 G → A nt 4136 A → G nt 4160 T → C nt 4216 T → C nt 4917 A → G nt 5244 G → A nt 11778 G → A nt 13708 G → A nt 15257 G → A nt 15812 G → A
Leigh syndrome/NARP (neuropathy, ataxia, retinitis pigmentosa, and ptosis)	Neonatal subacute sclerosing encephalopathy, seizures, dementia, ventilatory failure	nt 8993 T → G (encoding subunit 6 of mitochondrial ATP synthase)
MELAS (mitochondrial myopathy, encephalomyopathy, lactic acidosis, stroke-like symptoms)	As per acronym	7,436 bp deletion: nt 8637 and nt 16073
MERRF (myoclonic epilepsy with ragged red fibers)	Seizures	nt 8344 C → G
MNGIE (myoneurogenic gastrointestinal encephalopathy)	Gastrointestinal pseudo-obstruction, neuropathy	Multiple mtDNA deletions[b] nt 8482 → 13447 nt 6341 → 13994 nt 16263 → 572 nt 5795 → 13920 nt 4469 → 13923 nt 5797 → 16071

nt nucleotide, *mtDNA* mitochondrial DNA
[a] From Wallace [2, 7] and Douglas et al. [6]
[b] From Nishigaki et al. [8]

base substitutions during DNA replication. CBDs are the predominant type of DNA lesion found in skin irradiated with UVA [25]. UVR exposure of tissue also produces ROS, particularly singlet oxygen ($^1O_2$) and hydroxyl radical, which can damage DNA directly [26]. More than 20 base lesions resulting from hydroxyl radical attack on DNA have been identified [5]. The most abundant DNA modification produced by hydroxyl attack is 8-oxodeoxyguanine (8-oxodG), which results from the addition of HO· to the C-8 atom of guanine. In the *syn* conformation, 8-oxodG has been shown to cause GC → TA transversions [27].

Mitochondrial DNA Deletions

Mitochondrial genomes exhibit an unusual tendency to undergo spontaneous deletion that encompasses large DNA tracts. The frequency of deletion is greatly increased under conditions of oxidative stress [2]. MtDNA deletions accumulate with age and are associated with various disease states, a number of which are genetic and show a mitochondrial pattern of inheritance [2–8]. A particularly ubiquitous aberration, known as the common deletion (CD), involves deletion of 4,977 bp of mtDNA created by breaks within two

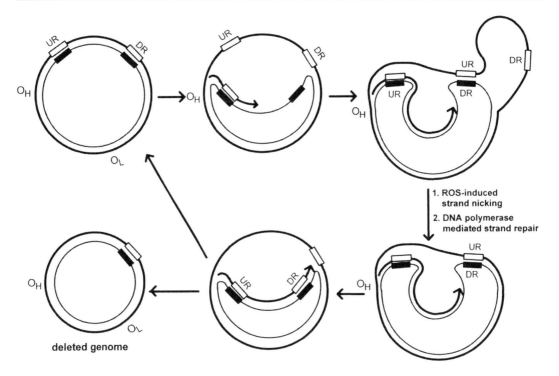

Fig. 11.2 Possible mechanism for formation of the common deletion (adapted from [30]). A slipstrand mispairing intermediate is shown, in which the H strand upstream repeat segment mispairs with the complementary sequences of its downstream counterpart. This leads to the formation of a single-stranded loop which is susceptible to attack by ROS, followed by exonucleolytic degradation. Recombination within the base-paired repeats completes the formation of the deleted strand. The *open box* (□) represents the 13 bp direct repeat ACCTCCCTCACCA and the *filled box* (■) represents its complement. The upstream repeat (UR) is located at nt 8470–8482 and the downstream repeat (DR) is located at nt 13447–13459. DNA replication initiated at the heavy strand replication origin (O_H) produces a large single-stranded loop, in which mispairing between the light strand UR and heavy strand DR is possible. The single-stranded loop is susceptible to strand breaking caused by ROS. Exonucleolytic degradation of the nicked loop is followed by DNA polymerase-mediated repair, completing the formation of the deletion on the unreplicated heavy strand. A round of replication, initiated from the light strand replication origin, produces a deleted genome

13 bp direct repeats [28]. It seems that formation of most, if not all, mtDNA deletions involve "slipstrand" base mispairing of repeat segments at or near the deletion cut sites [29]. According to the model proposed by Berneburg et al. [30], mispairing of direct repeats occurs during asymmetric replication of the DNA strands. This leads to the extrusion of a single-stranded loop that is susceptible to attack by ROS and which contains the segment that is deleted. Figure 11.2 illustrates this model for formation of the common deletion. The majority of the mtDNA deletions currently databased appear to involve direct repeats (see the Mitomap website for a database of mtDNA deletions; reference [31]), but deletion formation mediated by inverted complementary repeats has also been reported [32]. A modified slipstrand mechanism has been proposed, in which the cut site sequences are aligned in parallel and annealing of the aligned segments is stabilized by Hoogsteen base pairing. A duplex, in which the sequences are aligned in parallel, could be generated by mispairing of the cut sites via an intrastrand duplex or a triple helical intermediate with the double-stranded downstream cut site, similar to the model proposed by Rocher et al. [33]. There are also deletion variants that are less common, in which short insertions between inverted

repeats are seen [29]. These types of mtDNA deletions are not consistent with a slipstrand mispairing mechanism. Hwang et al. [29] have proposed template strand switching during DNA replication as a possible alternative mechanism for generation of these types of deletions. There is good evidence for deletion formation caused by template strand switching at segments containing both direct and palindromic repeats in viral and yeast systems [34–36], as well as in bacteria [37] and mitochondria [38]. Hairpin structures resulting from alignment of the inverted repeats offer a possible mechanism for generating single or dinucleotide insertions, similar to P insertions that are generated from hairpin intermediates during the process of VDJ recombination [39]. Mutation-bearing mitochondrial genomes can undergo clonal expansion as a result of selective replication [40, 41]. This mechanism has been proposed to explain why, in certain mitochondrial disease states, mitochondria bearing unique mutations come to predominate in a large proportion of cells in affected tissues.

Reactive Oxygen Species (ROS)

ROS Formation by Mitochondria in Cutaneous Tissues

It has been estimated that the mutation rate for mtDNA is ten times higher than that for nDNA [21, 42]. This is due, in large part, to the high levels of DNA-damaging ROS that exist in the mitochondrial matrix: singlet oxygen, hydroxide ion, hydroxyl radical, superoxide anion, and peroxynitrite ion (Fig. 11.3). These species are produced as a natural byproduct of electron flow in the mitochondrial electron transport chain. In particular, they are found in cases where the normal steady-state flow of electrons to molecular oxygen through complex IV is blocked, as a result of mutation in a gene(s) encoding one or more of the upstream carriers.

Perturbations in electron transport, that lead to accumulation of electrons on an intermediate carrier, can result in aberrant transfer of single

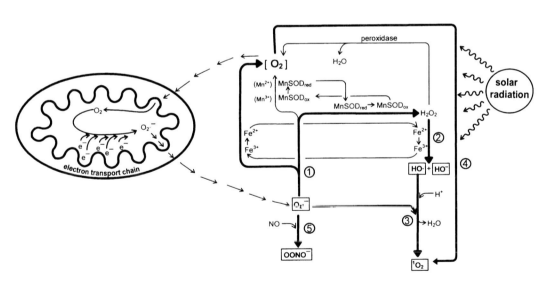

Fig. 11.3 Formation of reactive oxygen species (ROS) during mitochondrial respiration (adapted from [64]). Some of the oxygen that enters the mitochondrial matrix may be reduced by intermediate electron carriers to produce superoxide radical, instead of reduction via the normal pathway through complex IV. A summary of the major pathways (*thick lines*) for formation of ROS from superoxide is shown. (1) MnSOD catalyzes the formation of hydrogen peroxide from superoxide, (2) cleavage of the -O–O- bond in hydrogen peroxide by Fe^{+2} yields hydroxyl radical and hydroxide ion, (3) reaction of hydroxyl radical with superoxide produces singlet oxygen, which is also produced as a result of solar irradiation of molecular oxygen (4), and (5) superoxide can react with nitrous oxide to produce peroxynitrite ion

electrons directly to molecular oxygen from the individual electron carriers/donors within complexes I, III and IV; for example, ubiquinone (UQ) either in the semiquinone form (UQ·) or as the fully reduced quinol (UQH_2). It is estimated that approximately 1–5% of the oxygen (O_2) consumed in aerobic respiration becomes reduced to superoxide anion ($O_2^{·-}$) by aberrant electron transfer [43].

$$UQH· \longrightarrow UQ + H^+$$
$$UQH_2 \longrightarrow UQH· + H^+$$
$$O_2 \longrightarrow O_2^{·-}$$

Superoxide produced in the mitochondrial matrix is metabolized by manganese superoxide dismutase (MnSOD) in two steps. First, an electron from the superoxide is transferred to the manganese atom to produce molecular oxygen:

$$Mn^{3+} + O_2^{·-} \xrightarrow{MnSOD} Mn^{2+} + O_2 \quad (11.1)$$

A second superoxide ion together with an electron from the reduced manganese ion (Mn^{2+}) can then react with two protons ($2H^+$) to form hydrogen peroxide (H_2O_2):

$$Mn^{2+} + O_2^{·-} + 2H^+ \xrightarrow{MnSOD} Mn^{3+} + H_2O_2 \quad (11.2)$$

The hydrogen peroxide produced by the action of MnSOD can then be acted upon by a peroxidase (i.e., catalase or glutathione peroxidase) to complete the detoxification:

$$2H_2O_2 \longrightarrow 2H_2O + O_2 \quad (11.3)$$

Superoxide is released into the cytosol from the mitochondrion. In the cytosol, superoxide is also produced through the action of NADPH and P450 oxidases, and is then detoxified through essentially the same reactions shown in $(11.1) \rightarrow (11.3)$ above, but utilizing a cytosolic SOD co-factored by Zn and Cu (Cu-Zn-SOD).

In an alternative reaction catalyzed by iron, hydrogen peroxide can be decomposed into hydroxide ion (HO^-) and the highly reactive hydroxyl radical ($HO·$) (Fenton's reaction). In this reaction, ferric iron ion catalyzes the breakage of the oxygen–oxygen bond of hydrogen peroxide to produce the hydroxyl(–ide) species:

$$Fe^{2+} + H_2O_2 \longrightarrow Fe^{3+} + HO^- + HO· \quad (11.4)$$

Superoxide participates in this reaction by promoting the formation of Fe^{2+}, through the donation of an electron to Fe^{3+} to complete an $Fe^{2+} \leftrightarrow Fe^{3+}$ redox cycle:

$$Fe^{3+} + O_2^{·-} \longrightarrow Fe^{2+} + O_2 \quad (11.5)$$

Hydroxyl radical can react with superoxide to produce singlet oxygen ($^1O_2$), a highly reactive form of molecular oxygen that contains an unpaired electron, in contrast to the normal, relatively unreactive form (triplet oxygen):

$$H^+ + O_2^{·-} + HO· \longrightarrow {}^1O_2 + H_2O \quad (11.6)$$

Superoxide can also react with nitric oxide (NO) to produce peroxynitrite ($OONO^-$):

$$O_2^{·-} + NO \longrightarrow OONO^- \quad (11.7)$$

Role of Melanin in ROS Formation

Melanins are pigments composed of heterogeneous polymers of linked indolic monomers that are found in a wide variety of organisms throughout both the plant and animal kingdoms (Fig. 11.4). In humans, the association between the development of pigmentation and exposure to solar radiation evidences the photoprotective function of melanin; the conversion of absorbed UVR into heat (photon–phonon coupling) via the large network of conjugated double bonds. The fact that melanins are so widely distributed among organisms and tissues that are never exposed to sunlight argues strongly that melanins serve functions beyond photoprotection and camouflage that are yet to be discovered. There is now strong evidence that melanin may act as both a photoprotector and a photosensitizer [44–47]. The ability of melanin to sensitize cells to UVR has been linked to its redox properties. The similarity of the indolic quinone melanin precursors to quinone electron acceptor/donors has been

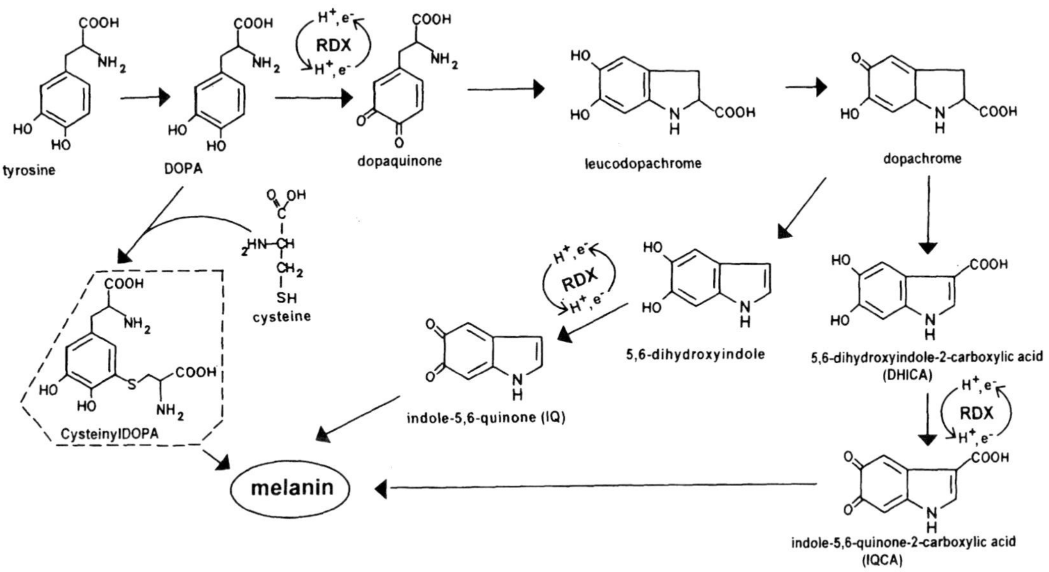

Fig. 11.4 Initiation of melanin synthesis – Pathways of melanin synthesis from tyrosine-derived precursors showing phenolic and indole intermediates (adapted from [44]). Cysteinyl DOPA (*dashed outline*) is an intermediate in the synthesis of pheomelanins. Redox cycling (RDX) is possible between the quinone and hydroxy forms of indolic and phenolic intermediates

widely noted, and this has lead to the suggestion that melanin may function as an electron carrier in cellular redox reactions [44]. If true, then it is predicted that single electron transfers would generate a semiquinone intermediate. The presence of the hypothesized semiquinone species in eumelanin was directly demonstrated by Sealy et al. nearly 30 years ago [48, 49], using electron spin resonance spectroscopy. Melanins are known to undergo photo-oxidation, a process during which the pigment undergoes darkening, that corresponds to an increase in carbonyl content caused by the transfer of electrons from the hydroxy intermediates [44]. Photo-oxidation carried out in the presence of oxygen generates superoxide [44], and oxidized melanin can react with O_2 to form H_2O_2, superoxide, and other radicals [50]. Thus melanin, as an electron transport molecule, could provide a direct cytosolic pathway for reduction of molecular oxygen, leading to the formation of superoxide and superoxide-derived ROS.

ROS are also known to be produced during the process of melanin formation. This occurs during the oxygen-dependent formation of the reactive dihydroxyindoles and the corresponding (semi) quinone intermediates (as well as the phenol/phenolic quinone precursors). ROS are generated as a result of redox cycling between the dihydroxy and quinone intermediates (Fig. 11.4) [51, 52]. Exposure of melanin and its precursors to UVR has also been shown to lead to the generation of ROS [53–55]. Hydrogen peroxide production, resulting from superoxide formation during melanin irradiation, has been measured directly [56]. In these experiments, the production of hydrogen peroxide was shown to be increased in the presence of superoxide dismutase. Increasing melanin content in cultured melanocytes using high tyrosine medium has been shown to lead to an increase in their sensitivity to UVA, as measured by single strand breaks in the Comet assay [57].

In a study in which melanin (from DOPA) was applied directly to calf thymus DNA, the switch from photoprotection to photosensitization was found to be dose-dependent, as measured by thymine glycol dimer formation after gamma irradiation [58]. In the same study, melanin was also shown to cause single-stranded breaks in ΦX174 DNA, as evidenced by the conversion of the supercoiled form (form I) to the nicked circular form (form II) following melanin treatment. This observation is consistent with the finding that high levels of mtDNA deletions are present in the substantia nigra of patients with Parkinson's disease [59].

Pheomelanin in particular has been shown to act a photosensitizer [60, 61]. For example, the cytotoxic effects of UVR exposure on Ehrlich ascites carcinoma cells were found to be enhanced in the presence of melanin, and more so by pheomelanin than eumelanin [62]. Ultraviolet irradiation of pheomelanin causes structural changes in catalase, resulting in a decrease in enzymatic activity and reflected in an increase in ROS levels [63]. Radiation-induced synthesis of pheomelanin uses large amounts of cysteine, which can deplete the precursor pool needed for synthesis of glutathione and thus reduce the activity of glutathione-cofactored peroxidases [64]. Dyplastic nevi which synthesize more pheomelanin than normal skin melanocytes also display more DNA fragmentation in Comet assays than either normal melanocytes or common nevi, and these differences are enhanced by UVB irradiation [65].

Mitochondrial DNA Alterations in Melanoma

Alterations in mtDNA derived from melanoma tumors have been studied for the purpose of identifying biomarkers that have utility for disease diagnosis and tumor progression. Putative tumor biomarkers from sequence analyses of the D-loop region in both tumor tissue and melanoma cell lines have been reported (Table 11.2) [42, 66, 67]. These studies have found mainly single nucleotide base substitutions, insertions, and deletions; almost 75% of which were located within a narrow segment of HVR2 spanning nucleotides 146–319. Of these, about half were C insertions within the polycytidine microsatellite region. Outside of the microsatellite region, the changes tend to be pyrimidine/pyrimidine or purine/purine substitutions rather than transversions. A clear correlation between the polymorphic changes observed in mtDNA and the stage of tumor progression has yet to be established; although, it was found that in advanced stages of melanoma, mtDNA fragments (carrying some of the alterations seen in the tumors) were also detectable in the peripheral blood of patients [67]. A large fraction of the nucleotide changes occur within the poly-C (nt 303–315) and CA repeat (nt 514–523) microsatellites, suggesting that mitochondrial microsatellite instability (mtMSI) may be a useful means of distinguishing less aggressive tumors from their more aggressive counterparts [42]. Despite the causal link between melanoma and exposure to solar radiation, only a small percentage of the nucleotide changes in melanoma tumors studied have been found to be the UVR "signature" C→T or CC→TT substitutions [24]. In addition to single nucleotide changes, the 4,977 bp common deletion was also found in about 10% of the melanoma tumor specimens examined [43].

Detailed studies on the occurrence of mtDNA deletions in melanoma tumors are lacking at present. However, there is abundant evidence that either solar radiation, or its ultraviolet component, which are causatively linked to melanoma, can also induce mtDNA deletions. Induction of the common deletion has been demonstrated in UVA-irradiated fibroblasts in culture [30], and following UVB irradiation of keratinocytes *in vitro* [29, 32]. The common deletion has also been shown to be a biomarker of sun exposure in skin [68–71]. More recently, several novel mtDNA deletions have also been characterized as biomarkers of exposure to solar radiation. For example, Krishnan et al. [72] have shown that the presence of a specific 3,895 bp deletion at different body sites corresponds to the degree of sun exposure. A similar finding was reported by Steinberg et al. [70] in skin specimens taken from the margins of melanoma tumors. In this study, the relative levels of a novel 5,128 bp mtDNA deletion (Δuv), derived from an *in vitro* keratinocyte system [32], were found to correlate with history of sun exposure and DNA damage (as measured in Comet assays), as well as induction

Table 11.2 Mitochondrial D-loop[a] nucleotide alterations in melanoma

Study	Microsatellite (MSI)[b,c]	HVR1[d,e]	HVR2[e,f]	Other D-loop regions[e]
Takeuchi et al. [67]				
Cell lines (n=20)	C ins (5)	G16042A	A251G	T64C
	C del (2)	A16300G	A263G	C433–438 ins
		T16362C		
Tumors (n=12)	C ins (2)	T16126C	C72T	C438T
		C16362T	C239T	T16366C
				G16482A
Poetsch et al. [42]				
Nodular type (n=32)	(4) ND	N/A	T152C	N/A
			T195C	
Metastatic (n=43)	(11) ND	N/A	C146T	A513G
			A189G	
			A189G	
			T195C	
			T310C	
Martin et al. [66]				
Nodular type (n=1)	C309T	N/A	N/A	C324T
	T310C			A374G
Metastatic (n=9)	C ins (3)	N/A	G316C	A384T
	TCC310 ins		T319C	C387T
	TC310 ins		T319C	
	A308 ins		A325 ins	
	T310C		326A del	
			329C del	
			C340T	

[a] The D-loop spans the region between nucleotides (nt) 16024 → 576
[b] (#); number of C insertions (ins) or deletions (del) within the microsatellite region (nt 303 → 315)
[c] ND; alterations not described
[d] HVR1 (hypervariable region 1; nt 16024–16365)
[e] N/A; no alterations found
[f] HVR2 (hypervariable region 2; nt 72–340)

of DNA repair genes in microarray analyses. Tests run in parallel, using primer sets that detect the common deletion, were found to correspond well to those obtained for the Δuv deletion. Eshaghian et al. [68] characterized a wide spectrum of mtDNA deletions in skin adjacent to non-melanoma skin cancers. The number of mtDNA deletions was strongly correlated with patient age, a finding consistent with the concept of large mtDNA deletions as markers of skin photoaging. Of the aberrations studied, the vast majority (28 of 37) were noted to be novel deletions, while the common deletion was found in eight sequenced cases. Most of the deletions identified were flanked by direct or indirect repeats and were located within the mitochondrial segment between the two replication origins.

Mitochondrial Resequencing Arrays (Mitochips)

Recent advances in chip microarray technology have made possible new hybridization-based techniques for high-throughput detection of sequence alterations in genomes, for which reference sequences are available. This field is rapidly evolving and several iterations of the chip array technology have been described over the past decade [73–77]. Since the reference sequence used as the hybridization target must be known in advance, information on base changes derived from chip hybridizations is referred to as "resequencing", and the chip arrays themselves are referred to as resequencing arrays/chips. In the standard procedure, labeled probes derived from a test DNA are hybridized at high stringency to the chip arrays (which consist of oligonucleotides attached to a solid support matrix, such as glass). Creation of the chip arrays by synthesis and attachment of the oligonucleotides is carried out using photolithography to create an ordered high-density array of oligonucleotides over the surface of the matrix; a cluster of identical oligonucleotides is called a feature of the array. Each oligonucleotide on the array represents a short segment of the reference sequence with a base alteration that is to be tested by hybridization against the query sequence. Each segment of the reference sequence is represented by eight features (four features for each strand), each containing a different nucleotide substitution at the same position in the sequence (Fig. 11.5). Hybridization targets, representing sequences to be queried, can be created in a variety of ways, but are commonly generated by polymerase chain reaction (PCR) using various fluorescent or chromogenic labels (such as fluorescein or biotin) that are attached to, or incorporated into, the PCR products by any of a number of standard procedures. Since each oligonucleotide is short (generally 15–35 bp), single nucleotide mismatches cause a significant reduction in the hybridization of the target to the arrayed oligonucleotide probes under stringent conditions. Thus relative levels of hybridization can be used to determine the presence of base (mis)matching for a given feature. Base calls at each queried nucleotide position are made using algorithms that compare the quantified signal intensities of target hybridization to the corresponding oligonucleotide probes(s) from the two complementary DNA strands. Averaging of results from replicate chips is usually required for high accuracy. It must be recognized that variations in hybridization signal, including mismatches between probe and target at positions flanking the interrogated nucleotide position, introduce complexities which must be taken into account by the base-calling algorithm. Based on comparison with standard dideoxy sequencing, success rates for base calls using resequencing chips can often exceed 99% for single nucleotide substitutions, insertions and deletions. However,

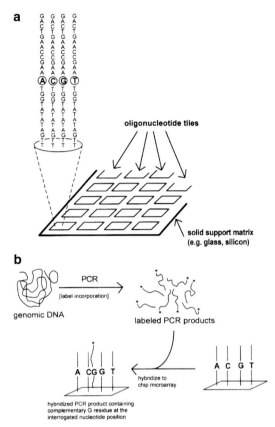

Fig. 11.5 Diagrammatic representation of a chip microarray. (**a**) Oligonucleotides representing a short segment of genomic sequences, containing all possible base substitutions at a defined nucleotide position, are covalently attached to a solid matrix by surface engineering. Oligonucleotides representing both strands of the same substituted segment are placed together in a localized cluster (feature). The feature outlined in (**a**) shows substituted 25-mers spanning nt 10391–10415 of the mitochondrial ND3 gene (Fig. 11.1) attached to the matrix at the 3′ end; only the substituted oligonucleotides for one strand are shown. (**b**) Chip hybridization strategy. Long-range PCR is used to create labeled PCR products that are then probed by hybridization to the oligonucleotides arrayed on the chip. Hybridization of a PCR product to an oligonucleotide containing the complementary base indicates the identity of that base at the interrogated position

resequencing chips cannot be practically applied to more complex DNA alterations, such as large deletions, insertions, and duplications.

Resequencing arrays covering the entire human mitochondrial genome (such as the GeneChip® Mitochondrial Resequencing 2.0 Array, Affymetrix) have been widely available to researchers for several years. In the first generation of mitochips, more than 29 kb of double-stranded DNA could be analyzed on a single chip [76]. Probes for the entire mitochondrial coding segment were created from three overlapping long PCR fragments, and more than two million base pairs of mtDNA were tested. Base calls were successfully assigned at 96.0% of the nucleotide positions and >99.99% reproducibility was found in replicate experiments. In a study of melanoma tumors using the Mitochip, polymorphic changes in mtDNA in 16 melanoma tumors from 14 patients were catalogued in a high-throughput analysis, in which 529,408 bases from 32 samples were sequenced [13]. One hundred and five single nucleotide changes were described, of which 32 were non-synonymous. Single nucleotide polymorphisms (SNPs) were distributed throughout the mitochondrial genome, but a much higher proportion were found in the D-loop region than would be expected from the length of the D-loop segment relative to the overall length of the mitochondrial genome. A large proportion of tumors (10/16) also exhibited mutations in the NADH dehydrogenase complex.

References

1. Druzhyna NM, Wilson GL, LeDoux SP. Mitochondrial DNA repair in aging and disease. Mech Ageing Dev. 2008;129:383–90.
2. Wallace DC. Mitochondrial genetics: a paradigm for aging and degenerative diseases? Science. 1992;256:628–32.
3. Larsen NB, Rasmussen M, Rasmussen LJ. Nuclear and mitochondrial DNA repair: similar pathways? Mitochondrion. 2005;5:89–108.
4. Croteau DL, Bohr VA. Repair of oxidative damage to nuclear and mitochondrial DNA in mammalian cells. J Biol Chem. 1997;272:25409–12.
5. Stuart JA, Brown MF. Mitochondrial DNA maintenance and bioenergetics. Biochim Biophys Acta. 2006;1757:79–89.
6. Douglas C, Wallace DC. Diseases of the mitochondrial DNA. Annu Rev Biochem. 1992;61:1175–212.
7. Wallace DC. Mitochondrial diseases in man and mouse. Science. 1999;283:1482–8.
8. Nishigaki Y, Martí R, Hirano M. ND5 is a hot-spot for multiple atypical mitochondrial DNA deletions in mitochondrial neurogastrointestinal encephalomyopathy. Hum Mol Genet. 2004;13:91–101.
9. Zeviani M, Di Donato S. Mitochondrial disorders. Brain. 2004;127:2153–72.
10. Martinez-Ruiz G, Maldonado V, Ceballos-Cancino G, et al. Role of Smac/DIABLO in cancer progression. J Exp Clin Cancer Res. 2008;26:27–48.
11. Ishikawa K, Takenaga K, Akimoto M, et al. ROS-generating mitochondrial DNA mutations can regulate tumor cell metastasis. Science. 2008;320:661–4.
12. Birch-Machin MA. The role of mitochondria in ageing and carcinogenesis. Clin Exp Dermatol. 2006;31:548–52.
13. Mithani SK, Smith IM, Topalian SL, et al. Nonsynonymous somatic mitochondrial mutations occur in the majority of cutaneous melanomas. Melanoma Res. 2008;18:214–9.
14. Mithani SK, Taube JM, Zhou S, et al. Mitochondrial mutations are a late event in the progression of head and neck squamous cell cancer. Clin Cancer Res. 2007;13:4331–5.
15. Zhu W, Qin W, Sauter ER. Large-scale mitochondrial DNA deletion mutations and nuclear genome instability in human breast cancer. Cancer Detect Prev. 2004;28:119–26.
16. Shieh DB, Chou WP, Wei YH, et al. Mitochondrial DNA 4,977-bp deletion in paired oral cancer and precancerous lesions revealed by laser microdissection and real-time quantitative PCR. Ann NY Acad Sci. 2004;1011:154–67.
17. Dai JG, Xiao YB, Min JX, et al. Mitochondrial DNA 4977 BP deletion mutations in lung carcinoma. Indian J Cancer. 2006;43:20–5.
18. Dasgupta S, Hoque MO, Upadhyay S, et al. Mitochondrial cytochrome B gene mutation promotes tumor growth in bladder cancer. Cancer Res. 2008;68:700–6.
19. Rigoli L, Di Bella C, Verginelli F, et al. Histological heterogeneity and somatic mtDNA mutations in gastric intraepithelial neoplasia. Mod Pathol. 2008;21:733–41.
20. Kamalidehghan B, Houshmand M, Ismail P, et al. Delta mtDNA4977 is more common in non-tumoral cells from gastric cancer sample. Arch Med Res. 2006;37:730–5.
21. Sharma H, Singh A, Sharma C, et al. Mutations in the mitochondrial DNA D-loop region are frequent in cervical cancer. Cancer Cell Int. 2005;5:34.
22. Wang Y, Liu VW, Ngan HY, et al. Frequent occurrence of mitochondrial microsatellite instability in the D-loop region of human cancers. Ann NY Acad Sci. 2005;1042:123–9.
23. Budowle B, Wilson MR, DiZinno JA, et al. Mitochondrial DNA regions HVI and HVII population data. Forensic Sci Int. 1999;103:23–35.
24. Nityanand M, Vijayasaradhi S. Role of UV in cutaneous melanoma. Photochem Photobiol. 2008;84:528–36.
25. Mouret S, Baudouin C, Charveron M, et al. Cyclobutane pyrimidine dimers are predominant DNA lesions in whole human skin exposed to UVA radiation. Proc Natl Acad Sci USA. 2006;103:13765–70.
26. Ravanat J-L, Saint-Pierre C, Di Mascio P, et al. Damage to isolated DNA mediated by singlet oxygen. Helv Chim Acta. 2002;84:3702–9.

27. Grollman AP, Moriya M. Mutagenesis by 8-oxoguanine: an enemy within. Trends Genet. 1993;9:246–9.
28. Soong NW, Arnheim N. Detection and quantification of mitochondrial DNA deletions. Methods Enzymol. 1996;264:421–31.
29. Hwang B-J, Kuttamperoor F, Wu J, et al. Spectrum of mitochondrial DNA deletions within the common deletion region induced by low levels of UVB irradiation of human keratinocytes in vitro. Gene. 2009;440:23–7.
30. Berneburg M, Grether-Beck S, Kürten V, et al. Singlet oxygen mediates the UVA-induced generation of the photoaging-associated mitochondrial common deletion. J Biol Chem. 1994;274:15345–9.
31. MITOMAP: a human mitochondrial genome database. 2011. http://www.mitomap.org. Accessed 20 Feb 2011.
32. Fang J, Pierre Z, Liu S, et al. Novel mitochondrial deletions in human epithelial cells irradiated with an FS20 ultraviolet light source in vitro. J Photochem Photobiol. 2006;184:340–6.
33. Rocher C, Letellier T, Copeland WC, et al. Base composition at mtDNA boundaries suggests a DNA triple helix model for human mitochondrial DNA large-scale rearrangements. Mol Genet Metab. 2002;76:123–32.
34. Cheung AK. Detection of template strand switching during initiation and termination of DNA replication of porcine circovirus. J Virol. 2004;78:4268–77.
35. Lewellyn EB, Loeb DD. Base pairing between cis-acting sequences contributes to template switching during plus-strand DNA synthesis in human hepatitis B virus. J Virol. 2007;81:6207–15.
36. Nag DK, Fasullo M, Dong Z, et al. Inverted repeat-stimulated sisterchromatid exchange events are RAD1-independent but reduced in a msh2 mutant. Nucleic Acids Res. 2005;33:5243–9.
37. Pinder DJ, Blake CE, Lindsey JC, et al. Replication strand preference for deletions associated with DNA palindromes. Mol Microbiol. 1998;28:719–27.
38. Mita S, Rizzuto R, Moraes CT, et al. Recombination via flanking direct repeats is a major cause of large-scale deletions of human mitochondrial DNA. Nucleic Acids Res. 1990;18:561–7.
39. Lewis SM. P nucleotide insertions and the resolution of hairpin DNA structures in mammalian cells. Proc Natl Acad Sci USA. 1994;91:1332–6.
40. Yoneda M, Chomyn A, Martinuzzi A, et al. Marked replicative advantage of human mtDNA carrying a point mutation that causes the MELAS encephalomyopathy. Proc Natl Acad Sci USA. 1992;89:11164–8.
41. Elson JL, Samuels DC, Turnbull DM, et al. Random intracellular drift explains the clonal expansion of mitochondrial DNA mutations with age. Am J Hum Genet. 2001;68:802–6.
42. Poetsch M, Dittberner T, Petersmann A, et al. Mitochondrial DNA instability in malignant melanoma of the skin is mostly restricted to nodular and metastatic stages. Melanoma Res. 2004;14:501–8.
43. Karihtala P, Soini Y. Reactive oxygen species and antioxidant mechanisms in human tissues and their relation to malignancies. APMIS. 2007;115:81–103.
44. Riley PA. Molecules in focus: melanin. Int J Biochem Cell Biol. 1997;29:1235–9.
45. Hill HZ. The function of melanin or six blind people examine an elephant. Bioessays. 1992;14:49–56.
46. Wang A, Marino AR, Gasyna Z, et al. Photoprotection by porcine eumelanin against singlet oxygen production. Photochem Photobiol. 2008;84:679–82.
47. Brenner M, Hearing VJ. The protective role of melanin against UV damage in human skin. Photochem Photobiol. 2008;84:539–49.
48. Sealy RC, Felix CC, Hyde JS, et al. Structure and reactivity of melanins: influence of free radicals and metal ions. In: Pryor WA, editor. Free radicals in biology, vol. 4. New York: Academic; 1980. p. 209–59.
49. Sarna T, Sealy RC. Photoinduced oxygen consumption in melanin systems. Action spectra and quantum yield for eumelanin and synthetic melanin. Photochem Photobiol. 1984;39:69–74.
50. Meyskens Jr FL, Farmer PJ, Anton-Culver H. Etiologic pathogenesis of melanoma: a unifying hypothesis for the missing attributable risk. Clin Cancer Res. 2004;10:2581–3.
51. Fridovich I. Superoxide dismutases. Annu Rev Biochem. 1975;44:147–59.
52. Nappi AJ, Vass E. Hydrogen peroxide generation associated with the oxidations of the eumelanin precursors 5,6-dihydroxyindole and 5,6-dihydroxyindole-2-carboxylic acid. Melanoma Res. 1996;6:341–9.
53. Koch WH, Chedekel MR. Photochemistry and photobiology of melanogenic metabolites: formation of free radicals. Photochem Photobiol. 1987;46:229–38.
54. Wenczl E, Pool S, Timmerman A, et al. Physiological doses of ultraviolet irradiation induce DNA strand breaks in cultured human melanocytes, as detected by means of an immunochemical assay. Photochem Photobiol. 1997;66:826–30.
55. Marrot L, Belaidi J, Meunier J, et al. The human melanocyte as a particular target for UVA radiation and an endpoint for photoprotection assessment. Photochem Photobiol. 1999;69:686–93.
56. Korytowski W, Pilas B, Sarna T, et al. Photoinduced generation of hydrogen peroxide and hydroxyl radicals in melanins. Photochem Photobiol. 1987;45:185–90.
57. Wenczl E, Van der Schans G, Roza L, et al. (Pheo) melanin photosensitizes UVA-induced DNA damage in cultured human melanocytes. J Invest Dermatol. 1998;111:678–82.
58. Hubbard-Smith K, Hill HZ, Hill GJ. Melanin both causes and prevents oxidative base damage in DNA: quantitation by anti-thymine glycol antibodies. Radiat Res. 1992;130:160–5.
59. Krishnan KJ, Morris CM, Taylor GA, et al. High levels of mitochondrial DNA deletions in substantia nigra neurons in aging and Parkinson disease. Nat Genet. 2006;38:515–7.
60. Chedekel MR, Smith SK, Post PW, et al. Photodestruction of pheomelanin: role of oxygen. Proc Natl Acad Sci USA. 1978;75:5395–9.
61. Ezzahir A. The influence of melanins on the photoperoxidation of lipids. J Photochem Photobiol B Biol. 1989;3:341–9.

62. Menon IA, Persad S, Ranadive NS, et al. Effects of ultraviolet-visible irradiation in the presence of melanin isolated from human black or red hair upon Ehrlich ascites carcinoma cells. Cancer Res. 1983;43:3165–9.
63. Wood JM, Schallreuter KU. UVA-irradiated pheomelanin alters the structure of catalase and decreases its activity in human skin. J Invest Dermatol. 2006;126:13–4.
64. Wittgen HG, van Kempen LC. Reactive oxygen species in melanoma and its therapeutic implications. Melanoma Res. 2007;17:400–9.
65. Noz KC, Bauwens M, van Buul PP, et al. Comet assay demonstrates a higher ultraviolet B sensitivity to DNA damage in dysplastic nevus cells than in common melanocytic nevus cells and foreskin melanocytes. J Invest Dermatol. 1996;106:1198–202.
66. Martin D, Birgit K, Axel B, et al. Somatic mitochondrial mutations in melanoma resection specimens. Int J Oncol. 2004;24:137–41.
67. Takeuchi H, Fujimoto A, Hoon DS. Detection of mitochondrial DNA alterations in plasma of malignant melanoma patients. Ann NY Acad Sci. 2004;1022:50–4.
68. Eshaghian A, Vleuge RA, Canter JA, et al. Mitochondrial DNA deletions serve as biomarkers of aging in the skin, but are typically absent in nonmelanoma skin cancers. J Invest Dermatol. 2006;126:336–44.
69. Hubbard K, Steinberg ML, Hill HZ, et al. Mitochondrial DNA deletions in skin from melanoma patients. Ethn Dis. 2008;18(S2):38–43.
70. Steinberg ML, Hubbard K, Utti C, et al. Patterns of persistent DNA damage associated with sun exposure and the glutathione S-transferase M1 genotype in melanoma patients. Photochem Photobiol. 2009;85:379–86.
71. Berneburg M, Plettenberg H, Medve-Konig K, et al. Induction of the photoaging-associated mitochondrial common deletion in vivo in normal human skin. J Invest Dermatol. 2004;122:1277–83.
72. Krishnan KJ, Harbottle A, Birch-Machin MA. The use of a 3895 bp mitochondrial DNA deletion as a marker for sunlight exposure in human skin. J Invest Dermatol. 2004;123:1020–4.
73. Hacia JG. Resequencing and mutational analysis using oligonucleotide microarrays. Nat Genet. 1999;21:42–7.
74. Bender A, Cutler DJ, Zwick ME, et al. High-throughput variation detection and genotyping using microarrays. Genome Res. 2001;11:1913–25.
75. Shendure J, Mitra RD, Varma C, et al. Advanced sequencing technologies: methods and goals. Nat Rev Genet. 2004;5:335–44.
76. Maitra A, Cohen Y, Gillespie SE, et al. The human mitoChip: a high-throughput sequencing microarray for mitochondrial mutation detection. Genome Res. 2004;14:812–9.
77. Zhou S, Kassauei K, Cutler DJ, et al. An oligonucleotide microarray for high-throughput sequencing of the mitochondrial genome. J Mol Diagn. 2006;8:476–82.

Tissue-Based Protein Biomarkers in Melanoma: Immunohistochemistry: (A) Diagnosis

Steven J. Ohsie, Basil A. Horst, Alistair Cochran, and Scott W. Binder

Melanocytic tumors are some of the most difficult neoplasms dealt with in the world of diagnostic pathology. While most melanocytic lesions are not diagnostically challenging, a significant minority show histopathological features that are ambiguous, making it difficult to assess their invasive and metastatic potential. Overdiagnosis of a benign nevus may cause significant morbidity; scarring following a wide excision in a cosmetically sensitive location such as the face, lymphedema secondary to lymph node dissection, and/or the adverse psychological impact of an erroneous malignant diagnosis. Underdiagnosis of a melanoma may provide the time during which a potentially curable malignancy advances to an untreatable illness.

S.J. Ohsie, M.D. (✉)
Affiliated Pathologists Medical Group/Pathology, Inc., Torrence, CA, USA
e-mail: sohsie@hotmail.com

B.A. Horst, M.D.
Departments of Dermatology, Pathology and Cell Biology, Columbia University Medical Center, New York, NY, USA

A. Cochran, M.D.
Departments of Pathology and Laboratory Medicine and Surgery, David Geffen School of Medicine at the University of California, Los Angeles, CA, USA

S.W. Binder, M.D.
Department of Pathology and Laboratory Medicine, David Geffen School of Medicine at the University of California, Los Angeles, CA, USA

This chapter discusses the evaluation of protein markers by immunohistochemistry, as an aid in the diagnosis of melanoma. Topics to be discussed are:
Histopathological features of melanoma
Immunohistochemical markers of melanocytic differentiation
Protein markers to distinguish benign and malignant melanocytic lesions
Protein markers in special situations
Summary/Conclusions

Histopathological Features of Melanoma

On microscopic examination, melanomas are distinguished from benign nevi by the presence of atypical histopathological features. Architectural abnormalities include: large size of the lesion, asymmetrical growth pattern and asymmetry of lymphocytic infiltrate, lack of circumscription, pagetoid upward spread of melanocytes, and predominance of single melanocytes over nests. Atypical cytologic features include: increased amounts of "dusky melanized" cytoplasm, enlarged nuclei with prominent nucleoli and irregular nuclear membranes, mitoses within the deep dermal component, and especially atypical mitotic figures. The majority of nevi should lack most of these features, while melanomas in general show several of them [1, 2].

Some benign melanocytic lesions can show atypical features, depending on the age of the patient or anatomic site of the lesion. Nevi in young patients may demonstrate an occasional mitotic figure in the dermal component, and nevi on acral sites may show a predominance of single cells over nests and even foci of pagetoid spread of melanocytes [1, 2].

Not all benign melanocytic lesions show the typical growth pattern of common nevi, but may exhibit features that could be regarded as "atypical", depending on the clinical context. In these cases, immunohistochemistry can be helpful. For example, congenital nevi show nevomelanocytes that dissect between collagen bundles and track down adnexal structures. Blue nevi are composed of irregular groups of heavily pigmented, spindle-shaped melanocytes, unlike common nevi where heavy pigmentation, if seen, is usually restricted to the superficial component. In addition, cellular blue nevi may not show maturation with dermal descent that is characteristic of common melanocytic nevi. Spitz tumors represent a special group of melanocytic lesions that are comprised of enlarged epithelioid and spindle-shaped melanocytes with enlarged nuclei, and can show focal intraepidermal pagetoid scatter of nested melanocytes as well as occasional mitotic figures in the dermal component, especially in young patients. Their clinical behavior may be difficult to predict on the basis of histopathological features alone, particularly in older individuals. Lastly, so-called dysplastic or atypical nevi are a somewhat ill-defined group of melanocytic lesions that show architectural and/or cytologic features that in a certain clinical context may be worrisome for malignancy [2].

In these challenging cases, adjunctive protein biomarkers can be of use in distinguishing nevi from melanomas.

Immunohistochemical Markers of Melanocytic Differentiation

Although the melanocytic origin of most melanomas is apparent on H&E-stained sections, melanomas can show an extremely wide spectrum of microscopic features. Melanomas may undergo schwannian, fibroblastic, myofibroblastic, rhabdoid, osteoid, cartilaginous, ganglionic, and smooth muscle differentiation and can mimic epithelial, hematologic, mesenchymal, and neural tumors [3]. Due to this extraordinary histopathologic heterogeneity, the differential diagnostic process can be complex and may necessitate the use of a wide range of immunohistochemical markers to confirm or exclude melanocytic histogenesis. The following proteins belong to the group of well-established markers of melanocytic differentiation (see Table 12.1).

S100 is a 21 kDa acidic calcium-binding protein that is present in the nucleus and cytoplasm of melanocytic cells. S100 shows the highest sensitivity for melanocytic tumors (97–100%), but has a relatively low specificity (75–87%), since it is also expressed by nerve sheath cells, myoepithelial cells, adipocytes, chondrocytes and Langerhans cells, as well as their respective tumors [4–6]. S100 is therefore generally used in conjunction with more specific markers of melanocytic lineage, and for most practical purposes ensures that a melanocytic lesion will not be missed.

HMB-45, a marker of the cytoplasmic premelanosomal glycoprotein gp100, is not as sensitive as S100 in this setting, but has greater specificity [6]. HMB-45 staining is cytoplasmic, and characteristically reflects "maturation" of benign melanocytic lesions, with strong staining of intraepidermal melanocytes and the more superficial dermal component in most nevi [7, 11–13, 34, 41]. Melanomas, in contrast to nevi, may retain strong staining even in cells located deep in the lesion [7, 8, 12]. Specificity is limited, since HMB-45 is also expressed by PEComas (i.e., angiomyolipomas, lymphangiomyomatosis, pulmonary "sugar" tumors), sweat gland tumors, meningeal melanocytomas, clear cell sarcoma of the tendons and aponeuroses, some ovarian steroid cell tumors, some breast cancers, and renal cell carcinomas with a t(6;11)(p21;q12) translocation [6, 12, 26–33]. Because of the characteristic staining pattern of HMB-45 in common nevi, this marker is especially helpful in evaluating the dermal component of melanocytic lesions (see below).

MART-1 (Melanoma Antigen Recognized by T-cells-1) is a cytoplasmic protein of melanosomal differentiation recognized by T-cells [6, 9, 10, 14]. This marker is widely used as both a confirmatory marker for melanocytic differentiation

Table 12.1 Melanocytic differentiation markers

Marker	Sensitivity/specificity	Also seen in	Comment
S100	Sensitivity – 97–100%; specificity – 75–87% [4]	Numerous tumors, including but not limited to those derived from nerve sheath cells, myoepithelial cells, adipocytes, chondrocytes, and Langerhans cells [5, 6]	Nuclear and cytoplasmic stain [5, 7–10]; most sensitive marker for spindle cell/desmoplastic melanomas [11–23]
HMB-45	Sensitivity – 69–93% (77–100% in primary melanomas, 56–83% in metastatic melanomas) [7, 8, 11–13, 15, 24, 25]	PEComas (angiomyolipomas, lymphangiomyomatosis, pulmonary "sugar" tumors), meningeal melanocytomas, clear cell sarcomas, some ovarian steroid cell tumors, sweat gland tumors, some breast cancers, renal cell carcinoma with a t(6;11)(p21;q12) translocation [6, 12, 26–33]	Cytoplasmic stain; decreased sensitivity in metastatic melanoma [6, 8, 10, 11, 34, 35]; can be used to help distinguish nevi from melanoma [7, 8, 12]
MART-1/Melan-A	Sensitivity – 75–92%; specificity – 95–100% [10, 12–17, 23, 34, 36]	PEComas (angiomyolipomas, lymphangiomyomatosis, pulmonary "sugar" tumors), some clear cell sarcomas [30, 32, 33]; clone A103 (Melan-A) also stains adrenal cortical tumors and gonadal steroid tumors [16, 36]	More intense and diffuse staining than HMB-45 [12, 13, 16, 34, 36]
Tyrosinase	Sensitivity – 84–94%; specificity – 97–100% [10, 12, 17–19, 37]	Rare angiolipomas, a minority of angiomyolipomas and clear cell sarcomas of the tendon sheath, and pigmented nerve sheath tumors [17, 19, 20, 38, 39]	Sensitivity decreases with increased clinical stage and in metastatic lesions [12, 17–19, 37]
MITF	Sensitivity – 81–100%; specificity – 88–100%; lower in spindle cell lesions [17, 18, 21–23, 40]	Spindle cell tumors, lymphoid neoplasms, angiomyolipomas, rare breast carcinomas and renal cell carcinomas [17, 22, 23, 38]; can also stain histiocytes, lymphocytes, fibroblasts, Schwann cells, smooth muscle cells and mast cells [17, 21, 22]	Nuclear stain – increased ease of interpretation, but stains tumors of many other lineages [9]

in S100-positive lesions and a primary marker to evaluate the extent of microscopically apparent melanocytic tumors. Two clones of the antibody to this protein are used: (1) M2-7C10, generally referred to as MART-1, and (2) A103, generally, but not exclusively, referred to as Melan-A [15, 16]. In addition to melanocytic lesions, the A103 clone also labels adrenal cortical tumors and gonadal steroid tumors, whereas the M2-7C10 clone does not [16, 36]. Both clones stain PEComas and can highlight clear cell sarcomas [30, 32, 33]. These antibodies generally show more diffuse and intense staining than HMB-45, without reduction in intensity in the deeper dermal components of melanocytic lesions [12, 13, 16, 34, 36].

Tyrosinase is an enzyme that hydroxylates tyrosine during the first step in melanin synthesis [9]. Melanocytic lesions stained for tyrosinase exhibit fine granular cytoplasmic staining, and melanocytic nevi show a similar staining pattern to HMB-45 [37, 41]. Positive staining tends to be strong and diffuse [12, 13]. The sensitivity of tyrosinase for melanoma is reportedly better than that of HMB-45 (84–94%), but sensitivity decreases with increasing clinical stage, as well as in metastatic lesions (79–93%) [10, 12, 17–19, 37]. The specificity of tyrosinase for melanoma is reported to be 97–100% [8, 17, 19]. Tyrosinase expression has rarely been found in angiolipomas, a minority of angiomyolipomas (a type of PEComa), clear cell sarcomas of the tendon sheath, and pigmented nerve sheath tumors [17, 19, 20, 38, 39].

MITF (Microphthalmia Transcription Factor) is a transcription factor protein necessary for the development of melanocytes during embryogenesis [9]. As a nuclear stain it may be easier to interpret, especially in cases where melanin pigment may overlay reaction product, making evaluation of cytoplasmic immunohistochemical stains difficult. It may be especially useful for the assessment of intraepidermal melanocytic lesions (see below) [9]. Apart from expression in melanocytic tumors, like other melanocytic markers, MITF is also positive in angiomyolipomas [38]. MITF has been reported to stain histocytes and mast cells in some studies [17, 21, 22], with Busam et al. [22] reporting MITF staining in histiocytes, lymphocytes, fibroblasts, Schwann cells, and smooth muscle cells; this relative non-specificity may represent a potentially troubling pitfall, especially in evaluating the extent of melanocytic lesions. The advantages of nuclear staining must therefore be weighed against the relative non-specificity of MITF as a marker in this setting.

Once the melanocytic nature of a lesion is confirmed, whether by histopathological features on H&E or with the aid of immunohistochemistry, the next step is to determine whether a lesion is benign or malignant. While microscopic changes allow differential diagnosis in most cases, immunohistochemical markers can be very helpful in making this distinction.

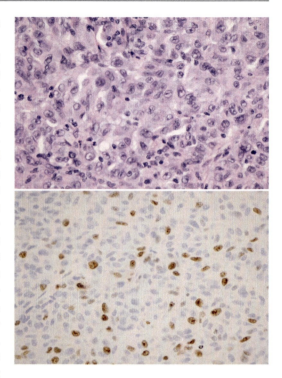

Fig. 12.1 Ki-67 immunohistochemical staining in an invasive melanoma

Protein Markers to Distinguish Benign and Malignant Melanocytic Lesions

Markers of Tumor Cell Proliferation

Mitotic activity is an important factor in the assessment of melanocytic lesions with a dermal component, and impacts the current American Joint Committee on Cancer (AJCC) staging criteria for thin melanomas. In general, the presence of several mitoses in dermal melanocytic lesions may be considered a feature worrisome for potential malignant behavior, depending on the clinical context (the major exception being melanocytic tumors in children/younger patients, as well as certain types of blue nevi). Protein markers that can aid in visualizing cells in the active stage of the cell cycle have therefore been intensely studied.

The proliferation marker most widely used is Ki-67, a nuclear antigen expressed in all active phases of the cell cycle (G_1, S, G_2, and M), but not in the quiescent phase (G_0) [42–49]. In multiple studies, Ki-67 staining has been found in <5% of nevomelanocytes in most common nevi; although, there have been reports of up to 15% positivity in Spitz and dysplastic nevi [42–44, 46, 50–54]. Conversely, Ki-67 is expressed in 13–30% of tumor cells in melanoma, and individual cases may show up to 100% nuclear positivity (Fig. 12.1) [42, 43, 45, 46, 50–54]. In addition to extent of staining, the location of cells positive for Ki-67 is helpful in differentiating benign and malignant lesions. Similar to HMB-45, melanoma cells tend to express Ki-67 in deeper portions of the lesion. In contrast, positive nuclear staining for Ki-67 is typically restricted to the superficial portions of melanocytic nevi [55]. The significant utility of Ki-67 will be elaborated later in this chapter.

Proliferating cell nuclear antigen (PCNA) is a 36 kDa protein and a co-factor of DNA polymerase δ that is expressed in all active phases of the cell cycle (G_1, S, G_2, and M) [43, 56–58]. There is increased expression of PCNA in melanomas relative to benign nevi, although Spitz nevi may also show relatively increased expression [43, 56–59]. Niezabitowski et al. [60] found increased PCNA expression to be an independent prognostic factor for decreased disease-free survival and increased mortality; however, other investigations have been unable to confirm this finding [56, 61, 62]. Whether PCNA provides additional diagnostically helpful information when used in conjunction with Ki-67 is less well studied.

Melanocytic Markers

Aside from being a marker for melanocytic differentiation, HMB-45 may help to distinguish benign from malignant melanocytic lesions. As outlined above, HMB-45 staining typically reflects "maturation" of benign melanocytic lesions, with strong staining of intraepidermal melanocytes as well as the more superficial dermal component in most nevi, and generally a loss of staining with increasing nevomelanocyte depth in the dermis [41]. Melanoma cells, on the other hand, generally retain HMB-45 staining, even in their deep dermal components [2]. Exceptions to this rule are deep penetrating nevi and blue nevi, which can show HMB-45 staining throughout the dermal component [2]. HMB-45 can be especially useful in evaluating a compound melanocytic lesion with an overt malignant epidermal component (melanoma in situ) and a dermal component of uncertain malignant potential. A retained HMB-45 staining pattern, in combination with atypical cytologic features, would be worrisome for malignancy and may influence extent of re-excision of the lesion or consideration for a possible sentinel lymph node biopsy.

Cell Cycle-Related/Anti-Apoptosis Proteins

Cyclins are proteins that bind and activate cyclin-dependent kinases, causing the cell to progress through the stages of the cell cycle [51, 53, 63–65]. Cyclins C, D1, D2, D3, and E help the cell progress from G_1 to S phase, cyclin A from S to G_2 phase, and cyclin B from G_2 to mitosis [51, 53, 64, 65]. Overall, cyclin D1 shows increased staining in melanomas as compared to nevi, but there is considerable overlap in individual cases [66–68]. Cyclin-dependent kinase inhibitors inhibit progression through the cell cycle [63]. P16 inactivates cyclin D/cdk4 complexes, inhibiting phosphorylation of the retinoblastoma (RB) protein that enables cell cycle progression from G_1 to S phase [69–75]. P16 staining is present in most benign nevi, but lost in 50–98% of melanomas [50, 71, 73–77]. P21 also inhibits cyclin/cdk complexes and binds PCNA to directly inhibit DNA polymerase δ (which is involved in DNA synthesis) [62, 78–80]. P27 inhibits cyclin D/cdk4 and cyclin E/cdk2 complexes, preventing cell cycle progression from G_1 to S phase [81–84]. Another marker related to p27 is Skp2, an Fbox protein that aids formation of a larger protein complex which ubiquitinates and degrades p27 [84]. P57, like p27, is a member of the CIP/KIP family of cyclin-dependent kinase inhibitors that prevent progression of the cell cycle from G_1 to S phase [85]. P53 is a 53 kDa tumor suppressor protein that promotes cell cycle arrest in G_1 and G_2 in response to DNA damage [42, 54, 83, 84]. P53 also induces the expression of p21, which helps inhibit DNA synthesis [76, 86]. The gene encoding p53 is the most commonly mutated gene in cancer [54, 83]. Mutations of the TP53 gene can result in the formation of abnormal p53 protein which is unable to inhibit the cell cycle [83]. Wild-type p53 has a very short half-life and is usually not detected by immunohistochemistry; however, the half-life of mutant p53 is much longer, and it can therefore be readily detected in this way [42, 54, 83, 84]. P53 does not stain most common nevi, but is present in 25–58% of melanomas [53, 54, 76, 84, 85].

Expression of the Bcl-2 family of anti-apoptotic proteins during melanoma progression has been studied by Zhuang et al. [87]. Bcl-2 staining was assessed using a panel of 100 compound and dysplastic nevi, in addition to primary and metastatic melanomas. Strong cytoplasmic staining for Bcl-2 was observed in compound nevi, dysplastic nevi, and thin primary melanomas (Breslow thickness <1.0 mm). Staining for Bcl-2 was significantly reduced in primary melanomas thicker than 1.0 mm and in metastatic tumors. The reverse staining pattern was observed for other members of the Bcl-2 family (Bcl-xL, Mcl-1); staining for these markers was significantly higher in primary melanomas thicker than 1.0 mm and metastatic tumors as compared to nevi and thin primary melanomas. Apart from possible use of these molecules in the distinction of benign from malignant melanocytic lesions, there may be important implications for treatment strategies that target anti-apoptotic pathways in melanoma [87]. The staining characteristics of cell cycle-related and other proteins in nevi vs. melanomas are outlined in Table 12.2.

Table 12.2 Protein markers to distinguish nevi from melanomas

Name	Type	Staining	Comment	References
Akt	S	• Limited potential to differentiate benign from malignant lesions • Does not distinguish dysplastic nevi or Spitz nevi from melanomas	The product of the oncogene Akt is a serine-threonine kinase that inhibits apoptosis through the phosphatidylinositol-3 kinase (PI3K) pathway	[88–90]
Bcl-2	C	• Strong, diffuse cytoplasmic staining in compound and dysplastic nevi and thin primary melanomas (<1.0 mm), weak diffuse/focal staining in thick primary melanomas (>1.0 mm) and metastatic melanoma	–	[87]
BMI-1	C	• Reported to be reduced in melanomas relative to nevi, but the specific numbers of lesions studied was not reported	A hematopoietic stem cell marker that helps to regulate p16	[91]
Cancer/testis antigens	I	• Panel of six markers shown to distinguish nevi from melanoma in 19 nevi and 38 primary melanomas	Proteins normally expressed only in the testis, but aberrantly expressed in many types of malignancy	[92–94]
CD26	I	• Increased staining in the radial growth phase of melanomas (22 of 66) relative to nevi (2 of 44)	An adenosine deaminase receptor	[95]
CD40	I	• Increased expression in melanomas relative to benign nevi	B-cell marker; also a tumor suppressor	[96, 97]
Cdk2	C	• Significantly increased staining for cdk2 in 46 primary cutaneous invasive melanomas relative to 17 benign nevi • No difference was noted between melanoma in situ and benign nevi	Study authors suggest that cdk2 may be useful in distinguishing nevi from early invasive melanomas	[98]
Cyclin A	C	• Rarely expressed in nevi, positive in 42–99% of melanomas	–	[51, 53, 77]
Cyclin B	C	• Rarely expressed in nevi, expressed in approximately 50% of melanomas	–	[53, 77]

(continued)

Table 12.2 (continued)

Name	Type	Staining	Comment	References
Cyclin D1	C	• Decreased expression in nevi relative to melanomas; however, individual cases may show considerable overlap in staining • Advanced lesions may show decreased staining • Demirkan et al. [67] suggested using p16 and cyclin D1 to differentiate some borderline melanocytic lesions, based on higher expression of cyclin D1 by melanomas relative to nevi	–	[66–68]
Cyclin D3	C	• Rarely expressed in benign nevi, commonly expressed in melanomas	–	[65, 77]
Ezrin	S	• No distinction between nevi and 95 melanomas studied	70 kDa protein involved in the phosphatidylinositol-3 kinase pathway	[99]
FAS and FAS-ligand	I	• Discrepancy between studies as to whether there is increased or decreased staining in melanomas relative to nevi • Bozdogan et al. [103] found positive membrane and cytoplasmic staining for FAS in 10/10 nevi and 12/12 primary melanomas and FAS-ligand in 6/10 nevi and 12/12 primary melanomas	Tumor suppressor proteins of the tumor necrosis family	[100–103]
FLIP	I	• Positive staining in 24/29 melanomas vs. 1/32 benign nevi	–	[104]
GADD	C	• Average staining of 82–92% of lesional cells in nevi vs. 19–31% of lesional cells in melanomas	GADD (Growth Arrest DNA Damage) proteins control transcription factors associated with cell cycle arrest, apoptosis, and cellular differentiation	[84]
HDM2	C	• >20% of lesional cells stained positive in 67/102 primary melanomas as opposed to 3/11 melanomas in situ and 1/16 dysplastic nevi	HDM2 is a 90 kDa zinc finger protein which binds to the transcription activation domain of p53, thereby inhibiting its function and targeting it for ubiquitination and degradation by proteasomes	[105–107]
HLA class I and II	I	• Increased positive staining in melanomas as compared to nevi	Follow-up studies are awaited	[108–110]
Jab1	C	• Similar levels of expression of Jab1 in nevi and primary melanomas, but significantly decreased expression in metastatic melanomas	It has been suggested that relocation of p27 to the cytoplasm may reduce its ability to act as a tumor suppressor, and that Jab1 (c-Jun activation domain-binding protein-1) is involved in translocation of p27 from the nucleus to the cytoplasm, and in its degradation	[79, 111]

(continued)

Table 12.2 (continued)

Name	Type	Staining	Comment	References
_Ki-67_	P	• <5% staining of cells in nevi and 13–30% in melanomas, although individual cases can be higher • Ki-67 is also increased in Spitz tumors	Distribution of staining in nevi is superficial, whereas melanomas show staining within deeper dermal component	[7–22, 26–34, 36–39, 41–46, 50–55]
_P16_	C	• Positive in nevi, loss of staining in 50–98% of melanomas	Melanoma cells tend to lose nuclear staining, but preserve cytoplasmic staining	[5, 71, 73–77, 112]
P21	C	• Rare staining in nevi, increased staining in melanomas	May be evidence of an "attempted inhibitory response" to the increased proliferation of melanoma cells	[55, 76, 77, 86, 113]
P27	C	• Conflicting reports as to its ability to distinguish benign nevi from melanomas • Some studies show decreased nuclear staining, but increased cytoplasmic staining in melanomas • Recurrent nevi tend to show lack of expression	Absence of p27 expression in blue nevi and in foci of neurotization within benign nevi	[79–82, 111, 114, 115]
P53	C	• Many reports show lack of staining in nevi, positive staining in 25–58% of melanomas • Stefanski et al. [55] also noted the presence of staining within deeper portions of melanomas, in contrast to nevi which may show rare superficial staining	Chorny et al. [42] reported that Spitz neoplasms and minimal deviation melanomas both show approximately 9% staining	[42, 53–55, 76, 84, 85]
P57	C	• Recurrent nevi retain nuclear expression of p57 in contrast to melanomas, cytoplasmic staining is similar in both lesions	p57, like p27, is a member of the CIP/KIP family of cyclin-dependent kinase inhibitors that prevent progression of the cell cycle from G_1 to S phase	[82]
PCNA	P	• Increased staining in melanomas and Spitz tumors vs. nevi	Proliferating cell nuclear antigen (PCNA) is a 36 kDa protein, a co-factor of DNA polymerase δ, that is expressed in all phases of cell cycle proliferation (G_1, S, G_2, M)	[43, 56–58]
PTEN	S	• Generally not considered to distinguish nevi from melanomas • However, recent study showed no cytoplasmic expression in 41 nevi vs. positive cytoplasmic expression in 87.7% of 162 primary melanomas	A tumor suppressor that is also involved in the phosphatidylinositol-3 kinase pathway and is the main antagonist of phosphoinositide 3-kinase (PI3K)	[60, 61, 69, 77, 116–118]
Retinoblastoma protein (RB)	C	• Statistically significant increase in nuclear staining in melanomas relative to nevi, but difference too narrow to be practical in a clinical setting	Retinoblastoma protein (RB) interacts with cyclin-dependent kinases and p16 to regulate cell cycle progression from G_1 to S phase	[55, 66]

(continued)

Table 12.2 (continued)

Name	Type	Staining	Comment	References
Skp2	C	• Increased nuclear staining for Skp2 in melanomas relative to nevi, but increase may be slight • Conflicting results with regards to cytoplasmic staining	An Fbox protein which aids formation of a larger protein complex that ubiquitinizes and degrades p27	[81, 115]
Trk-A	S	• Nuclear staining may be seen in both nevi and melanomas • Cytoplasmic and membrane staining in 21.7% of 152 melanomas vs. no staining in eight nevi	Trk-A is a nerve growth factor receptor tyrosine kinase that is involved in activation of major oncogenic signaling pathways in melanoma, including the Ras/MAPK and phosphatidylinositol-3 kinase pathways	[119]

Italics and underlined – Markers which may be most useful in routine clinical practice
S signaling molecule, *C* cell cycle-related/anti-apoptosis markers, *I* immune modulatory marker, *P* proliferation marker

Immune Modulatory Markers and Signaling Molecules

Several smaller studies have investigated the use of immune modulatory and signaling molecules for the distinction of melanocytic nevi from melanomas. A summary of findings is provided in Table 12.2.

In most instances in current clinical practice, the decision to treat a melanocytic lesion as either benign or malignant does not generally depend on the staining profile of a specific immunohistochemical marker. Many studies are limited by sample size and lack of information on clinical outcome/recurrence. Ki-67 may be regarded as the most reliable immunohistochemical marker currently applied in the clinical setting, since it is one of the very few markers for which there is considerable data supporting its use in the differentiation of nevi and melanomas. Numerous studies encompassing several hundreds of cases have advocated the use of Ki-67 as an adjunctive marker. Importantly, to our knowledge, there are no significant counter studies that have questioned its role in this setting (see Table 12.2). P16 also appears to have diagnostic utility, based on the results of several larger studies that document a decrease in nuclear staining within melanomas versus nevi. Since evidence of significant capacity to separate malignant and benign melanocytic lesions is scarce for most potential markers, large-scale studies are required before reliable clinical application becomes possible. Diagnostic utility will likely be enhanced by the employment of panels of markers, possibly in combination with digital imaging techniques.

Protein Markers in Special Situations

A recent review by Prieto and Shea [41] points out that immunohistochemistry, using combinations of relatively well-established protein markers, can be especially helpful in the setting of specific differential diagnostic challenges encountered in routine dermatopathology. Such special situations can include distinction of nevoid melanomas from either atypical nevi or melanomas arising in association with melanocytic nevi. The distinction of desmoplastic melanomas from desmoplastic nevi or scar tissue, as well as the differentiation of atypical keratinocytes of sun-damaged skin from atypical melanocytes can also be challenging. Some of these scenarios will be discussed below. Key immunohistochemical characteristics are listed in Table 12.3.

Spitz Tumors

Spitz tumors typically occur in children and young adults, arising as pink papules/nodules, often on the face. These lesions are characterized by large

Table 12.3 Protein markers in special situations

Situation	Marker	Results	References
Spitzoid lesions	Cyclin D1	• Increased staining in Spitz tumors and melanomas relative to nevi, but Spitz nevi show "zonal distribution" as opposed to "heterogenous pattern" in melanomas • Garrido-Ruiz et al. [121] found increased staining in Spitz tumors compared with conventional melanomas	[120, 121]
	HMB-45	• Loss of staining in the deeper component of Spitz nevi as opposed to spitzoid melanomas	[41]
	Ki-67	• Increased staining in Spitz tumors and melanomas relative to nevi, but Spitz nevi show "zonal distribution" as opposed to "heterogenous pattern" in melanomas • Studies conflict as to whether melanomas show increased staining vs. Spitz tumors overall	[41, 120–123]
	P16	• One study showed retained staining in dermal component of Spitz tumors vs. loss of dermal staining in melanomas, but another study did not show significant difference	[120, 121]
	P21	• Increased staining in Spitz tumors and melanomas relative to nevi, but Spitz nevi show "zonal distribution" as opposed to "heterogenous pattern" in melanomas • Increased staining in Spitz tumors relative to melanomas, but difference is not large enough to be clinically useful	[120, 121, 123]
	P27	• Retained staining in dermal component of Spitz tumors vs. loss of dermal staining in melanomas	[120]
	P53	• Increased staining noted in a subset of both Spitz tumors and melanomas	[120, 121]
	RB	• No difference between 28 Spitz tumors and 62 melanomas studied	[121]
	Survivin	• No difference between 28 Spitz tumors and 62 melanomas studied • 69% positive staining in melanomas vs. no staining in Spitz tumors in 28 Spitz tumors and 62 melanomas studied	[121]
	Topoisomerase IIα	• Marked increase in staining of melanomas vs. Spitz tumors with retained deep staining in 28 Spitz tumors and 62 melanomas studied	[121]
Proliferation nodules	Ki-67, P16, P21, P27	• 30 compound nevi with proliferation nodules showed no difference in staining within the nodules	[124]
	P53	• 30 compound nevi with proliferation nodules showed significantly increased staining within the nodules	[124]
Nevoid melanoma vs. compound/intradermal nevi	HMB-45	• Loss of staining in the deeper component of nevi as opposed to nevoid melanomas	[41]
	Ki-67	• Increased staining in nevoid melanomas vs. nevi • Loss of staining in the deeper component of nevi as opposed to nevoid melanomas	[41, 42]
	P53	• Increased staining in nevoid melanomas vs. nevi	[42]

Melanoma arising in association with a nevus	HMB-45	• Loss of staining in the deeper component of nevi associated with melanoma as opposed to dermal component of melanoma	[41]
	Ki-67	• Loss of staining in the deeper component of nevi associated with melanoma as opposed to dermal component of melanoma	[41]
Cellular blue nevi and melanoma	Ki-67	• Increased staining as well as prominent deep staining in melanomas as opposed to cellular blue nevi	[41]
Desmoplastic melanoma vs. desmoplastic nevus	Ki-67	• Increased staining of desmoplastic melanomas vs. desmoplastic nevi • The staining pattern is NOT helpful in distinguishing these entities	[41, 125]
	HMB-45	• Diffuse positivity in desmoplastic nevi vs. only rare staining in desmoplastic melanoma	[41, 125]
	Melan-A	• Diffuse positivity in desmoplastic nevi vs. only rare staining in desmoplastic melanoma	[41, 125]
Desmoplastic melanoma vs. scar tissue	S100	• Sensitivity – 98.7% • Scars may show focally positive fibroblasts, but do not show diffuse positivity as seen in desmoplastic melanoma	[11–23, 41]
	HMB-45	• Sensitivity – 17.6%	[11–23, 41]
	MART-1/Melan-A	• Sensitivity – 21.6%	[11–23, 41]
	Tyrosinase	• Sensitivity – 26.4%	[11–23, 41]
	MITF	• Sensitivity – 15.5%	[11–23, 41]
	P75	• Stained 26/29 spindle cell melanomas combined in two studies • Marker has low specificity, may also stain peripheral nerve sheath tumors, dermatofibrosarcoma protuberans, synovial sarcomas, rhabdomyosarcomas, and "neurotized" nevi	[41, 126–128]
	SOX10	• Sensitivity – 100% • Staining intensity in spindle fibroblasts of scars was weak	[129, 130]
Solar-damaged skin/actinic keratosis vs. melanoma in situ, lentigo maligna type	Melanocytic markers	• Look for clustering of melanocytes in melanoma in situ as well as extension of atypical melanocytes down hair follicles vs. dispersed single melanocytes in actinic keratosis • MART-1/Melan-A may mimic clustering of melanocytes due to staining of melanocytic dendrites • MITF may serve to be the most useful stain in these cases, as it is a nuclear stain which eases the definitive identification of distinct melanocytic cells	[9, 41]

spindle-shaped and epithelioid melanocytes with abundant cytoplasm, and enlarged nuclei with prominent nucleoli. Some tumors show focal pagetoid spread, may contain dermal mitotic figures, and can be accompanied by an inflammatory infiltrate; the combination of these features may pose challenges to their distinction from melanoma [2]. Furthermore, lesions may arise in older patients where their clinical behavior is uncertain. Some Spitz tumors have been shown to metastasize; however, these lesions still may not necessarily possess the same potential for extensive metastatic spread as conventional melanomas.

Since the histopathological features of these lesions may not definitively indicate their behavior, immunohistochemistry in atypical cases can be helpful. As reviewed by Prieto and Shea [41], Ki-67 and HMB-45 are typically expressed at lower levels within the deeper dermal components of Spitz nevi as compared to spitzoid melanomas. A summary of characteristic expression patterns of other immunohistochemical markers is outlined in Table 12.3. In addition, the assessment of spitzoid lesions may also include adjunctive genomic techniques, such as fluorescence in-situ hybridization (FISH).

Proliferation Nodules

Melanocytic nevi may contain proliferation nodules; nodular aggregates of nevomelanocytes that are different from the cells in the remainder of the lesion and which may resemble nodular melanoma, with increased cellularity, cellular enlargment, prominent nucleoli, and occasional mitoses [124]. Herron et al. [124] reported that benign nevi and both "normal" and "atypical" proliferation nodules show similar staining patterns for Ki-67, p16, p21, p27, c-myc, Bax, CD95, and Bcl-2. They found an increase in staining for p53 in proliferation nodules relative to adjacent nevomelanocytes and a prominent increase in staining for c-kit (CD117) in the cells comprising the proliferation nodules [124]. However, staining for Ki-67 was still low, suggesting a role for Ki-67 in the distinction of a proliferation nodule from melanoma arising within a melanocytic nevus.

Nevoid Melanoma vs. Compound/Intradermal Nevi

Nevoid melanomas, similar to melanomas in general, are reported to have increased Ki-67 nuclear staining compared to nevi, and retain higher nuclear positivity in their deeper dermal components [41]. Prieto and Shea [41] advocate the use of HMB-45, in combination with Ki-67, to determine if there is a staining gradient between the upper and lower dermal components of a melanocytic tumor; this would favor a benign lesion in the appropriate clinical context [41]. Nevi tend to show "top heavy" staining, while nevoid melanomas would be expected to show similar staining patterns in their superficial and deep dermal components [41].

Melanoma Arising in Association with a Nevus

Ki-67 and HMB-45 are useful markers for distinguishing the dermal component of invasive melanoma from dermal nevomelanocytes present in association with an overlying melanoma in situ [41]. The dermal nevus component would not express, or expresses at a truly low level, these two markers that are well conserved in melanomas [41].

Cellular Blue Nevi and Melanoma

Scattered cells throughout melanomas demonstrate Ki-67 positivity, whereas cellular blue nevi typically show both rare and superficial reactive cells [41]. HMB-45 will strongly and diffusely label the majority of cells in cellular blue nevi, while melanomas demonstrate patchy reactivity [41]. Melanomas that arise in cellular blue nevi show differences in Ki-67 and HMB-45 staining patterns between the benign and malignant components [41].

Distinction of Desmoplastic Melanoma from Desmoplastic Nevus

Prieto and Shea [41] advocate the use of Ki-67 and HMB-45 to distinguish desmoplastic nevi from melanomas. HMB-45 tends to be diffusely positive in desmoplastic nevi, but is usually not seen in desmoplastic melanomas. The extent of Ki-67 staining is critical in distinguishing desmoplastic nevi (low frequency of Ki-67 positive nuclei) from melanomas (high frequency of Ki-67 positive nuclei) [41].

Distinction of Desmoplastic Melanoma from Scar Tissue

A particular diagnostic dilemma is posed by spindle cell and desmoplastic melanomas, especially in cases which lack an epidermal component. These lesions may be mistaken for scar tissue. Although most desmoplastic melanomas are positive for S100, many of these lesions lack expression of HMB-45, tyrosinase and Melan-A (the melanocytic differentiation markers). Prieto and Shea [41] note that while scars may show some S100-positive fibroblasts, they do not show the widely distributed positive nuclear staining seen in melanomas [41]. The use of p75 (nerve growth factor receptor) in conjunction with S100 protein has been suggested as an alternative tool if more conventional melanocytic markers fail to assist in making a conclusive diagnosis [41, 126]. However, specificity of p75 is limited, since p75 also stains other malignant spindle cell tumors, including malignant peripheral nerve sheath tumors, dermatofibrosarcoma protuberans, synovial sarcomas, and rhabdomyosarcomas [131].

Distinction Between Solar-Damaged Skin/Actinic Keratosis and Melanoma In Situ, Lentigo Maligna Type

On rare occasions, it may be difficult to distinguish actinic keratosis from lentigo maligna (or the two conditions may co-exist). Careful evaluation using a melanocytic differentiation marker (examples: Melan-A, HMB-45, MITF) can be helpful in making this distinction [41]. A confluent pattern of atypical melanocytes (seen at least focally) in melanoma in situ contrasts with scattered enlarged, so-called "solar-activated" melanocytes of solar-damaged skin.

Summary/Conclusions

In summary, most melanomas are readily diagnosed by routine light microscopy. However, in borderline lesions a definite diagnosis may not be reached through the review of histopathological features alone, as indicated by the considerable lack of consensus on the malignant potential of equivocal melanocytic lesions among expert dermatopathologists [132]. Despite the accepted usefulness of established markers such as S100, HMB-45, Melan-A/MART-1, MITF and Ki-67, no single marker, or set of markers, can be expected to reliably distinguish benign from malignant lesions across the wide spectrum of melanocytic tumors. However, immunohistochemical analysis, used as an adjunct tool with clinical and histomorphologic findings, has a definite and powerful role in the evaluation of melanocytic lesions.

A wide array of protein markers has been evaluated for their capacity to differentiate between nevi and melanomas. Most of these, used as single markers, cannot reliably distinguish these two entities. However, one interesting and potentially useful approach is the simultaneous assessment of multiple protein markers. An algorithmic approach that makes use of a multimarker assay has recently been described by Kashani-Sabet et al. [133]. Using five protein markers identified in genomic screens, greater than 90% sensitivity and specificity for melanomas were achieved [133]. A composite algorithm of intensity scores for these five different protein markers (ARPC2, FN1, RGS1, SPP1, WNT2), assessed individually in the superficial and deep portions of the lesion by a pathologist, generates a diagnostic output in the form of a simple binary conclusion (benign vs. malignant). Although this latter report demonstrates the potential of more complex immunohistochemical analyses, further validation in different patient cohorts as well as demonstration of practicality in routine diagnostics will be necessary before such methods can be more widely applied.

References

1. Markovic SN, Erickson LA, Rao RD, et al. Malignant melanoma in the 21st century, part 1: epidemiology, risk factors, screening, prevention, and diagnosis. Mayo Clin Proc. 2007;82:364–80.
2. Elder DE. Lever's histopathology of the skin. 10th ed. Philadelphia: Lippincott, Williams and Wilkins; 2009.
3. Banerjee SS, Harris M. Morphological and immunophenotypic variations in malignant melanoma. Histopathology. 2000;36:387–402.
4. Ohsie SJ, Sarantoupolous GP, Cochran AJ, Binder SW. Immunohistochemical characterstics of melanoma. J Cutan Pathol. 2008;35:433–44.
5. Cochran AJ, Wen DR. S-100 protein as a marker for melanocytic and other tumours. Pathology. 1985; 17:340–5.
6. McKee PH, Calonje E, Granter SR. Pathology of the skin with clinical correlations. 3rd ed. Philadelphia: Elsevier Mosby; 2005.
7. Sujatha SEF, Johnson S, Bate J. Immunohistochemical analysis of cutaneous malignant melanoma: comparison of S-100 protein, HMB-45 monoclonal antibody and NKI/C3 monoclonal antibody. Pathology. 1994;26:16–9.
8. Bishop PW, Menasce LP, Yates AJ, Win NA, Banerjee SS. An immunophenotypic survey of malignant melanomas. Histopathology. 1993;23:159–66.
9. Dabbs DJ. Diagnostic immunohistochemistry. Philadelphia: Churchill Livingstone; 2002.
10. Kaufmann O, Koch S, Burghardt J, Audring H, Dietel M. Tyrosinase, Melan-A, and KBA62 as markers for the immunohistochemical identification of metastatic amelanotic melanomas on paraffin sections. Mod Pathol. 1998;11:740–6.
11. Ordonez NG, Xiaolong J, Hickey RC. Comparison of HMB-45 monoclonal antibody and S-100 protein in the immunohistochemical diagnosis of melanoma. Am J Clin Pathol. 1988;90:385–90.
12. Orchard GE. Comparison of immunohistochemical labeling of melanocyte differentiation antibodies melan-A, tyrosinase and HMB45 with NKIC3 and S100 protein in the evaluation of benign naevi and malignant melanoma. Histochem J. 2000;32:475–81.
13. Clarkson KS, Sturdgess IC, Molyneux AJ. The usefulness of tyrosinase in the immunohistochemical assessment of melanocytic lesions: a comparison of the novel T311 antibody (anti-tyrosinase) with S-100, HMB45, and A103 (anti-melan-A). J Clin Pathol. 2001;54:196–200.
14. Jungbluth AA, Busam KJ, Gerald WL, et al. A103: an anti-Melan-A monoclonal antibody for the detection of malignant melanoma in paraffin-embedded tissues. Am J Surg Pathol. 1998;22:595–602.
15. Sundram U, Harvell JD, Rouse RV, Natkunam Y. Expression of the B-cell proliferation marker MUM1 by melanocytic lesions and comparison with S100, gp100 (HMB45), and MelanA. Mod Pathol. 2003;16: 802–10.
16. Fetsch PA, Marincola FM, Abati A. The new melanoma markers: MART-1 and Melan-A (the NIH experience). Am J Surg Pathol. 1999;23:607–9.
17. Miettinen M, Fernandez M, Franssila K, Gatalica Z, Lasota J, Sarlomo-Rikala M. Microphthalmia transcription factor in the immunohistochemical diagnosis of metastatic melanoma: comparison with four other melanoma markers. Am J Surg Pathol. 2001;25: 205–11.
18. Busam KJ, Kucukgol D, Sato E, Frosina D, Teruya-Feldstein J, Jungbluth AA. Immunohistochemical analysis of novel monoclonal antibody PNL2 and comparison with other melanocyte differentiation markers. Am J Surg Pathol. 2005;29:400–6.
19. Jungbluth AA, Iversen K, Coplan K, et al. T311 – an anti-tyrosinase monoclonal antibody for the detection of melanocytic lesions in paraffin embedded tissues. Pathol Res Pract. 2000;196:235–42.
20. Boyle JL, Haupt HM, Stern JB, Multhaupt HAB. Tyrosinase expression in malignant melanoma, desmoplastic melanoma, and peripheral nerve tumors: an immunohistochemical study. Arch Pathol Lab Med. 2002;126:816–22.
21. King R, Googe PB, Weilbacher KN, Mihm Jr MC, Fisher DE. Microphthalmia transcription factor expression in cutaneous benign, malignant melanocytic, and nonmelanocytic tumors. Am J Surg Pathol. 2001;25:51–7.
22. Busam KJ, Iversen K, Coplan KC, Jungbluth AA. Analysis of microphthalmia transcription factor expression in normal tissues and tumors, and comparison of its expression with S-100 protein, gp100, and tyrosinase in desmoplastic malignant melanoma. Am J Surg Pathol. 2001;25:197–204.
23. Granter SR, Weilbaecher KN, Quigley C, Fisher DE. Role for microphthalmia transcription factor in the diagnosis of metastatic malignant melanoma. Appl Immunohistochem Mol Morphol. 2002;10:47–51.
24. Trefzer U, Rietz N, Chen Y, et al. SM5-1: a new monoclonal antibody which is highly sensitive and specific for melanocytic lesions. Arch Dermatol Res. 2000;292:583–9.
25. Wick MR, Swanson PE, Rocamora A. Recognition of malignant melanoma by monoclonal antibody HMB-45. An immunohistochemical study of 200 paraffin-embedded cutaneous tumors. J Cutan Pathol. 1988;15:201–7.

26. Argani P, Lae M, Hutchinson B, et al. Renal carcinomas with the t(6;11)(p21;q12): clinicopathologic features and demonstration of the specific alpha-TFEB gene fusion by immunohistochemistry, RT-PCR, and DNA PCR. Am J Surg Pathol. 2005;29: 230–40.
27. Turhan T, Oner K, Yurtseven T, Akalin T, Ovul I. Spinal meningeal melanocytoma. Report of two cases and review of the literature. J Neurosurg. 2004;100(3 Suppl Spine):287–90.
28. O'Brien DF, Crooks D, Mallucci C, et al. Meningeal melanocytoma. Childs Nerv Syst. 2006;22:556–61.
29. Deavers MT, Malpica A, Ordonez NG, Silva EG. Ovarian steroid cell tumors: an immunohistochemical study including a comparison of calretinin with inhibin. Int J Gynecol Pathol. 2003;22:162–7.
30. Dim DC, Cooley LD, Miranda RN. Clear cell sarcoma of tendons and aponeuroses: a review. Arch Pathol Lab Med. 2007;131:152–6.
31. Swanson PE, Wick MR. Clear cell sarcoma: an immunohistochemical analysis of six cases and comparison with other epithelioid neoplasms of soft tissue. Arch Pathol Lab Med. 1989;113:55–60.
32. Mai KT, Belanger EC. Perivascular epithelioid cell tumour (PEComa) of the soft tissue. Pathology. 2006;38:415–20.
33. Hornick JL, Fletcher CDM. PEComa: what do we know so far? Histopathology. 2006;48:75–82.
34. Zubovits J, Buzney E, Yu L, Duncan LM. HMB-45, S-100, NK1/C3, and MART-1 in metastatic melanoma. Hum Pathol. 2004;35:217–23.
35. Chorny JA, Barr RJ. S100-positive spindle cells in scars: a diagnostic pitfall in the re-excision of desmoplastic melanoma. Am J Dermatopathol. 2002;24: 309–12.
36. Busam K, Jungbluth A. The new melanoma markers: MART-1 and Melan-A (the NIH experience): author's response. Am J Surg Pathol. 1999;23:610.
37. Hofbauer GFL, Kamarashev J, Geertsen R, Boni R, Dummer R. Tyrosinase immunoreactivity in formalin-fixed, paraffin-embedded primary and metastatic melanoma: frequency and distribution. J Cutan Pathol. 1998;25:204–9.
38. Makhlouf HR, Ishak KG, Shekar R, Sesterhenn IA, Young DY, Fanburg-Smith JC. Melanoma markers in angiomyolipoma of the liver and kidney. Arch Pathol Lab Med. 2002;126:49–55.
39. Roma AA, Magi-Galluzzi C, Zhou M. Differential expression of melanocytic markers in myoid, lipomatous, and vascular components of renal angiomyolipomas. Arch Pathol Lab Med. 2007;131:122–5.
40. King R, Weilbaecher KN, McGill G, Cooley E, Mihm M, Fisher DE. Microphthalmia transcription factor: a sensitive and specific melanocyte marker for melanoma diagnosis. Am J Pathol. 1999;155:731–8.
41. Prieto VG, Shea CR. Use of immunohistochemistry in melanocytic lesions. J Cutan Pathol. 2008;35(Suppl 10):1–10.
42. Chorny JA, Barr RJ, Kyshtoobayeva A, Jakowatz J, Reed RJ. Ki-67 and p53 expression in minimal deviation melanomas as compared with other nevomelanocytic lesions. Mod Pathol. 2003;16:525–9.
43. Rieger E, Hoffman-Wellenhof R, Soyer HP, et al. Comparison of proliferative activity as assessed by proliferating cell nuclear antigen (PCNA) and Ki-67 monoclonal antibodies in melanocytic skin lesions. J Cutan Pathol. 1993;20:229–36.
44. Vogt T, Zipperer KH, Vogt A, Holzel D, Landthaler M, Stolz W. P53-protein and Ki-67 antigen expression are both reliable biomarkers of prognosis in thick stage I nodular melanomas of the skin. Histopathology. 1997;30:57–63.
45. Korabiowska M, Brinck U, Middel P, et al. Proliferative activity in the progression of pigmented skin lesions, diagnostic and prognostic significance. Anticancer Res. 2000;20:1781–6.
46. Li LXL, Crotty KA, McCarthy SW, Palmer AA, Kril JJ. A zonal comparison of MIB1-Ki67 immunoreactivity in benign and malignant melanocytic lesions. Am J Dermatopathol. 2000;22:489–95.
47. Hazan C, Melzer K, Panageas KS, et al. Evaluation of the proliferation marker MIB-1 in the prognosis of cutaneous malignant melanoma. Cancer. 2002;95: 634–40.
48. Henrique R, Azevedo R, Bento MJ, Domingues JC, Silva C, Jeronimo C. Prognostic value of Ki-67 expression in localized cutaneous malignant melanoma. J Am Acad Dermatol. 2000;43:991–1000.
49. Moretti S, Spallanzani A, Chiarugi A, Fabiani M, Pinzi C. Correlation of Ki-67 expression in cutaneous primary melanoma with prognosis in a prospective study: different correlation according to thickness. J Am Acad Dermatol. 2001;44:188–92.
50. Mihic-Probst D, Mnich CD, Oberholzer PA, et al. p16 status in primary malignant melanoma is associated with prognosis and lymph node status. Int J Cancer. 2006;118:2262–8.
51. Florenes VA, Maelandsmo GM, Faye R, Nesland JM, Holm R. Cyclin A expression in superficial spreading malignant melanomas correlates with clinical outcome. J Pathol. 2001;195:530–6.
52. Kanter-Lewensohn L, Hedblad MA, Wejde J, Larsson O. Immunohistochemical markers for distinguishing spitz nevi from malignant melanomas. Mod Pathol. 1997;10:917–20.
53. Tran TA, Ross JS, Carlson JA, Mihm Jr MC. Mitotic cyclins and cyclin dependent kinases in melanocytic lesions. Hum Pathol. 1998;29:1085–90.
54. Saenz-Santamaria MC, McNutt NS, Bogdany JK, Shea CR. P53 expression is rare in cutaneous melanomas. Am J Dermatopathol. 1995;17:344–9.
55. Stefanski C, Stefanski K, Antoniou C, et al. G1 cell cycle regulators in congenital melanocytic nevi. Comparison with acquired nevi and melanomas. J Cutan Pathol. 2008;35:799–808.
56. Woosley JT, Dietrich DR. Prognostic significance of PCNA grade in malignant melanoma. J Cutan Pathol. 1993;20:498–503.
57. Kanoko M, Ueda M, Ichihashi M. PCNA expression and nucleolar organizer regions in

malignant melanoma and nevus cell nevus. Kobe J Med Sci. 1994;40:107–23.
58. Niemann TH, Argenyi ZB. Immunohistochemical study of spitz nevi and malignant melanoma with use of antibody to proliferating cell nuclear antigen. Am J Dermatopathol. 1993;15:441–5.
59. Florell SR, Bowen AR, Hanks AN, et al. Proliferation, apoptosis, and surviving expression in a spectrum of melanocytic nevi. J Cutan Pathol. 2005;32:45–9.
60. Niezabitowski A, Czajecki K, Rys J, et al. Prognostic evaluation of cutaneous malignant melanoma: a clinicopathologic and immunohistochemical study. J Surg Oncol. 1999;70:150–60.
61. Reddy VB, Gattuso P, Aranha G, Carson HJ. Cell proliferation markers in predicting metastases in malignant melanoma. J Cutan Pathol. 1995;22:248–51.
62. Karjalainen JM, Eskelinen MJ, Kellokoski JK, Reinikainen M, Alhava EM, Kosma VM. P21$^{WAF1/CIP1}$ expression in stage I cutaneous malignant melanoma: its relationship with p53, cell proliferation and survival. Br J Cancer. 1999;79:895–902.
63. Bales ES, Dietrich C, Bandyopadhyay D, et al. High levels of expression of p27^{KIP1} and cyclin E in invasive primary malignant melanomas. J Invest Dermatol. 1999;113:1039–46.
64. Georgieva J, Sinha P, Schadendorf D. Expression of cyclins and cyclin dependent kinases in human benign and malignant melanocytic lesions. J Clin Pathol. 2001;54:229–35.
65. Florenes VA, Faye RS, Maelandsmo GM, Nesland JM, Holm R. Levels of cyclin D1 and D3 in malignant melanoma: deregulated cyclin D3 expression is associated with poor clinical outcome in superficial melanoma. Clin Cancer Res. 2000;6:3614–20.
66. Karim RZ, Li W, Sanki A, et al. Reduced p16 and increased cyclin D1 and pRb expression are correlated with progression in cutaneous melanocytic tumors. Int J Surg Pathol. 2009;17:361–7.
67. Demirkin NC, Kesen Z, Akdag B, Larue L, Delmas V. The effect of the sun on expression of β–catenin, p16, and cyclin D1 proteins in melanocytic lesions. Clin Exp Dermatol. 2007;32:733–9.
68. Ramirez JA, Guitart J, Rao MS, Diaz LK. Cyclin D1 expression in melanocytic lesions of the skin. Ann Diagn Pathol. 2005;9:185–8.
69. Straume O, Sviland L, Akslen LA. Loss of nuclear p16 protein expression correlates with increased tumor cell proliferation (Ki-67) and poor prognosis in patients with vertical growth phase melanoma. Clin Cancer Res. 2000;6:1845–53.
70. Bachmann IM, Straume O, Akslen LA. Altered expression of cell cycle regulators cyclin D1, p14, p16, CDK4 and Rb in nodular melanomas. Int J Oncol. 2004;25:1559–65.
71. Talve L, Sauroja I, Collan Y, Punnonen K, Ekfors T. Loss of expression of the p16^{INK4}/CDKN2 gene in cutaneous malignant melanoma correlates with tumor cell proliferation and invasive stage. Int J Cancer. 1997;74:255–9.
72. Pavey SJ, Cummings MC, Whiteman DC, et al. Loss of p16 expression is associated with histological features of melanoma invasion. Melanoma Res. 2002;12:539–47.
73. Mihic-Probst D, Saremaslani P, Komminoth P, Heitz PU. Immunostaining for the tumour suppressor gene p16 product is a useful marker to differentiate melanoma metastasis from lymph-node nevus. Virchows Arch. 2003;443:745–51.
74. Funk JO, Schiller PI, Barrett MT, Wong DJ, Kind P, Sander CA. P16^{INK4a} expression is frequently decreased and associated with 9p21 loss of heterozygosity in sporadic melanoma. J Cutan Pathol. 1998;25:291–6.
75. Wang YL, Uhara H, Yamazaki Y, Nikaido T, Saida T. Immunohistochemical detection of CDK4 and p16^{INK4} proteins in cutaneous malignant melanoma. Br J Dermatol. 1996;134:269–75.
76. Sparrow LE, Eldon MJ, English DR, Heenan PJ. P16 and p21^{WAF1} protein expression in melanocytic tumors by immunohistochemistry. Am J Dermatopathol. 1998;20:255–61.
77. Alonso SR, Ortiz P, Pollan M, et al. Progression in cutaneous malignant melanoma is associated with distinct expression profiles. Am J Pathol. 2004;164:193–203.
78. Florenes VA, Maelandsmo GM, Kerbel RS, Slingerland JM, Nesland JM, Holm R. Protein expression of the cell-cycle inhibitor p27^{Kip1} in malignant melanoma: inverse correlation with disease-free survival. Am J Pathol. 1998;153:305–12.
79. Ivan D, Diwan AH, Esteva FJ, Prieto VG. Expression of cell cycle inhibitor p27^{Kip1} and its inactivator Jab1 in melanocytic lesions. Mod Pathol. 2004;17:811–8.
80. Morgan MB, Cowper SE. Expression of p-27 (kip1) in nevi and melanomas. Am J Dermatopathol. 1999;21:121–4.
81. Li Q, Murphy M, Ross J, Sheehan C, Carlson JA. Skp2 and p27^{kip1} expression in melanocytic nevi and melanoma: an inverse relationship. J Cutan Pathol. 2004;31:633–42.
82. Curry JL, Richards HW, Huttenbach YT, Medrano EE, Reed JA. Different expression patterns of p27^{KIP1} and p57^{KIP2} in benign and malignant neoplasms and in cultured human melanocytes. J Cutan Pathol. 2009;36:197–205.
83. Talve K, Kainu J, Collan Y, Ekfors T. Immunohistochemical expression of p53 protein, mitotic index and nuclear morphometry in primary malignant melanoma of the skin. Pathol Res Pract. 1996;192:825–33.
84. Korabiowska M, Betke H, Kellner S, Stachura J, Schauer A. Differential expression of growth arrest, DNA damage genes and tumour suppressor gene p53 in naevi and malignant melanomas. Anticancer Res. 1997;17:3697–700.
85. Korabiowska M, Brinck U, Hoenig JF, et al. Significance of p-53 antigen in malignant melanomas and naevi of the head and neck area. Anticancer Res. 1995;15:885–90.

86. Trotter MJ, Tang L, Tron VA. Overexpression of the cyclin-dependent kinase inhibitor p21$^{WAF1/CIP1}$ in human cutaneous malignant melanoma. J Cutan Pathol. 1997;24:265–71.
87. Zhuang L, Lee CS, Scolyer RA, et al. Mcl-1, Bcl-XL and Stat3 expression are associated with progression of melanoma whereas Bcl-2, AP-2 and MITF levels decrease during progression of melanoma. Mod Pathol. 2007;20:416–26.
88. Dai DL, Martinka M, Li G. Prognostic significance of activated Akt expression in melanoma: a clinicopathologic study of 292 cases. J Clin Oncol. 2005;23:1473–82.
89. Dhawan P, Singh AB, Ellis DL, Richmond A. Constitutive activation of Akt/protein kinase B in melanoma leads to up-regulation of nuclear factor-κB and tumor progression. Cancer Res. 2002;62:7335–42.
90. Kantrow SM, Boyd AS, Ellis DL, et al. Expression of activated Akt in benign nevi, Spitz nevi and melanomas. J Cutan Pathol. 2007;34:593–6.
91. Bachmann IM, Puntervoll HE, Otte AP, Akslen LA. Los of BMI-1 expression is associated with clinical progress of malignant melanoma. Mod Pathol. 2008;21:583–90.
92. Jungbluth AA, Chen YT, Stockert E, et al. Immunohistochemical analysis of NY-ESO-1 antigen expression in normal and malignant human tissues. Int J Cancer. 2001;92:856–60.
93. Prasad ML, Jungbluth AA, Patel SG, Iversen K, Hoshaw-Woodard S, Busam KJ. Expression and significance of cancer testis antigens in primary mucosal melanoma of the head and neck. Head Neck. 2004;26:1053–7.
94. Luftl M, Schuler G, Jungbluth AA. Melanoma or not? Cancer testis antigens may help. Br J Dermatol. 2004;151:1213–8.
95. van den Oord JJ. Expression of CD26/dipeptidylpeptidase IV in benign and malignant pigment-cell lesions of the skin. Br J Dermatol. 1998;138:615–21.
96. Sviatoha V, Rundgren A, Tani E, Hansson J, Kleina R, Skoog L. Expression of CD40, CD44, bcl-2 antigens and rate of cell proliferation on fine needle aspirates from metastatic melanoma. Cytopathology. 2002;13:11–21.
97. van den Oord JJ, Maes A, Stas M, et al. CD40 is a prognostic marker in primary cutaneous malignant melanoma. Am J Pathol. 1996;149:1953–61.
98. Kuźbicki Ł, Aładowicz E, Chwirot B. Cyclin-dependent kinase 2 expression in human melanomas and benign melanocytic skin lesions. Melanoma Res. 2006;16:435–44.
99. Ilmonen S, Vaheri A, Asko-Seljavaara S, Carpen O. Ezrin in primary cutaneous melanoma. Mod Pathol. 2005;18:503–10.
100. Anastassiou G, Coupland SE, Stang A, Boeloeni R, Schilling H, Bornfeld N. Expression of Fas and Fas ligand in uveal melanoma: biological implication and prognostic value. J Pathol. 2001;194:466–72.
101. Redondo P, Solano T, Vazquez B, Bauza A, Idoate M. Fas and Fas ligand: expression and soluble circulating levels in cutaneous malignant melanoma. Br J Dermatol. 2002;147:80–6.
102. Bullani RR, Wehrli P, Viard-Leveugle I, et al. Frequent downregulation of Fas (CD95) expression and function in melanoma. Melanoma Res. 2002;12:263–70.
103. Bozdogan N, Bozdogan O, Pak I, Atasoy P. FAS, FAS ligand, tumor infiltrating lymphocytes, and macrophages in malignant melanoma: an immunohistochemical study. Int J Dermatol. 2010;49:761–7.
104. Bullani RR, Huard B, Viard-Leveugle I, et al. Selective expression of FLIP in malignant melanocytic skin lesions. J Invest Dermatol. 2001;117:360–4.
105. Gelsleichter L, Gown AM, Zarbo RJ, Wang E, Coltrera MD. P53 and mdm-2 expression in malignant melanoma: an immunohistochemical study of expression of p53, mdm-2, and markers of cell proliferation in primary versus metastatic tumors. Mod Pathol. 1995;8:530–5.
106. Polsky D, Bastian BC, Hazan C, et al. HDM2 protein overexpression, but not gene amplification, is related to tumorigenesis of cutaneous melanoma. Cancer Res. 2001;61:7642–6.
107. Polsky D, Melzer K, Hazan C, et al. HDM2 protein overexpression and prognosis in primary malignant melanoma. J Natl Cancer Inst. 2002;94:1803–6.
108. Kageshita T, Hirai S, Ono T, Hicklin DJ, Ferrone S. Down-regulation of HLA class I antigen-processing molecules in malignant melanoma: association with disease progression. Am J Pathol. 1999;154:745–54.
109. Kageshita T, Kawakami Y, Ono T. Clinical significance of MART-1 and HLA-A2 expression and CD8+ T cell infiltration in melanocytic lesions in HLA-A2 phenotype patients. J Dermatol Sci. 2001;25:36–44.
110. Ruiter DJ, Bergman W, Welvaart K, et al. Immunohistochemical analysis of malignant melanomas and nevocellular nevi with monoclonal antibodies to distinct monomorphic determinants of HLA antigens. Cancer Res. 1984;44:3930–5.
111. Denicourt C, Saenz CC, Datnow B, Cui XS, Dowdy SF. Relocalized p27^{Kip1} tumor suppressor functions as a cytoplasmic metastatic oncogene in melanoma. Cancer Res. 2007;67:9238–43.
112. Hilliard NJ, Krahl D, Sellhayer K. p16 expression differentiates between desmoplastic Spitz nevus and desmoplastic melanoma. J Cutan Pathol. 2009;36:753–9.
113. Maelandsmo GM, Holm R, Fodstad O, Kerbel RS, Florenes VA. Cyclin kinase inhibitor p21$^{WAF1/CIP1}$ in malignant melanoma: reduced expression in metastatic lesions. Am J Pathol. 1996;149:1813–22.
114. Sanki A, Li W, Colman M, et al. Reduced expression of p16 and p27 is correlated with tumor progression in cutaneous melanoma. Pathology. 2007;39:551–7.
115. Woenckhaus C, Maile S, Uffmann S, et al. Expression of Skp2 and p27KIP1 in naevi and malignant

116. Sparrow LE, English DR, Taran JM, Heenan PJ. Prognostic significance of MIB-1 proliferative activity in thin melanomas and immunohistochemical analysis of MIB-1 proliferative activity in melanocytic tumors. Am J Dermatopathol. 1998;20:12–6.
117. Cantley LC. The phosphoinositide 3-kinase pathway. Science. 2002;296:1655–7.
118. Slipicevic A, Holm R, Nguyen MT, et al. Expression of activated Akt and PTEN in malignant melanomas: relationship with clinical outcome. Am J Clin Pathol. 2005;124:528–36.
119. Flørenes VA, Mælandsmo GM, Holm R. Expression of activated TrkA protein in melanocytic tumors: relationship to cell proliferation and clinical outcome. Am J Clin Pathol. 2004;122:412–20.
120. Stefanski C, Stefanski K, Antoniou C, et al. Cell cycle and apoptosis regulators in Spitz nevi: comparison with melanomas and common nevi. J Am Acad Dermatol. 2007;56:815–24.
121. Garrido-Ruiz MC, Requena L, Ortiz P, et al. The immunohistochemical profile of Spitz nevi and conventional (non-Spitzoid) melanomas: a baseline study. Mod Pathol. 2010;23:1–10.
122. Vollmer RT. Use of bayes rule and MIB-1 proliferation index to discriminate Spitz nevus from malignant melanoma. Am J Clin Pathol. 2004;122:499–505.
123. Kapur P, Selim MA, Roy LC, et al. Spitz nevi and atypical Spitz nevi/tumors: a histologic and immunohistochemical analysis. Mod Pathol. 2005;18:197–204.
124. Herron MD, Vanderhooft SL, Smock K, et al. Proliferative nodules in congenital melanocytic nevi: a clinicopathologic and immunohistochemical analysis. Am J Surg Pathol. 2004;28:1017–25.
125. Kucher C, Zhang PJ, Pasha T, et al. Expression of Melan-A and Ki-67 in desmoplastic melanoma and desmoplastic nevi. Am J Dermatopathol. 2004;26:452–7.
126. Radfar A, Stefanato CM, Ghosn S, Bhawan J. NGFR-positive desmoplastic melanomas with focal or absent S-100 staining: further evidence supporting the use of both NGFR and S-100 as a primary immunohistochemical panel for the diagnosis of desmoplastic melanomas. Am J Dermatopathol. 2006;28:162–7.
127. Kanik AB, Yaar M, Bhawan J. p75 nerve growth factor receptor staining helps identify desmoplastic and neurotropic melanoma. J Cutan Pathol. 1996;23:205–10.
128. Satori I, Burrows R, Agoff SN, Piepkorn M, Bothwell M, Schmidt R. The p75 neurotrophin receptor, relative to other schwann cell and melanoma markers, is abundantly expressed in spindled melanomas. Am J Dermatopathol. 2001;23:288–94.
129. Nonaka D, Chiriboga L, Rubin BP. Sox10: a pan-schwannian and melanocytic marker. Am J Surg Pathol. 2008;32:1291–8.
130. Ramos-Herberth FI, Karamchandani J, Kim J, Dadras SS. SOX10 immunostaining distinguishes desmoplastic melanoma from excision scar. J Cutan Pathol. 2010;37:944–52.
131. Fanburg-Smith JC, Miettinen M. Low affinity nerve growth factor receptor (p75) in dermatofibrosarcoma protuberans and other nonneural tumors: a study of 1,150 tumors and fetal and adult normal tissues. Hum Pathol. 2001;32:976–83.
132. Carlson JA, Ross JS, Slominski AJ. New techniques in dermatopathology that help to diagnose and prognosticate melanoma. Clin Dermatol. 2009;27:75–102.
133. Kashani-Sabet M, Rangela J, Torabian S, et al. A multi-marker assay to distinguish malignant melanomas from benign nevi. Proc Natl Acad Sci USA. 2009;106:6268–72.

Tissue-Based Protein Biomarkers in Melanoma: Immunohistochemistry: (B) Prognostication

Basil A. Horst, Steven J. Ohsie, Alistair Cochran, and Scott W. Binder

Current Melanoma Risk Stratification: Challenges for Melanoma Biology-Based Prognostication

Protein biomarkers for primary melanoma are discussed in two separate chapters: markers used to differentiate melanoma from other melanocytic tumors (Chap. 12), and markers that aid prognostication, as discussed here. As melanocytic lesions fall into three categories (benign, malignant, and those of uncertain biological potential), overlap exists when trying to distinguish benign from malignant lesions, and in the assessment of how biologically aggressive a specific tumor will be. Placement in these three categories makes an important statement regarding the risk of metastatic disease and is used to guide clinical management.

The development of protein biomarkers which are based on the molecular profile of a primary melanoma and help determine risk for the individual patient is the focus of intense investigation. In this chapter, we discuss the extent to which protein biomarkers, detectable by routine immunohistochemical assessment, may facilitate prediction of outcome for individual melanoma patients. Serum-based protein biomarkers and those that predict the likelihood of response to a particular treatment are discussed elsewhere.

In current clinical practice, a light microscopic diagnosis of melanoma is followed by risk assessment for regional and systemic disease, using clinicopathologic criteria that are defined by the TNM classification for tumor staging (2009 American Joint Committee on Cancer [AJCC] guidelines, seventh edition [1]). The most important prognostic factors for primary melanoma (in the absence of regional or systemic disease) are Breslow thickness, presence versus absence of ulceration, and mitotic rate/mm^2 [1]. Sentinel lymph node (SLN) tumor status, as a marker for regional and systemic disease, remains the single most important parameter for outcome, and includes detection of micrometastases by immunohistochemistry [1–6].

While this evidence-based clinicopathologic staging system assigns patients to risk categories, it does not predict outcome for individual patients.

B.A. Horst, M.D. (✉)
Departments of Dermatology, Pathology and Cell Biology, Columbia University Medical Center, New York, NY, USA
e-mail: bh2179@columbia.edu

S.J. Ohsie, M.D.
Affiliated Pathologists Medical Group/Pathology, Inc., Torrence, CA, USA

A. Cochran, M.D.
Departments of Pathology and Laboratory Medicine and Surgery, David Geffen School of Medicine at the University of California, Los Angeles, CA, USA

S.W. Binder, M.D.
Department of Pathology and Laboratory Medicine, David Geffen School of Medicine at the University of California, Los Angeles, CA, USA

Some thin (≤1 mm) melanomas eventually metastasize, whereas other patients with thick primary tumors may never advance to systemic disease. The identification of early-stage tumors with risk of metastasis is of particular importance. Stage I tumors account for ~78% of all cutaneous melanomas reported to the National Cancer Institute Surveillance Epidemiology and End Results (SEER) cancer registry, more than 80% of which are thin tumors [7, 8]. However, according to SEER, a significant proportion (~15%) of melanoma deaths results from metastases of thin primary tumors [8].

Therefore, in melanoma as in other cancers, there is an urgent need to identify precise predictors of outcome. This will facilitate a move towards personalized management of patients through marker-assisted diagnosis and targeted therapy, based on the molecular profile of the individual lesion. To achieve this goal, many studies are correlating clinical and histopathologic features of melanomas with genetic findings in an attempt to develop a molecular classification of melanocytic tumors. Melanomas can be classified on the basis of genomic aberrations that correlate with level of sun-exposure, evidenced by alterations in the surrounding skin [9], suggesting that subsets of melanoma develop along distinctly different genetic pathways. Melanomas with identical clinical and histopathogical parameters may have markedly different mRNA expression profiles, which could be used to classify tumors into subgroups that correlate with differing patient outcomes [10, 11]. The identification of specific gene-signatures in formalin-fixed paraffin-embedded (FFPE) tissue demonstrates the utility of combining molecular diagnostic testing with light microscopy in the evaluation of diagnostically challenging melanocytic lesions [12]. Such molecular genetic classifications may be reflected by unique expression profiles of cytoplasmic and/or nuclear proteins (post-translational modifications aside) amenable to rapid assessment by immunohistochemistry, thus avoiding more complex and expensive molecular genetic analysis.

A "role-model" for defining disease on the molecular level is provided by hematologic malignancies. The current WHO classification of this group of diseases is based on their characteristic translocations [13]. In solid tumors, molecular and cytogenetic studies have also become useful adjuncts for the diagnosis of soft-tissue sarcomas through the identification of signature translocations [14]. Increasingly detailed knowledge of tumorigenesis is now becoming the basis of both molecular diagnosis and the development of new techniques for management of melanocytic tumors [15, 16], and calls for tools to rapidly identify biologically distinct lesions which are morphologically similar. However, the incorporation of immunophenotypic and molecular genetic features of melanoma subtypes is complicated by (1) the diversity of genetic alterations encountered and (2) the occurrence of these changes in both benign and malignant melanocytic proliferations. It has become evident that melanoma is not a uniform disease, but comprises several genetically and mechanistically distinct entities. Evidence for this heterogeneity comes from studies of melanoma-prone families, candidate-gene searches of sporadic melanomas (based on functionally relevant cellular processes), and recent genome-wide studies of gene expression, copy number alterations and allelic imbalances [17]. This diversity greatly complicates the use of expressed biomarkers at the protein level for differential diagnosis and prognostication.

The wide molecular heterogeneity of melanoma is indicated by the literally hundreds of immunohistochemical studies that have attempted to correlate clinical outcome with biomarker expression in primary tumors. Markers studied derive from all classes of molecules known to impact tumorigenesis; cell cycle-associated proteins, tumor suppressors/oncogenes, and regulators of apoptosis, cell adhesion, tissue invasion and metastasis (for reviews, see references [18–23]). Despite these extensive efforts, no immunohistochemistry-based protein biomarker is currently recommended in the authoritative guidelines for routine assessment of metastatic risk.

The absence of a practical immunohistochemically detectable marker is in fact attributable to a lack of robust, reproducible and validated results across broad tumor collectives. The bar for a new biomarker to be acceptable for routine clinical use is high: current AJCC recommendations are based on cohort studies of more than 30,000 patients with extensive follow-up data [1]. Any new biomarker must be measured against tumor status of the SLN, which represents the current "gold standard" and most accurate available indicator of prognosis for patients with localized disease [3]. In multivariate analysis, few of the numerous immunohistochemical markers tested for their ability to identify risk of metastasis improved on the performance of morphologic phenotypic markers, particularly Breslow's measure of tumor thickness [4, 20, 24].

Mitotic Rate/Proliferation Biomarkers

Mitotic rate is a powerful prognostic indicator in primary cutaneous melanoma [1, 25, 26]. The 2009 (seventh edition) AJCC melanoma staging system recognizes mitotic rate as an important primary tumor prognostic factor. This significantly changes classification of thin (≤1 mm), non-ulcerated melanomas, which are defined as T1b if one or more mitoses are present/mm^2, replacing Clark level of invasion as a staging criterion in this tumor category (AJCC sixth edition, 2002). For tumors in which the invasive component is <1 mm^2 in area, the mitotic count is given for 1 mm^2 of dermal tissue that includes the tumor; alternatively, the presence or absence of mitoses may be recorded as "at least 1/mm^2" or "0/mm^2", respectively. These changes are the result of analysis of several large multicenter studies, including >10,000 patients with clinically localized melanoma, that showed correlation of survival outcome with mitotic activity [1]. Mitotic rate is the most powerful predictor after tumor thickness [1].

In light of these data, an immunohistochemical marker that visualizes cells in the active stages of the cell cycle could be a useful prognostic adjunct (Fig. 12.1). Potentially more sensitive than mitotic index, especially in thin melanomas, an ideal marker of "proliferative" cells would relate closely to clinical outcome and be rapidly assessable using standardized techniques. Statistically sound data from substantial studies, stringent adherence to clearly defined staining protocols and cut-off levels, and demonstration of limitations would be necessary prerequisites for routine clinical application.

The following example illustrates the challenges to be overcome if an immunohistochemical marker is to be accepted for routine application. Human Ki-67 protein was identified in 1983 [27] as a nuclear protein associated with proliferating cells. It is expressed during all active phases of the cell cycle (G1, S, G2, and M [mitosis]), but absent from resting cells (G0). Ki-67 is an excellent marker for determining the growth-fraction of a cell population [28]. MIB-1 antibody is the equivalent of Ki-67 antibody, but can be used on FFPE tissue following antigen retrieval [29]. Immunohistochemically, Ki-67 is among the most widely-studied proteins in human malignancies, and its expression has been shown to correlate with outcome in a variety of neoplasms, including breast and prostate carcinoma, as well as hematologic malignancies (for review, see reference [28]). The use of Ki-67 expression as a reference variable in multivariate regression analyses further attests to its established role as a reliable proliferation marker within experimental settings [30, 31].

Rudolph et al. [32] reported the use of Ki-S5 antibody in melanocytic lesions with equivocal histopathology. This antibody is reactive against a formalin-resistant epitope of Ki-67 antigen, but with no cross-reaction with cytoplasmic structures of epithelial cells, as may be observed with MIB-1. A cut-off of 5% positivity was selected for a diagnosis of malignancy, and 70% of cases classified as malignant on the basis of their fraction of proliferative cells showed systemic disease progression, suggesting a role for proliferative index as a diagnostic and prognostic tool for melanocytic lesions. Ostmeier et al. [33] described the independent prognostic significance of Ki-67 staining in a multivariate analysis of 399 primary melanomas, with increased metastasis-free survival being associated with tumors showing lower Ki-67 rates (<75 Ki-67 positive melanoma cells/mm^2). Numerous other studies have assessed a possible correlation between Ki-67 expression and outcome in melanoma [30, 34–38]; however, results from studies using Ki-67 as a prognostic marker vary [19], and in some cases a variable pattern of Ki-67 staining between different areas within the same tumor can complicate assessment [30]. Several studies have shown a correlation between Ki-67 staining and metastatic potential or mortality in thick melanomas [36, 38, 39]. Other studies have reported an association between MIB-1 reactivity and outcome in thick (>1.5 mm), but not in thin (≤0.75 mm) melanomas [37]. Others have shown a correlation between proliferation and outcome in thin tumors [40, 41], and proposed a prognostic tree based on analysis of 396 thin primary melanomas [40]. These authors demonstrated an association between metastasis and ≥20% Ki-67 expression in dermal melanoma cells of tumors ≤1.0 mm in thickness. Though many studies have shown increased recurrences and mortality directly correlated with increasing Ki-67 positivity, this association was not independent of Breslow thickness in several small cohorts [30, 31, 39, 42–45]. Henrique et al. [34] defined a "proliferation-based prognostic index" by combining Ki-67 index with tumor thickness. This showed independent prognostic significance (in contrast to the Ki-67 index alone), but only for melanomas thicker than 4 mm [34].

From these divergent results, it is not clear whether a possible correlation of Ki-67 with outcome is linear across different melanoma thicknesses. This difficulty in validating consistent prognostic relevance for Ki-67, a marker with wide and longstanding application, demonstrates how substantial the challenges are for the establishment of biomarkers of this disease.

As reviewed by Haass et al. [20], other factors associated with cell proliferation correlate with outcome. Expression of proliferating cell nuclear antigen (PCNA), a cofactor of DNA-polymerase expressed during the DNA synthesis-phase of the cell cycle, correlates with decreased survival when expressed in ≥35% of tumor cell nuclei [39] (see Table 13.1). Minichromosome maintenance proteins 4 and 6, part of a protein complex which unwinds DNA at the replication fork origins during cell division [46], are also associated with poor survival when expressed at higher levels [11]. Patients whose primary melanomas retain expression of microtubule-associated protein-2 (MAP-2) were found to have significantly improved disease-free survival [47] (see Table 13.1).

Human double minute-2 (HDM2) and growth arrest DNA-damage (GADD) are two other proteins involved in regulation of cell proliferation which are reported to have prognostic significance in melanoma [48–50].

Additional markers associated with the replicative potential of melanoma cells, shown to have prognostic significance independent of other variables, are discussed below.

Emerging Protein Biomarkers: Need for Systematic Study Design

Several recent reviews have examined the use of protein biomarkers in melanoma [18–23]. The meta-analysis by Gould Rothberg et al. [23] provides an excellent overview of the hurdles to be overcome before routine application of prognostic biomarkers in clinical practice. This analysis, based on a PubMed medical literature database search on January 15, 2008, was restricted to studies that rigorously adhered to guidelines recommended by the National Cancer Institute and the European Organization for Research and Treatment of Cancer, the REMARK criteria ("REporting recommendations for tumor MARKer prognostic studies" [51]). Adherence to these guidelines is also viewed as critical in translational studies of other cancers [52].

Six criteria had to be met (for details, see references [21, 53]): (1) Cohort study design; (2) Evaluation of primary cutaneous melanomas; (3) Detailed description of methods, including; (4) Details of positive and negative controls; (5) Use of a multivariable proportional hazards analysis that adjusted for clinical prognostic factors; and (6) Reported data include hazard ratios and 95% confidence intervals. Table 13.1 outlines potentially applicable protein markers with independent prognostic significance that have emerged from

Table 13.1 Proteins showing statistically significant ($P \leq 0.05$) associations in multivariate analyses with all-cause mortality (ACM), melanoma-specific mortality (MSM), or disease-free survival (DFS), in cohort studies that conform to REMARK criteria[a]

Protein	Functional class[b]	Study size (n)	Associated outcome	Staining characteristics of reference group	Antibody (concentration)	HR; P	Reference
AP-2α (alpha)	1	214	MSM	ratio cytoplasmic/nuclear AQUA score ≤25%ile	Santa Cruz polyclonal C18 (1:1,600)	2.14; 0.008	[69]
	1	273	DFS	Strong staining	Santa Cruz polyclonal C18	3.12, moderate/ 2.52, weak; 0.01	[70]
ATF-2	1	269	MSM	High nuclear with low cytoplasmic AQUA score	Santa Cruz polyclonal (1:50)	0.55; <0.001	[71]
Bcl-2	3	159	MSM	≤50%ile AQUA score	DAKO monoclonal 124 (1:30)	0.64; 0.03	[72]
Bcl-xL	3	60	ACM	<10% cells positive	Zymed monoclonal 2 H12 (1:10)	8.07; 0.007	[45]
CEACAM-1	6	100	DFS	<20% cells positive	U. Schumacher lab monoclonal 4D1/C2 (8 μg/mL)	7.17; <0.001	[73]
CD44	6	282	DFS	≤90% cells positive	R&D Systems monoclonal 2 C5 (1:2,000)	0.57; 0.03	[74]
Cyclin A	4	172	DFS	<5% cells positive	Novocastra monoclonal 6E6 (1:50)	3.7; 0.001	[31]
Cyclin E	4	60	ACM	<10% cells positive	Novocastra monoclonal 13A3 (1:10)	2.89; 0.03	[45]
CXCR4	6	71	ACM	No staining	R&D Systems monoclonal 44,716 (dilution N/A)	2.07; 0.02	[75]
	6	71	DFS	No staining	R&D Systems monoclonal 44,716 (dilution N/A)	1.65; 0.01	[75]
gp100	7	93	DFS	≤90% cells positive	Biogenex monoclonal HMB45 (1:80)	1.86; 0.01	[39]
iNOS	5	132	MSM	<5% cells positive	Transduction Labs monoclonal (dilution N/A)	4.63; <0.001	[76]
Ki-67	4	187	MSM	<16% cells positive	Dako polyclonal A047 (1:50)	3.7; 0.003	[30]
	4	153	ACM	<20% cells positive	Dako monoclonal MIB-1 (1:100) [45]; Immunotech monoclonal MIB-1 [39]	2.66; 0.002	[39, 45]
Ku70	4	76	ACM	No staining	Santa Cruz polyclonal M19 (1:50)	0.87; <0.001	[77]
Ku80	4	76	ACM	No staining	Santa Cruz polyclonal M20 (1:50)	0.85; <0.001	[77]
L1-CAM	6	100	DFS	<20% cells positive	U. Schumacher lab polyclonal (1:100)	4.38; <0.001	[78]
MAP-2	4	37	DFS	<70% cells positive	Zymed monoclonal	0.18; 0.003	[47]
MCAM/MUC18	6	76	ACM	No staining	Novocastra monoclonal N1238 (1:50)	16.34; <0.001	[79]
	6	76	DFS	No staining	Novocastra monoclonal N1238 (1:50)	14.83; 0.01	[80]
Metallothionein	4	1,428	MSM	<10% cells positive	Dako monoclonal E9	3.08; <0.001	[81, 82]
	4	1,428	DFS	<10% cells positive	Dako monoclonal E9	3.77; <0.001	[81, 82]

(continued)

Table 13.1 (continued)

Protein	Functional class[b]	Study size (n)	Associated outcome	Staining characteristics of reference group	Antibody (concentration)	HR; P	Reference
MMP-2	6	157	MSM	<20% cells positive	Diabor monoclonal CA-4001 (5 μg/mL)	2.6; 0.006	[83]
	6	50	ACM	<34% cells positive	T. THpolyclonal (dilution N/A)	4.5; 0.006	[84]
NCOA3	1	343	MSM	Negative/weak staining	Abcam monoclonal Ab14139 (1:10)	1.91; 0.021	[85]
	1	343	DFS	Negative/weak staining	Abcam monoclonal Ab14139 (1:10)	1.69; 0.001	[85]
OPN	6	345	MSM	Weak staining	Abcam polyclonal ab8448 (1:200)	1.55; 0.049	[56]
p16/INK4a	2	187	MSM	Weak staining (no antigen retrieval)	Santa Cruz polyclonal SC-468 (1:500)	0.4; 0.007	[30]
p27/KIP1	2	60	ACM	<50% cells positive	Santa Cruz monoclonal F12 (1:50)	0.29; 0.02	[45]
	2	60	ACM	<10% cells positive	Transduction Labs monoclonal 57 (1:1000)	3.08; 0.02	[45]
p53	4	187	MSM	No staining	Dako monoclonal DO-7 (1:100)	8.9; <0.001	[30]
PCNA	4	93	ACM	≤35% cells positive	Dako monoclonal PC10 (1:200)	2.27; 0.03	[39]
	4	93	DFS	≤15% cells positive	Dako monoclonal PC10 (1:200)	4.00; 0.039	[39]
PRKCA	1	127	DFS	<50% cells positive	Santa Cruz monoclonal H7 (1:25)	2.03; 0.009	[86]
Survivin	3	50	DFS	No nuclear stain	Novus rabbit polyclonal (1:200)	7.32; 0.017	[87]
Tenascin-C	6	98	DFS	No staining	Biohit monoclonal 143DB7	1.20; 0.04	[88]
tPA	6	214	ACM	<5% cells positive	American Diagnostica polyclonal (dilution N/A)	1.90, 6%–50%; 0.04, >50%	[89]

%ile percentile, HR hazard ratio, P p-value, AP-2α (alpha) transcription factor AP-2 alpha, ATF-2 activating transcription factor-2, Bcl-2 B-cell CLL/lymphoma 2, Bcl-xL BCL2-like 1, CEACAM-1 carcinoembryonic antigen-related cell adhesion molecule-1, CXCR4 chemokine (C-X-C motif) receptor 4, gp100 HMB45, iNOS nitric oxide synthase 2, inducible, L1-CAM L1 cell adhesion molecule, MAP-2 microtubule-associated protein-2, MCAM/MUC18 melanoma cell adhesion molecule, MMP-2 matrix metalloproteinase-2, NCOA3 nuclear receptor coactivator 3, OPN osteopontin/secreted phosphoprotein 1, PCNA proliferating cell nuclear antigen, PRKCA protein kinase C, alpha, tPA plasminogen activator, tissue

[a]Adapted from Gould Rothberg et al. [23]

[b](1) Self-sufficiency in growth signals, (2) Insensitivity to anti-growth signals, (3) Evasion of apoptosis, (4) Limitless replicative potential, (5) Sustained angiogenesis, (6) Tissue invasion and metastasis, (7) Melanoma-associated antigens, (8) Altered immunocompetence (not shown in this table)

cohort studies performed with rigorous methodology, as reported by Gould Rothberg et al. [23]. The authors categorized biomarkers according to the six acquired capabilities of cancer, as defined by Hanahan and Weinberg [53], and supplemented by two additional functional categories, melanocyte differentiation and altered immunocompetence (see Table 13.1). However, well-defined biological function is not a pre-requisite for a predictive marker, and some biological phenomena with prognostic impact remain poorly understood, such as the correlation of ulceration with metastasis. As our knowledge of cancer biology increases, overlap between functional classes of molecules will become more apparent. Even though sample numbers are small in many of the studies outlined in Table 13.1, the rationale for their inclusion is strict adherence to published protocol guidelines, facilitating their independent validation. This stringency applies not only to molecular targets and study methodology, but also to specific antibody clones, staining protocols, and the cut-off points chosen for evaluation.

As shown in Table 13.1, data from two or more eligible studies on Ki-67 and Metallothionein staining were available for calculation of a combined hazard ratio. Other promising markers include melanoma cell adhesion molecule (MCAM, MUC18), matrix metalloproteinase-2 (MMP-2), proliferating cell nuclear antigen (PCNA) and p16/INK4a [20, 23]. For example, the expression of p16/INK4a was found to be associated with decreased risk of recurrence in a recent study [54]. Microtubule-associated protein-2, a neuron-specific protein involved in mitotic spindle assembly and induced in primary melanomas [55], also distinguishes primary tumors with significantly different prognoses, independent of other variables (Table 13.1, and references [18, 47]). Another interesting candidate protein involved in several mechanistic pathways, including proliferation and tissue invasion, is osteopontin [56]. The expression of this protein predicted SLN disease and was associated with reduced disease-specific survival in melanoma patients (Table 13.1, and reference [56]). Osteopontin was also identified as the gene most predictive of relapse-free survival in a recent RNA-expression study of more than 200 primary melanomas [57].

As Gould Rothberg et al. [23] point out, only a small subset of studies (37/455) that reported immunohistochemical results from primary melanomas met all the above inclusion criteria, and consequently only 62/387 collectively studied proteins could be reviewed for prognostic significance. Among assays excluded due to inadequate study design or methodology were studies of several signal transduction components considered critical for melanoma progression, such as c-Met, EGFR, FGFR-1, trk-C, Akt, PTEN, p42/22, p38, c-Jun and c-Myc. Eligible data were also lacking for VEGF, VEGF-receptors and hypoxia-inducible transcription factors. The main reasons for exclusion were (1) cross-sectional study design limited to determining the association between levels of marker expression with either melanocytic lesion progression or clinicopathologic parameters (284 studies), (2) case series without information on source population or sampling strategy (53 studies), (3) incomplete reporting of immunohistochemistry methods (27 studies), and (4) reporting of only univariate risk estimates (21 studies) [23]. Studies of non-Caucasian populations and those focusing on stromal/vascular markers were not included [23]. Of note, promising markers associated with the tumor microenvironment include connexins, which may have expression patterns in the epidermis adjacent to melanocytic lesions that relate to prognosis [20, 58].

The prognostic utility of some of the proteins listed in Table 13.1 may be overestimated, since many of the ineligible/excluded studies reported results with a range of markers that were not statistically significant. Their inclusion would likely have cancelled some of the identified statistical associations (publication bias).

The significant shortcomings of published prognostic biomarker data, derived from immunohistochemical assessment of primary melanomas, must be overcome. This will permit the use of this data to improve risk stratification in clinical practice. The combination of multiple, independent studies with acceptably comparable design has the potential to increase the impact of prognosis research.

Outlook

Given the genetic heterogeneity of melanoma, it is likely that no single protein marker will have sufficient predictive strength to supplant traditional primary melanoma-derived prognostic criteria. Current experimental efforts focus on the identification of biomarkers that stratify patients for SLN biopsy and identify high-risk groups who may benefit from adjuvant therapy. A recent example is the report by Kashani-Sabet et al. [59], describing a multimarker prognostic assay that achieved statistical significance in predicting disease-specific survival, independent of standard clinical or histopathologic factors, including SLN biopsy. In this study, expression levels and cut-off points for three markers (NCOA3, SPP1 [osteopontin], RGS1) were assessed in a cohort of 365 melanoma patients, and validated using an independent cohort of 141 patients. In another study of 438 primary melanomas by Gould Rothberg et al. [60], a multimarker prognostic model stratified patients into low- and high-risk groups based on the expression levels of five proteins: ATF2, p21, p16, β-catenin, and fibronectin. From this study, disease-specific survival was significantly better for patients assigned to the low-risk group (requiring elevated levels of overall β-catenin and nuclear p21, decreased levels of fibronectin, increased nuclear/cytoplasmic ratio of p16 and decreased nuclear/cytoplasmic ratio of ATF2, as assessed by automated quantitative imaging analysis). Winnepenninckx et al. [11] identified 254 genes in a set of 58 primary melanomas that were differentially expressed in tumors with a relatively favorable outcome. Immunohistochemical testing for the expression of related proteins, for which commercial antibodies were available, yielded a set of five markers whose expression levels correlated with survival. Two of these proteins (minichromosome maintenance proteins 6 and 4) demonstrated statistical significance, independent of standard clinical and histopathologic parameters (tumor thickness, ulceration, age, and gender).

These recent examples of multimarker studies demonstrate the enormous potential for biomarker assays as adjunctive tests for use in parallel with traditional prognosticators, such as Breslow thickness and SLN status. However, authors of these studies acknowledge that applying such tests in routine clinical practice and accepting their results as a basis for treatment decisions will require independent validation in larger melanoma cohorts. Validation will be greatly facilitated by strict adherence to standardized study guidelines such as the REMARK criteria, and will depend on consistent application of statistical methods to analyze the inter-dependence of multiple differentially expressed variables.

Finally, in addressing the important constraint of limited sample size on translational studies, tissue microarrays (TMAs) are a popular tool for validating (multiple) differentially expressed proteins. These platforms expand on the concept of simultaneous study of multi-tumor tissue blocks described by Battifora et al. [61]. TMAs are now widely used to validate expression patterns and correlate biomarker levels with clinical outcome in human cancers [62], including melanoma [59, 60]. TMAs are commercially available for a variety of neoplasms [63, 64]. Their expanded use allows for the simultaneous study of melanoma cohorts comprised of hundreds or even thousands of tumors. This will help to overcome the limiting factor of small sample size and facilitate the identification of biomarkers that may complement traditional prognostic criteria. Recent examples include the finding of an association of increased RGS1 (regulator of G protein signaling 1) expression with decreased disease-specific survival in primary melanoma patients [65]. Similarly, levels of HER3 [66], Osteopontin [56], and ING4 (inhibitor of growth 4) [67] had independent prognostic significance in multivariate analyses of expression patterns, as assessed on TMAs of melanoma cohorts [68]. However, access to sizeable cohorts of primary melanomas with detailed annotated clinical data remains a challenge.

Concluding Remarks

Despite major advances in our understanding of melanoma biology, tumor thickness, mitotic rate, and presence or absence of ulceration (based on histopathologic assessment) remain the critical primary melanoma parameters for prognostication. SLN status as a marker of regional or systemic disease is still the single most important factor for overall outcome.

Molecular biologic studies have yielded potential candidates for protein biomarkers which may emerge as valuable adjunct prognostic tools. The expectation is that such markers of tumor biology will enable a shift from assigning patients to broad risk categories toward a more individualized risk assessment. Importantly, these markers are expected to identify lesions which show more aggressive behavior than predicted from their conventionally assumed risk category, such as thin melanomas with risk of metastasis.

Among promising proteins which have shown independent prognostic value are factors impacting on cell-cycle progression (Ki-67, MAP-2, and Metallothionein) and tissue invasion (Osteopontin and MMP-2) (see Table 13.1).

Significant challenges remain, as exemplified by the difficulties of establishing a reliable clinical role even for protein markers with a record of widespread use. The need for statistically and methodologically sound study design in prognosis research is clear.

We believe that a concerted effort by the melanoma research community to produce and validate data in a rigorous manner will be the most promising and rewarding approach to the establishment of clinically useful biomarkers. High-throughput methods to search for differentially expressed genes, in addition to TMAs which can be shared among different institutions for independent validation, represent currently available powerful tools. Because of the heterogeneity of melanoma, it is likely that no single immunohistochemical marker will predict outcome for the majority of patients. Rather, different sets of biomarkers may be relevant for different tumor subclasses (possibly based on histopathologic subtypes, the mutational spectrum associated with the level of sun-exposure, or yet undefined groupings). The interpretation of expression data of any marker (panel) will depend on the clinical context and require correlation with routine histopathologic findings. As noted earlier, strict adherence to general study guidelines, such as the REMARK criteria, should allow for validation of biomarkers. This will facilitate the development of a prognostic tool with sufficient impact, and eventually increase confidence in its predictive value within the broader clinical community.

References

1. Balch CM, Gershenwald JE, Soong SJ, et al. Final version of 2009 AJCC melanoma staging and classification. J Clin Oncol. 2009;27:6199–206.
2. Chakera AH, Hesse B, Burak Z, et al. EANM-EORTC general recommendations for sentinel node diagnostics in melanoma. Eur J Nucl Med Mol Imaging. 2009;36:1713–42.
3. Cochran AJ. A glimpse of future management of melanoma. Arch Dermatol. 2009;145:1176–7.
4. Carlson JA, Ross JS, Slominski AJ. New techniques in dermatopathology that help to diagnose and prognosticate melanoma. Clin Dermatol. 2009;27:75–102.
5. Morton DL, Cochran AJ, Thompson JF, et al. Sentinel node biopsy for early-stage melanoma: accuracy and morbidity in MSLT-I, an international multicenter trial. Ann Surg. 2005;242:302–11. discussion 11–3.
6. Gershenwald JE, Thompson W, Mansfield PF, et al. Multi-institutional melanoma lymphatic mapping experience: the prognostic value of sentinel lymph node status in 612 stage I or II melanoma patients. J Clin Oncol. 1999;17:976–83.
7. Gimotty PA, Botbyl J, Soong SJ, Guerry D. A population-based validation of the American Joint Committee on Cancer melanoma staging system. J Clin Oncol. 2005;23:8065–75.
8. Gimotty PA, Elder DE, Fraker DL, et al. Identification of high-risk patients among those diagnosed with thin cutaneous melanomas. J Clin Oncol. 2007;25:1129–34.
9. Curtin JA, Fridlyand J, Kageshita T, et al. Distinct sets of genetic alterations in melanoma. N Engl J Med. 2005;353:2135–47.
10. Bittner M, Meltzer P, Chen Y, et al. Molecular classification of cutaneous malignant melanoma by gene expression profiling. Nature. 2000;406:536–40.
11. Winnepenninckx V, Lazar V, Michiels S, et al. Gene expression profiling of primary cutaneous melanoma and clinical outcome. J Natl Cancer Inst. 2006;98: 472–82.
12. Koh SS, Opel ML, Wei JP, et al. Molecular classification of melanomas and nevi using gene expression microarray signatures and formalin-fixed and paraffin-embedded tissue. Mod Pathol. 2009;22:538–46.
13. Hsi ED. Towards a molecular classification of hematolymphoid neoplasms: where are we now? Where are we going? J Histochem Cytochem. 2001;49:1323–4.
14. Iwasaki H, Nabeshima K, Nishio J, et al. Pathology of soft-tissue tumors: daily diagnosis, molecular cytogenetics and experimental approach. Pathol Int. 2009;59: 501–21.

15. Sekulic A, Haluska Jr P, Miller AJ, et al. Malignant melanoma in the 21st century: the emerging molecular landscape. Mayo Clin Proc. 2008;83:825–46.
16. Chin L, Garraway LA, Fisher DE. Malignant melanoma: genetics and therapeutics in the genomic era. Genes Dev. 2006;20:2149–82.
17. de Snoo FA, Hayward NK. Cutaneous melanoma susceptibility and progression genes. Cancer Lett. 2005;230:153–86.
18. Larson AR, Konat E, Alani RM. Melanoma biomarkers: current status and vision for the future. Nat Clin Pract Oncol. 2009;6:105–17.
19. Ohsie SJ, Sarantopoulos GP, Cochran AJ, Binder SW. Immunohistochemical characteristics of melanoma. J Cutan Pathol. 2008;35:433–44.
20. Haass NK, Smalley KS. Melanoma biomarkers: current status and utility in diagnosis, prognosis, and response to therapy. Mol Diagn Ther. 2009;13:283–96.
21. Bosserhoff AK. Novel biomarkers in malignant melanoma. Clin Chim Acta. 2006;367:28–35.
22. Ugurel S, Utikal J, Becker JC. Tumor biomarkers in melanoma. Cancer Control. 2009;16:219–24.
23. Gould Rothberg BE, Bracken MB, Rimm DL. Tissue biomarkers for prognosis in cutaneous melanoma: a systematic review and meta-analysis. J Natl Cancer Inst. 2009;101:452–74.
24. Carlson JA, Ross JS, Slominski A, et al. Molecular diagnostics in melanoma. J Am Acad Dermatol. 2005;52:743–75. quiz 75–8.
25. Azzola MF, Shaw HM, Thompson JF, et al. Tumor mitotic rate is a more powerful prognostic indicator than ulceration in patients with primary cutaneous melanoma: an analysis of 3661 patients from a single center. Cancer. 2003;97:1488–98.
26. Francken AB, Shaw HM, Thompson JF, et al. The prognostic importance of tumor mitotic rate confirmed in 1317 patients with primary cutaneous melanoma and long follow-up. Ann Surg Oncol. 2004;11:426–33.
27. Gerdes J, Schwab U, Lemke H, Stein H. Production of a mouse monoclonal antibody reactive with a human nuclear antigen associated with cell proliferation. Int J Cancer. 1983;31:13–20.
28. Scholzen T, Gerdes J. The Ki-67 protein: from the known and the unknown. J Cell Physiol. 2000;182:311–22.
29. Cattoretti G, Becker MH, Key G, et al. Monoclonal antibodies against recombinant parts of the Ki-67 antigen (MIB 1 and MIB 3) detect proliferating cells in microwave-processed formalin-fixed paraffin sections. J Pathol. 1992;168:357–63.
30. Straume O, Sviland L, Akslen LA. Loss of nuclear p16 protein expression correlates with increased tumor cell proliferation (Ki-67) and poor prognosis in patients with vertical growth phase melanoma. Clin Cancer Res. 2000;6:1845–53.
31. Florenes VA, Maelandsmo GM, Faye R, et al. Cyclin A expression in superficial spreading malignant melanomas correlates with clinical outcome. J Pathol. 2001;195:530–6.
32. Rudolph P, Schubert C, Schubert B, Parwaresch R. Proliferation marker Ki-S5 as a diagnostic tool in melanocytic lesions. J Am Acad Dermatol. 1997;37:169–78.
33. Ostmeier H, Fuchs B, Otto F, et al. Prognostic immunohistochemical markers of primary human melanomas. Br J Dermatol. 2001;145:203–9.
34. Henrique R, Azevedo R, Bento MJ, et al. Prognostic value of Ki-67 expression in localized cutaneous malignant melanoma. J Am Acad Dermatol. 2000;43:991–1000.
35. Korabiowska M, Brinck U, Middel P, et al. Proliferative activity in the progression of pigmented skin lesions, diagnostic and prognostic significance. Anticancer Res. 2000;20:1781–5.
36. Vogt T, Zipperer KH, Vogt A, et al. p53-protein and Ki-67-antigen expression are both reliable biomarkers of prognosis in thick stage I nodular melanomas of the skin. Histopathology. 1997;30:57–63.
37. Boni R, Doguoglu A, Burg G, et al. MIB-1 immunoreactivity correlates with metastatic dissemination in primary thick cutaneous melanoma. J Am Acad Dermatol. 1996;35:416–8.
38. Ramsay JA, From L, Iscoe NA, Kahn HJ. MIB-1 proliferative activity is a significant prognostic factor in primary thick cutaneous melanomas. J Invest Dermatol. 1995;105:22–6.
39. Niezabitowski A, Czajecki K, Rys J, et al. Prognostic evaluation of cutaneous malignant melanoma: a clinicopathologic and immunohistochemical study. J Surg Oncol. 1999;70:150–60.
40. Gimotty PA, Van Belle P, Elder DE, et al. Biologic and prognostic significance of dermal Ki67 expression, mitoses, and tumorigenicity in thin invasive cutaneous melanoma. J Clin Oncol. 2005;23:8048–56.
41. Moretti S, Spallanzani A, Chiarugi A, et al. Correlation of Ki-67 expression in cutaneous primary melanoma with prognosis in a prospective study: different correlation according to thickness. J Am Acad Dermatol. 2001;44:188–92.
42. Hazan C, Melzer K, Panageas KS, et al. Evaluation of the proliferation marker MIB-1 in the prognosis of cutaneous malignant melanoma. Cancer. 2002;95:634–40.
43. Frahm SO, Schubert C, Parwaresch R, Rudolph P. High proliferative activity may predict early metastasis of thin melanomas. Hum Pathol. 2001;32:1376–81.
44. Sparrow LE, English DR, Taran JM, Heenan PJ. Prognostic significance of MIB-1 proliferative activity in thin melanomas and immunohistochemical analysis of MIB-1 proliferative activity in melanocytic tumors. Am J Dermatopathol. 1998;20:12–6.
45. Alonso SR, Ortiz P, Pollan M, et al. Progression in cutaneous malignant melanoma is associated with distinct expression profiles: a tissue microarray-based study. Am J Pathol. 2004;164:193–203.
46. Calzada A, Hodgson B, Kanemaki M, et al. Molecular anatomy and regulation of a stable replisome at a paused eukaryotic DNA replication fork. Genes Dev. 2005;19:1905–19.

47. Soltani MH, Pichardo R, Song Z, et al. Microtubule-associated protein 2, a marker of neuronal differentiation, induces mitotic defects, inhibits growth of melanoma cells, and predicts metastatic potential of cutaneous melanoma. Am J Pathol. 2005;166:1841–50.
48. Berger AJ, Camp RL, Divito KA, et al. Automated quantitative analysis of HDM2 expression in malignant melanoma shows association with early-stage disease and improved outcome. Cancer Res. 2004;64:8767–72.
49. Polsky D, Melzer K, Hazan C, et al. HDM2 protein overexpression and prognosis in primary malignant melanoma. J Natl Cancer Inst. 2002;94:1803–6.
50. Korabiowska M, Cordon-Cardo C, Betke H, et al. GADD153 is an independent prognostic factor in melanoma: immunohistochemical and molecular genetic analysis. Histol Histopathol. 2002;17:805–11.
51. McShane LM, Altman DG, Sauerbrei W, et al. REporting recommendations for tumor MARKer prognostic studies (REMARK). Nat Clin Pract Oncol. 2005;2:416–22.
52. Mallett S, Timmer A, Sauerbrei W, Altman DG. Reporting of prognostic studies of tumour markers: a review of published articles in relation to REMARK guidelines. Br J Cancer. 2010;102:173–80.
53. Hanahan D, Weinberg RA. The hallmarks of cancer. Cell. 2000;100:57–70.
54. Karim RZ, Li W, Sanki A, et al. Reduced p16 and increased cyclin D1 and pRb expression are correlated with progression in cutaneous melanocytic tumors. Int J Surg Pathol. 2009;17:361–7.
55. Fang D, Hallman J, Sangha N, et al. Expression of microtubule-associated protein 2 in benign and malignant melanocytes: implications for differentiation and progression of cutaneous melanoma. Am J Pathol. 2001;158:2107–15.
56. Rangel J, Nosrati M, Torabian S, et al. Osteopontin as a molecular prognostic marker for melanoma. Cancer. 2008;112:144–50.
57. Conway C, Mitra A, Jewell R, et al. Gene expression profiling of paraffin-embedded primary melanoma using the DASL assay identifies increased osteopontin expression as predictive of reduced relapse-free survival. Clin Cancer Res. 2009;15:6939–46.
58. Haass NK, Wladykowski E, Kief S, et al. Differential induction of connexins 26 and 30 in skin tumors and their adjacent epidermis. J Histochem Cytochem. 2006;54:171–82.
59. Kashani Sabet M, Venna S, Nosrati M, et al. A multimarker prognostic assay for primary cutaneous melanoma. Clin Cancer Res. 2009;15:6987–92.
60. Gould Rothberg BE, Berger AJ, Molinaro AM, et al. Melanoma prognostic model using tissue microarrays and genetic algorithms. J Clin Oncol. 2009;27:5772–80.
61. Battifora H. The multitumor (sausage) tissue block: novel method for immunohistochemical antibody testing. Lab Invest. 1986;55:244–8.
62. Kononen J, Bubendorf L, Kallioniemi A, et al. Tissue microarrays for high-throughput molecular profiling of tumor specimens. Nat Med. 1998;4:844–7.
63. Datta MW, True LD, Nelson PS, Amin MB. The role of tissue microarrays in prostate cancer biomarker discovery. Adv Anat Pathol. 2007;14:408–18.
64. Fedor HL, De Marzo AM. Practical methods for tissue microarray construction. Methods Mol Med. 2005;103:89–101.
65. Rangel J, Nosrati M, Leong SP, et al. Novel role for RGS1 in melanoma progression. Am J Surg Pathol. 2008;32:1207–12.
66. Reschke M, Mihic-Probst D, van der Horst EH, et al. HER3 is a determinant for poor prognosis in melanoma. Clin Cancer Res. 2008;14:5188–97.
67. Li J, Martinka M, Li G. Role of ING4 in human melanoma cell migration, invasion and patient survival. Carcinogenesis. 2008;29:1373–9.
68. Gogas H, Eggermont AM, Hauschild A, et al. Biomarkers in melanoma. Ann Oncol. 2009;20 Suppl 6:vi8–13.
69. Berger AJ, Davis DW, Tellez C, et al. Automated quantitative analysis of activator protein-2alpha subcellular expression in melanoma tissue microarrays correlates with survival prediction. Cancer Res. 2005;65:11185–92.
70. Karjalainen JM, Kellokoski JK, Eskelinen MJ, et al. Downregulation of transcription factor AP-2 predicts poor survival in stage I cutaneous malignant melanoma. J Clin Oncol. 1998;16:3584–91.
71. Berger AJ, Kluger HM, Li N, et al. Subcellular localization of activating transcription factor 2 in melanoma specimens predicts patient survival. Cancer Res. 2003;63:8103–7.
72. Divito KA, Berger AJ, Camp RL, et al. Automated quantitative analysis of tissue microarrays reveals an association between high Bcl-2 expression and improved outcome in melanoma. Cancer Res. 2004;64:8773–7.
73. Thies A, Moll I, Berger J, et al. CEACAM1 expression in cutaneous malignant melanoma predicts the development of metastatic disease. J Clin Oncol. 2002;20:2530–6.
74. Karjalainen JM, Tammi RH, Tammi MI, et al. Reduced level of CD44 and hyaluronan associated with unfavorable prognosis in clinical stage I cutaneous melanoma. Am J Pathol. 2000;157:957–65.
75. Scala S, Ottaiano A, Ascierto PA, et al. Expression of CXCR4 predicts poor prognosis in patients with malignant melanoma. Clin Cancer Res. 2005;11:1835–41.
76. Ekmekcioglu S, Ellerhorst JA, Prieto VG, et al. Tumor iNOS predicts poor survival for stage III melanoma patients. Int J Cancer. 2006;119:861–6.
77. Korabiowska M, Tscherny M, Stachura J, et al. Differential expression of DNA nonhomologous end-joining proteins Ku70 and Ku80 in melanoma progression. Mod Pathol. 2002;15:426–33.
78. Thies A, Schachner M, Moll I, et al. Overexpression of the cell adhesion molecule L1 is associated with metastasis in cutaneous malignant melanoma. Eur J Cancer. 2002;38:1708–16.

79. Pacifico MD, Grover R, Richman PI, et al. Development of a tissue array for primary melanoma with long-term follow-up: discovering melanoma cell adhesion molecule as an important prognostic marker. Plast Reconstr Surg. 2005;115:367–75.
80. Pearl RA, Pacifico MD, Richman PI, et al. Stratification of patients by melanoma cell adhesion molecule (MCAM) expression on the basis of risk: implications for sentinel lymph node biopsy. J Plast Reconstr Aesthet Surg. 2008;61:265–71.
81. Weinlich G, Eisendle K, Hassler E, et al. Metallothionein – overexpression as a highly significant prognostic factor in melanoma: a prospective study on 1270 patients. Br J Cancer. 2006;94:835–41.
82. Weinlich G, Topar G, Eisendle K, et al. Comparison of metallothionein-overexpression with sentinel lymph node biopsy as prognostic factors in melanoma. J Eur Acad Dermatol Venereol. 2007;21:669–77.
83. Vaisanen AH, Kallioinen M, Turpeenniemi-Hujanen T. Comparison of the prognostic value of matrix metalloproteinases 2 and 9 in cutaneous melanoma. Hum Pathol. 2008;39:377–85.
84. Vaisanen A, Kallioinen M, Taskinen PJ, Turpeenniemi-Hujanen T. Prognostic value of MMP-2 immunoreactive protein (72 kD type IV collagenase) in primary skin melanoma. J Pathol. 1998;186:51–8.
85. Rangel J, Torabian S, Shaikh L, et al. Prognostic significance of nuclear receptor coactivator-3 overexpression in primary cutaneous melanoma. J Clin Oncol. 2006;24:4565–9.
86. Alonso SR, Tracey L, Ortiz P, et al. A high-throughput study in melanoma identifies epithelial-mesenchymal transition as a major determinant of metastasis. Cancer Res. 2007;67:3450–60.
87. Piras F, Murtas D, Minerba L, et al. Nuclear survivin is associated with disease recurrence and poor survival in patients with cutaneous malignant melanoma. Histopathology. 2007;50:835–42.
88. Ilmonen S, Jahkola T, Turunen JP, et al. Tenascin-C in primary malignant melanoma of the skin. Histopathology. 2004;45:405–11.
89. Ferrier CM, Suciu S, van Geloof WL, et al. High tPA-expression in primary melanoma of the limb correlates with good prognosis. Br J Cancer. 2000;83:1351–9.

Tissue-Based Protein Biomarkers in Melanoma: Mass Spectrometry-Based Strategies

Michael J. Murphy, Karim Rezaul, and David K. Han

Melanoma is considered an epidemic cancer as its incidence has increased 697% between 1950 and 2000, and continues to increase, faster than any other cancer subtype [1, 2]. Each year, over 53,000 Americans will be diagnosed with melanoma and over 7,000 will die from their disease. While representing <7% of all skin malignancies, melanoma accounts for ~75% of all deaths from skin tumors [1, 2].

Recent developments in proteomic and genomic technologies, coupled with advances in biocomputing, have motivated the effort to identify biomarkers in melanoma [3, 4]. These are tumor- or host-derived factors that are detectable in biological specimens, and which correlate with biological behavior of the tumor and patient prognosis. A number of putative biomarkers in melanoma have been identified, but their relevance to tumor progression, treatment selection and clinical outcome remains to be established [3, 4]. Recent genomic studies indicate that melanoma has distinct genetic defects (i.e., BRAF mutations) [5], but it is difficult to determine the functional consequence of any particular mutation on disease pathogenesis, progression or response to treatment. While genes contain the instructions for cellular assembly, it is through the actions of their encoded proteins that the functional characteristics and phenotype of any tumor, including melanoma, are manifest [6, 7]. Changes at the protein level do not always correlate with changes at the mRNA transcript level, and genomic methodologies cannot accurately predict the status of post-translational protein modifications, localization of proteins in tissues and cells, their association with other proteins, or protein release into the plasma [6, 7]. Moreover, there are genetic aberrations common to both melanoma and their benign counterparts (i.e., benign melanocytic nevi), limiting the diagnostic utility of some genomic analyses [5]. Therefore, the study of the proteome (i.e., 'proteomics') can provide unique information that is not available by other 'omic' technologies and holds great promise for the identification of protein biomarkers of clinical value in patients with melanoma. Currently, no tissue-based protein biomarker has become a standard part of recommended clinical practice in patients with melanoma [3, 4]. The study of the proteome in melanocytic lesions, and in particular solid tumor samples, is both relatively recent and limited [8–16]. This is in contrast to the more extensive and longstanding genomic investigations of these tumors been undertaken [5].

M.J. Murphy, M.D. (✉)
Department of Dermatology,
University of Connecticut Health Center,
Farmington, CT, USA
e-mail: drmichaelmurphy@netscape.net

K. Rezaul, Ph.D. • D.K. Han, Ph.D.
Department of Cell Biology, Center for Vascular Biology, University of Connecticut Health Center,
Farmington, CT, USA

In many respects, the challenge of proteomic studies may be greater than that of genomic analyses. The human genome, which has been sequenced, consists of approximately 21,000 protein-encoding genes [6]. In contrast, the total number of proteins in human cells is estimated to be between 250,000 and 1,000,000, of which only a small percentage has been identified or sequenced [6]. This 10–50 fold difference in abundance between protein-encoding genes and actual protein species is predominantly a result of alternative splicing, sequence deletions, and post-translational modifications that occur during protein production [6]. In addition, cellular proteins are continually moving and undergoing changes such as binding to cell membranes, interacting with other proteins, gaining or losing chemical groups, or breaking into smaller proteins or peptides [6]. Several other properties of proteins vary among individuals, between cell types, and even within the same cell under different conditions. One gene can produce multiple protein species (even up to 1,000), and any one particular protein may be modified in multiple ways, which can change its activity [6]. Moreover, the quantity of different proteins can also vary greatly. With some proteins expressed abundantly and others expressed at only a few copies per cell, coupled with differences in the half-lives of expression, proteins can be both difficult to isolate and characterize [4, 6]. Constantly improving mass spectrometry (MS)-based peptide-sequencing capabilities have led to in-depth analysis of highly complex protein mixtures, and the proteomics view has brought about a better understanding of malignant disease [4, 6, 7].

Unlike other protein identification strategies (such as immunohistochemistry [IHC]), MS-based proteomic technologies allow for the analysis of hundreds-to-thousands of proteins within a single assay, without the requirement for *a priori* knowledge of the proteins identified, and without the need for commercially available antibodies or antibody development for biomarker discovery [4, 6–16]. An MS analyzer consists essentially of three components: (1) an ion source to create ionized species; (2) a mass analyzer to measure the mass to charge (m/z) ratio; and (3) a detector to count the number of ions at each m/z value. For a given protein, an MS analyzer will produce a characteristic peptide spectrum, and the measured mass for each of these peptides can be used to infer the identity of the original protein [4, 6–16]. The protein and peptide profiles of clinical samples identified by MS-based techniques can then be analyzed by statistical programs to identify specific patterns that may correlate with the characteristics of the disease [4, 6–16]. While tumor pathways may be activated by different genetic abnormalities, proteomics methods allow for the study of common downstream effects at a protein level. In addition, proteomics offers the possibility to identify and assess changes in important tumor-regulatory proteins whose encoding genes may not be targets for mutation in melanoma.

Archival formalin-fixed paraffin-embedded (FFPE) tissue samples represent a potentially valuable resource for retrospective biomarker discovery studies in melanoma [4, 11–14, 17–19]. FFPE melanoma specimens are abundantly available in pathology archives worldwide and are linked to a wealth of patient data, including clinical outcomes related to disease course and/or response to treatment regimens. Fixation of tissue in formalin leads to significant protein-protein and protein-nucleic acid cross-linking [4, 20–22]. While these formalin-induced cross-links act to stabilize the cellular and morphological details of cells in tissue sections, they hinder the efficient extraction of full-length protein species, thereby rendering FFPE samples incompatible with many protein identification strategies, such as Western blot or protein microarrays [4, 20–22]. Accordingly, the identification of proteins within FFPE melanocytic tumor samples has largely been limited to IHC-based studies [17–19]. This methodology has been greatly enhanced by enzymatic and heat-induced antigen retrieval techniques, which 'unmask' cross-linked epitopes, and dramatically reduce the detection thresholds of IHC reactivity for a wide range of antibodies [17–19]. However, IHC-based studies have been limited to the analysis of one or a few proteins at a time, due to the nature of the technology [17–19]. Another major drawback with IHC analysis is that it requires *a priori* knowledge of the protein under investigation [17–19]. In addition, many proteins are still not detectable by IHC-methods, partly because antibodies to formalin-resistant epitopes are not available for all proteins. We and others have recently reviewed the published data on hundreds of proteins analyzed by IHC methods with respect to their possible diagnostic and/or prognostic applications in melanocytic tumors [17–19]. Unfortunately, aside from a small number of melanocytic-differentiation (i.e., HMB-45) and cellular proliferation (i.e., Ki-67) markers, to date no other proliferation, immunoregulatory or signaling proteins have proven to significantly improve diagnostic or prognostic accuracy in melanocytic tumors as a whole [17–19].

Proteomic studies of melanoma using MS-based strategies have generally been limited to cultured melanoma cell lines and serum samples of patients with melanoma [15, 16]. In only a handful of cases have solid tumor melanoma specimens been studied by MS-based approaches [8–14]. Of these, two studies have utilized xenografts from melanoma cell lines or solid murine melanoma [8, 9], one study employed laser microdissected melanoma cells from skin organ cultures [10], and four studies analyzed solid tumor samples from patients with melanoma [11–14], including a report by our group [13]. Of note, MS-based testing of archival cytologic (fine needle aspirate) melanoma samples has been employed to determine a distinct, reproducible protein fingerprint in melanoma, that could be used for potential diagnostic purposes in blinded specimens [11]. The ability to perform MS-based proteomic analysis on FFPE melanocytic tumor specimens would provide significant opportunities for biomarker and therapeutic target discovery in archival samples with well-documented clinical follow-up. A major challenge for MS-based strategies has been overcome with the development of novel methods to extract peptides, and not intact proteins, from FFPE tissue. Prior to our report, proteomic analysis of archival FFPE melanoma specimens had been performed in only one other study [12]. In this latter study, 120 proteins that were differentially expressed in FFPE specimens of primary and metastatic melanoma were identified [12]. While all of the proteins uncovered in the latter study are known to be implicated in the pathobiology of a variety of human cancers, only some of them have been previously reported to be associated with melanoma progression and metastasis by other protein analytical methodologies [12]. More recently, another group has reported that MS analysis of FFPE tissue may be useful in the differentiation of Spitz nevi from spitzoid melanoma [14].

Recent work in our laboratory has confirmed that cross-linked proteins in FFPE tissue samples can be efficiently extracted and digested for subsequent MS-based analysis [4, 13, 20, 21]. It is known that tumor cells and normal cells share high abundance commonly-expressed housekeeping proteins, whereas tumor-specific protein biomarkers are typically expressed at much lower abundance levels [4]. Therefore, it is critical that efficient protein extraction/identification methods with high coverage are employed to determine expressed proteins in tumor studies. The ability to achieve adequate amounts of proteins from FFPE tissue for proteomic analysis is attributable to the use of heating in combination with a detergent (such as SDS or acetonitrile), analogous to the heat-induced antigen retrieval methodologies for protein cross-link reversal commonly utilized for IHC. In addition, we have confirmed the feasibility of a method known as liquid chromatography-tandem mass spectrometry (LC-MS/MS) shotgun proteomics to characterize proteins in a variety of FFPE human tissue samples [4, 13, 20, 21]. With the LC-MS/MS shotgun proteomic method applied to FFPE tissue, the entire proteome is first digested into a highly complex mixture of peptides, followed by multidimensional chromatographic separation of the peptides, which are then sequenced by automated MS/MS analysis. Tandem MS involves the identification of a particular ion species (peptide) of interest by the first mass analyzer, which is then subjected to collision-induced-dissociation (CID) to generate a series of peptide fragments, that are then evaluated in the second mass analyzer. The peaks in the resulting MS/MS spectra from these peptide fragments provide additional information to infer the amino acid sequence of the protein and potentially the site and nature of specific post-translational modifications. Protein identification with this approach relies on searching against protein sequence databases using one or

a

MEGCMGEESFQMWELNRRLEAYLARVKALEEQNELLSAELGGLRAQSADTSWRAHADDELAALRALVDQRWREKHAAEVARDNLAEELEGVAGRCQQLRLARER
TTEEVARNRRAVEAEKCARAWLSSQVAELERELEALRVAHEEERVGLNAQAACAPRCPAPPRGPPAPEVEELARRLGEAWRGAVRGYQERVAHMETSLGQARE
RLGRAVQGAREGRLELQQLQAERGGLLERRAALEQRLEGRWQERLRATEKFQLAVEALEQEKQGLQSQIAQVLEGRQQLAHLKMSLSLEVATYRTLLEAENSRLQTP
GGGSKTSLSFQDPKLELQFPRTPEGRRLGSLLPVLSPTSLPSPLPATLETPVPAFLKNQEFLQARTPTLASTPIPPTPQAPSPAVDAEIRAQDAPLSLLQTQGGRKQAPEP
LRAEARVAIPASVLPGPEEPGGQRQEASTGQSPEDHASLAPPLSPDHSSLEAKDGESGGSRVFSICRGEGEGQIWGLVEKETAIEGKVVSSLQQEIWEEEDLNRKEIQD
SQVPLEKETLKSLGEEIQESLKTLENQSHETLERENQECPRSLEEDLETLKSLEKENKELLKDVEVVRPLEKEAVGQLKPTGKEDTQTLQSLQKENQELMKSLEGNLETF
LFPGTENQELVSSLQENLESLTALEKENQEPLRSPEVGDEEALRPLTKENQEPLRSLEDENKEAFRSLEKENQEPLKTLEEEDQSIVRPLETENHKSLRSLEEQDQETLT
LEKETQQRRRSLGEQDQMTLRPPEKVDLEPLKSLDQEIARPLENENQEFLKSLKEESVEAVKSLETEILESLKSAGQENLETLKSPETQAPLWTPEEINQGAMNPLEKEI
QEPLESVEVNQETFRLLEEENQESLRSGAWNLENLRSPEEVDKESQRNLEEEENLGKGEYQESLRSLEEEGQELPQSADVQRWEDTVEKDQELAQESPPGMAGVEE
DEAELNLREQDGFTGKEEVVEQGELNAT..TQREGDRESWSSGED

b

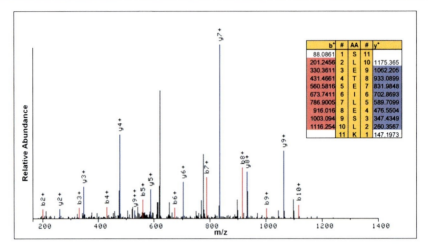

Fig. 14.1 Identification of Nestin in formalin-fixed paraffin-embedded melanoma tumor using mass spectrometry (MS). (**a**) A total of 15 tryptic peptides matched to the Nestin protein sequence, shown in bold and pink colored (partial). (**b**) MS/MS spectrum from m/z 1262.4430 [M+H]+, corresponding to the peptide SLETEILESLK from Nestin. Detected *b*- and *y*-series ions are highlighted in red and blue colors, respectively. See Fig. 14.2 for validation of Nestin expression

more algorithms, for which established guidelines and statistical tools to ensure consistency and confidence in the identified proteins are available [4, 13, 20, 21]. Because the connection between the peptides and the proteins from which they were derived is 'lost' using this approach, it is analogous to the shotgun genome sequencing strategy that was used to sequence the human genome. A number of studies using a similar shotgun proteomic approach have demonstrated: (1) a remarkable overlap (83–95%) in the number and identities of proteins between FFPE and frozen tissue; (2) no bias in protein identification based on sub-cellular localization (i.e., nuclear, cytoplasmic, membranous, extracellular); (3) identified proteins cover a wide variety of biological functions and gene ontology categories (i.e., structural, transcriptional, translational, binding, signaling, etc.); and (4) variations in the duration of formalin fixation (up to 14 days) and storage (even up to 10 years) have a minimal effect on protein inventories [23, 24]. Therefore, the equivalence of proteome inventories obtained from FFPE and corresponding frozen tissue samples validates the use of FFPE tissue as the starting material for retrospective MS-based methods of protein biomarker discovery [23, 24].

In our recent study, we described a protocol for the extraction of proteins from FFPE melanoma samples for subsequent sequencing, identification and validation, using a MS-, bioinformatics-, and IHC-based approach [13]. In this study, 250 μg of protein was successfully extracted from six 10 μm-thick tissue sections of a 0.8 cm×0.8 cm in-diameter melanoma tumor sample. Fifty μg of protein was subsequently analyzed by LC-MS/MS. We identified 935 proteins with high confidence (false discovery rate of <1%) using multiple sequence criteria (based on >2 peptide hits). Proteins were noted to cover all sub-cellular localizations and a wide variety of biological functions. The expression of a number of identified proteins was then validated by IHC on the same tissue block. Results are illustrated in Figs. 14.1 and 14.2.

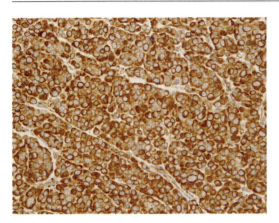

Fig. 14.2 Validation of Nestin expression in formalin-fixed paraffin-embedded melanoma tumor using immunohistochemistry. Based on data from Fig. 14.1

Nestin is a 177 kDa protein of 1621 amino acids. It is an intermediate filament that is also considered as a hair follicle stem cell and neural stem cell marker [25, 26]. Recent studies have demonstrated that tumor cells may behave as stem cells and show re-expression of progenitor cell proteins [25, 26]. Nuclear, cytoplasmic and/or membranous expression of nestin has been previously reported in 35–57% of primary and metastatic melanoma, suggesting that stem cells or at least the expression of stem cell markers may play a role in melanoma pathogenesis and progression [26–28]. A number of studies have suggested that nestin expression may be a predictor of poor prognosis in patients with melanoma [27, 28]. In our study, MS identified peptides belonging to the full-length protein nestin in the FFPE melanoma sample [13], as shown in Fig. 14.1. Follow-up IHC confirmed strong diffuse cytoplasmic staining for nestin within tumor cells [13], as shown in Fig. 14.2. Stromal cells were found to be negative for this protein by IHC.

An integrated MS- and IHC-based approach on the same tissue blocks can be used to: (1) confirm the validity of the protocol, by documenting the presence of previously known melanoma-related proteins; (2) identify novel proteins expressed in melanoma; and (3) correlate the MS-identification of proteins with their cellular/tissue distribution in tumor samples (i.e., tumor cells versus stroma). MS-based proteomic profiling of archival FFPE melanoma tumor samples could potentially be utilized to discover novel protein biomarkers in this disease. Subsequent IHC can be employed to correlate protein identification with the tissue distribution and intracellular localization of particular molecules.

References

1. Demierre MF, Sabel MS, Margolin KA, et al. State of the science 60th anniversary review: 60 years of advances in cutaneous melanoma epidemiology, diagnosis, and treatment, as reported in the journal Cancer. Cancer. 2008;113(7 Suppl):1728–43.
2. Linos E, Swetter SM, Cockburn MG, et al. Increasing burden of melanoma in the United States. J Invest Dermatol. 2009;129:1666–74.
3. Larson AR, Konat E, Alani RM. Melanoma biomarkers: current status and vision for the future. Nat Clin Pract Oncol. 2009;6:105–17.
4. Rezaul K, Wilson LL, Han DK. Direct tissue proteomics in human diseases: potential applications to melanoma research. Expert Rev Proteomics. 2008;5:405–12.
5. Takata M, Saida T. Genetic alterations in melanocytic tumors. J Dermatol Sci. 2006;43:1–10.
6. Clinical proteomic technologies for cancer. http://proteomics.cancer.gov/. Accessed 5 March 2011.
7. Kondo T. Tissue proteomics for cancer biomarker development: laser microdissection and 2D-DIGE. BMB Rep. 2008;41:626–34.
8. Zanivan S, Gnad F, Wickström SA, et al. Solid tumor proteome and phosphoproteome analysis by high resolution mass spectrometry. J Proteome Res. 2008;7:5314–26.
9. Culp WD, Neal R, Massey R, et al. Proteomic analysis of tumor establishment and growth in the B16-F10 mouse melanoma model. J Proteome Res. 2006;5:1332–43.
10. Hood BL, Grahovac J, Flint MS, et al. Proteomic analysis of laser microdissected melanoma cells from skin organ cultures. J Proteome Res. 2010;9:3656–63.
11. Fetsch PA, Simone NL, Bryant-Greenwood PK, et al. Proteomic evaluation of archival cytologic material using SELDI affinity mass spectrometry: potential for diagnostic applications. Am J Clin Pathol. 2002;118:870–6.
12. Huang SK, Darfler MM, Nicholl MB, et al. LC/MS-based quantitative proteomic analysis of paraffin-embedded archival melanomas reveals potential proteomic biomarkers associated with metastasis. PLoS One. 2009;4:e4430.
13. Rezaul K, Murphy M, Lundgren DH, et al. Combined mass spectrometry- and immunohistochemistry-based approach to determine protein expression in archival

melanoma–proof of principle. Pigment Cell Melanoma Res. 2010;23:849–52.
14. Lazova R, Seeley E, Keenan M, et al. Mass spectrometry – a promising method to differentiate spitz nevi for spitzoid malignant melanoma [abstract]. Am J Dermatopathol. 2011;33:418.
15. Paulitschke V, Kunstfeld R, Mohr T, et al. Entering a new era of rational biomarker discovery for early detection of melanoma metastases: secretome analysis of associated stroma cells. J Proteome Res. 2009;8:2501–10.
16. Findeisen P, Peccerella T, Neumaier M, Schadendorf D. Proteomics for biomarker discovery in malignant melanoma. Expert Rev Dermatol. 2008;3:209–20.
17. Rothberg BE, Bracken MB, Rimm DL. Tissue biomarkers for prognosis in cutaneous melanoma: a systematic review and meta-analysis. J Natl Cancer Inst. 2009;101:452–74.
18. Ohsie SJ, Sarantopoulos GP, Cochran AJ, Binder SW. Immunohistochemical characteristics of melanoma. J Cutan Pathol. 2008;35:433–44.
19. Carlson JA, Ross J, Murphy M. Markers of high-risk cutaneous melanoma: is there a winning combination for individualized prognosis? J Cutan Pathol. 2005;32:700–3.
20. Bagnato C, Thumar J, Hwang S, et al. Proteomics analysis of human coronary atherosclerotic plaque: a feasibility study of direct tissue proteomics by liquid-chromatography and tandem mass spectrometry. Mol Cell Proteomics. 2007;6:1088–102.
21. Hwang S-I, Thumar J, Lundgren DH, et al. Direct cancer tissue proteomics: a method to identify candidate cancer biomarkers from formalin-fixed paraffin embedded archival tissues. Oncogene. 2007;26:65–76.
22. Fowler CB, Cunningham RE, O'Leary TJ, Mason JT. 'Tissue surrogates' as a model for archival formalin-fixed paraffin-embedded tissues. Lab Invest. 2007;87:836–46.
23. Sprung Jr RW, Brock JW, Tanksley JP, et al. Equivalence of protein inventories obtained from formalin-fixed paraffin-embedded and frozen tissue in multidimensional liquid chromatography-tandem mass spectrometry shotgun proteomic analysis. Mol Cell Proteomics. 2009;8:1988–98.
24. Guo T, Wang W, Rudnick PA, et al. Proteome analysis of microdissected formalin-fixed and paraffin-embedded tissue specimens. J Histochem Cytochem. 2007;55:763–72.
25. Nestin: human protein atlas. http://www.proteinatlas.org/tissue_profile.php?antibody_id=5889&g_no=ENSG00000132688. Accessed 5 March 2011.
26. Bakos RM, Maier T, Besch R, et al. Nestin and SOX9 and SOX10 transcription factors are coexpressed in melanoma. Exp Dermatol. 2010;19:e89–94.
27. Tanabe K, Amoh Y, Kanoh M, et al. Prognostic significance of the hair follicle stem cell marker nestin in patients with malignant melanoma. Eur J Dermatol. 2010;20:283–8.
28. Piras F, Perra MT, Murtas D, et al. The stem cell marker nestin predicts poor prognosis in human melanoma. Oncol Rep. 2010;23:17–24.

Serological Biomarkers in Melanoma

Mel Ziman, Michael Millward, Robert Pearce, and Mark Lee

Introduction

Mortality rates for melanoma have remained constant in all age groups, largely due to frequent, drug-resistant tumor metastasis, for which the cure rate is currently less than 20%. A great deal of information has been compiled in an attempt to identify prognostic factors that correlate with clinical outcomes. However, current clinical staging system parameters, based upon histopathological evaluation of the primary tumor, lymph node and distant metastases [1], as well as serum Lactate Dehyorogenase (LDH) levels and genomic changes within the primary tumor [2–5], are not sufficient for predicting the risk and outcome of metastatic disease in an individual patient.

M. Ziman, Ph.D. (✉)
School of Pathology and Laboratory Medicine,
University of Western Australia,
Joondalup, WA, Australia

School of Exercise, Biomedical and Health Science,
Edith Cowan University, Joondalup, WA, Australia
e-mail: m.ziman@ecu.edu.au

M. Millward, M.D.
School of Medicine and Pharmacology,
University of Western Australia, Perth, WA, Australia

R. Pearce, M.D.
School of Exercise, Biomedical and Health Science,
Edith Cowan University, Joondalup, WA, Australia

M. Lee, M.D.
Plastic Surgery, Sir Charles Gairdner Hospital, Perth, WA, Australia

To date, metastases remains undiagnosed in ~30% of cases [6, 7], with the result that recurrences transpire within a year, or even several years, after removal of the primary tumor. Metastases at ten or more years after surgery indicate that disseminated tumor cells can remain quiescent for decades and change their biological behavior at any time [8]. The inability to accurately predict melanoma progression, and thus the low cure rates, may be related to the fact that the majority of studies use primary and, less often, metastatic tumor tissue to stratify patients and delineate prognostic markers. Very few studies investigate the circulating Tumor Cell (CTC) phenotype that actually gives rise to metastatic disease. Accordingly, there is an urgent need for detailed analyses of CTCs to provide early identification of metastatic risk, determine prognosis, and evaluate response to adjuvant therapies.

Metastatic Melanoma

Although metastasis is widely regarded as an inefficient process, most cancer patients die as a result of metastatic spread rather than from their primary tumors [9, 10]. Metastatic inefficiency of the primary tumor is likely overcome by the large number of malignant cells that may enter the systemic circulation daily, estimated to be up to ~4×10^6 cells per gram of primary tumor [11, 12]. CTCs may invade the venous or lymphatic circulation very early in the disease course

[13–16], and this being an obligate event in systemic metastasis, it is likely to be associated with disease progression [17]. In fact, a recent meta-analysis showed that the number of CTCs in patient peripheral blood increases with advancing stages of melanoma [18]. However, the variety and phenotype of these CTCs, their ability to remain in the circulation for many years (thus evading the immune system), and their subsequent re-activation to produce metastatic deposits, remain largely unexplored, particularly for melanoma.

The Process of Melanoma Cell Metastasis

Cell metastasis requires several steps, including loss of adhesion, dermal invasion, migration from the primary site, intravasation and survival in the bloodstream, migration into target tissues, and increased proliferation in the new tissue microenvironment, followed by orchestration of angiogenesis at the new site [19].

Melanoma cells arise in the epidermis, tethered tightly to other melanoma cells and surrounding keratinocytes by cell surface molecules [20]. On entering the invasive stage, melanoma cells may lose many of the cell surface proteins responsible for tight epithelial cell-cell adhesive interactions [6]. One of the key cell surface proteins, CDH1 (Cadherin 1, E-cadherin), is bound via its cytoplasmic tail to α-catenin and β-catenin, and thus to the actin cytoskeleton, maintaining tight cell junctions [21]. In fact, the replacement of CDH1 with CDH5 (V-cadherin) or CDH2 (N-cadherin) indicates the start of an epithelial-to-mesenchymal transition (EMT) [22]. The EMT process, also utilized by migrating cells during embryonic development, involves switching of polarized cells to contractile, motile mesenchymal progenitor cells, and is triggered by secretion of growth factors, such as EGF (epithelial growth factor), FGF (fibroblast growth factor), and chemotactic/pro-migratory factors SF/HGF (hepatocyte growth factor) and chemokines from stromal fibroblasts and macrophages. This secretion induces intracellular transduction pathways (Wnt, Notch), which in turn activate transcription factors (Twist, SNAI1 and 2) [23, 24], bringing about the invasion of melanoma cells into the circulation and tumor progression [14, 25].

When cancer cells detach from the primary tumor and intravasate into blood vessels or lymphatics, they can do so either actively or passively [7]. Passive cell intravasation, where cells are simply dislodged from the primary tumor, occurs as a result of increased hemodynamic flow and low CDH1 levels [10, 26, 27]. In contrast, active migration defines a process whereby cells separate from their neighbors as a result of an EMT transition and migrate as a result of activated signaling cascades, such as the NEDD9-DOCK3-Rac (Neural precursor cell expressed developmentally down-regulated protein 9-Dorsocross 3-Rac) pathway. The highly plastic movement of these cells through the extracellular matrix and their migration toward blood vessels is assisted by integrin and matrix metalloproteinase expression [14, 28, 29]. The next step in the active migration process is the attraction of tumor cells to lymphatics and blood vessels, a process mediated by ligand-receptor interactions between tumor cells and stromal and/or endothelial cells. Tumor cells secrete CSF1 (colony stimulating factor 1) and growth factors (such as EGF) which activate the formation and proliferation of tumor-associated macrophages in the stroma. These cells in turn secrete chemokines, including SDF-1 (stromal-cell-derived factor 1), SCL/CCL21 (chemokine C-C motif ligand 21) and I309/CCL1 (chemokine C-C motif ligand 1), which assist with the chemotaxis into blood vessels of tumor cells expressing the appropriate receptors (CXCR4, CCR7 and CCR8) [14, 30, 31].

Whether cells actively move toward and into nearby blood vessels, or whether the process is passive and coincidental, may be of some significance (Fig. 15.1). The expression of specific genes that assist entry into the circulation, either passively or actively, may determine cell survival and metastatic capability. That is, cells expressing genes associated with EMT or cell migration may be more prone to tumorigenesis and metastasis. Therefore, markers that delineate actively

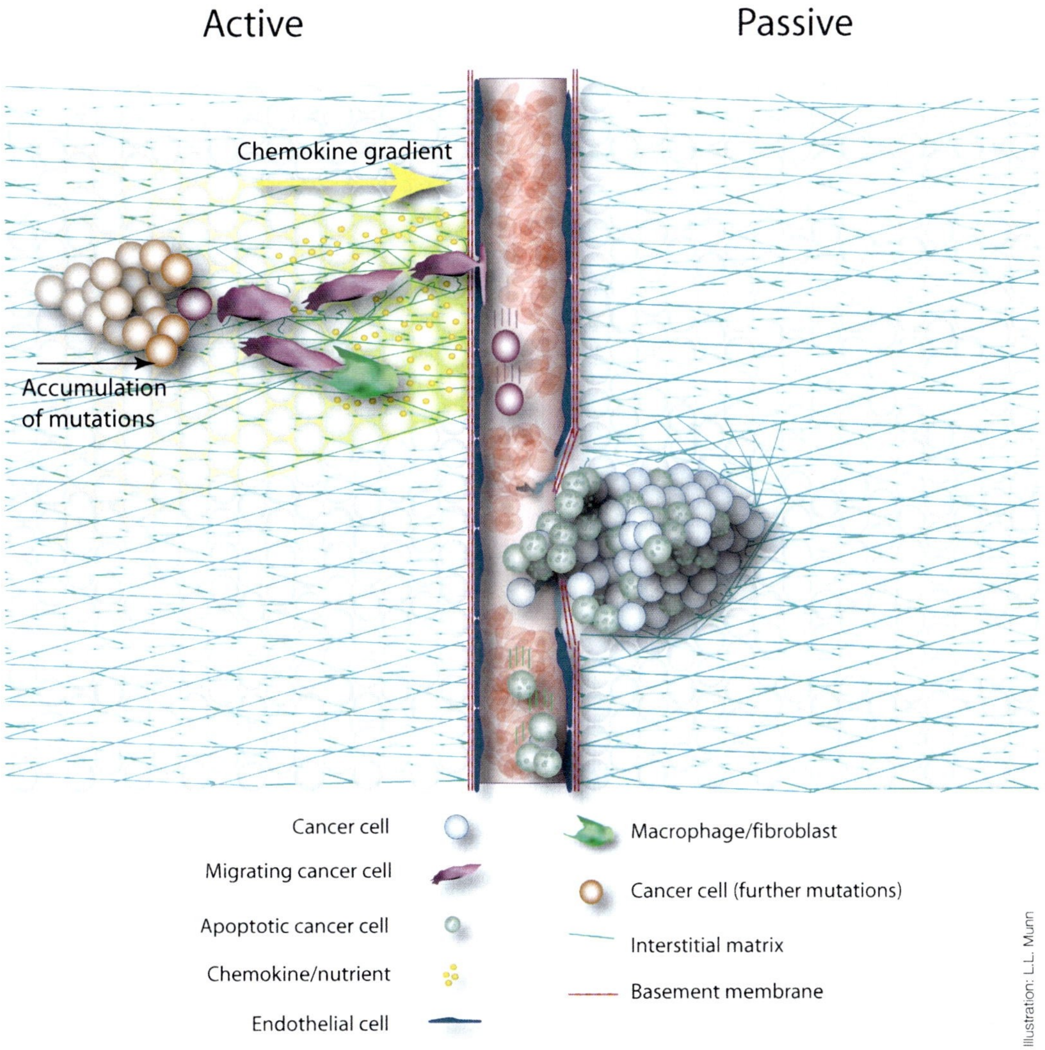

Fig. 15.1 A schematic representation of active versus passive melanoma cell migration and intravasation into blood vessels. An actively migrating melanoma cell would acquire mutations that assist it to actively migrate into the circulatory system and survive. In contrast, cells that are passively sloughed off the tumor, and pass into the bloodstream, would be predominantly apoptotic and necrotic and not survive for long periods of time in the circulation (Courtesy of Dr. Lance L. Munn, Massachusetts General Hospital & Harvard Medical School, Charlestown, MA, USA)

migrating, metastasizing cells could provide better measures of progression than those which measure cells that are merely sloughed off the tumor.

In order to investigate CTCs in more detail, models have been developed in which a tumor and its vascular system are isolated, and blood vessels are monitored so as to quantify and characterize cells entering and leaving the tumor mass [11, 32, 33]. Notably, a high rate of cancer cell shedding is observed ($3–4 \times 10^6$ malignant cells/day per gram of tumor), confirming that millions of cells are shed from a tumor every day, yet relatively few establish clinically detectable metastases. Characterization of these CTCs indicates that they are predominantly apoptotic or necrotic and unlikely to survive [34, 35], as evidenced in patients with advanced breast and prostate cancer [36, 37]. Furthermore, it is thought that shear stress and immune cells in the circulation destroy the bulk of CTCs and prevent all but the most proficient from producing secondary colonies [6, 38]. Recent evidence suggests that self-seeding of the original tumor by CTCs may also contribute to tumor progression [39].

Nevertheless, some cells do survive for long periods of time in the vasculature where, with the exception of cells from hematopoietic cancers, they do not typically circulate as independent entities (as depicted in Fig. 15.1) [6, 40]. Rather, they are usually found in clumps or clusters known as circulating tumor microemboli [41–43]. These may be surrounded by a "cloak" of platelets and leukocytes which assist in tumor cell survival [41–43].

Melanoma cell survival in the bloodstream can be attributed to mechanisms that ensure evasion from attack by natural killer (NK)-cells, the most potent mode of host defence against cancers. One such mechanism, which provides immune privilege and prevents NK-cell-mediated cytotoxicity, is the intracellular localization within melanoma cells of the ligand that typically activates NKD2D receptors on NK-cells [44]. Metastatic melanoma cells also develop resistance to inhibitory cytokines through the modification of oncostatin M receptors [45, 46]. A melanoma cell may invade the circulation and survive even without clinical evidence of a primary tumor; not infrequently, a patient may have metastatic melanoma without a known cutaneous primary site [47, 48]. A recent case of lethal melanoma in a patient with defective tumor angiogenesis resulted from CTC proliferation and survival in the complete absence of large solid tumor masses (either primary or secondary) [49]. As ~15% of patients whose lymph nodes are negative for melanoma at the time of surgical intervention eventually develop metastatic disease [7, 50–53], it is clear that CTCs are a significant prognostic factor.

Differential Gene Expression Profiles of CTCs

The question remains then, how do we differentiate those cells that are able to survive in the circulation and metastasize from those that cannot? Fundamentally, the genetic factors and mutations that prompt a melanoma cell to proliferate in situ must be different from those that permit a cell to proliferate and survive as a CTC, and these may be different again from events required to establish a secondary tumor. Analysis of the gene expression signature of CTCs relative to cells of respective primary and secondary solid tumors is likely to shed light on their phenotype, adaptability and association with disease progression. Some support for this approach is provided by observations of differential gene expression patterns in primary versus circulating cells from the same melanoma patient [15, 16].

The evolution theory of cancer development depicts malignant progression as a series of changes in the genome of tumor cells through amplification, translocation, or loss of heterozygosity. These changes produce a subpopulation of cells capable of overcoming all barriers to successful metastasis. Of note, different gene expression patterns have been observed within a subset of primary tumor cells that are predictive of metastatic potential [54]. A cancer cell could acquire the ability to disseminate at any time, even prior to overt tumor formation [51, 55]. For heterogeneous tumors, such as melanoma, an unstable, genetically-variant, invasive cell could intravasate and prevail in the circulating cell population, but not exist in great abundance in the primary tumor [14, 56]. Metastasis-promoting genes that provide an aggressive edge in survival during both intravasation and extravasation at the new metastatic site may not be advantageous to the primary tumor, and too rare to influence its population-averaged, gene expression profile [14].

In recent years, a number of researchers have demonstrated the existence of a subset of tumor-initiating or melanoma stem cells within the primary tumor that possess two important features. Firstly, they are capable of asymmetric cell division, allowing both self-renewal to maintain the subset and differentiation into cancer progenitor cells. Secondly, they are inherently resistant to both chemotherapy and radiotherapy [57–61]. These cells are believed to be responsible for relapse and metastasis by virtue of their ability to survive treatment and initiate new tumor formation. Rare cancer stem cells would therefore be capable of effectively managing the metastatic process [62]. The few melanoma stem cells that escape the primary tumor and invade the circulation would evade therapy due to their stem cell properties of slow turnover and chemotherapy resistance, and upon reaching their homing organ, act as a seed for metastasis formation [63]. Melanoma stem cells have been identified in both primary tumors and cell lines. Recently identified melanoma stem cell markers include JARID1B (jumonji, AT-rich interactive domain 1B) [64], ABCB5 (ATP-binding cassette subfamily B (MDR/TAP) member 5), ABCG2 (ATP-binding cassette subfamily G member 2), and MDR1 (multi-drug resistance 1) [58, 65–71]. A recent study reported that melanoma cells in peripheral blood expressed stem cell-associated markers nestin and CD133 [72]. Higher expression of nestin by CTCs might represent an index of poor prognosis [72]. Reports of disseminated tumor cells with stem cell-like phenotypes have been confirmed in the bone marrow of patients with other cancers [73].

Methods of Detecting CTCs

Since very few tumor cells survive in the circulation, CTCs are expected to be present at relatively low concentrations; one tumor cell per 10^6–10^7 normal blood cells [63, 74] or, on average, 60 cells in 7.5 mL of blood. When quantified in 2,183 blood samples from 964 metastatic carcinoma patients, CTC levels ranged from 0 to 23,618 CTCs per 7.5 mL of blood, with a mean of 60 ± 693 CTCs per 7.5 mL of blood [75]. Consequently, a technique that can accurately detect low levels of CTCs is required for accurate prognostic analysis. Over the past 40 years, several techniques have been developed, but few have withstood the scrutiny required to confirm their reproducibility and significance. To date, the most promising techniques include (1) indirect analysis of CTC gene expression in peripheral blood by quantitative reverse transcription-polymerase chain reaction (RT-PCR) [18, 53, 76–78] and (2) direct analysis using immunomagnetic bead capture, microscopic cell labeling, fiber-optic array scanning technology or photoacoustics [15, 16, 79–81].

Quantitative RT-PCR (qPCR) appears to be the most sensitive and extensively studied technique for circulating melanoma cell analysis [53, 76, 77, 82, 83]. Typically, assays are designed to detect expression of melanocyte-differentiation genes, such as tyrosinase (TYR) [84, 85]. Since normal melanocytes are not thought to circulate in peripheral blood, detection of melanocytic gene transcripts should correlate with identification of CTCs [86, 87]. The sensitivity and specificity of qPCR for circulating melanoma cells is increased by analysis of multiple markers [87], including melan-A (MLANA), beta-1,4-N-acetyl-galactosaminyltransferase 1 (B4GALNT1), silver homolog (SILV), melanoma cell adhesion molecule (MCAM), melanoma associated antigen p97 (MFI2), melanoma antigen family A3 (MAGEA3) and microphthalmia-associated transcription factor 4 (MITF4) [76, 77, 88, 89]. Several studies, albeit with relatively few patients, have shown that melanoma CTCs detected by multimarker qPCR correlate to AJCC stage, survival and disease recurrence [18, 86, 90]. Additionally, serial monitoring of CTC levels by qPCR can be used to assess the efficacy of therapy for metastatic melanoma [90, 91]. For example, a change in CTC positivity from 23% to 11% of patients was noted 5 months after vaccine treatment [18, 76, 88].

To date, there is no consensus on which markers are the most appropriate for analysis of melanoma CTCs. Results are often highly inconsistent and confounded by false-positive and false-negative results [92, 93]. For example, samples may be positive and negative, or even have substantially different gene expression levels, within the same day for an individual patient [94]. False-positive results, indicated by the expression of melanocyte-specific markers in the blood of non-cancer patients, often arise as a result of the capture of normal melanocytes during epidermal puncture for blood sample collection. Discarding the first few millilitres of blood draw can alleviate melanocyte cell contamination [18]. PCR product carry-over is a much more common cause of statistical inaccuracy. Nowadays, commercial PCR mixtures often contain UDG (Uracil-DNA-glycosylase) to ensure destruction of contaminating PCR products [95]. In addition, the preparation of PCR reactions in flow cabinets containing decontaminating ultraviolet (UV) light are considered mandatory. Furthermore, nucleic acids are fragile and susceptible to degradation, if not stabilized and stored at −80°C immediately after isolation [92]. The use of PAX blood tubes has largely alleviated this problem, but often causes another compounding issues, including the unlikelihood of obtaining the same number of circulating cells for a patient at any given time point from the small amount of blood collected for analysis [87]. Standardization of sample quality can be achieved by concurrent analysis of "house-keeping genes" [96], including hydroxymethylbilane synthase (HMBS), beta-2-microglobulin (B2M) and glyceraldehyde-3-phosphate dehydrogenase (GAPDH).

Two recent meta-analyses highlight the inconsistencies obtained with RT-PCR testing [18, 82]. Tsao et al. [82] analyzed RT-PCR detection of CTCs in 1,799 melanoma patients and reported an overall CTC positivity rate of 18% for stage I, 28% for stage II, 30% for stage III, and 45% for stage IV disease. Similar numbers have been found in other studies [78, 97–99]. In contrast, a meta-analysis by Mocellin et al. [18] reported >80% positivity in patient peripheral blood regardless of clinical stage. While gene expression analysis remains extremely promising, stringent technical measures must be routinely adopted before qPCR measures of patient CTC levels can be considered clinically relevant [100].

Alternatively, detection of whole CTCs in peripheral blood is possible by a variety of techniques. Automated digital microscopy and fiber-optic array scanning technology (FAST) rely on advanced optics to detect labeled CTCs, by locating immunofluorescently labeled rare cells on glass substrates at scan rates 500 times faster than conventional automated digital microscopy. These high scan rates are achieved by collecting fluorescent emissions using a fiber bundle with a large (50 mm) field of view [101]. FAST can detect rare epithelial cells with a sensitivity of 98% and a specificity of 99.99%, in a background of 25 million total cells in 2 min. During a scan, the locations of fluorescent objects are recorded, enabling the relocation of CTCs for automated digital fluorescent microscopy for additional viewing or analysis.

The selection of CTCs from a background of normal hematopoietic cells can also be achieved with the use of immunomagnetic beads [79]. This technology is used in the CellSearch system (Veridex LLC), which was recently approved by the USA FDA for breast cancer CTC detection. With this system, which employs a combination of immunomagnetic labeling and automated digital microscopy, CTCs are shown to be an independent prognostic indicator and a predictor of progression-free and overall survival [102]. To date, the CellSearch system applied to analysis of melanoma patient peripheral blood has only detected CTCs in those with stage IV disease [103].

An immunomagnetic bead technology has been developed specifically for enrichment of tumor cells from peripheral blood, bone marrow, and lymphoid tissue of melanoma patients – the anti-Melanoma-Associated Chondroitin Sulphate Proteoglycan 4 (CSPG4) MicroBead kit. The CSPG4 antigen is expressed on melanoma cells, but not on carcinoma cells, mesenchymal cells, or cells of hematopoietic origin. The kit provides an FcR-blocking reagent to prevent nonspecific binding to Fc receptor-containing cells, including B-cells, monocytes and macrophages [80, 104]. With this kit, spiking of peripheral blood cells (PBCs) with melanoma cells showed that the bead-based detection assay can identify ~1 melanoma cell in 5×10^6 PBCs [104]. Moreover, using immunomagnetic beads to isolate CTCs, an association with prognosis was firmly established for melanoma [15], as it has been for many other cancers [75].

Recent advances in technology suggest that highly selective and sensitive detection of rare cancer cells may be possible using multi-wavelength photoacoustic imaging and molecular-specific gold nanoparticles [105, 106]. Gold nanoparticles targeting epidermal growth factor receptor (EGFR) via antibody conjugation undergo molecular-specific aggregation when they bind to receptors on cancer cell surfaces, leading to a red shift in their plasmon resonance frequency [106].

In summary, it seems likely that one or more of these highly sensitive techniques will allow the problems and issues associated with detection of rare CTCs to be overcome and provide highly specific analysis of CTCs for clinical use. It remains for researchers to identify the most reliable, informative melanoma markers for use in conjunction with any of these methods of CTC analysis.

Melanoma Markers: Which to Use?

A plethora of studies have focused on identification of markers with sufficient specificity to accurately predict melanoma progression. Although many of these markers were initially identified using primary tissue or melanoma cell lines, they have been employed in the multitude of CTC studies conducted thus far [86, 107–109]. As mentioned above, melanocytic and melanoma cell markers commonly used for qPCR analysis of CTCs include SILV, MLANA, TYR, MAGEA3 and MAGEA10 [18, 53, 76, 77, 86, 110], and, more recently, ABCB5 [57, 58]. From high-throughput analyses of melanoma, several key progression pathways have been identified [109, 111–114], but remain to be tested and validated as informative for CTC analysis. Key amongst these pathways are: receptor tyrosine kinase (RTK) pathways (i.e., VEGFR, ERBB2, TGF-betaR), the Ras/Raf/MEK/ERK pathway, the PI3K/Akt/PTEN/mTOR pathway, cell cycle regulation pathways (Rb/p53/p16INKA/p14ARF/HDM2), epigenetic gene expression regulation (DNA methylation, histone modifications, microRNA expression), DNA repair pathways, apoptotic pathways (FAS, TRAILR, TNFR, Bcl-2 family), common apoptosis effectors, protein chaperoning, and degradation mediators (HSP, proteasome) [18, 115, 116], and EMT (reviewed in [117]). A thorough screening for these activated pathways in CTCs from patients with metastatic melanoma is required. This will establish their involvement in CTC survival, proliferation, intravasation and extravasation. By detecting additional markers specific for melanoma stem cells and metastatic pathways, RT-PCR analyses might be significantly enhanced, particularly when detecting CTCs from amelanotic tumors which have significantly lower expression of melanocyte-differentiation genes [118].

Due to the fact that the metastatic process requires dissemination of tumor stem cells and/or tumor cells showing EMT, it seems likely that such cells should be detectable amongst CTCs in cancer patients [119, 120]. The detection and characterization of CTCs with EMT and/or stem cell-like signatures may assist with earlier therapeutic intervention, selection of more targeted treatment strategies, and/or provide evidence of resistance to a given therapeutic intervention.

Other Serological Markers of Melanoma

Recent studies provide strong evidence that microRNA (miRNA) expression signatures in peripheral blood may be useful diagnostic biomarkers for melanoma [121, 122]. MiRNAs are endogenous, small (~22 nucleotide in length), noncoding RNAs that regulate gene transcription and translation. Using a microarray-based approach, 51 differentially regulated miRNAs, including 21 downregulated miRNAs and 30 upregulated miRNAs, were identified in the peripheral blood of melanoma patients as compared with healthy controls [121]. A subset of 16 significantly deregulated miRNAs distinguished melanoma patients from healthy individuals with an accuracy of 97.4% [121]. In another study, circulating levels of five cancer-associated miRNAs (let-7a, miR-10b, miR-145, miR-155, and miR-21) were deregulated in the presence of several cancers (including melanoma), with no specific one of these five markers denoting a particular malignancy [122]. The usefulness of miRNA signatures as prognostic, predictive, or early detection biomarkers in melanoma patients requires further study.

Intact circulating tumor-related DNA has also been identified in the peripheral blood of patients with melanoma [104, 123]. This can result from tumor cell turnover, physical disruption of tumor cells, and/or tumor necrosis or apoptosis. Its detection appears to have some clinical utility as a marker of disease stage, therapeutic response and disease recurrence in melanoma patients [76, 124–126]. However, DNA from non-malignant cells is also commonly found in peripheral blood, probably as a result of normal cellular apoptosis. Therefore, the challenge has been to find DNA markers specific for melanoma cells, in order to distinguish between non-malignant and melanoma-related DNA. A number of studies have now identified an association between detectable circulating microsatellite loss, methylated DNA, mitochondrial DNA alterations, and mutant BRAF with disease stage and progression, response to therapy, and overall survival in melanoma patients [76, 124–129]. Prospective studies, combining serial peripheral blood analyses with long-term clinical follow-up, are needed to fully evaluate the clinical utility of these assays.

Circulating Melanoma Cells as a Prognostic Measure: Précis

In summary, conventional prognostic measures and treatment regimens are based on clinical and histopathological staging, but would be more precise and dramatically improved by analyses that measure molecular and cellular markers/pathways which play key roles in tumor progression. Such markers could include proteolytic enzymes, such as proteinases of the plasmin system, serine proteinases, and matrix metalloproteinases (MMPs), which degrade the extracellular matrix (ECM). Analysis of superficial glycoproteins and factors responsible for cell adhesion (integrins) and intercellular communication (cadherins) could also be undertaken. Neoangiogenesis markers, including vascular endothelial growth factor (VEGF), endoglin (CD105, a transmembranous glycoprotein and component of the receptor for transforming growth factor beta [TGF-beta]), and neuropilin (NRP1, the coreceptor for VEGF), may be included [22]. As previously described, markers of EMT transition and stem cell phenotype are also important.

Several reports also suggest that altered regulation of melanocyte developmental pathways in melanoma cells is key to the acquisition of metastatic potential [130–135]. Indeed, melanoma metastases reflect to some extent the migratory capacity of melanoblast developmental precursors, the neural crest cells. Moreover, genes that are critical for melanocyte development have been recognized as important factors of melanoma growth; for example, MITF, DCT and SOX10 all function to maintain the stem or progenitor cell population of melanoblasts during migration from the neural crest and promote melanoblast survival in the hair follicle niche [86, 117, 136–138]. These genes may be equally important in melanoma cell maintenance and migration.

From our own studies [139] (Fig. 15.2) and other reports [6, 35–38], it is clear that positivity *per se* is not a prognostic indicator (i.e., it may be that observable gene expression does not arise from circulating melanoma cells or that not all circulating melanoma cells establish successful tissue metastases). Of note, in uveal melanoma, measures of quantity and quality of CTCs, not presence, are required for prognosis [80]. Moreover, it requires

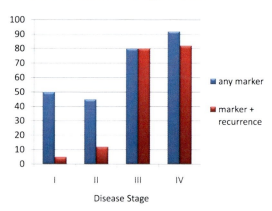

Fig. 15.2 A graphical representation of real-time quantitative reverse transcription-polymerase chain reaction (qPCR) results indicating circulating melanoma cell positivity in patients with respect to clinical stage and tumor recurrence. Peripheral blood RNA was analyzed by qPCR, using a number of melanoma markers. Samples were collected from 217 patients at the time of surgery and 6 monthly over the following 3 years. Marker detection was found to significantly correlate with disease recurrence only at advanced disease stages (p=0.001) (From Ziman et al. [139])

confirmation whether increased marker levels equate to increased CTC numbers in more advanced tumors. A thorough investigation of circulating melanoma cells requires that these cells be isolated and quantified, so as to assess the association of CTC numbers and phenotype with melanoma progression. Increased marker levels may arise from an altered phenotype rather than an increase in cell numbers. A more comprehensive set of experiments using newly identified markers is required to better understand the diagnostic and prognostic significance of circulating melanoma cells [86, 91]. For example, improved isolation, characterization and quantification of circulating melanoma cells will reduce the risk of false-positive results due to the detection of non-melanoma cells.

Serial evaluations for the presence of CTCs during the post-operative period or following adjuvant therapy are recommended rather than the performance of a single test, since the prolonged presence of CTCs is strongly associated with disease progression and poor outcome in melanoma patients [140]. Sequential assays to detect CTCs would also provide: (1) earlier evidence of the effectiveness of therapy and (2) earlier indication of disease recurrence. The detection of CTCs in peripheral blood both at baseline and during follow-up could be correlated with response to treatment, development of new metastatic sites, time to progression and survival.

Conclusion

This chapter addresses one of the most perplexing questions of biomedical science, namely how cells switch from a quiescent to a metastatic proliferating phenotype. We hypothesize that the ability of circulating melanoma cells to become activated, proliferative and migratory depends on the expression of several key genes. An alternative hypothesis is that malignant cells disseminate from the primary tumor early in the disease course and remain in a clinically latent state until either the cells themselves or the host environment is receptive to the development of metastases.

Both Quintana et al. [141] and Roesch et al. [64] have shown that single human melanoma cells with no specifically identifiable gene signature can re-establish melanoma tumors when xenotransplanted into severely immunocompromised mice. Therefore, it is of paramount importance that we identify pathways associated with metastasis of CTCs (i.e., those pathways that confer metastatic properties on quiescent melanoma stem cells capable of evading human anti-tumor immune responses). Furthermore, it is necessary to identify whether CTC numbers, gene expression profiles, or a combination of both, are key factors in patient outcome. It also remains to be seen whether other serological biomarkers, such as microRNAs, tumor-related DNA and/or proteins, provide more accurate measures of melanoma progression. A combination of biomarker types may yet prove to be more accurate than measures of CTCs alone. Future multi-institutional collaborations will likely identify serological biomarkers that can be incorporated into the routine clinical management of melanoma patients.

Acknowledgement The authors would like to thank Mr. Peter Matthews for thoughtful discussion and valuable suggestions.

References

1. Balch CM, Gershenwald JE, Soong SJ, et al. Final version of 2009 AJCC melanoma staging and classification. J Clin Oncol. 2009;27:6199–206.
2. Eton O, Legha SS, Moon TE, et al. Prognostic factors for survival of patients treated systemically for disseminated melanoma. J Clin Oncol. 1998;16:1103–11.
3. Francken AB, Accortt NA, Shaw HM, et al. Prognosis and determinants of outcome following locoregional or distant recurrence in patients with cutaneous melanoma. Ann Surg Oncol. 2008;15:1476–84.
4. Leiter U, Meier F, Schittek B, Garbe C. The natural course of cutaneous melanoma. J Surg Oncol. 2004;86:172–8.
5. Thompson JF, Scolyer RA, Kefford RF. Cutaneous melanoma in the era of molecular profiling. Lancet. 2009;374:362–5.
6. Paterlini-Brechot P, Benali NL. Circulating tumor cells (CTC) detection: clinical impact and future directions. Cancer Lett. 2007;253:180–204.
7. Michaelson JS, Cheongsiatmoy JA, Dewey F, et al. Spread of human cancer cells occurs with probabilities indicative of a nongenetic mechanism. Br J Cancer. 2005;93:1244–9.

8. Singh AD, Rennie IG, Kivela T, Seregard S, Grossniklaus H. The Zimmerman-McLean-Foster hypothesis: 25 years later. Br J Ophthalmol. 2004; 88:962–7.
9. Chen LL, Blumm N, Christakis NA, Barabasi AL, Deisboeck TS. Cancer metastasis networks and the prediction of progression patterns. Br J Cancer. 2009;101:749–58.
10. Bockhorn M, Jain RK, Munn LL. Active versus passive mechanisms in metastasis: do cancer cells crawl into vessels, or are they pushed? Lancet Oncol. 2007;8:444–8.
11. Butler TP, Gullino PM. Quantitation of cell shedding into efferent blood of mammary adenocarcinoma. Cancer Res. 1975;35:512–6.
12. Fidler IJ, Yano S, Zhang RD, Fujimaki T, Bucana CD. The seed and soil hypothesis: vascularisation and brain metastases. Lancet Oncol. 2002;3:53–7.
13. Ikuta Y, Nakatsura T, Kageshita T, et al. Highly sensitive detection of melanoma at an early stage based on the increased serum secreted protein acidic and rich in cysteine and glypican-3 levels. Clin Cancer Res. 2005;11:8079–88.
14. Chiang AC, Massague J. Molecular basis of metastasis. N Engl J Med. 2008;359:2814–23.
15. Ulmer A, Schmidt-Kittler O, Fischer J, et al. Immunomagnetic enrichment, genomic characterization, and prognostic impact of circulating melanoma cells. Clin Cancer Res. 2004;10:531–7.
16. Ulmer A, Beutel J, Susskind D, et al. Visualization of circulating melanoma cells in peripheral blood of patients with primary uveal melanoma. Clin Cancer Res. 2008;14:4469–74.
17. Husemann Y, Geigl JB, Schubert F, et al. Systemic spread is an early step in breast cancer. Cancer Cell. 2008;13:58–68.
18. Mocellin S, Hoon D, Ambrosi A, Nitti D, Rossi CR. The prognostic value of circulating tumor cells in patients with melanoma: a systematic review and meta-analysis. Clin Cancer Res. 2006;12:4605–13.
19. Mazzocca A, Carloni V. The metastatic process: methodological advances and pharmacological challenges. Curr Med Chem. 2009;16:1704–17.
20. Van Den Bossche K, Naeyaert JM, Lambert J. The quest for the mechanism of melanin transfer. Traffic. 2006;7:769–78.
21. Vogelmann R, Nguyen-Tat MD, Giehl K, Adler G, Wedlich D, Menke A. TGFbeta-induced downregulation of E-cadherin-based cell-cell adhesion depends on PI3-kinase and PTEN. J Cell Sci. 2005;118: 4901–12.
22. Moustakas A, Heldin CH. Signaling networks guiding epithelial-mesenchymal transitions during embryogenesis and cancer progression. Cancer Sci. 2007;98:1512–20.
23. Peinado H, Portillo F, Cano A. Transcriptional regulation of cadherins during development and carcinogenesis. Int J Dev Biol. 2004;48:365–75.
24. Cheng GZ, Chan J, Wang Q, Zhang W, Sun CD, Wang LH. Twist transcriptionally up-regulates AKT2 in breast cancer cells leading to increased migration, invasion, and resistance to paclitaxel. Cancer Res. 2007;67:1979–87.
25. Hsu MY, Meier FE, Nesbit M, et al. E-cadherin expression in melanoma cells restores keratinocyte-mediated growth control and down-regulates expression of invasion-related adhesion receptors. Am J Pathol. 2000;156:1515–25.
26. Dvorak HF. Tumors: wounds that do not heal. Similarities between tumor stroma generation and wound healing. N Engl J Med. 1986;315:1650–9.
27. Liang S, Slattery MJ, Wagner D, Simon SI, Dong C. Hydrodynamic shear rate regulates melanoma-leukocyte aggregation, melanoma adhesion to the endothelium, and subsequent extravasation. Ann Biomed Eng. 2008;36:661–71.
28. Bartolome RA, Galvez BG, Longo N, et al. Stromal cell-derived factor-1alpha promotes melanoma cell invasion across basement membranes involving stimulation of membrane-type 1 matrix metalloproteinase and Rho GTPase activities. Cancer Res. 2004;64:2534–43.
29. Sanz-Moreno V, Gadea G, Ahn J, et al. Rac activation and inactivation control plasticity of tumor cell movement. Cell. 2008;135:510–23.
30. Lewis CE, Pollard JW. Distinct role of macrophages in different tumor microenvironments. Cancer Res. 2006;66:605–12.
31. Pittet MJ. Behavior of immune players in the tumor microenvironment. Curr Opin Oncol. 2009;21:53–9.
32. Liotta LA, Kleinerman J, Saidel GM. Quantitative relationships of intravascular tumor cells, tumor vessels, and pulmonary metastases following tumor implantation. Cancer Res. 1974;34:997–1004.
33. Bockhorn M, Roberge S, Sousa C, Jain RK, Munn LL. Differential gene expression in metastasizing cells shed from kidney tumors. Cancer Res. 2004; 64:2469–73.
34. Glinsky GV. Apoptosis in metastatic cancer cells. Crit Rev Oncol Hematol. 1997;25:175–86.
35. Swartz MA, Kristensen CA, Melder RJ, et al. Cells shed from tumours show reduced clonogenicity, resistance to apoptosis, and in vivo tumorigenicity. Br J Cancer. 1999;81:756–9.
36. Mehes G, Witt A, Kubista E, Ambros PF. Circulating breast cancer cells are frequently apoptotic. Am J Pathol. 2001;159:17–20.
37. Larson CJ, Moreno JG, Pienta KJ, et al. Apoptosis of circulating tumor cells in prostate cancer patients. Cytometry A. 2004;62:46–53.
38. Holmgren L, O'Reilly MS, Folkman J. Dormancy of micrometastases: balanced proliferation and apoptosis in the presence of angiogenesis suppression. Nat Med. 1995;1:149–53.
39. Kim MY, Oskarsson T, Acharyya S, et al. Tumor self-seeding by circulating cancer cells. Cell. 2009; 139:1315–26.
40. Nguyen DX, Bos PD, Massague J. Metastasis: from dissemination to organ-specific colonization. Nat Rev Cancer. 2009;9:274–84.

41. Al-Mehdi AB, Tozawa K, Fisher AB, Shientag L, Lee A, Muschel RJ. Intravascular origin of metastasis from the proliferation of endothelium-attached tumor cells: a new model for metastasis. Nat Med. 2000;6:100–2.
42. Borsig L, Wong R, Hynes RO, Varki NM, Varki A. Synergistic effects of L- and P-selectin in facilitating tumor metastasis can involve non-mucin ligands and implicate leukocytes as enhancers of metastasis. Proc Natl Acad Sci USA. 2002;99:2193–8.
43. Laubli H, Stevenson JL, Varki A, Varki NM, Borsig L. L-selectin facilitation of metastasis involves temporal induction of Fut7-dependent ligands at sites of tumor cell arrest. Cancer Res. 2006;66:1536–42.
44. Fuertes MB, Girart MV, Molinero LL, et al. Intracellular retention of the NKG2D ligand MHC class I chain-related gene A in human melanomas confers immune privilege and prevents NK cell-mediated cytotoxicity. J Immunol. 2008;180: 4606–14.
45. Lacreusette A, Nguyen JM, Pandolfino MC, et al. Loss of oncostatin M receptor beta in metastatic melanoma cells. Oncogene. 2007;26:881–92.
46. Zbytek B, Carlson JA, Granese J, Ross J, Mihm MC, Slominski A. Current concepts of metastasis in melanoma. Expert Rev Dermatol. 2008;3:569–85.
47. Vijuk G, Coates AS. Survival of patients with visceral metastatic melanoma from an occult primary lesion: a retrospective matched cohort study. Ann Oncol. 1998;9:419–22.
48. Lee CC, Faries MB, Wanek LA, Morton DL. Improved survival after lymphadenectomy for nodal metastasis from an unknown primary melanoma. J Clin Oncol. 2008;26:535–41.
49. Lee RT, Fallarino F, Ashikari A, Gajewski TF. Melanoma presenting as circulating tumor cells associated with failed angiogenesis. Melanoma Res. 2008;18:289–94.
50. Jack A, Boyes C, Aydin N, Alam K, Wallack M. The treatment of melanoma with an emphasis on immunotherapeutic strategies. Surg Oncol. 2006;15: 13–24.
51. Weight RM, Viator JA, Dale PS, Caldwell CW, Lisle AE. Photoacoustic detection of metastatic melanoma cells in the human circulatory system. Opt Lett. 2006;31:2998–3000.
52. Zalaudek I, Horn M, Richtig E, Hodl S, Kerl H, Smolle J. Local recurrence in melanoma in situ: influence of sex, age, site of involvement and therapeutic modalities. Br J Dermatol. 2003;148:703–8.
53. Koyanagi K, O'Day SJ, Gonzalez R, et al. Serial monitoring of circulating melanoma cells during neoadjuvant biochemotherapy for stage III melanoma: outcome prediction in a multicenter trial. J Clin Oncol. 2005;23:8057–64.
54. Ramaswamy S, Ross KN, Lander ES, Golub TR. A molecular signature of metastasis in primary solid tumors. Nat Genet. 2003;33:49–54.
55. Bernards R, Weinberg RA. A progression puzzle. Nature. 2002;418:823.
56. Waghorne C, Thomas M, Lagarde A, Kerbel RS, Breitman ML. Genetic evidence for progressive selection and overgrowth of primary tumors by metastatic cell subpopulations. Cancer Res. 1988;48: 6109–14.
57. Schatton T, Frank MH. Cancer stem cells and human malignant melanoma. Pigment Cell Melanoma Res. 2008;21:39–55.
58. Schatton T, Murphy GF, Frank NY, et al. Identification of cells initiating human melanomas. Nature. 2008; 451:345–9.
59. Grichnik JM, Burch JA, Schulteis RD, et al. Melanoma, a tumor based on a mutant stem cell? J Invest Dermatol. 2006;126:142–53.
60. Monzani E, Facchetti F, Galmozzi E, et al. Melanoma contains CD133 and ABCG2 positive cells with enhanced tumourigenic potential. Eur J Cancer. 2007;43:935–46.
61. Zabierowski SE, Herlyn M. Melanoma stem cells: the dark seed of melanoma. J Clin Oncol. 2008;26: 2890–4.
62. Wicha MS. Cancer stem cells and metastasis: lethal seeds. Clin Cancer Res. 2006;12:5606–7.
63. Pantel K, Brakenhoff RH, Brandt B. Detection, clinical relevance and specific biological properties of disseminating tumour cells. Nat Rev Cancer. 2008;8: 329–40.
64. Roesch A, Fukunaga-Kalabis M, Schmidt EC, et al. A temporarily distinct subpopulation of slow-cycling melanoma cells is required for continuous tumor growth. Cell. 2010;141:583–94.
65. Herlyn M. Driving in the melanoma landscape. Exp Dermatol. 2009;18:506–8.
66. Passegue E, Rafii S, Herlyn M. Cancer stem cells are everywhere. Nat Med. 2009;15:23.
67. Smalley KS, Herlyn M. Integrating tumor-initiating cells into the paradigm for melanoma targeted therapy. Int J Cancer. 2009;124:1245–50.
68. Vultur A, Herlyn M. Cracking the system: melanoma complexity demands new therapeutic approaches. Pigment Cell Melanoma Res. 2009;22:4–5.
69. Keshet GI, Goldstein I, Itzhaki O, et al. MDR1 expression identifies human melanoma stem cells. Biochem Biophys Res Commun. 2008;368:930–6.
70. Fang D, Nguyen TK, Leishear K, et al. A tumorigenic subpopulation with stem cell properties in melanomas. Cancer Res. 2005;65:9328–37.
71. La Porta C. Cancer stem cells: lessons from melanoma. Stem Cell Rev. 2009;5:61–5.
72. Fusi A, Reichelt U, Busse A, Ochsenreither S, et al. Correlation of stem cell marker nestin expression on circulating melanoma cells with extension of disease and survival [abstract 8551]. J Clin Oncol. 2010;28: 15s.
73. Balic M, Lin H, Young L, et al. Most early disseminated cancer cells detected in bone marrow of breast cancer patients have a putative breast cancer stem cell phenotype. Clin Cancer Res. 2006;12:5615–21.
74. Pantel K, Otte M. Occult micrometastasis: enrichment, identification and characterization of single

disseminated tumour cells. Semin Cancer Biol. 2001;11:327–37.
75. Allard WJ, Matera J, Miller MC, et al. Tumor cells circulate in the peripheral blood of all major carcinomas but not in healthy subjects or patients with nonmalignant diseases. Clin Cancer Res. 2004;10: 6897–904.
76. Koyanagi K, Mori T, O'Day SJ, Martinez SR, Wang HJ, Hoon DS. Association of circulating tumor cells with serum tumor-related methylated DNA in peripheral blood of melanoma patients. Cancer Res. 2006;66:6111–7.
77. Koyanagi K, O'Day SJ, Gonzalez R, et al. Microphthalmia transcription factor as a molecular marker for circulating tumor cell detection in blood of melanoma patients. Clin Cancer Res. 2006;12: 1137–43.
78. Voit CA, Schafer-Hesterberg G, Kron M, et al. Impact of molecular staging methods in primary melanoma: reverse-transcriptase polymerase chain reaction (RT-PCR) of ultrasound-guided aspirate of the sentinel node does not improve diagnostic accuracy, but RT-PCR of peripheral blood does predict survival. J Clin Oncol. 2008;26:5742–7.
79. Krivacic RT, Ladanyi A, Curry DN, et al. A rare-cell detector for cancer. Proc Natl Acad Sci USA. 2004; 101:10501–4.
80. Cools-Lartigue JJ, McCauley CS, Marshall JC, et al. Immunomagnetic isolation and in vitro expansion of human uveal melanoma cell lines. Mol Vis. 2008;14: 50–5.
81. Weight RM, Dale PS, Viator JA. Detection of circulating melanoma cells in human blood using photoacoustic flowmetry. Conf Proc IEEE Eng Med Biol Soc. 2009;2009:106–9.
82. Tsao H, Nadiminti U, Sober AJ, Bigby M. A meta-analysis of reverse transcriptase-polymerase chain reaction for tyrosinase mRNA as a marker for circulating tumor cells in cutaneous melanoma. Arch Dermatol. 2001;137:325–30.
83. Van der Auwera I, Peeters D, Benoy IH, et al. Circulating tumour cell detection: a direct comparison between the Cell Search System, the AdnaTest and CK-19/mammaglobin RT-PCR in patients with metastatic breast cancer. Br J Cancer. 2010;102: 276–84.
84. Palmieri G, Ascierto PA, Perrone F, et al. Prognostic value of circulating melanoma cells detected by reverse transcriptase-polymerase chain reaction. J Clin Oncol. 2003;21:767–73.
85. Gradilone A, Cigna E, Agliano AM, Frati L. Tyrosinase expression as a molecular marker for investigating the presence of circulating tumor cells in melanoma patients. Curr Cancer Drug Targets. 2010;10:529–38.
86. Medic S, Pearce RL, Heenan PJ, Ziman M. Molecular markers of circulating melanoma cells. Pigment Cell Res. 2007;20:80–91.
87. Keilholz U, Goldin-Lang P, Bechrakis NE, et al. Quantitative detection of circulating tumor cells in cutaneous and ocular melanoma and quality assessment by real-time reverse transcriptase-polymerase chain reaction. Clin Cancer Res. 2004;10:1605–12.
88. Reynolds SR, Albrecht J, Shapiro RL, et al. Changes in the presence of multiple markers of circulating melanoma cells correlate with clinical outcome in patients with melanoma. Clin Cancer Res. 2003;9: 1497–502.
89. Samija I, Lukac J, Maric-Brozic J, et al. Prognostic value of microphthalmia-associated transcription factor and tyrosinase as markers for circulating tumor cells detection in patients with melanoma. Melanoma Res. 2010;20:293–302.
90. Koyanagi K, O'Day SJ, Boasberg P, et al. Serial monitoring of circulating tumor cells predicts outcome of induction biochemotherapy plus maintenance biotherapy for metastatic melanoma. Clin Cancer Res. 2010;16:2402–8.
91. Fusi A, Collette S, Busse A, et al. Circulating melanoma cells and distant metastasis-free survival in stage III melanoma patients with or without adjuvant interferon treatment (EORTC 18991 side study). Eur J Cancer. 2009;45:3189–97.
92. Reinhold U, Berkin C, Bosserhoff AK, et al. Interlaboratory evaluation of a new reverse transcriptase polymerase chain reaction-based enzyme-linked immunosorbent assay for the detection of circulating melanoma cells: a multicenter study of the Dermatologic Cooperative Oncology Group. J Clin Oncol. 2001;19:1723–7.
93. Gradilone A, Gazzaniga P, Silvestri I, et al. Detection of CK19, CK20 and EGFR mRNAs in peripheral blood of carcinoma patients: correlation with clinical stage of disease. Oncol Rep. 2003;10:217–22.
94. Blaheta HJ, Paul T, Sotlar K, et al. Detection of melanoma cells in sentinel lymph nodes, bone marrow and peripheral blood by a reverse transcription-polymerase chain reaction assay in patients with primary cutaneous melanoma: association with Breslow's tumour thickness. Br J Dermatol. 2001;145:195–202.
95. Thornton CG, Hartley JL, Rashtchian A. Utilizing uracil DNA glycosylase to control carryover contamination in PCR: characterization of residual UDG activity following thermal cycling. Biotechniques. 1992;13:180–4.
96. Hoon DS, Bostick P, Kuo C, et al. Molecular markers in blood as surrogate prognostic indicators of melanoma recurrence. Cancer Res. 2000;60:2253–7.
97. Voit C, Schoengen A, Schwurzer M, Weber L, Mayer T, Proebstle TM. Detection of regional melanoma metastases by ultrasound B-scan, cytology or tyrosinase RT-PCR of fine-needle aspirates. Br J Cancer. 1999;80:1672–7.
98. Curry BJ, Myers K, Hersey P. MART-1 is expressed less frequently on circulating melanoma cells in patients who develop distant compared with locoregional metastases. J Clin Oncol. 1999;17:2562–71.
99. Kopreski MS, Benko FA, Kwak LW, Gocke CD. Detection of tumor messenger RNA in the serum of

patients with malignant melanoma. Clin Cancer Res. 1999;5:1961–5.
100. Nezos A, Lembessis P, Sourla A, Pissimissis N, Gogas H, Koutsilieris M. Molecular markers detecting circulating melanoma cells by reverse transcription polymerase chain reaction: methodological pitfalls and clinical relevance. Clin Chem Lab Med. 2009;47:1–11.
101. Hsieh HB, Marrinucci D, Bethel K, et al. High speed detection of circulating tumor cells. Biosens Bioelectron. 2006;21:1893–9.
102. Cristofanilli M, Budd GT, Ellis MJ, et al. Circulating tumor cells, disease progression, and survival in metastatic breast cancer. N Engl J Med. 2004;351:781–91.
103. Steen S, Nemunaitis J, Fisher T, Kuhn J. Circulating tumor cells in melanoma: a review of the literature and description of a novel technique. Proc (Bayl Univ Med Cent). 2008;21:127–32.
104. Kitago M, Koyanagi K, Nakamura T, et al. mRNA expression and BRAF mutation in circulating melanoma cells isolated from peripheral blood with high molecular weight melanoma-associated antigen-specific monoclonal antibody beads. Clin Chem. 2009;55:757–64.
105. Holan SH, Viator JA. Automated wavelet denoising of photoacoustic signals for circulating melanoma cell detection and burn image reconstruction. Phys Med Biol. 2008;53:N227–36.
106. Mallidi S, Larson T, Tam J, et al. Multiwavelength photoacoustic imaging and plasmon resonance coupling of gold nanoparticles for selective detection of cancer. Nano Lett. 2009;9:2825–31.
107. Bosserhoff AK. Novel biomarkers in malignant melanoma. Clin Chim Acta. 2006;367:28–35.
108. Bennett DC. How to make a melanoma: what do we know of the primary clonal events? Pigment Cell Melanoma Res. 2008;21:27–38.
109. Gogas H, Eggermont AM, Hauschild A, et al. Biomarkers in melanoma. Ann Oncol. 2009;20(Suppl 6):vi8–13.
110. Xi L, Nicastri DG, El-Hefnawy T, Hughes SJ, Luketich JD, Godfrey TE. Optimal markers for real-time quantitative reverse transcription PCR detection of circulating tumor cells from melanoma, breast, colon, esophageal, head and neck, and lung cancers. Clin Chem. 2007;53:1206–15.
111. Hoek KS, Schlegel NC, Brafford P, et al. Metastatic potential of melanomas defined by specific gene expression profiles with no BRAF signature. Pigment Cell Res. 2006;19:290–302.
112. Talantov D, Mazumder A, Yu JX, et al. Novel genes associated with malignant melanoma but not benign melanocytic lesions. Clin Cancer Res. 2005;11:7234–42.
113. Mandruzzato S, Callegaro A, Turcatel G, et al. A gene expression signature associated with survival in metastatic melanoma. J Transl Med. 2006;4:50.
114. Alonso SR, Tracey L, Ortiz P, et al. A high-throughput study in melanoma identifies epithelial-mesenchymal transition as a major determinant of metastasis. Cancer Res. 2007;67:3450–60.
115. Winnepenninckx V, Lazar V, Michiels S, et al. Gene expression profiling of primary cutaneous melanoma and clinical outcome. J Natl Cancer Inst. 2006;98:472–82.
116. Kauffmann A, Rosselli F, Lazar V, et al. High expression of DNA repair pathways is associated with metastasis in melanoma patients. Oncogene. 2008;27:565–73.
117. Medic S, Ziman M. PAX3 across the spectrum: from melanoblast to melanoma. Crit Rev Biochem Mol Biol. 2009;44:85–97.
118. Orlow SJ, Silvers WK, Zhou BK, Mintz B. Comparative decreases in tyrosinase, TRP-1, TRP-2, and Pmel 17/silver antigenic proteins from melanotic to amelanotic stages of syngeneic mouse cutaneous melanomas and metastases. Cancer Res. 1998;58:1521–3.
119. Aktas B, Tewes M, Fehm T, Hauch S, Kimmig R, Kasimir-Bauer S. Stem cell and epithelial-mesenchymal transition markers are frequently overexpressed in circulating tumor cells of metastatic breast cancer patients. Breast Cancer Res. 2009;11:R46.
120. Tewes M, Aktas B, Welt A, et al. Molecular profiling and predictive value of circulating tumor cells in patients with metastatic breast cancer: an option for monitoring response to breast cancer related therapies. Breast Cancer Res Treat. 2009;115:581–90.
121. Leidinger P, Keller A, Borries A, et al. High-throughput miRNA profiling of human melanoma blood samples. BMC Cancer. 2010;10:262.
122. Heneghan HM, Miller N, Kelly R, et al. Systemic miRNA-195 differentiates breast cancer from other malignancies and is a potential biomarker for detecting noninvasive and early stage disease. Oncologist. 2010;15:673–82.
123. Ziegler A, Zangemeister-Wittke U, Stahel RA. Circulating DNA: a new diagnostic gold mine? Cancer Treat Rev. 2002;28:255–71.
124. Taback B, O'Day SJ, Boasberg PD, et al. Circulating DNA microsatellites: molecular determinants of response to biochemotherapy in patients with metastatic melanoma. J Natl Cancer Inst. 2004;96:152–6.
125. Nakayama T, Taback B, Nguyen DH, et al. Clinical significance of circulating DNA microsatellite markers in plasma of melanoma patients. Ann N Y Acad Sci. 2000;906:87–98.
126. Shinozaki M, O'Day SJ, Kitago M, et al. Utility of circulating B-RAF DNA mutation in serum for monitoring melanoma patients receiving biochemotherapy. Clin Cancer Res. 2007;13:2068–74.
127. Daniotti M, Vallacchi V, Rivoltini L, et al. Detection of mutated BRAFV600E variant in circulating DNA of stage III-IV melanoma patients. Int J Cancer. 2007;120:2439–44.
128. Mori T, O'Day SJ, Umetani N, et al. Predictive utility of circulating methylated DNA in serum of melanoma patients receiving biochemotherapy. J Clin Oncol. 2005;23:9351–8.

129. Fujimoto A, O'Day SJ, Taback B, Elashoff D, Hoon DS. Allelic imbalance on 12q22-23 in serum circulating DNA of melanoma patients predicts disease outcome. Cancer Res. 2004;64:4085–8.
130. Gupta PB, Kuperwasser C, Brunet JP, et al. The melanocyte differentiation program predisposes to metastasis after neoplastic transformation. Nat Genet. 2005;37:1047–54.
131. Gupta PB, Mani S, Yang J, Hartwell K, Weinberg RA. The evolving portrait of cancer metastasis. Cold Spring Harb Symp Quant Biol. 2005;70:291–7.
132. White RM, Zon LI. Melanocytes in development, regeneration, and cancer. Cell Stem Cell. 2008;3: 242–52.
133. Topczewska JM, Postovit LM, Margaryan NV, et al. Embryonic and tumorigenic pathways converge via Nodal signaling: role in melanoma aggressiveness. Nat Med. 2006;12:925–32.
134. McArdle L, Rafferty MM, Satyamoorthy K, et al. Microarray analysis of phosphatase gene expression in human melanoma. Br J Dermatol. 2005;152:925–30.
135. Carreira S, Goodall J, Denat L, et al. Mitf regulation of Dia1 controls melanoma proliferation and invasiveness. Genes Dev. 2006;20:3426–39.
136. Kubic JD, Young KP, Plummer RS, Ludvik AE, Lang D. Pigmentation PAX-ways: the role of Pax3 in melanogenesis, melanocyte stem cell maintenance, and disease. Pigment Cell Melanoma Res. 2008;21:627–45.
137. Plummer RS, Shea CR, Nelson M, et al. PAX3 expression in primary melanomas and nevi. Mod Pathol. 2008;21:525–30.
138. Lang D, Lu MM, Huang L, et al. Pax3 functions at a nodal point in melanocyte stem cell differentiation. Nature. 2005;433:884–7.
139. Ziman M, Millward M, Medic S, et al. Blood test for cutaneous malignant melanoma. Proceedings of the 8th anticancer research conference, 2008. Anticancer Res. 2008;28:3552.
140. Palmieri G, Satriano SM, Budroni M, et al. Serial detection of circulating tumour cells by reverse transcriptase-polymerase chain reaction assays is a marker for poor outcome in patients with malignant melanoma. BMC Cancer. 2006;6:266.
141. Quintana E, Shackleton M, Sabel MS, Fullen DR, Johnson TM, Morrison SJ. Efficient tumour formation by single human melanoma cells. Nature. 2008;456:593–8.

Molecular Markers of Lymph Node Disease in Melanoma

Sandro Pasquali, Augustinus P.T. van der Ploeg, and Simone Mocellin

The molecular profiling of primary melanoma tumors and sentinel lymph node (SLN) specimens might improve patients' stratification according to their risk of disease progression, and thus the selection for surgical (e.g., radical lymph node dissection) and medical (e.g., interferon-alpha and molecular-targeted strategies) therapies. SLN status represents the most important prognostic factor in early-stage melanoma patients. Approximately 80% of patients undergoing sentinel lymph node biopsy (SLNB) will have negative results. Molecular profiling of primary melanomas might add important predictive information to the currently used clinico-histopathological features for predicting SLN status. Herein, the role of lymph-angiogenic biomarkers in identifying patients at high risk of harboring lymph node metastasis is discussed. Following lymphadenectomy for SLN disease, more than 80% of patients demonstrate negative non-SLNs. Micromorphometric evaluation of SLN tumor burden shows meaningful results for predicting non-SLN status and prognosis. A number of studies have investigated the molecular characterization of SLNs using polymerase chain reaction (PCR). To date, however, results have been inconclusive, and further evaluations are currently in progress.

Sentinel Lymph Node Biopsy (SNLB) in Melanoma: Current Standard and Open Issues

In the 1970s and 1980s, randomized controlled trials failed to demonstrate a positive impact on survival using elective lymph node dissection compared to radical lymph node dissection performed in melanoma patients with clinically evident lymph node metastases [1, 2]. During this period, a new procedure, the sentinel lymph node (SLN) biopsy (SLNB), was developed by Donald Morton and Alistair Cochran at the John Wayne Cancer Institute [3]. This minimally invasive procedure for the initial treatment of early-stage melanoma patients has gained favor with surgical oncologists around the world, and has now been extended to other solid malignancies, including breast cancer [4].

SLN status is the most important prognostic factor in patients with stage I–II melanoma and has been included in the TNM staging system since its 6th edition in 2001 [5, 6]. SLNB is characterized by a high negative predictive value (NPV) (i.e., when the SLN is negative, there is likelihood approaching 95% that the remaining lymph nodes in the regional basin are disease-free). SLNB leads to early identification and

S. Pasquali, M.D. • S. Mocellin, M.D., Ph.D. (✉)
Surgery Branch, Department of Oncological and Surgical Sciences, University of Padova, Padova, Italy
e-mail: mocellins@hotmail.com

A.P.T. van der Ploeg, M.Sc.
Erasmus University Medical Center,
Daniel den Hoed Cancer Center, Rotterdam,
The Netherlands

removal of involved lymph nodes at a subclinical stage (i.e., microscopic disease), maximizing the likelihood of survival benefit for patients receiving lymphadenectomy.

However, there are several controversies regarding the actual role of SLNB in the management of patients with melanoma, particularly from the therapeutic point of view, but also with a view to selection criteria and technical aspects of the procedure. The predominant unanswered question on SLNB regards its impact on patient survival. Interim results from the only conducted randomized controlled trial comparing SLNB and observation (Multicenter Selective Lymphadenectomy Trial-I, MSLT-I) reported that the procedure impacted disease-free survival, but not overall survival, in melanoma patients [7]. In this study, patients undergoing lymphadenectomy for SLN-positive disease showed a better prognosis compared to those who underwent delayed lymphadenectomy for clinically-evident disease that developed during follow-up. This survival benefit is consistent with findings from non-randomized studies, and recent meta-analysis has confirmed that the early removal of metastasis using SLNB and complete lymph node dissection (CLND) might provide patients with the best survival opportunity [8]. Further analysis of MSLT-I patients after longer follow-up, MSLT-II (a randomized trial comparing CLND versus observation in patients with positive SLNs), and the MINITUB study (a prospective single-arm study within the EORTC Melanoma Group Network) will provide more evidence-based information. In addition to the possible survival benefit, SLNB fails to identify metastases in approximately one of five-to-ten patients with positive lymph nodes (i.e., the false-negative rate), with patients developing later lymph node recurrence [9–18].

Current indications for SLNB are based on staging parameters (mainly tumor thickness greater than 1 mm or other adverse prognosticators, such as the presence of ulceration and/or mitoses in the case of thin melanomas), and ~80% of patients will have a negative SLN [19]. Considering the lack of definitive evidence of a survival benefit for melanoma patients discussed above, in addition to the low, but defined morbidity (~10%) [20], and the cost to the health care system of SLNB [21], SLN-negative patients might be considered as "over-treated". With the aim of improving the selection of patients for SLNB, researchers have tried to assess the statistical association between clinico-histopathological variables and SLN status in an effort to stratify patients into a predictive model according to their different risks of harboring lymph node metastases [22, 23]. In addition, the introduction of molecular biomarkers of primary tumors seems to be a promising approach to improve the selection of patients for SLNB [24, 25]. In particular, lymphangiogenic markers, as identified by immunohistochemistry (IHC), appear to be reliable and promising predictive and prognostic factors and are advocated as more meaningful than current histopathological parameters, such as tumor thickness [26, 27]. Unfortunately, putative biomarkers for SLN status prediction have not been widely implemented in the clinical setting to date. This is as a result of controversial findings from studies conducted thus far [28].

Another highly discussed topic is the management of patients with positive SLNs [29]. Patients with SLN disease are eligible for CLND. Approximately one in five patients shows additional non-SLN metastases in the CLND specimen. The optimal identification of this group might spare the remaining ~80% of SLN-positive patients an unnecessary and morbid CLND [30, 31]. Many melanoma researchers and specialists around the world have tried to determine criteria which identify this latter group of patients who do not develop additional non-SLN metastases and have good prognostic outcomes [32–37]. These criteria are based on a number of different factors regarding primary tumor characteristics and SLN tumor burden with similar or different cut-off values for the assessment of these micro-morphometric parameters [29]. The conclusion of all these studies, despite different measurements, methods and concepts, is that SLN tumor burden is of high predictive and prognostic value. However, although there is a high level of agreement between pathologists in the evaluation of overall histopathologic stage, the significant level of inter-observer discordance in histopathologic substaging suggests that accurate and reliable substage-based prognostic prediction might not be possible in all cases of melanoma [38].

Standard histopathological examination with light microscopic and IHC assessment still represents the gold standard for the diagnosis of SLN metastasis in patients with melanoma. The use of polymerase chain reaction (PCR) is a novel molecular approach, based on the hypothesis that the presence of melanoma deposits in the SLN can be identified through the detection of mRNA for melanoma-specific markers [39–41]. The PCR technique is performed using the following steps: mRNA isolation from SLN; complementary DNA (cDNA) synthesis by reverse transcription; the gene of interest (i.e., tyrosinase, MART-1, MAGE-3) is amplified by a primer in a polymerase-driven reaction; and finally, identification of the PCR product. Using several targets, numerous studies have been performed and thousands of patients have been enrolled; however, there is no consensus on the diagnostic and/or prognostic role of the PCR status of SLNs in patients with melanoma, and thus on the routine use of this molecular biology tool in the clinical setting [42–46]. Results support, at least in part, the use of PCR to improve metastatic detection; however, available evidence is not sufficient to conclude that PCR status is a prognostic indicator reliable enough to be clinically implemented in the therapeutic decision-making process [47].

In this chapter, the current standard for predicting SLN and non-SLN status is discussed. Primary melanoma biomarkers, and in particular molecules involved in lymphangiogenesis, are reported as promising descriptors for improving patients' selection for SLNB. Finally, PCR analysis of SLNs represents a tool to improve the detection of SLN metastasis and evaluate the potential prognostic implications of molecularly-evident metastatic disease.

Prediction of SLN Status from Primary Melanoma Analysis

Pathological Parameters

Nowadays the indications for SLNB are based mainly on tumor thickness and TNM staging parameters. SLNB is considered when Breslow thickness is greater than 1 mm [19, 48]. Patients with melanoma thicknesses of less than 1 mm have a ~5% probability of having lymph node metastases [49]. While it is difficult to predict the behavior of these latter thin lesions, SLNB may be appropriate when other adverse histopathologic prognostic features, such as ulceration, high Clark level and/or mitoses are present [19, 48].

Using these selection criteria, most patients have negative SLNs after SLNB. With the aim of improving selection criteria, several studies have investigated the ability of different statistical methods (especially logistic regression) to predict SLN status based on common clinico-histopathological features of the primary tumor [10, 15, 50–55]. However, most of these studies simply addressed the issue of whether or not each variable is statistically associated with SLN status. Although this approach is useful in proving the concept, it does not answer the question of whether clinico-histopathological variables have predictive power(s) of clinical significance [22, 23, 52, 56].

Nomograms, which are statistical models generally based on multivariate logistic regression analysis, allow for the study of simultaneously interacting variables, that are identified as relevant factors in defining the probability of an event; in this case, SLN status [57]. In this regard, investigators from Memorial Sloan-Kettering Cancer Center have developed ($n = 979$) and validated ($n = 3,108$) a nomogram for improved risk estimation of SLN positivity, which might lead to the optimization of patient counseling and treatment selection [23]. The accuracy of this nomogram in predicting SLN status approached 70%, which is a superior result to the one obtained using the AJCC TNM staging system (6th edition) parameters (66%) [6, 23]. However, it must be noted that accuracy is a global measure of the performance of a diagnostic test that simply describes the proportion of correct predictions among all tested patients (positive and negative). This approach is predominantly oriented towards enhancing patient counseling (i.e., the risk of having a positive SLN). The nomogram is unable to provide any decisional "rule" that might help in the selection of newly diagnosed melanoma patients for SLNB. The NPV is the parameter that could better address this issue. In the case of

SLNB, NPV represents the proportion of patients who test negative and are truly negative on histopathological examination. The use of a test with a high NPV, performed before SLNB, might safely identify patients with low risk of SLN metastasis who could avoid the procedure. "Safely" indicates the test as having a low rate of false-negative prediction (i.e., patients predicted as negative by the test, but with a positive SLN).

In the light of these considerations and based on commonly available clinico-histopathological variables (patient age and sex, tumor thickness, Clark level of invasion, presence of regression and/or ulceration, mitotic index and histological subtype), different statistical models have been evaluated for their ability to improve the selection of patients for SLNB [22]. For instance, logistic regression achieved a NPV of 93.6%, resulting in a SLNB reduction rate of 27.5% and an overall error rate of 1.8%. Further steps are required to assess the suitability of predictive models in improving patient selection for SLNB. Of note, the accuracy and NPV of these models might prove to be meaningful when biomarkers are added, as reported for other cancers [58].

Biomarkers: The Case of Lymphangiogenesis

In the last decade, several biomarkers of primary melanoma have been assessed for their ability to stratify melanoma patients according to their risk of SLN metastasis and melanoma death [59]. Promising biomarkers include those related to cell cycle regulation (p16 and Ki-67) [60], invasiveness (such as osteopontin [61], CCR10 [62], Tenascin-C [63], nuclear receptor coactivator-3 (NCOA3) [64, 65], melanoma cell adhesion molecules (MCAM) [64], metallothioneins [66, 67], c-ski [68], SnoN [68], and RGS1 [69]), and lymphangiogenesis [26, 27, 70–76].

Since the development of monoclonal antibodies for the detection of angiolymphatic vessels, the significance of lymphangiogenesis in melanoma and other solid tumors has been studied [77]. The vascular endothelial growth factor (VEGF)-related gene family of angiogenic and lymphangiogenic growth factors comprises seven secreted glycoproteins, referred to as VEGF-A, VEGF-B, VEGF-C, VEGF-D, VEGF-E, and placenta growth factor (PGF)-1 and -2 [77]. VEGF-A (commonly referred to as VEGF) was the first factor identified, capable of coupling both VEGFR-1 and -2 receptors and contributing to the neoangiogenesis phenomenon [78]. VEGF-C and VEGF-D and their receptor VEGFR-3 are the most relevant factors for the lymphangiogenic process in cancer [77]. In cutaneous melanoma, lymphangiogenic biomarkers, particularly VEGF-C, VEGF-D and VEGFR-3 are over-expressed when compared to normal melanocytic nevi [79, 80]. Interestingly, these biomarkers are expressed in the early stages of melanoma progression, underlying the important role of lymphangiogenesis in the first steps of melanomagenesis [80].

Using monoclonal antibodies, hundreds of melanoma samples have been evaluated to assess the relationship between lymphangiogenesis and lymph node status (Table 16.1: LYVE-1, CD31 and D2-40) [26, 27, 70–72, 75, 76, 81–87]. Several studies have suggested a significant correlation between the presence of lymphangiogenic vessels in the primary tumor and lymph node status [26, 27, 70, 71, 83, 84, 87]. In two separate studies, Dadras et al. [26, 27] reported that lymphangiogenesis can be used as an accurate predictor of SLN status; the lymphatic vascular area of primary melanomas, an index of tumor lymphangiogenesis, was found to be a highly sensitive (83%) and specific (89%) prognostic marker of SLN metastasis. The authors suggested that the evaluation of primary tumor lymphangiogenesis status might be considered as an alternative to SLNB. However, as SLNB may have a potential therapeutic benefit for melanoma patients, we think that lymphangiogenesis has to be considered as a predictive/prognostic marker and not a surrogate for this procedure. Emmett et al. [87] reported that the Shields' index (combined measurements of lymphatic density, Breslow thickness, and the presence or absence of lymphatic invasion) accurately predicted outcome in 90% of patients with metastases and 84% without metastases. In these patients, the Shields' index was noted to be more predictive than tumor thickness or lymphatic density. In another study of 45 melanoma patients, the identification of high peritumorous and intra-

Table 16.1 Studies on lymphangiogenesis biomarkers of primary melanoma for prediction of lymph node status and patient prognosis

Author, year	Reference	Factors	Methods	Antibody	Pts n	Lymph node status	Sentinel lymph node biopsy conducted	Patient prognosis
Dadras, 2003	[27]	LVI	IHC	LYVE-1; CD31	37	Significant	Yes	Significant
		VEGF-C	IHC; ISH	VEGF-C		Not significant		NR
Straume, 2003	[81]	LVI	IHC	D2-40; LYVE-1	202	Not significant	NR	Significant
Wobser, 2005	[75]	LVI	IHC	CD31	26	NR	Yes	NR
		VEGFR-3		VEGFR-3		NR		
Dadras, 2005	[26]	LVI	IHC	LYVE-1; CD31; D2-40	45	Significant	Yes	NR
		VEGF-C		VEGF-C		Significant		
		VEGF-D		VEGF-D		Not significant		
Sahni, 2005	[72]	LVI	IHC	LYVE-1	36	Not significant	Yes	NR
Massi, 2006	[71]	LVI	IHC	D2-40	45	Significant	Yes	Significant
		VEGF-C		VEGF-C		Not significant		
Brychtova, 2008	[82]	VEGF-A	IHC	VEGF-A	130	Not significant	Yes	–
		VEGF-C		VEGF-C		Not significant		–
		VEGFR-1		VEGFR-1		Not significant		–
		VEGFR-2		VEGFR-2		Not significant		–
		VEGFR-3		VEGFR-3		Not significant		–
Liu, 2008	[70]	LVI	IHC; PCR	LYVE-1	56	Unclear	NR	Not significant
		VEGF-C		VEGF-C		Significant		Significant
		VEGF-D		VEGF-D		Significant		Significant
		VEGFR-3		VEGFR-3		Significant		Not significant
Niakosari, 2008	[83]	LVI	IHC	D2-40	96	Significant	Yes	NR
Boone, 2008	[84]	VEGF-C	IHC	VEGF-C	113	Significant	Yes	Not significant
Xu, 2008	[76]	LVI	IHC	D2-40	106	NR	Yes	Significant[a]
Depasquale, 2008	[85]	VEGF	IHC	VEGF	204	–	–	Not significant[b]
Chua, 2009	[86]	CD31	IHC	CD31	77	–	–	Not significant
		VEGF		VEGF				
Emmett, 2010	[87]	Shields' index[c]	IHC	LYVE-1	18	Significant	Yes	NR

LVI lymphovascular invasion, *IHC* immunohistochemistry, *ISH* in situ hybridization, *PCR* polymerase chain reaction, *NR* not reported

[a]Time to regional lymph node metastasis was considered as well as disease-free and overall survival
[b]Time to recurrences only
[c]The Shields' index represents combined tumor thickness, lymphatic vessel density and lymphovascular invasion

tumorous lymphatic vessel density was found to be associated with SLN metastasis and reduced survival [71]. Interestingly, the intratumorous lymphatic vessel area was reported as the most significant predictive factor for SLN disease [71]. Similarly, Niakosari et al. [83] reported that lymphovascular invasion (absent or present) remained a significant predictive factor for SLN status when adjusted for other predictive factors in a multivariate model [83]. The detection of lymphangiogenesis biomarkers by PCR has demonstrated results that are comparable with those achieved by IHC [70]. However, two studies failed to identify any significant correlation between lymphangiogenesis and lymph node status, either by counting the absolute number of lymphatic vessels [72] or the number of vessels per mm^2 [81]. Interestingly, the latter study by Straume et al. [81] did not clearly state which procedure was implemented for the assessment of lymph node involvement. It is well established that SLNB can detect subclinical metastatic deposits. Therefore, the presence of lymphatic metastasis could have been underestimated in this study [81], probably explaining the lack of a statistical association between the presence of lymphovascular invasion and lymph node status.

The results of studies that utilized the lymphangiogenic markers VEGF-C and VEGF-D and their receptor VEGFR-3 are controversial. A study of 130 patients which assessed the expression of VEGF-A and -C, as well as the three receptors VEGFR-1, -2 and -3, did not find any relationship between lymphangiogenesis and SLN status (positive SLNB rate of 33%) [82]. Dadras et al. [26] identified VEGF-C, but not VEGF-D, as a significant predictor of lymph node involvement. In another study, VEGF-C, VEGF-D and VEGFR-3 were found to significantly predict lymph node status following IHC and PCR analysis [70]. Boone et al. [84] also reported a significant association between lymph node metastasis and VEGF-C expression in the primary tumor.

In conclusion, lymphangiogenic markers appear to have some promise in stratifying patients according to their risk of harboring lymphatic disease. However, further work needs to be done before their routine assessment can enter the clinical setting.

SLN and Non-SLN Metastasis

Pathological Parameters

Protocols used for SLNB assessment vary worldwide [88–91]. Since the area close to the central meridian of the SLN is regarded as the most common site for melanoma metastasis, most authors recommend that the SLN be bi-valved through the longest dimension of the hilum. Each part of the SLN is then serially sectioned for review of hematoxylin-eosin (H&E) and IHC stained slides. Among the different protocols, there is a general lack of consensus concerning both the number and thickness of the tissue sections that should be evaluated. In this setting, S-100, HMB-45, Melan-A/MART-1 and/or tyrosinase are the most frequently used antibodies for IHC. Different protocols have resulted in metastatic detection rates ranging from 15–20% to ~34% [37, 88]. This is lower than that reported using reverse transcription (RT)-PCR methodologies (up to 38%); however, the detailed histopathology work-up protocol proposed by Cook et al. [88] was found to be virtually free of false-positive results, as compared with RT-PCR, which was subject to a false-positive rate of 7% in their study.

The presence of metastatic disease in the SLN (~20% of patients undergoing SLNB) is an indication for follow-up CLND. Approximately 80% of these patients will not have non-SLN disease. Numerous studies have tried to identify those patients with good prognostic outcome and low risk of developing non-SLN metastasis who might avoid CLND and its potentially high morbidity [30]. Lymph node disease is the most important prognostic factor for patients with early-stage melanoma [7]. Therefore, tumor burden in the SLN has been evaluated as a possible risk stratification factor in order to identify those patients who might benefit from follow-up CLND. Important in this assessment would be the ability to address both predictive and prognostic data with appropriate statistical methodology; although, most studies provide results for one or the other outcome (Table 16.2). A number of markers of SLN tumor load have been studied, including:

Table 16.2 Different parameters evaluated as predictive factors for non-sentinel lymph node (non-SLN) involvement

Parameters	Author, year	Parameter subgroup	Non-SLN positivity (%)	5-year overall survival (%)
Size as largest diameter of largest lesion	Ranieri 2002 [92]	≤3 mm	–	86 (3 year)
	Carlson 2003 [93]	Isolated tumor cells	–	86 (3 year)
		≤2 mm	–	90 (3 year)
	Lee 2004 [94]	<2 mm	16	–
	Sabel 2005 [95]	Micrometastasis	2	–
	Pearlman 2006 [96]	≤2 mm	6	85
	van Akkooi 2006 [97]	<0.1 mm	0[a]	100
	Govindarajan 2007 [98]	≤0.2 mm	0	–
	Debarbieux 2007 [99]	≤2 mm	18[a]	±80
		≤1 mm	13	–
		(smallest diameter)	12	87
	Scheri 2007 [100]	≤0.2 mm	8[a]	–
	Roka 2008 [101]	≥2 mm	16[a]	–
	Rossi 2008 [33]	≤2 mm	0[a]	–
	Satzger 2008 [102]	<0.1 mm	9[a]	–
		<1 mm	11[a]	–
	Guggenheim 2008 [103]	<2 mm	16[a]	–
	Gershenwald 2008 [32]	≤2 mm	5	–
		≤0.5 mm	8	–
	van Akkooi 2008 [35]	≤2 mm	3	91
	van der Ploeg 2009 [36]	<0.1 mm	0[a]	100[a]
	Glumac 2008 [104]	≤2 mm	0	–
Penetrative depth	Starz 2004 [105]	≤0.3 mm	8	±80
		0.3–1.0 mm	–	±90
	Scolyer 2004 [34]	≤2 mm	12[b]	–
	Fink 2005 [106]	≤1.0 mm	0[b]	–
	van Akkooi 2006 [97]	0.3–1.0 mm	8[a]	–
		≤1.5 mm	14[a]	–
	Debarbieux 2007 [99]	<2 mm	–	±80
	Satzger 2007 [102]	≤0.3 mm	0[a]	–
	Rossi 2008 [33]	≤1 mm	6[a]	–
	Satzger 2008 [107]	≤2 mm	9[a]	–
	van der Ploeg 2009 [108]	≤0.3 mm	0	92
Location	Dewar 2004 [109]	Subcapsular	0	–
	van Akkooi 2006 [97]	Combined	9[a]	–
	Govindarajan 2007 [98]	Sinusoidal	0[a]	–
	Roka 2008 [101]	Non-extensive	13	–
	Rossi 2008 [33]	Subcapsular	0[a]	–
	Gershenwald 2008 [32]	Subcapsular	10	–
	Frankel 2008 [110]	Subcapsular	10[a]	–
	van Akkooi 2008 [35]	Subcapsular	8[a]	–
	van der Ploeg 2009 [36]	Subcapsular	3[a]	83
Area	Cochran 2004 [111]	<4%	3	–
	Scolyer 2004 [34]	≤10 mm²	13[b]	–
		≤10%	15[a]	–
	Vuylsteke 2005 [112]	<0.03 mm²	0	–
	Satzger 2008 [102]	≤10%	9	–
	Frankel 2008 [107]	≤1%	9	–
	Gershenwald 2008 [32]	≤10 mm²	10	–

(continued)

Table 16.2 (continued)

Parameters	Author, year	Parameter subgroup	Non-SLN positivity (%)	5-year overall survival (%)
Combinations of different parameters	Reeves 2003 [113]	SU score = 0[c]	0	–
	Vuylsteke 2005 [110]	Group A[d]	0	94
	Satzger 2007 [102]	Score = 0[e]	–	±100
	Satzger 2008 [106]	Risk score = 0[f]	5	100
	Roka 2008 [101]	SU score = 0[c]	12	–
	Gershenwald 2008 [32]	Total score = 0[g]	0	–

[a]Variable is not significant for non-SLN positivity in multivariate analyses
[b]Multivariate analyses were not performed
[c]SU Score = Size/Ulceration Score; 1 point is given when largest diameter of metastasis is ≥2 mm and 1 point is given for the presence of ulceration
[d]Group A consists of patients with Breslow thickness <2.5 mm and a tumor area of <0.3 mm²
[e]Capsular invasion; tumor infiltrative depth (<2 or ≥2 mm); size of largest tumor deposit (<30 cells or ≥30 cells)
[f]Risk score = 1 point for perinodal intralymphatic tumor, 1 point for relative tumor burden >10%, and 1 point for positivity by H&E staining
[g]Total Score = Sum of scores for tumor thickness (0 for tumor thickness ≤2 mm and 1 for >2 mm), largest SLN metastatic focus (0, 1, 2 or 3 for ≤0.5 mm, >0.5 to ≤2 mm, >2 to ≤10 mm or >10 mm, respectively), and number of SLNs harvested (0, 1 or 2 for ≥3, 2, or 1, respectively)

size as maximum diameter of the largest lesion; site of the tumor deposit; tumor penetrative depth; and, more recently, the percentage or square area of the tumor burden [7, 34, 35, 37, 105, 109, 111, 114]. Other parameters assessed include the number of positive SLNs, number of metastatic foci, extracapsular spread and capsular invasion [33, 111, 115]. Some studies have combined primary melanoma and SLN features into working models for prediction of survival and/or non-SLN status [32, 116].

A number of authors have suggested that patients with low tumor burden in the SLN (i.e., a small amount of metastatic deposit) might be spared CLND. In this respect, some studies report minimal tumor burden as highly predictive for non-SLN negativity and good prognostic outcome. For instance, van Akkooi et al. [35, 97] demonstrated that patients with SLN disease of less than 0.1 mm have an excellent prognosis comparable to SLN-negative cases and could probably be referred to as having "false-positive" disease. However, these results have not been confirmed by other investigators, who suggest that these patients do not represent a subgroup with different biological behavior [100]. Other authors have suggested that a subcapsular localization [109]; a thin penetrative depth of invasion into the lymph node [23, 36, 108, 114]; or models generated using several parameters [32] might identify patients who will not benefit from CLND. A recent study, that included seven pathologists who are experts in the melanoma field, reported that there was excellent inter-observer agreement concerning: the maximal size of the largest deposit; estimated percentage area occupied by metastases; and tumor penetrative depth [117]. While there is no international agreement as to which parameter shows the best prognostic and predictive value and/or the best accuracy and reproducibility, on-going prospective studies (i.e., MINITUB and MSLT-II) may provide additional data.

Some authors have suggested that features of the primary tumor, such as Breslow thickness, are not predictive of non-SLN status [33, 34]. Instead, tumor migration to additional lymph nodes might be related to some biological characteristics of the SLN metastasis (e.g., microanatomy of individual lymph nodes, expression of adhesion molecules that promote malignant cell homing within the SLN, and/or patient immune response). As described previously, some investigators have reported that biomarkers of lymphangiogenesis might have a greater predictive efficacy than primary tumor staging features [26, 27]. Moreover, findings from melanoma and breast cancer studies suggest that tumor cells express chemokine receptors (e.g., CXCR4 and CCR7) which bind to cognate ligands (e.g., CXCL12 and CCL21) present on cells in lymph nodes, lung, liver, and bone marrow, promoting metastases to these sites [118, 119]. Moreover, the expression of these factors has been shown to correlate with patient prognosis [118, 119]. Therefore, it would appear that the arrest of malignant cells in a given target organ or tissue hinges not only on primary tumor features, but also on the molecular characteristics of the microenvironment of the metastatic site.

Molecular Markers: The Case of Polymerase Chain Reaction

As stated previously, SLNB is associated with false-negative results in approximately one of five-to-ten patients with lymph node metastasis. We have observed locoregional disease recurrence in about 10–20% of patients [9, 11, 12, 18]. Of course, the reliability of nodal staging depends on the accuracy of the procedure utilized for melanoma cell identification. Although the most appropriate protocol is still a matter of debate (e.g., SLN sampling, type/number of target antigens), IHC has been shown to increase the detection rate of micrometastatic disease as compared to standard H&E staining [120].

It has been suggested that the use of PCR could improve the detection of SLN metastases in patients with melanoma [16, 47]. Moreover, PCR analysis of SLNs could provide clinicians with a powerful tool with which to identify patients with very low tumor burden and allow for the stratification of patients for medical and surgical therapies. However, despite this potential, the many studies conducted to date have provided conflicting results [42, 46]. Early studies with limited follow-up suggested that patients with histopathologically-negative SLNs could be stratified into those at high or low risk for metastasis on the basis of the PCR results (i.e., positive vs. negative) [42, 43]. However, a prospective randomized trial, designed to assess the role of SLNB, CLND and adjuvant therapy with interferon-alpha in the treatment of patients with early-stage melanoma, failed to demonstrate a significant prognostic difference between patients on the basis of SLN status following PCR analysis [46].

We performed a recent meta-analysis of the findings from 22 studies, encompassing 4,019 patients who underwent SLNB for clinical stage I or II cutaneous melanoma (Table 16.3) [47]. Histopathological examination of SLNs consisted of H&E staining combined with IHC in virtually all studies. IHC protocols utilized antibodies specific for S-100 and gp100 (HMB-45), in addition to tyrosinase and MART-1/Melan-A (melanoma antigen recognized by T cells-1). With regard to molecular biology methods, a number of different PCR-based techniques (i.e., standard PCR, nested PCR and quantitative real-time PCR) were employed and directed to amplify genes coding for different melanoma-associated markers, including tyrosinase, MART-1, melanoma antigen gene family (MAGE-3), β-N-acetylgalactosaminyl-transferase, TRP1, TRP2, and paired box homeotic gene transcription factor-3 (PAX3). Histopathology-based and PCR-based positivity rates were 20.3% and 51.1%, respectively [47]. Interestingly, among patients with histopathologically-positive SLNs, PCR was found to be negative in 49% of cases (PCR false-negative rate); while among patients with histopathologically-negative SLNs, PCR was reported as positive in 42.3% of cases (PCR false-positive rate). If melanoma patients with positive findings for both histopathology and PCR were considered as true-positive results, and those non-melanoma patients negative for both histopathology and

Table 16.3 Studies on polymerase chain reaction (PCR) analysis of sentinel lymph nodes (SLNs) in melanoma

Author	Year	Reference	Pts n	SLN positivity (%)	PCR type	PCR target(s)	PCR positivity (%)	Median FU (months)
Goydos et al.	1998	[121]	50	30.0	Nested	Tyr, MART-1	36.0	–
Shivers et al.	1998	[40]	114	20.2	Nested	Tyr	61.4	28
Blaheta et al.	1999	[122]	73	17.8	Standard	Tyr	49.3	–
Bostick et al.	1999	[42]	72	23.6	Standard	Tyr, MART-1, MAGE-3	50.0	12
Blaheta et al.	2000	[123]	116	12.9	Nested	Tyr	44.0	19
Li et al.	2000	[43]	233	22.3	Nested	Tyr	70.0	20
Palmieri et al.	2001	[124]	75	18.7	Nested	Tyr, MART-1	53.3	29
Boi et al.	2002	[125]	88	15.9	Nested	Tyr	45.5	–
Goydos et al.	2003	[126]	175	19.4	Standard	Tyr	58.3	34
Kuo et al.	2003	[127]	77	48.1	Standard	Tyr, MART-1, TRP1, TRP2	74.0	55
Ribuffo et al.	2003	[44]	134	11.2	Nested	Tyr, MART-1	63.4	42
Rimoldi et al.	2003	[128]	71	23.9	Standard	Tyr, MART-1	57.7	36
Starz et al.	2003	[129]	63	58.7	Nested	Tyr	68.3	–
Blaheta et al.	2004	[130]	59	11.9	Standard	Tyr, MART-1	67.8	–
Kammula et al.	2004	[45]	112	13.4	Nested	Tyr	65.2	67
Takeuchi et al.	2004	[131]	215	24.7	qrtPCR	MART-1, MAGE-A3, GalNAc-T, PAX3	46.0	60
Ulrich et al.	2004	[132]	322	10.6	Standard	Tyr	12.1	37
Abrahamsen et al.	2005	[133]	95	28.4	qrtPCR	Tyr, MART-1	67.4	–
Giese et al.	2005	[134]	139	18.0	qrtPCR	Tyr, MART-1	44.6	29
Romanini et al.	2005	[135]	124	18.5	Standard	Tyr, MART-1	31.5	30
Mangas et al.	2006	[136]	180	21.1	Nested	Tyr	68.9	45
Scoggins et al.	2006	[46]	1446	–	Standard	Tyr, MART-1, MAGE-3, gp100	42.9	30
Mocellin et al.	2007	[47]	Meta-analysis: overall and disease-free survival significantly higher for patients with negative SLN by PCR; albeit with significant heterogeneity					
Denninghoff et al.	2008	[137]	60	NA	qrtPCR	Tyr	84	>24
Riber-Hansen et al.	2008	[138]	93	29	qrtPCR	Tyr, MART-1	74	43.5
Nowecki et al.	2008	[139]	114	100	qrtPCR	Tyr, MART-1, MAGE-3	41.5	–
Hilari et al.	2009	[140]	195	–	qrtPCR	Tyr, MART-1, SSX2, MAGE-3, PAX3, GalNAc-T	–	64

FU follow-up, *qrtPCR* quantitative real-time PCR, *NA* not available

PCR were considered as true-negative results, molecular analysis sensitivity, specificity, accuracy, positive predictive value (PPV), and NPV were found to be 94.9%, 95.9%, 95.2%, 98.0%, and 89.9%, respectively [47]. Upon investigating the potential prognostic value of PCR status, both false-positive and true-negative results were identified among melanoma patients who experienced disease recurrence. Under these conditions, molecular analysis sensitivity, specificity, accuracy, PPV, and NPV were found to be 57.4%, 61.1%, 60.6%, 16.8%, and 91.3%, respectively [47]. With regard to overall survival, meta-analysis of pooled data showed a significantly increased risk of death in patients with PCR positivity (hazard ratio, HR: 5.08, 95% confidence interval, CI: 1.83–14.08; P=0.002) [47]. Considering disease-free survival, meta-analysis of pooled data indicated a significantly increased risk of disease progression in patients with PCR positivity (HR: 3.41, CI: 1.86–6.24; P<0.0001) [47]. These results support the hypothesis that PCR status may play a clinically useful prognostic role in patients with melanoma. In fact, most investigators have reported a significant correlation between PCR status and patient survival, with many studies demonstrating the independent prognostic value of PCR on multivariate analysis. Most importantly, meta-analysis of pooled data has confirmed that PCR status represents a significant meta-risk for both overall and disease-free survival [47]. These findings could support the incorporation of SLN molecular ultrastaging into the TNM melanoma staging system. Nevertheless, caution is required. PCR appears better as a diagnostic (95.2% accuracy) rather than prognostic test (60.6% accuracy); although, it must be taken into consideration that these data come from pooled series in which the disease recurrence rate was 12.1% after a mean follow-up of 35.4 months, a time that may not be sufficient to observe the expected disease recurrence rate (~30%, according to 10-year survival data from TNM stage I–IIIA patients) [47]. This finding is corroborated by the satisfactory NPV of PCR (91.3%); the only parameter potentially not affected by time (if a patient is destined not to recur, the length of follow-up will not change the classification in that particular instance). The significant heterogeneity found in this meta-analysis for both overall and disease-free survival is likely to result from a number of differences that exist between the studies, including: PCR methods used (standard vs. nested vs. quantitative real-time); SLN sampling (bi-valved vs. alternate vs. paraffin-embedded sections); type of tumor marker analyzed (up to eight different genes were utilized); number of tumor markers amplified per study (from one to four); definition of risk [PCR positivity/negativity vs. number of positive markers vs. mRNA cut-off values (quantitative real-time PCR)]; clinical end-points (correlation with disease stage or survival); and statistical analysis (univariate vs. multivariate survival analysis, different covariates investigated using multivariate analysis). Moreover, intra-study variability with regard to the enrollment of patients with different treatment regimens made it impossible to assess the potential impact of this important variable.

In addition, although the incidence of lymph node metastasis during the natural history of clinical stage I and II melanoma patients is known to be up to 30%, the mean PCR positivity rate in this meta-analysis was noted to be 51.4% [47]. Technical limitations of PCR-based analysis (e.g., contamination or carryover events, amplification of pseudogenes, illegitimate transcription) might underlie some false-positive results. In this regard, the use of quantitative real-time PCR methods has been advocated as a means to set cut-off values that distinguish illegitimate transcription from marker expression by malignant cells. The MSLT-II trial is currently assessing the potential significance of quantitative real-time PCR-based molecular ultrastaging of melanoma SLNs. In addition, PCR false-positivity may result from the use of gene markers that are not specific for melanoma, but also identify melanocytic nevus cells in SLNs [129]. Some investigators have observed that the risk of disease recurrence or death significantly increases with the number of transcripts found to be expressed in the SLN [131], suggesting that the low specificity of PCR (due to a relatively high false-positivity rate) might be counterbalanced through the use of a multimarker assay.

Aside from these technical issues, it is important to consider a biological hypothesis which suggests that the presence of melanoma cells in the SLN might be a reliable marker of cancer aggressiveness and dissemination [which correlates with disease recurrence (any site) and patient survival], rather than a sign of lymph node colonization (which correlates strictly with locoregional disease recurrence). In other words, as for the detection of melanoma cells circulating in the peripheral blood which appears to correlate with patient clinical outcome [141], the presence of melanoma cells in the lymphatic system (and in particular, within the SLN) might reflect the metastatic potential of the primary tumor, as discussed above with regard to lymphangiogenesis. If this concept holds true, the correlation between PCR status and survival (instead of lymph node metastasis rate) might be explained: of note, 10-year survival data indicate that 5–60% of patients with clinical stage I–II melanoma will recur at any site [5, 142, 143], underscoring the fact that a significant proportion of patients can experience disease recurrence in the absence of regional lymph node metastasis [15]. This hypothesis has been supported by the results of two different studies [16, 140], which show that patients experiencing regional lymph node recurrence after being reported as SLN-negative (i.e., false-negative SLNB) could be positive by PCR examination.

Whether the PCR status of the SLN is a potential marker for adjuvant treatment selection remains unclear. In a recent systematic analysis and meta-analysis, we reported that interferon-alpha (IFN-α) adjuvant treatment was associated with statistically significant improvement in disease-free and overall survival in patients with high-risk cutaneous melanoma (i.e., radically resected TNM stages II–III disease) [144]. A search for predictive markers of drug response might identify those patients who would benefit from this treatment. In this regard, several randomized controlled trials have reported IFN-α to be more effective in cases of low tumor burden [145–147]. Of note, the Sunbelt Melanoma Trial is the only study that has addressed the role of IFN-α in patients with histopathologically-negative, but PCR-positive SLNs [148]. This subgroup of patients was randomized to receive observation only (180 patients), CLND (192 patients), or CLND and high dose IFN-α (184 patients). No differences in either disease-free or overall survival were demonstrated among these cohorts [148].

In conclusion, the role of PCR analysis in the assessment of SLN status and patient prognosis seems promising, but requires further investigation; as is being undertaken in the side study of the MSLT-II trials.

Final Remarks

The molecular characterization of primary melanomas and SLNs represents an important step towards improved stratification of patients according to their risk of tumor progression. Primary tumor biomarkers, such as those belonging to the lymphangiogenic family, and PCR analysis of SLN metastases provide reliable information to improve upon the histopathological parameters currently used in the evaluation of primary melanomas and SLNs, respectively. Further studies must be encouraged. These should incorporate large prospective tumor specimen collections to be analysed with standardized methodologies in order to assess the true role of these biomarkers in the management of melanoma patients.

References

1. Veronesi U, Adamus J, Bandiera DC, et al. Inefficacy of immediate node dissection in stage I melanoma of the limbs. N Engl J Med. 1977;297(12):627–30.
2. Sim FH, Taylor WF, Pritchard DJ, Soule EH. Lymphadenectomy in the management of stage I malignant melanoma: a prospective randomized study. Mayo Clin Proc. 1986;61(9):697–705.
3. Morton DL, Wen DR, Wong JH, et al. Technical details of intraoperative lymphatic mapping for early stage melanoma. Arch Surg. 1992;127(4):392–9.
4. Chen SL, Iddings DM, Scheri RP, Bilchik AJ. Lymphatic mapping and sentinel node analysis: current concepts and applications. CA Cancer J Clin. 2006;56(5):292–309. quiz 316–297.

5. Balch CM, Soong SJ, Gershenwald JE, et al. Prognostic factors analysis of 17,600 melanoma patients: validation of the American Joint Committee on Cancer Melanoma Staging system. J Clin Oncol. 2001;19(16):3622–34.
6. Balch CM, Buzaid AC, Soong SJ, et al. Final version of the American Joint Committee on Cancer Staging system for cutaneous melanoma. J Clin Oncol. 2001;19(16):3635–48.
7. Morton DL, Thompson JF, Cochran AJ, et al. Sentinel-node biopsy or nodal observation in melanoma. N Engl J Med. 2006;355(13):1307–17.
8. Pasquali S, Mocellin S, Campana LG, et al. Early (sentinel lymph node biopsy-guided) versus delayed lymphadenectomy in melanoma patients with lymph node metastases: personal experience and literature meta-analysis. Cancer. 2010;116(5):1201–9.
9. Rossi CR, Pasquali S, Mocellin S. Actual false-negative rate prompts the routine use of ultrasound scan before and after sentinel node biopsy in melanoma. Ann Surg Oncol. 2008;15(10):2976–7.
10. Testori A, De Salvo GL, Montesco MC, et al. Italian Melanoma I. Clinical considerations on sentinel node biopsy in melanoma from an Italian multicentric study on 1,313 patients (SOLISM-IMI). Ann Surg Oncol. 2009;16(7):2018–27.
11. Nieweg OE. False-negative sentinel node biopsy. Ann Surg Oncol. 2009;16(8):2089–91.
12. Nieweg OE, Estourgie SH. What is a sentinel node and what is a false-negative sentinel node? Ann Surg Oncol. 2004;11(3 Suppl):169S–73.
13. Thompson JF, Stretch JR, Uren RF, Ka VS, Scolyer RA. Sentinel node biopsy for melanoma: where have we been and where are we going? Ann Surg Oncol. 2004;11(3 Suppl):147S–51.
14. Scolyer RA, Thompson JF, Li LX, et al. Failure to remove true sentinel nodes can cause failure of the sentinel node biopsy technique: evidence from antimony concentrations in false-negative sentinel nodes from melanoma patients. Ann Surg Oncol. 2004;11(3 Suppl):174S–8.
15. Yee VS, Thompson JF, McKinnon JG, et al. Outcome in 846 cutaneous melanoma patients from a single center after a negative sentinel node biopsy. Ann Surg Oncol. 2005;12(6):429–39.
16. Karim RZ, Scolyer RA, Li W, et al. False negative sentinel lymph node biopsies in melanoma may result from deficiencies in nuclear medicine, surgery, or pathology. Ann Surg. 2008;247(6):1003–10.
17. Lam TK, Uren RF, Scolyer RA, Quinn MJ, Shannon KF, Thompson JF. False-negative sentinel node biopsy because of obstruction of lymphatics by metastatic melanoma: the value of ultrasound in conjunction with preoperative lymphoscintigraphy. Melanoma Res. 2009;19(2):94–9.
18. Sondak VK, Zager JS. Who is to blame for false-negative sentinel node biopsies in melanoma? Ann Surg Oncol. 2010;17(3):670–3.
19. Thompson JF, Scolyer RA, Kefford RF. Cutaneous melanoma. Lancet. 2005;365(9460):687–701.
20. Morton DL, Cochran AJ, Thompson JF, et al. Sentinel node biopsy for early-stage melanoma: accuracy and morbidity in MSLT-I, an international multicenter trial. Ann Surg. 2005;242(3):302–11. discussion 311–303.
21. Morton RL, Howard K, Thompson JF. The cost-effectiveness of sentinel node biopsy in patients with intermediate thickness primary cutaneous melanoma. Ann Surg Oncol. 2009;16(4):929–40.
22. Mocellin S, Thompson JF, Pasquali S, et al. Sentinel node status prediction by four statistical models: results from a large bi-institutional series (n = 1132). Ann Surg. 2009;250(6):964–9.
23. Wong SL, Kattan MW, McMasters KM, Coit DG. A nomogram that predicts the presence of sentinel node metastasis in melanoma with better discrimination than the American Joint Committee on Cancer staging system. Ann Surg Oncol. 2005;12(4):282–8.
24. Thompson JF, Scolyer RA, Kefford RF. Cutaneous melanoma in the era of molecular profiling. Lancet. 2009;374(9687):362–5.
25. Kashani-Sabet M, Venna S, Nosrati M, et al. A multimarker prognostic assay for primary cutaneous melanoma. Clin Cancer Res. 2009;15(22):6987–92.
26. Dadras SS, Lange-Asschenfeldt B, Velasco P, et al. Tumor lymphangiogenesis predicts melanoma metastasis to sentinel lymph nodes. Mod Pathol. 2005;18(9):1232–42.
27. Dadras SS, Paul T, Bertoncini J, et al. Tumor lymphangiogenesis: a novel prognostic indicator for cutaneous melanoma metastasis and survival. Am J Pathol. 2003;162(6):1951–60.
28. Gould Rothberg BE, Bracken MB, Rimm DL. Tissue biomarkers for prognosis in cutaneous melanoma: a systematic review and meta-analysis. J Natl Cancer Inst. 2009;101(7):452–74.
29. van Akkooi AC, Voit CA, Verhoef C, Eggermont AM. New developments in sentinel node staging in melanoma: controversies and alternatives. Curr Opin Oncol. 2010;22(3):169–77.
30. Guggenheim MM, Hug U, Jung FJ, et al. Morbidity and recurrence after completion lymph node dissection following sentinel lymph node biopsy in cutaneous malignant melanoma. Ann Surg. 2008;247(4):687–93.
31. Wrightson WR, Wong SL, Edwards MJ, et al. Complications associated with sentinel lymph node biopsy for melanoma. Ann Surg Oncol. 2003;10(6):676–80.
32. Gershenwald JE, Andtbacka RH, Prieto VG, et al. Microscopic tumor burden in sentinel lymph nodes predicts synchronous nonsentinel lymph node involvement in patients with melanoma. J Clin Oncol. 2008;26(26):4296–303.
33. Rossi CR, De Salvo GL, Bonandini E, et al. Factors predictive of nonsentinel lymph node involvement and clinical outcome in melanoma patients with metastatic sentinel lymph node. Ann Surg Oncol. 2008;15(4):1202–10.

34. Scolyer RA, Li LX, McCarthy SW, et al. Micromorphometric features of positive sentinel lymph nodes predict involvement of nonsentinel nodes in patients with melanoma. Am J Clin Pathol. 2004;122(4):532–9.
35. van Akkooi AC, Nowecki ZI, Voit C, et al. Sentinel node tumor burden according to the Rotterdam criteria is the most important prognostic factor for survival in melanoma patients: a multicenter study in 388 patients with positive sentinel nodes. Ann Surg. 2008;248(6):949–55.
36. van der Ploeg IM, Kroon BB, Antonini N, Valdes Olmos RA, Nieweg OE. Comparison of three micromorphometric pathology classifications of melanoma metastases in the sentinel node. Ann Surg. 2009;250(2):301–4.
37. van der Ploeg AP, van Akkooi AC, Schmitz PI, Koljenovic S, Verhoef C, Eggermont AM. EORTC melanoma group sentinel node protocol identifies high rate of submicrometastases according to Rotterdam Criteria. Eur J Cancer. 2010;46(13):2414–21.
38. Murali R, Hughes MT, Fitzgerald P, Thompson JF, Scolyer RA. Interobserver variation in the histopathologic reporting of key prognostic parameters, particularly Clark level, affects pathologic staging of primary cutaneous melanoma. Ann Surg. 2009;249(4):641–7.
39. Smith B, Selby P, Southgate J, Pittman K, Bradley C, Blair GE. Detection of melanoma cells in peripheral blood by means of reverse transcriptase and polymerase chain reaction. Lancet. 1991;338(8777):1227–9.
40. Shivers SC, Wang X, Li W, et al. Molecular staging of malignant melanoma: correlation with clinical outcome. JAMA. 1998;280(16):1410–5.
41. Wang X, Heller R, VanVoorhis N, et al. Detection of submicroscopic lymph node metastases with polymerase chain reaction in patients with malignant melanoma. Ann Surg. 1994;220(6):768–74.
42. Bostick PJ, Morton DL, Turner RR, et al. Prognostic significance of occult metastases detected by sentinel lymphadenectomy and reverse transcriptase-polymerase chain reaction in early-stage melanoma patients. J Clin Oncol. 1999;17(10):3238–44.
43. Li W, Stall A, Shivers SC, et al. Clinical relevance of molecular staging for melanoma: comparison of RT-PCR and immunohistochemistry staining in sentinel lymph nodes of patients with melanoma. Ann Surg. 2000;231(6):795–803.
44. Ribuffo D, Gradilone A, Vonella M, et al. Prognostic significance of reverse transcriptase-polymerase chain reaction-negative sentinel nodes in malignant melanoma. Ann Surg Oncol. 2003;10(4):396–402.
45. Kammula US, Ghossein R, Bhattacharya S, Coit DG. Serial follow-up and the prognostic significance of reverse transcriptase-polymerase chain reaction–staged sentinel lymph nodes from melanoma patients. J Clin Oncol. 2004;22(19):3989–96.
46. Scoggins CR, Ross MI, Reintgen DS, et al. Prospective multi-institutional study of reverse transcriptase polymerase chain reaction for molecular staging of melanoma. J Clin Oncol. 2006;24(18):2849–57.
47. Mocellin S, Hoon DS, Pilati P, Rossi CR, Nitti D. Sentinel lymph node molecular ultrastaging in patients with melanoma: a systematic review and meta-analysis of prognosis. J Clin Oncol. 2007;25(12):1588–95.
48. Australian Cancer Network Melanoma Guidelines Revision Working Party. Clinical Practice Guidelines for the Management of Melanoma in Australia and New Zealand. Cancer Council Australia and Australian Cancer Network, Sydney and New Zealand Guidelines Group. Wellington, 2008.
49. Warycha MA, Zakrzewski J, Ni Q, et al. Meta-analysis of sentinel lymph node positivity in thin melanoma (<or=1 mm). Cancer. 2009;115(4):869–79.
50. Cascinelli N, Bombardieri E, Bufalino R, et al. Sentinel and nonsentinel node status in stage Ib and II melanoma patients: two-step prognostic indicators of survival. J Clin Oncol. 2006;24(27):4464–71.
51. Sondak VK, Taylor JM, Sabel MS, et al. Mitotic rate and younger age are predictors of sentinel lymph node positivity: lessons learned from the generation of a probabilistic model. Ann Surg Oncol. 2004;11(3):247–58.
52. Mocellin S, Ambrosi A, Montesco MC, et al. Support vector machine learning model for the prediction of sentinel node status in patients with cutaneous melanoma. Ann Surg Oncol. 2006;13(8):1113–22.
53. Paek SC, Griffith KA, Johnson TM, et al. The impact of factors beyond Breslow depth on predicting sentinel lymph node positivity in melanoma. Cancer. 2007;109(1):100–8.
54. Taylor RC, Patel A, Panageas KS, Busam KJ, Brady MS. Tumor-infiltrating lymphocytes predict sentinel lymph node positivity in patients with cutaneous melanoma. J Clin Oncol. 2007;25(7):869–75.
55. Kunte C, Geimer T, Baumert J, et al. Prognostic factors associated with sentinel lymph node positivity and effect of sentinel status on survival: an analysis of 1049 patients with cutaneous melanoma. Melanoma Res. 2010;20(4):330–7.
56. Faries MB, Wanek LA, Elashoff D, Wright BE, Morton DL. Predictors of occult nodal metastasis in patients with thin melanoma. Arch Surg. 2010;145(2):137–42.
57. Iasonos A, Schrag D, Raj GV, Panageas KS. How to build and interpret a nomogram for cancer prognosis. J Clin Oncol. 2008;26(8):1364–70.
58. Kattan MW, Shariat SF, Andrews B, et al. The addition of interleukin-6 soluble receptor and transforming growth factor beta1 improves a preoperative nomogram for predicting biochemical progression in patients with clinically localized prostate cancer. J Clin Oncol. 2003;21(19):3573–9.

59. Grimm EA, Hoon DSB, McDivitt Duncan L. Biomarkers for melanoma. In: Balch CM, Houghton AN, Sober AJ, Soong S, Atkins MB, Thompson JF, editors. Cutaneous melanoma. St. Louis: Quality Medical Publishing; 2009. p. 883–95.
60. Mihic-Probst D, Mnich CD, Oberholzer PA, et al. P16 expression in primary malignant melanoma is associated with prognosis and lymph node status. Int J Cancer. 2006;118(9):2262–8.
61. Rangel J, Nosrati M, Torabian S, et al. Osteopontin as a molecular prognostic marker for melanoma. Cancer. 2008;112(1):144–50.
62. Simonetti O, Goteri G, Lucarini G, et al. Potential role of CCL27 and CCR10 expression in melanoma progression and immune escape. Eur J Cancer. 2006;42(8):1181–7.
63. Kaariainen E, Nummela P, Soikkeli J, et al. Switch to an invasive growth phase in melanoma is associated with tenascin-C, fibronectin, and procollagen-I forming specific channel structures for invasion. J Pathol. 2006;210(2):181–91.
64. Pearl RA, Pacifico MD, Richman PI, Wilson GD, Grover R. Stratification of patients by melanoma cell adhesion molecule (MCAM) expression on the basis of risk: implications for sentinel lymph node biopsy. J Plast Reconstr Aesthet Surg. 2008;61(3):265–71.
65. Rangel J, Torabian S, Shaikh L, et al. Prognostic significance of nuclear receptor coactivator-3 overexpression in primary cutaneous melanoma. J Clin Oncol. 2006;24(28):4565–9.
66. Weinlich G, Zelger B. Metallothionein overexpression, a highly significant prognostic factor in thin melanoma. Histopathology. 2007;51(2):280–3.
67. Weinlich G, Topar G, Eisendle K, Fritsch PO, Zelger B. Comparison of metallothionein-overexpression with sentinel lymph node biopsy as prognostic factors in melanoma. J Eur Acad Dermatol Venereol. 2007;21(5):669–77.
68. Boone B, Haspeslagh M, Brochez L. Clinical significance of the expression of c-Ski and SnoN, possible mediators in TGF-beta resistance, in primary cutaneous melanoma. J Dermatol Sci. 2009;53(1):26–33.
69. Rangel J, Nosrati M, Leong SP, et al. Novel role for RGS1 in melanoma progression. Am J Surg Pathol. 2008;32(8):1207–12.
70. Liu B, Ma J, Wang X, et al. Lymphangiogenesis and its relationship with lymphatic metastasis and prognosis in malignant melanoma. Anat Rec (Hoboken). 2008;291(10):1227–35.
71. Massi D, Puig S, Franchi A, et al. Tumor lymphangiogenesis is a possible predictor of sentinel lymph node status in cutaneous melanoma: a case-control study. J Clin Pathol. 2006;59(2):166–73.
72. Sahni D, Robson A, Orchard G, Szydlo R, Evans AV, Russell-Jones R. The use of LYVE-1 antibody for detecting lymphatic involvement in patients with malignant melanoma of known sentinel node status. J Clin Pathol. 2005;58(7):715–21.
73. Schacht V, Dadras SS, Johnson LA, Jackson DG, Hong YK, Detmar M. Up-regulation of the lymphatic marker podoplanin, a mucin-type transmembrane glycoprotein, in human squamous cell carcinomas and germ cell tumors. Am J Pathol. 2005;166(3):913–21.
74. Schietroma C, Cianfarani F, Lacal PM, et al. Vascular endothelial growth factor-C expression correlates with lymph node localization of human melanoma metastases. Cancer. 2003;98(4):789–97.
75. Wobser M, Siedel C, Schrama D, Brocker EB, Becker JC, Vetter-Kauczok CS. Expression pattern of the lymphatic and vascular markers VEGFR-3 and CD31 does not predict regional lymph node metastasis in cutaneous melanoma. Arch Dermatol Res. 2006;297(8):352–7.
76. Xu X, Gimotty PA, Guerry D, et al. Lymphatic invasion revealed by multispectral imaging is common in primary melanomas and associates with prognosis. Hum Pathol. 2008;39(6):901–9.
77. Hicklin DJ, Ellis LM. Role of the vascular endothelial growth factor pathway in tumor growth and angiogenesis. J Clin Oncol. 2005;23(5):1011–27.
78. Senger DR, Galli SJ, Dvorak AM, Perruzzi CA, Harvey VS, Dvorak HF. Tumor cells secrete a vascular permeability factor that promotes accumulation of ascites fluid. Science. 1983;219(4587):983–5.
79. Giorgadze TA, Zhang PJ, Pasha T, et al. Lymphatic vessel density is significantly increased in melanoma. J Cutan Pathol. 2004;31(10):672–7.
80. Mehnert JM, McCarthy MM, Jilaveanu L, et al. Quantitative expression of VEGF, VEGFR-1, VEGFR-2, and VEGFR-3 in melanoma tissue microarrays. Hum Pathol. 2010;41(3):375–84.
81. Straume O, Jackson DG, Akslen LA. Independent prognostic impact of lymphatic vessel density and presence of low-grade lymphangiogenesis in cutaneous melanoma. Clin Cancer Res. 2003;9(1):250–6.
82. Brychtova S, Bezdekova M, Brychta T, Tichy M. The role of vascular endothelial growth factors and their receptors in malignant melanomas. Neoplasma. 2008;55(4):273–9.
83. Niakosari F, Kahn HJ, McCready D, et al. Lymphatic invasion identified by monoclonal antibody D2-40, younger age, and ulceration: predictors of sentinel lymph node involvement in primary cutaneous melanoma. Arch Dermatol. 2008;144(4):462–7.
84. Boone B, Blokx W, De Bacquer D, Lambert J, Ruiter D, Brochez L. The role of VEGF-C staining in predicting regional metastasis in melanoma. Virchows Arch. 2008;453(3):257–65.
85. Depasquale I, Thompson WD. Prognosis in human melanoma: Par-1 expression is superior to other coagulation components and VEGF. Histopathology. 2008;52(4):500–9.
86. Chua R, Setzer S, Govindarajan B, Sexton D, Cohen C, Arbiser JL. Maspin expression, angiogenesis, prognostic parameters, and outcome in malignant melanoma. J Am Acad Dermatol. 2009;60(5):758–66.
87. Emmett MS, Symonds KE, Rigby H, et al. Prediction of melanoma metastasis by the Shields index based on lymphatic vessel density. BMC Cancer. 2010;10(1):208.

88. Cook MG, Green MA, Anderson B, et al. The development of optimal pathological assessment of sentinel lymph nodes for melanoma. J Pathol. 2003;200(3):314–9.
89. Scolyer RA, Murali R, McCarthy SW, Thompson JF. Pathologic examination of sentinel lymph nodes from melanoma patients. Semin Diagn Pathol. 2008;25(2):100–11.
90. Cochran AJ, Roberts A, Wen DR, et al. Update on lymphatic mapping and sentinel node biopsy in the management of patients with melanocytic tumors. Pathology. 2004;36(5):478–84.
91. Roberts AA, Cochran AJ. Pathologic analysis of sentinel lymph nodes in melanoma patients: current and future trends. J Surg Oncol. 2004;85(3):152–61.
92. Ranieri JM, Wagner JD, Azuaje R, et al. Prognostic importance of lymph node tumor burden in melanoma patients staged by sentinel node biopsy. Ann Surg Oncol. 2002;9(10):975–81.
93. Carlson GW, Murray DR, Lyles RH, Staley CA, Hestley A, Cohen C. The amount of metastatic melanoma in a sentinel lymph node: does it have prognostic significance? Ann Surg Oncol. 2003;10(5):575–81.
94. Lee JH, Essner R, Torisu-Itakura H, Wanek L, Wang H, Morton DL. Factors predictive of tumor-positive nonsentinel lymph nodes after tumor-positive sentinel lymph node dissection for melanoma. J Clin Oncol. 2004;22(18):3677–84.
95. Sabel MS, Griffith K, Sondak VK, et al. Predictors of nonsentinel lymph node positivity in patients with a positive sentinel node for melanoma. J Am Coll Surg. 2005;201(1):37–47.
96. Pearlman NW, McCarter MD, Frank M, et al. Size of sentinel node metastases predicts other nodal disease and survival in malignant melanoma. Am J Surg. 2006;192(6):878–81.
97. van Akkooi AC, de Wilt JH, Verhoef C, et al. Clinical relevance of melanoma micrometastases (<0.1 mm) in sentinel nodes: are these nodes to be considered negative? Ann Oncol. 2006;17(10):1578–85.
98. Govindarajan A, Ghazarian DM, McCready DR, Leong WL. Histological features of melanoma sentinel lymph node metastases associated with status of the completion lymphadenectomy and rate of subsequent relapse. Ann Surg Oncol. 2007;14(2):906–12.
99. Debarbieux S, Duru G, Dalle S, Beatrix O, Balme B, Thomas L. Sentinel lymph node biopsy in melanoma: a micromorphometric study relating to prognosis and completion lymph node dissection. Br J Dermatol. 2007;157(1):58–67.
100. Scheri RP, Essner R, Turner RR, Ye X, Morton DL. Isolated tumor cells in the sentinel node affect long-term prognosis of patients with melanoma. Ann Surg Oncol. 2007;14(10):2861–6.
101. Roka F, Mastan P, Binder M, et al. Prediction of nonsentinel node status and outcome in sentinel node-positive melanoma patients. Eur J Surg Oncol. 2008;34(1):82–8.
102. Satzger I, Volker B, Al Ghazal M, Meier A, Kapp A, Gutzmer R. Prognostic significance of histopathological parameters in sentinel nodes of melanoma patients. Histopathology. 2007;50(6):764–72.
103. Guggenheim M, Dummer R, Jung FJ, et al. The influence of sentinel lymph node tumor burden on additional lymph node involvement and disease-free survival in cutaneous melanoma–a retrospective analysis of 392 cases. Br J Cancer. 2008;98(12):1922–8.
104. Glumac N, Hocevar M, Zadnik V, Snoj M. Sentinel lymph node micrometastasis may predict non-sentinel involvement in cutaneous melanoma patients. J Surg Oncol. 2008;98(1):46–8.
105. Starz H, Siedlecki K, Balda BR. Sentinel lymphadenectomy and S-classification: a successful strategy for better prediction and improvement of outcome of melanoma. Ann Surg Oncol. 2004;11(3 Suppl):162S–8.
106. Fink AM, Weihsengruber F, Spangl B, et al. S-classification of sentinel lymph node biopsy predicts the results of complete regional lymph node dissection. Melanoma Res. 2005;15(4):267–71.
107. Satzger I, Volker B, Meier A, Kapp A, Gutzmer R. Criteria in sentinel lymph nodes of melanoma patients that predict involvement of nonsentinel lymph nodes. Ann Surg Oncol. 2008;15(6):1723–32.
108. van der Ploeg IM, Kroon BB, Antonini N, Valdes Olmos RA, Nieweg OE. Is completion lymph node dissection needed in case of minimal melanoma metastasis in the sentinel node? Ann Surg. 2009;249(6):1003–7.
109. Dewar DJ, Newell B, Green MA, Topping AP, Powell BW, Cook MG. The microanatomic location of metastatic melanoma in sentinel lymph nodes predicts nonsentinel lymph node involvement. J Clin Oncol. 2004;22(16):3345–9.
110. Frankel TL, Griffith KA, Lowe L, et al. Do micromorphometric features of metastatic deposits within sentinel nodes predict nonsentinel lymph node involvement in melanoma? Ann Surg Oncol. 2008;15(9):2403–11.
111. Cochran AJ, Wen DR, Huang RR, Wang HJ, Elashoff R, Morton DL. Prediction of metastatic melanoma in nonsentinel nodes and clinical outcome based on the primary melanoma and the sentinel node. Mod Pathol. 2004;17(7):747–55.
112. Vuylsteke RJ, Borgstein PJ, van Leeuwen PA, et al. Sentinel lymph node tumor load: an independent predictor of additional lymph node involvement and survival in melanoma. Ann Surg Oncol. 2005;12(6):440–8.
113. Reeves ME, Delgado R, Busam KJ, Brady MS, Coit DG. Prediction of nonsentinel lymph node status in melanoma. Ann Surg Oncol. 2003;10(1):27–31.
114. Starz H, Balda BR, Kramer KU, Buchels H, Wang H. A micromorphometry-based concept for routine classification of sentinel lymph node metastases and its clinical relevance for patients with melanoma. Cancer. 2001;91(11):2110–21.

115. Spillane AJ, Winstanley J, Thompson JF. Lymph node ratio in melanoma: a marker of variation in surgical quality? Cancer. 2009;115(11):2384–7.
116. Wiener M, Acland KM, Shaw HM, et al. Sentinel node positive melanoma patients: prediction and prognostic significance of nonsentinel node metastases and development of a survival tree model. Ann Surg Oncol. 2010;17(8):1995–2005.
117. Murali R, Cochran AJ, Cook MG, et al. Interobserver reproducibility of histologic parameters of melanoma deposits in sentinel lymph nodes: implications for management of patients with melanoma. Cancer. 2009;115(21):5026–37.
118. Di Tommaso L, Arizzi C, Rahal D, et al. Anatomic location of breast cancer micrometastasis in sentinel lymph node predicts axillary status. Ann Surg. 2006;243(5):706–7. author reply 706–707.
119. Franco R, Cantile M, Scala S, et al. Histomorphologic parameters and CXCR4 mRNA and protein expression in sentinel node melanoma metastasis are correlated to clinical outcome. Cancer Biol Ther. 2010;9(6):423–9.
120. Scolyer RA, Mihm MC, Cochran AJ, Busam KJ, McCarthy MM. Pathology of melanoma. In: Balch CM, Houghton AB, Sober A, Soong S, Atkins MB, Thompson JF, editors. Cutaneous melanoma. St. Louis: Quality Medical Publishing; 2009. p. 205–48.
121. Goydos JS, Ravikumar TS, Germino FJ, Yudd A, Bancila E. Minimally invasive staging of patients with melanoma: sentinel lymphadenectomy and detection of the melanoma-specific proteins MART-1 and tyrosinase by reverse transcriptase polymerase chain reaction. J Am Coll Surg. 1998;187(2):182–8. discussion 188–190.
122. Blaheta HJ, Schittek B, Breuninger H, et al. Detection of melanoma micrometastasis in sentinel nodes by reverse transcription-polymerase chain reaction correlates with tumor thickness and is predictive of micrometastatic disease in the lymph node basin. Am J Surg Pathol. 1999;23(7):822–8.
123. Blaheta HJ, Ellwanger U, Schittek B, et al. Examination of regional lymph nodes by sentinel node biopsy and molecular analysis provides new staging facilities in primary cutaneous melanoma. J Invest Dermatol. 2000;114(4):637–42.
124. Palmieri G, Ascierto PA, Cossu A, et al. Detection of occult melanoma cells in paraffin-embedded histologically negative sentinel lymph nodes using a reverse transcriptase polymerase chain reaction assay. J Clin Oncol. 2001;19(5):1437–43.
125. Boi S, Cristofolini P, Togni R, et al. Detection of nodal micrometastases using immunohistochemistry and PCR in melanoma of the arm and trunk. Melanoma Res. 2002;12(2):147–53.
126. Goydos JS. Prevention and early diagnosis of cutaneous melanoma. N J Med. 2000;97(5):37–40.
127. Kuo CT, Hoon DS, Takeuchi H, et al. Prediction of disease outcome in melanoma patients by molecular analysis of paraffin-embedded sentinel lymph nodes. J Clin Oncol. 2003;21(19):3566–72.
128. Rimoldi D, Lemoine R, Kurt AM, et al. Detection of micrometastases in sentinel lymph nodes from melanoma patients: direct comparison of multimarker molecular and immunopathological methods. Melanoma Res. 2003;13(5):511–20.
129. Starz H, Haas CJ, Schulz GM, Balda BR. Tyrosinase RT-PCR as a supplement to histology for detecting melanoma and nevus cells in paraffin sections of sentinel lymph nodes. Mod Pathol. 2003;16(9):920–9.
130. Blaheta HJ, Roeger S, Sotlar K, et al. Additional reverse transcription-polymerase chain reaction of peripheral slices is not superior to analysis of the central slice in sentinel lymph nodes from melanoma patients. Br J Dermatol. 2004;150(3):477–83.
131. Takeuchi H, Morton DL, Kuo C, et al. Prognostic significance of molecular upstaging of paraffin-embedded sentinel lymph nodes in melanoma patients. J Clin Oncol. 2004;22(13):2671–80.
132. Ulrich J, Bonnekoh B, Bockelmann R, et al. Prognostic significance of detecting micrometastases by tyrosinase RT/PCR in sentinel lymph node biopsies: lessons from 322 consecutive melanoma patients. Eur J Cancer. 2004;40(18):2812–9.
133. Abrahamsen HN, Sorensen BS, Nexo E, Hamilton-Dutoit SJ, Larsen J, Steiniche T. Pathologic assessment of melanoma sentinel nodes: a role for molecular analysis using quantitative real-time reverse transcription-PCR for MART-1 and tyrosinase messenger RNA. Clin Cancer Res. 2005;11(4):1425–33.
134. Giese T, Engstner M, Mansmann U, Hartschuh W, Arden B. Quantification of melanoma micrometastases in sentinel lymph nodes using real-time RT-PCR. J Invest Dermatol. 2005;124(3):633–7.
135. Romanini A, Manca G, Pellegrino D, et al. Molecular staging of the sentinel lymph node in melanoma patients: correlation with clinical outcome. Ann Oncol. 2005;16(11):1832–40.
136. Mangas C, Hilari JM, Paradelo C, et al. Prognostic significance of molecular staging study of sentinel lymph nodes by reverse transcriptase-polymerase chain reaction for tyrosinase in melanoma patients. Ann Surg Oncol. 2006;13(7):910–8.
137. Denninghoff VC, Falco J, Kahn AG, Trouchot V, Curutchet HP, Elsner B. Sentinel node in melanoma patients: triple negativity with routine techniques and PCR as positive prognostic factor for survival. Mod Pathol. 2008;21(4):438–44.
138. Riber-Hansen R, Abrahamsen HN, Sorensen BS, Hamilton-Dutoit SJ, Steiniche T. Quantitative real-time RT-PCR in sentinel lymph nodes from melanoma patients. Detection of melanocytic mRNA predicts disease-free survival. APMIS. 2008;116(3):199–205.
139. Nowecki ZI, Rutkowski P, Kulik J, Siedlecki JA, Ruka W. Molecular and biochemical testing in stage III melanoma: multimarker reverse transcriptase-polymerase chain reaction assay of lymph fluid after lymph node dissection and preoperative serum lactate dehydrogenase level. Br J Dermatol. 2008;159(3):597–605.

140. Hilari JM, Mangas C, Xi L, et al. Molecular staging of pathologically negative sentinel lymph nodes from melanoma patients using multimarker, quantitative real-time RT-PCR. Ann Surg Oncol. 2009; 16(1):177–85.
141. Mocellin S, Hoon D, Ambrosi A, Nitti D, Rossi CR. The prognostic value of circulating tumor cells in patients with melanoma: a systematic review and meta-analysis. Clin Cancer Res. 2006;12(15): 4605–13.
142. Balch CM, Gershenwald JE, Soong SJ, et al. Final version of 2009 AJCC melanoma staging and classification. J Clin Oncol. 2009;27(36):6199–206.
143. Balch CM, Gershenwald JE, Soong SJ, et al. Multivariate analysis of prognostic factors among 2,313 patients with stage III melanoma: comparison of nodal micrometastases versus macrometastases. J Clin Oncol. 2010;28(14):2452–9.
144. Mocellin S, Pasquali S, Rossi CR, Nitti D. Interferon alpha adjuvant therapy in patients with high-risk melanoma: a systematic review and meta-analysis. J Natl Cancer Inst. 2010;102(7):493–501.
145. Eggermont AM, Suciu S, Santinami M, et al. Adjuvant therapy with pegylated interferon alfa-2b versus observation alone in resected stage III melanoma: final results of EORTC 18991, a randomised phase III trial. Lancet. 2008;372(9633): 117–26.
146. Grob JJ, Dreno B, de la Salmoniere P, et al. Randomised trial of interferon alpha-2a as adjuvant therapy in resected primary melanoma thicker than 1.5 mm without clinically detectable node metastases. French Cooperative Group on Melanoma. Lancet. 1998;351(9120):1905–10.
147. Pehamberger H, Soyer HP, Steiner A, et al. Adjuvant interferon alfa-2a treatment in resected primary stage II cutaneous melanoma. Austrian Malignant Melanoma Cooperative Group. J Clin Oncol. 1998; 16(4):1425–9.
148. McMasters KM, Ross MI, Reintgen DS, et al. Final results of the Sunbelt Melanoma Trial. 2008 ASCO Annual Meeting Proceedings. J Clin Oncol. 2008;26(Suppl):9003.

Melanoma Cell Propagation: Cancer Stem Cell, Clonal Evolution and Interconversion Models of Tumorigenicity

Qiuzhen Liu, Marianna Sabatino, David F. Stroncek, Ping Jin, Francesco M. Marincola, and Ena Wang

Melanoma is a significant health problem worldwide. Available treatments can induce transient tumor regression in a small percentage of patients; however, these responses are not always associated with improved long-term survival. The mechanisms underlying therapeutic resistance and tumor recurrence in melanoma are still elusive. Tumor escape as a result of cancer cell heterogeneity and genomic instability may explain the persistence of disease despite an apparent primary response to therapy. For a long time, the accumulation of random mutations was believed to be associated with progressive transformation of normal cells into malignant cells, based on a classic "survival of the fittest" evolutionary model. Among other factors, these genetic alterations were also believed to be responsible for the acquisition of drug resistance during treatment. Recent progress in cancer research suggests that melanomas, as for other solid tumors, contain a subpopulation of cells which have unlimited self-renewal capability, based on their direct descent from an original founder cell and characterized by relatively stable genetic properties throughout disease evolution. This model also applies to the development of each individual metastasis and, as we will discuss, may be responsible for drug resistance and cancer recurrence. These cells with tumor-initiating ability are termed cancer stem cells (CSCs). However, with few exceptions, no universal CSC marker has been identified. Different technologies and methods employed to identify biomarkers characterizing CSCs have produced inconsistent results, even in those instances when the same cancer type was being investigated. Therefore, there is a need to reevaluate the criteria and models used to identify CSCs in order to advance this field of research. This chapter provides an overview of the advances and challenges in melanoma stem cell (MSC) research. In addition, the clonal evolution and interconversion (cancer cell plasticity) models for tumorigenicity will be discussed. Current evidence suggests that all these models of cancer progression may be relevant to melanoma pathobiology.

Q. Liu, M.D., Ph.D. • F.M. Marincola, M.D.
• E. Wang, M.D. (✉)
Infectious Disease and Immunogenetics Section (IDIS),
Clinical Center, National Institutes of Health,
Bethesda, MD, USA
e-mail: ewang@mail.nih.gov

M. Sabatino, M.D. • D.F. Stroncek, M.D. • P. Jin, Ph.D.
Cell Processing Section, Department of Transfusion Medicine, Clinical Center, National Institutes of Health,
Bethesda, MD, USA

Introduction

The incidence of melanoma has been increasing over the past several decades. In USA, the lifetime risk of melanoma in the year 2000 was estimated at 1 in 75 individuals [1]. Patients with advanced disease have a poor prognosis, with a reported median survival ranging between 3 and

11 months. For these patients, immunotherapy [systemic high-dose interleukin (IL)-2 or interferon (IFN)-α], antigen-specific immunization and/or chemotherapy (dacarbazine or temozolomide) show responses in only 5–20% of cases [2, 3]. Adoptive transfer of autologous tumor-infiltrating lymphocytes following myeloablative/lymphodepleting regimens has been reported to induce objective tumor regression in ~60% of selected patients [4–6]. However, in most cases, these responses do not result in overall survival benefit, as the large majority of patients die with relapsing disease that is often resistant to further therapeutic intervention. It has been hypothesized that the stubborn recurrence of cancer, following a primary response to treatment, is likely due to the survival of a subset of tumor cells that display an intrinsic resistance to treatment-induced cell apoptosis [7, 8]. The existence of cancer stem cells (CSCs), which are characterized by a less differentiated state and lower immunogenicity (i.e., resistance to immune rejection) [9], might explain cancer relapse and resistance to therapy [8, 10]. It is important to note that the term "cancer stem cells" is more of a functional definition, created to define a subgroup of cancer cells which can self-renew, initiate tumors, and differentiate into a heterogeneous progeny that maintain some similarity to the original tissue from which they derived. Unlike normal stem cells, CSCs share the accumulated genomic instability that is responsible for tumor development and acquire additional genetic alterations required to promote malignant progression [11].

The concept of CSCs and the hierarchical model of tumorigenesis have implications for our understanding of tumor biology and the development of more effective anti-cancer treatments. However, different methods employing distinct putative biomarkers for the identification of CSCs, particularly in melanoma, have yielded conflicting results. It is important to understand the criteria and models used for the identification of CSCs in melanoma and the reasons for the variable results reported by different studies. The purpose of this chapter is to provide an overview of advances in melanoma stem cell (MSC) research and highlight unresolved issues. The potential relevance of MSCs to the initiation, progression, and response to treatment in melanoma will be discussed. The concepts of clonal evolution and interconversion as they relate to melanoma propagation will also be described.

Research on Cancer Stem Cells (CSCs)

Identification of CSCs

As a reflection of their genomic instability, cancer cells are both phenotypically and functionally heterogeneous. Individual clones with higher survival and proliferation potential eventually become dominant within a given tumor population (clonal evolution model of cancer development) [12]. In recent years, CSCs have been described in several human tumors, including melanoma. This term refers to a subset of tumor cells that have the ability to self-renew and generate diverse progenies with decreasing proliferative potential. Both CSCs and their progenies contribute to tumor heterogeneity and the differential responses seen with anti-cancer therapy.

With the availability of a broad range of differentiation markers for hematopoietic cells, CSCs were first identified in hematopoietic malignant disease. Normal hematopoietic cell development is organized according to a hierarchical model that is sustained by a small population of quiescent, multi-potential stem cells which are capable of self-renewal and differentiation into all cell types of the hematopoietic system. Hematopoietic cells can be characterized by a panel of markers that are distinctive for each cell type. Using an animal model of bone marrow radio-ablation, Goodell et al. [13] observed that only $CD34^+/CD38^-$ cells could regenerate whole blood cells, providing a basis for more detailed phenotypic and functional characterization of hematopoietic stem cells (HSCs). This animal model also facilitated the identification of CSCs in leukemia and other malignant hematopoietic diseases. Lapidot et al. [14] subsequently observed that a subset of human acute myeloid leukemia cells with a $CD34^+/CD38^-$ phenotype could initiate disease when engrafted in severe combined immunodeficiency (SCID) mice. Others investigators have confirmed that engrafted $CD34^+/CD38^-/Lin^-$ cells could differentiate and reconstitute the heterogeneous phenotype that was observed in the original tumor [15]. Moreover, serial transplantations have demonstrated that these cells possess self-renewal capacity. Such studies have provided evidence of the existence of cells with stem cell-like properties in leukemia. The presence of malignancy-initiating cells, termed leukemia stem cells, was subsequently demonstrated in other malignant hematopoietic diseases [14–19].

The isolation of CSCs from the metastatic pleural effusions of a breast cancer patient by Al-Hajj et al. [16] represented the first demonstration of CSCs in a solid tumor. These investigators observed that $CD44^+/CD24^-/ESA^+$ cells, but not $CD44^+/CD24^+/ESA^+$ cells, had tumor-initiating capacity in immunodeficient mice, with regenerated tumors recapturing the phenotypic heterogeneity of the original tumor. Moreover, only $CD44^+/CD24^-/ESA^+$ cells demonstrated the potential for self-renewal following serial transplantation in immunodeficient mice. This finding might explain why CSCs within breast cancers, although infrequently found among malignant cells, may be responsible for the initiation and maintenance of tumor masses. Subsequently, Hemmati et al. [20] identified brain tumor-derived progenitor cells. Neuron stem cells were successfully cultured *in vitro* using specific culture media, growing and expanding as undifferentiated neurospheres. With the same culture media, it was found that brain tumor cells could also grow as neurospheres. Of note, the enrichment of cancer cell neurospheres with $CD133^+$ cells resulted in a high potential for proliferation *in vitro* and tumorigenicity in immunodeficient mice. $CD133^+$ cells were also noted to produce both $CD133^+$ and $CD133^-$ cells, but only passed on the potential for tumorigenicity to their $CD133^+$ progeny [21]. CSCs have been subsequently identified in variety of human tumors, including glioblastoma, medulloblastoma, squamous cell carcinoma, pancreatic cancer, colon cancer, lung cancer, liver cancer, and melanoma [22–29].

Methods for the Identification of CSCs

Candidate CSCs are often isolated from fresh human tumor samples, where they appear to be more hierarchically structured and more phenotypically stable than under *in vitro* cell culture conditions. Surface markers are essential for candidate CSC isolation and are similar to those used to identify their normal counterparts. For example, CD34 expression is shared by normal and malignant hematopoietic stem cells [30, 31]. CD133 is the most common biomarker employed for the isolation of normal adult stem cells and CSCs [32, 33]. $CD133^+$ cells have high proliferative capacity and are often observed to be in the G_2/M phases of the cell cycle. Accordingly, fluorescence-activated cell sorting (FACS) is the most commonly employed enrichment method to distinguish $CD133^+$ from $CD133^-$ cells in CSC studies. Most biomarkers for adult stem cells or candidate CSCs in human tissues have not been conclusively validated. Therefore, other methods for CSC enrichment are often employed. These include the use of special culture media, which favor the growth of CSCs among other cancer cell types and prevent cellular differentiation and/or apoptosis.

Flow cytometric analysis, based on the expression of ATP-binding cassette (ABC) transporters, has also been used for CSC isolation. This method identifies a side population (SP), as first observed by Goodell et al. [13]. Using the DNA dye Hoechst 33342, two populations of hematopoietic cells can be identified: one which is stained strongly by the dye and another with minimal staining. The latter is referred to as an SP. The SP is dependent upon the expression of ABC transporter family members, such as ABCG2. ABC transporters are transmembrane molecules which translocate a broad spectrum of molecules across the cell membrane and participate in diverse cellular processes, including drug resistance and metabolism [34]. Stem cells express higher levels of the ABC transporters than their differentiated counterparts. This may represent a mechanism by which CSCs are protected from the action of cytotoxic agents. This SP represents a fraction of the whole cancer cell population, but it is highly enriched with stem cells. FACS-based identification of CSCs as an SP is now widely employed as it does not require the use of specific biomarkers. Obviously, this is particularly useful in instances where a validated biomarker is unavailable, such as in MSC isolation studies [35].

The sphere cell formation assay (SCA) is another technique employed in many normal stem cell and CSC studies [36, 37]. Fang et al. [38] reported that both fresh melanoma specimens and melanoma cell lines could grow and propagate as non-adherent spherical aggregates. Unlike their counterparts cultured in RPMI 1640, multi-potential sphere melanoma cells can differentiate along multiple mesenchymal lineages (i.e., adipogenic, chondrogenic and osteogenic), suggesting that these cells possess certain mesenchymal stem cell properties. Moreover, melanoma cells grown as spheres in culture could also form xenografts when injected into immunodeficient mice, suggesting an MSC phenotype. However, as a caveat, non-sphere forming cells were not investigated for their potential ability to initiate xenografts in these experiments.

By demonstrating their self-renewal capacities, the cancer-initiating capability of isolated candidate CSCs can be confirmed (i.e., functional validation). This is commonly performed by testing their potential to initiate xenografts following serial transplantation in immunodeficient mice. Limiting dilutions of transplanted cells are used to evaluate CSC frequency in a given tumor cell population. Theoretically, no xenografts should grow following the injection of any concentration of non-CSCs. However, technical limitations in the purification of non-CSCs often do not allow for the isolation of a pure non-CSC population. Therefore, in the CSC model, only a high rate of xenograft initiation by CSCs compared to non-CSCs in considered significant.

Animal Models for the Identification of CSCs

Since the molecular characteristics and unique biomarkers specific for CSCs are still in discovery phases, the identification of CSCs remains heavily dependent on functional assays [39]. To effectively exert their properties of self-renewal and generation of differentiated progeny, both normal stem cells and CSCs require a favorable local environment, commonly referred to as a "niche". Niches are specific anatomical locations that provide a nurturing microenvironment for stem cell growth, by nourishing them, protecting them from apoptosis, and regulating the differentiation of their progeny. Niches are comprised of fibroblasts, endothelial cells and extracellular matrix; with each type of stem cell possessing a distinct relationship with its own niche cell population [40]. Stem cells, their progeny, and other components of the niche work together as a functional unit. Stem cells either cannot function or function less effectively in the absence of a niche [41]. Although, niches have been well characterized in different model systems of normal stem cells, little is known about the microenvironmental requirements that are conducive to CSC niche development [42].

Attempts to create a self-organizing niche in mice xenograft experiments, which could favor the establishment of CSC-initiated tumors, have been made through the co-infusion of potential "helper" cells [43]. An infusion of breast cancer cells together with human mesenchymal cells can greatly reduce the number of cells required to initiate tumors, suggesting that this co-injection may provide a tool to develop a "niche-like" environment in the mouse recipient. In fact, the cancer microenvironment is characterized by an intricate network of distinct supporting cells, including fibroblasts, endothelial cells, macrophages, mesenchymal stem cells, and their products, including cytokines and their respective receptors. However, the tumor microenvironment, a putative CSC niche, remains different from a normal stem cell niche; the latter supporting a steady-state number of stem cells and their progeny. In normal tissues, the niche maintains an organized structure where the self-renewal capabilities of stem cells are highly regulated. In contrast, the cancer microenvironment has no capacity to regulate the growth, differentiation and/or self-renewal capacity of CSCs. It is hypothesized that tissue niches, which are responsible for normal stem cell growth and behavior, could nurture early CSCs in primary tumors; while in metastatic lesions, migrating CSCs may be able to prime the target tissue and re-establish a surrogate niche that facilitates their growth and differentiation. Such a surrogate might not have the complete repertoire of factors which regulate the function of a normal stem cell niche.

In CSC validation models, immunodeficient mice provide an environment that is conducive to their engraftment. This environment, however, cannot be equated to that of normal stem cell niches. Cancer cells with greater survival potential, proliferative capacity and autocrine growth factor production are likely to preferentially grow and form tumors in immunodeficient mice. The frequency of xenograft tumor initiation depends not only on the intrinsic self-renewal capabilities of CSCs, but also on the anti-apoptotic status of cancer cells and their autocrine production of growth factors [44]. Tumor growth alone cannot be used as surrogate proof that the implant contained populations of CSCs. Animal models may be used to test the functional properties of putative CSCs (i.e., their self-renewal and tumor-initiation capacity), when injected under controlled experimental conditions. However, they are not useful in the qualitative identification of pure CSC populations.

Three Theories for the Phenotypic and Functional Heterogeneity of Tumor Cells

Tumor heterogeneity may be one reason for the differential responses to treatment and the survival of some, but not all, cancer cells following a given therapy [44–46]. A number of models have been proposed to explain the phenotypic and functional heterogeneity that is found among the cells within a given malignant neoplasm, including melanoma. These include (1) the clonal evolution model; (2) CSC model; and (3) the concept of cancer cell plasticity, also known as interconversion [45].

According to the clonal evolution model, tumor heterogeneity results from the continuous development of different clones as a function of cancer cell genomic instability [45, 46]. Clones with high potential for proliferation and survival are preferentially selected, and demonstrate enhanced growth and/or metastatic potential. While clonal populations are being established, the ancestral clone gradually disappears and the original genetics of the progenitor cell that initiated the cancer are lost. According to this theory, drug resistance is due to the stochastic development of a clonal population bearing genetic and/or epigenetic aberrations. Therefore, evolution theory-based strategies to prevent cancer recurrence focus on the discovery of a putative drug resistance gene or an epigenetic alteration that could be targeted, and assume its presence in all cancer cells.

According to the CSC theory, cancer cells are hierarchically organized, with CSCs sitting at the top. In contrast to the clonal evolution model, CSCs have a relatively stable genome; thereby, maintaining more faithfully the genetic makeup of the ancestral founder cell. At the same time, drug resistance is an intrinsic property of these cells that is related to their functional status and not a result of selection during a specific therapy. Based on the CSC theory, drug resistance should be considered at the outset of any therapy, if tumor eradication is to be achieved. According to this model, heterogeneity in the cancer cell population is dependent predominantly on differentiation of the CSC progeny and is somewhat irrelevant to resistance development, since these diverse cancer cells have limited self-renewal capacity and their long-term survival and colony formation is unlikely. This is a relatively well-recognized phenomenon *in vitro*, where individual cell cultures at a given time are less genetically similar compared with cultures of the same cell lines after multiple passages [47].

Cancer cell plasticity or interconversion describes the ability of cancer cells to "switch" between different phenotypic states that may be associated with more or less aggressive behaviors and differential responses to treatment [45]. The development of a population of cancer cells with limited self-renewal capability is conceptualized by a stepwise progression from CSCs, to transit-amplifying (TA) cells, to differentiated cancer cells. These three-cell stages are similar at the genomic level, but differ in their transcriptional and translational profiles [48]. In addition, these stages may have different sensitivities to drug treatment, and cooperate within their niche to survive cytotoxic agents.

As described by Shackleton et al. [45], it is likely that these three proposed models of tumor cell heterogeneity are not mutually exclusive. An individual cancer, including melanoma, may employ one or more of them, either simultaneously or at different times, during its evolution and progression. For example, if differentiated cancer cells and/or TA cells are eliminated by an anticancer agent, the CSCs can regenerate new cells. As discussed in a later section, should CSCs be destroyed, TA cells might dedifferentiate to regenerate them. Importantly, CSCs are believed to be more resistant to chemotherapeutic agents, as they are more frequently found in the G_0 phase of the cell cycle and display constitutively activated drug resistance mechanisms [49].

Melanoma Stem Cells (MSCs)

The Development of Melanoma

Stem cells of melanocytic lineage are derived from the neural crest and migrate to the hair follicle or the basal layer of the epidermis during embryonic development. At these sites, they remain in a quiescent state or asymmetrically divide when required; with one remaining as a steady-state stem cell, while the other becomes a TA cell which proliferates and eventually produces a progeny of differentiated melanocytes. TA melanocytes further differentiate into pigmented melanocytes, which are interspersed among basilar keratinocytes in the epidermis at a ratio of approximately 1:35, forming "epidermal-melanin units" [50]. TA melanocytes maintain a partial self-renewal capability, and can return to a quiescent state in the hair bulge area if the original stem cells are absent. Although they have similar properties, TA cells are different from the originating stem cells [51]. In fact, in contrast to TA cells, melanocyte stem cells globally suppress transcription, including that of "melanocyte-specific" genes, such as MLANA and SILV, but express embryonic stem cells markers, such as NESTIN, SLUG, SNAIL, TWIST, SOX9, BMP4, NANOG, and OCT4, which are less consistently expressed by TA cells [50, 52, 53]. Furthermore, under appropriate conditions, melanocyte stem cells are capable of differentiating not only into melanocytes, but also into neuronal and smooth muscle cells, demonstrating their potential plasticity.

Cancer arises as result of the accumulation of genetic and/or epigenetic alterations. Importantly, mutations of critical growth regulatory genes contribute to tumor initiation and progression [54, 55]. Ras/Raf/MEK/ERK signaling is one of the most critical signaling pathways for melanoma proliferation, with hyper-activation of ERK identified in up to 90% of melanomas. BRAF mutations are found in 50–70% of melanomas and drive ERK signaling activation. Besides this common initiation mechanism, the transforming cell needs to accumulate additional genetic and/or epigenetic changes in order to develop its full malignant potential, with this process taking years or even decades to occur. There are two models that have been proposed to explain how transformed cells retain their genetic code, while at the same time sequentially accumulating further genetic mutations that could be relevant or irrelevant to their survival: (1) one model describes the long-term survival of the founder(s) cell, and (2) the other suggests the continuous passage of genetic alterations through serial cell divisions that proceed vertically, generation by generation. Because of their intrinsic long-term survival in the host and ability to generate a progeny, adult melanocyte stem cells and TA melanocytes are the critical target cells for melanoma development, since mature differentiated melanocytes are the least likely to survive long enough to accumulate the required repertoire of genetic alterations for fully fledged malignant transformation [56]. Mutated melanocyte stem cells transform into MSCs and pass their self-renewal capacity on to them [56].

CSCs derived from normal stem cells would be expected to bear markers similar to those borne by the latter, whereas CSCs derived from differentiated cells might express differentiation-related markers. In fact, CSCs identified in different types of cancers have been found to share several phenotypic characteristics with their normal counterparts [57]. For example, mouse leukemias (induced by the fusion gene products MLL-AF9 and MOA-TIR2) are reported to contain leukemogenic cells with a phenotype closer to differentiated hematopoietic cells than HSCs [58]. However, this may not always be the case. In mouse models, mammary CSCs display lower expression of CD29 compared to normal mouse mammary stem cells [59]. As we will see later, the situation in the case of melanoma remains unclear.

It has been suggested that a reversal of genetic and/or epigenetic alterations could allow terminally differentiated cells to dedifferentiate back into stem cells. For instance, quail embryo melanocytic cells can dedifferentiate into multipotential stem cells [60]. Furthermore, it is possible to transform cultured differentiated normal melanocytes into MSCs through the introduction of oncogenes [61, 62]. However, the question remains whether these populations of differentiated melanocytes contained a small percentage of normal melanocytic stem cells or TA cells that could account for their plasticity. Clarification of this point is difficult because the cancer genome may be characterized by sporadic alterations which do not necessarily contribute to malignant transformation, but are rather due to the stochastic accumulation of mutations related to genomic instability. These "irrelevant" genetic patterns confound our understanding of tumor progression according to the CSC hypothesis, as it is difficult to distinguish variable phenotypes derived from random genetic alteration from unidirectional progression. Genomic analysis of metachronous melanoma metastases from a single patient, who underwent repeated treatments and experienced several recurrences over a decade, demonstrated that all metastatic lesions shared a core genetic pattern derived from the original progenitor cell, in addition to unique genetic alterations which appeared and disappeared over time without following a sequential pattern [63, 64]. Thus, only a small proportion of the molecular and cellular make-up of any cancer is likely due to alterations that promote its malignant behavior. However, these specific "driver" mutations may be difficult to identify unless the long-term progression of the disease can be followed, as was possible in this rare case [63, 64].

It may be that the driving genetics of cancer are regulated by key transcription factors which control the pluripotent state [65, 66]. Mouse and human somatic cells can be reprogrammed to a pluripotent-like state by ectopic expression of a variety of proteins, such as OCT4, SOX2, KLF4, c-MYC, NANOG and LIN28 [67–72]. However, successful reprogramming could include the sequential accumulation of epigenetic alterations that are acquired during culture and are similar to those arising during normal stem cell development. Though genetic and epigenetic changes are essential to the development of melanoma, a distinction between pure normal stem cells, CSCs and differentiated cells with pluripotent-like phenotypes may be difficult, as all these cells overlap within a continuum of molecular alterations of hierarchically decreasing relevance.

MSC Markers and Limitations

In many cases, CSC marker profiles are similar to those of their normal stem cell counterparts. For example, both human mammary stem cells and mammary CSCs lack CD24 expression [16, 57, 73]. Similarly, human acute myeloid leukemia stem cells and normal HSCs are enriched in the $CD34^+/CD38^-$ fraction of the bone marrow [14]. Markers of normal melanocyte stem cells have not yet been identified. Therefore, putative markers for MSCs have been deduced, based on our knowledge of prevalent stem cell markers and common methods used for identifying CSCs in other cancer systems. As we will discuss later in this chapter, the adoption of neuronal crest markers points to CD271 (neural crest nerve growth factor receptor) as a useful MSC marker [74].

The SCA assay used by Fang et al. [38] demonstrated that melanoma spheres are negative for embryonic, endothelial, neural and hematopoietic stem cells markers, such as SSEA-3, TRA-1-80, TRA-1-60, vWF, CD31, CD34, VEGFR2, GAP-43, CD56/NCAM, CD3, CD4, CD8, and CD45; but positive for melanoma-associated markers, including MCAM, SOX10 and MITF. This study also found that melanoma spheres are enriched with CD20+ cells [38]. CD20 is present in ~20% of human melanoma specimens and it is possible that this marker identifies a subpopulation of melanoma-initiating cells. Na et al. [75] reported that melanoma sphere cells from WM-266-4 (a highly metastatic melanoma cell line) express stem cell markers, such as ABCG2, BMI1, WNT5A, CD133, NESTIN, SCF, PROX1 and VEGFR3. However, the authors were unable to demonstrate differential tumorigenicity between WM-266-4 sphere cells and their non-sphere counterparts, since this cell line is characterized by high intrinsic tumorigenicity.

MSCs Identified According to Tumorigenic Potential

As a result of insufficient validated MSC markers, the distinction of MSCs from non-MSCs relies on their tumor-initiation capability. Monzani et al. [76] demonstrated that distinct subsets of CD133+ cells (0.2–0.8% of the overall melanoma cell population) existed in seven human melanoma specimens. Following injection of a nonobese diabetic (NOD)-SCID mouse with 1×10^5 CD133+ melanoma cells on one side and the same number of CD133− melanoma cells on the other, the authors determined that tumor growth only occurred in the former. Monzani et al. [76] also reported that the WM115 melanoma cell line, which shows 100% positivity for CD133+, possesses many stem cell-like properties, including the expression of neurogenic markers and an ability to differentiate into various mesenchymal lineages. Moreover, WM155 cells can grow as spheres in serum-free media. More importantly, when injected into immunodeficient mice, they form tumors that include a progeny of differentiated CD133− cells [76]. CD133 is a commonly used marker of normal stem cells and CSCs, including MSCs [77]. It has been reported that CD133+ melanoma cells not only have enhanced tumorigenic potential in mice, but also express higher levels of angiogenic and lymphangiogenic genes, promoting melanoma initiation and metastasis [77]. Klein et al. [78] observed that CD133+ melanoma cells show over-expression of both CD166 and NESTIN compared with melanocytic nevus cells.

MDR1, a multi-drug resistance gene and member of the ABC transporter family, has been reported to be enriched in melanoma sphere cells, representing 1.3–9.7% of the entire cellular population [79]. These multi-drug resistance gene-expressing cells show co-expression of a number of stem cell markers, such as ABCB5, NANOG and hTERT, but interestingly are negative for CD133. The expression of multi-drug resistance-associated genes may have significant implications regarding the responsiveness of MSCs to therapy [8].

Schatton et al. [25] suggested that ABCB5 (an ABC transporter that mediates resistance to doxorubicin) is an MSC marker and demonstrated that its expression correlated with clinical progression in melanoma patients. This marker is reported to be expressed by 1.6–20.4% of cells in melanoma specimens. Isolated ABCB5+ or ABCB5− melanoma cells display significantly different levels of tumorigenicity, with cells bearing this marker found to be more effective in initiating tumors in immunodeficient mice [25]. Of note, 14/23 mice formed tumors when ABCB5+ cells were injected compared with only 1/23 mice in the ABCB5− group [25]. In addition, the tumorigenic competence of ABCB5+ cells could be inhibited by the use of anti-ABCB5 antibodies [25]. ABCB5+ cell-derived xenografts re-established tumor heterogeneity (i.e., both ABCB5+ and ABCB5− progenies developed). By light microscopy, ABCB5-positivity correlated with non-pigmented, undifferentiated regions of human tumor samples, whereas pigmentation was more frequent in areas of ABCB5-negativity. ABCB5+ cells also co-expressed other melanoma progression-related markers, such as TIE1, CD144, CD133 and BMPR1. While ABCB5 may represent an essential component of the MSC repertoire, purified ABCB5+ cell populations do not invariably lead to tumor formation in animal models, suggesting that not every ABCB5+ cell represents an MSC or has tumor-initiation capability. Other factors may be necessary to achieve the complete stem cell phenotype.

ABCG2, another member of the ABC transporter family, has also been found to be expressed by a subpopulation (~4%) of melanoma cells with CD133-positivity [76]. However, any putative role for ABCG2 in the self-renewal capacity of MSCs remains to be investigated.

In one important study, Quintana et al. [80] were able to improve the conditions that favor engraftment, and thereby significantly reduce the number of cells required for xenograft initiation. Using a highly immune-compromised NOD/SCID IL-2R$\gamma^{-/-}$ mouse model, these investigators demonstrated that melanoma cells co-injected with matrigel grow faster than when injected alone. Moreover, a substantial difference in tumorigenicity was not observed between cells bearing stem cell markers (i.e., CD133, CD166, CD20, and ABCB5) and those that did not. In fact, a marker characteristic of melanoma-initiating ability was not identifiable. This study demonstrated that the number of cells required to propagate melanoma is determined to a large extent by the environment in which cells are placed, and not the frequency of CSCs [80]. In fact, in this and a subsequent study, Quintana et al. [80, 81] demonstrated that up to one quarter of cells obtained directly from human primary cutaneous or metastatic melanoma samples are capable of forming tumors following injection into immunodeficient mice. The authors were unable to find any large subpopulation of melanoma cells that lacked tumorigenic potential [81]. Moreover, results suggested that any single cell within a melanoma population can form a xenograft and, therefore, tumorigenic cells might be more common in melanoma than previously believed. In this regard, unlimited proliferation is an intrinsic property of all cancer cells and each cell maintains similar growth kinetics under favorable environmental conditions. Importantly, this study questioned some of the methods previously used to study CSCs/MSCs and suggested that the characterization of self-renewal properties may be biased through the provision of an environment which is not representative of natural conditions in human subjects [80].

Recently, Boiko et al. [74] reported that MSCs could be isolated prospectively according to their expression of the neural crest nerve growth factor receptor CD271. In this study, both CD271$^+$ and CD271$^-$ melanoma cells were re-suspended in a matrigel and implanted into T-, B- and NK-deficient Rag2$^{-/-}$ γc$^{-/-}$ mice. CD271$^+$ subsets formed xenografts at 90% of injected sites and were considered MSCs. At the same time, CD271$^-$ subsets did not develop tumors. Interestingly, CD271$^+$ melanoma cells lacked expression of TYR, MART-1 and MAGE (known melanocyte differentiation markers). This may help to explain why T-cell therapies directed against these antigens result in only temporary tumor shrinkage. To date, this is the most convincing characterization of MSCs and may have some application in the future analysis of subcategories of melanoma and their responsiveness to treatment. However, in their recent study, Quintana et al. [81] determined that both CD271$^-$ and CD271$^+$ melanoma cells, both CD133$^-$ and CD133$^+$ melanoma cells, and both ABCB5$^-$ and ABCB5$^+$ melanoma cells can form tumors in NOD/SCID IL2R$\gamma^{-/-}$ mice. In addition, CD133 appeared to be reversibly expressed by tumorigenic melanoma cells and could not be used to differentiate cells at different levels of hierarchy [81]. The conflicting results from the studies by Boiko et al. [74] and Quintana et al. [81] may be due to different assay conditions employed.

Plasticity of MSCs

The variable MSC frequency reported in many studies might be accounted for by their plasticity (i.e., phenotype switching potential) under different conditions. Highly aggressive melanoma cells have molecular signatures that are reminiscent of pluripotent stem cells [82, 83]. The concept of interconversion between tumorigenic and non-tumorigenic cells was recently proposed (i.e., a cell which is non-tumorigenic in one context could become tumorigenic in another) [84]. The majority of melanoma cells might be in a state of TA and share some degree of self-renewal potential, but could be easily dedifferentiated back to an MSC state under favorable environmental conditions [51]. Using different melanoma mouse models, Held et al. [85] identified three subsets of melanoma cells that could be segregated by surface marker expression and function: a CD34+/p75− subset acted as stem cells, a CD34−/p75− subset as TA ("intermediate") cells, and a CD34−/p75+ subset representing differentiated cells. Tumor formation occurred at high rates when CD34+/p75− melanoma cells were injected, while intermediate and low rates of growth were observed when CD34−/p75− or CD34−/p75+ cells were injected, respectively [85]. Similar to the studies by Quintana et al. [80, 81], these findings suggest that tumorigenic melanoma cells may be more common than previously believed and support the existence of multiple distinct populations of melanoma-propagating cells within a single tumor. Interestingly, individual CD34−/p75− cells could regenerate cellular heterogeneity after tumor formation in mice, whereas CD34+/p75− cells underwent self-renewal only [85].

The plasticity and TA dedifferentiation of melanoma cells might also contribute to the variable expression of MSC biomarkers. Melanoma cells cultured in vitro are noted to be heterogeneous, even when derived from a single cell expansion [86]. Therefore, a high degree of heterogeneity that exists in long-term dense cultures may confound the detection of MSC-to-TA cell conversion, and vice versa. It will be important to evaluate the stability of the CSC (and MSC) immunophenotype over time, in order to confidently determine the significance of expressed biomarkers as stable predictors of self-renewal capacity within a continuously evolving and chaotic cancer cell population. If some markers prove to be transiently expressed, prospective isolation of CSCs will be an approach of limited validity.

Metastasis and CSCs

The metastatic capability of a tumor depends on a number of factors, including tumor cell growth, survival, angiogenesis, and tissue invasion. Not every cell in a malignant tumor has the ability to metastasize to other organs. Similarly, the majority of circulating tumor cells are incapable of forming metastatic tumor deposits. It is possible that only CSCs can give rise to metastatic disease. Both CD44+/CD24−/low cells and CD44+/CD24+ cells can be isolated from metastatic pleural effusions of breast cancer patients [16]. However, only CD44+/CD24−/low cells show potential for tumor initiation in xenograft models [16]. Although a substantial percentage of CD44+/CD24+ cells can be found in metastatic foci, it is possible that they arise via in situ differentiation of their CSC counterparts. Hermann et al. [21] observed that a distinct subset of CD133+/CXCR4+ pancreatic CSCs exhibited significantly stronger migratory activity in vitro than CD133+/CXCR4− CSCs; thus, identifying another potential CSC marker relevant to the metastatic process (i.e., CXCR4). However, despite numerous publications and reports, no clear markers that specify the metastatic potential of MSCs have been identified, beyond those molecules already known to be functionally relevant to the general process of melanoma metastasization.

It is possible that a niche is required in order for CSCs to initiate a metastatic deposit, possibly explaining why some tumors show preferential development of metastases in particular tissues. It has also been hypothesized that primary tumors may influence the development of a niche, even before the onset of metastasis [87, 88]. Cancer cells may improve the efficiency of metastasis formation through the recruitment of mesenchymal and endothelial cells from the bone marrow [44, 89, 90]. Moreover, fibroblasts actively cooperate in the process of cancer development and progression within the niche [91]. It has also been observed that the early spread of cancer occurs through direct migration of CSC-like progenitors to the bone marrow, where they retain a quiescent phenotype and asymmetrical self-renewal capacity within a bone marrow niche, and only later migrate to metastatic foci [92]. Whether this concept applies to melanoma remains to be determined.

CSCs and Drug Design for Treatment of Melanoma

Melanoma is characterized by resistance to chemotherapy and immunotherapy. One reason could be a particular resistance of MSCs to these therapeutic modalities. As for other CSCs, MSCs might maintain properties of normal stem cells, including drug resistance mechanisms.

Limitations of Drug Testing Against CSCs

It is possible that the successful treatment of cancer rests on the use of multiple therapeutic approaches which target different cell types within the same tumor population. Cancer as a functional unit includes CSCs, TA cells, and differentiated cells. Each one of these cell types may have variable sensitivities to different drugs. If an agent is effective against CSCs, then as a function of the previously discussed system plasticity, resistant TA cells may restore the CSC populations, and vice versa. Therefore, the testing of drug efficacy cannot be limited to the elimination of CSCs.

Currently, drug testing relies heavily on the sensitivity of cancer cell lines cultured *in vitro*. These cell lines are almost all monoclonal in nature and may not recapitulate *in vivo* human tumor complexity with its variable subpopulations of CSCs, TA cells and differentiated cells. In addition, heterogeneity of drug resistance within cells of each cultured cell line, potentially due to CSCs (i.e., SP), is also often ignored. Similarly, *in vivo* xenograft models may not accurately predict drug efficacy, as they may not fully represent the niche-like environment (i.e., complex interactions between CSCs and other cells) in human tumors which both fosters cancer growth and protects against therapeutic intervention. Thus, a primary tumor model may better test drug effects. In this regard, drug evaluation studies performed on primary human glioblastomas seem to have greater accuracy in predicting treatment results in the preclinical setting [93].

There is no good experimental model with which to study the interactions between therapeutic modalities and different tumor subpopulations. The mechanisms of asymmetric cell division, TA cell dedifferentiation, and self-renewal capacity will require better understanding before a rational approach to the identification of effective drugs can be applied.

Targeting Pathways that Regulate CSC Growth

Many self-renewal pathways involved in the propagation of CSCs appear to be shared by normal stem cells, raising the possibility that CSC-targeted therapies will also destroy their normal counterparts. Therefore, it is important to determine unique targets that are not present on normal stem cells; some of which have indeed been identified. For example, leukemia stem cells show loss of PTEN tumor-suppressor activity necessary for their self-renewal capacity, while normal HSCs employ different mechanisms for their survival [94, 95]. Of note, rapamycin, which targets mTOR, eradicates leukemia-initiating cells in mice, and further restores normal HSC function [94, 95]. Moreover, parthenolide selectively targets human leukemia stem cells and not normal stem/progenitor cells [96]. Unfortunately, with the exception of NOTCH signaling which appears to be required for the maintenance of MSCs within a niche, no known pathways that are specific to MSCs as compared to normal stem cells have been identified to date.

In addition, it has been proposed that CSCs (and MSCs) may function to promote tumor growth and immunologic tolerance by inhibiting host anti-tumor immune effector responses. In this regard, Schatton et al. [97] have identified that ABCB5$^+$ subpopulations of melanoma cells possess distinct T-cell-modulatory functions.

Conclusion

Following the publication of our last review of MSCs [98], significant progress has been made in their characterization, particularly at the basic experimental level. Since the development of the CSC hypothesis more than 100 years ago [99], evidence is now growing for the existence of a virtual subpopulation of cancer cells that is responsible for tumor initiation, maintenance, growth and metastasis. These CSCs may demonstrate dramatically different biological properties compared with the broader population of cancer cells. Such changes could explain the poor efficacy of current therapies; given the fact that most were originally developed for their effect against "the bulk" of cancer cells and not functional subsets.

Many other questions remain. For example, the characterization of CSCs, including MSCs, has largely rested on: (1) the expression of surface stem cell markers; (2) the ability to form spherical aggregates under non-adherent culture conditions; and (3) the capacity to self-renew, proliferate, differentiate and initiate tumors when injected into immunodeficient mice. These arbitrary criteria have some limitations. For instance, markers that are used to isolate CSCs are not unique to these cell types, and are often expressed by somatic cells in normal tissues [100]. In addition, the expression levels of these markers can be modulated by different experimental and environmental conditions; for example, hypoxia interferes with the gene expression machinery of cancer cells and induces increased expression of stem cell-like surface markers [101]. Therefore, the detection of surface markers might not specifically identify a pure population of CSCs; however, it could be potentially used to enrich for a specific subpopulation of cells that bear stem cell-like properties, which are then tested for their ability to initiate tumors in animal models. However, the results of such *in vivo* assays may be difficult to interpret, because of the extreme variability of experimental conditions and the host microenvironment [102]. The ability of tumor cells to survive and regenerate in xenografts may be unrelated to stem cell-like features. Instead, it could be due to random alterations in cell cycle and/or apoptotic pathway regulators, or, indeed, aberrant methylation patterns.

Research on MSCs suffers for the same limitations as those experienced in other tumor models. It is also hampered by the high plasticity of melanoma, its unpredictable behavior and its unique resistance to current therapeutic modalities. As other aspects of cancer biology are being discovered, including "driver" mutations that promote tumor growth and immune system interactions responsible for tumor survival/rejection, it is becoming increasingly clear that combination therapies likely represent the best approach to disease eradication [103, 104]. It is possible that another level of complexity should be added to the current algorithm used to design anti-melanoma therapies; that is, the "plastic" interaction within each tumor of distinct subpopulations of cells with differential drug responses. For instance, the development of novel immunotherapies might take into consideration alternate target antigens unrelated to tissue differentiation [97], such as (1) cancer/testis antigens whose expression is increasingly stabilized in the later stages of cancer progression [105] or (2) mutated neoantigens that are associated with the oncogenic process and which identify CSCs [106, 107]. However, even these antigens may not always represent good MSC targets due to their differential sensitivities to cytotoxic agents and/or their intrinsic downregulation in some instances [74]. Future chemotherapeutic strategies may target pathways that are less strictly associated with rapidly-dividing differentiated melanoma cell populations and more closely related to the metabolism of resting MSCs [108].

References

1. Beddingfield III FC. The melanoma epidemic: res ipsa loquitur. Oncologist. 2003;8:459–65.
2. Gogas HJ, Kirkwood JM, Sondak VK. Chemotherapy for metastatic melanoma: time for a change? Cancer. 2007;109:455–64.
3. Rietschel P, Wolchok JD, Krown S, et al. Phase II study of extended-dose temozolomide in patients with melanoma. J Clin Oncol. 2008;26:2299–304.
4. Dudley ME, Wunderlich JR, Robbins PF, et al. Cancer regression and autoimmunity in patients after clonal repopulation with antitumor lymphocytes. Science. 2002;298:850–4.
5. Dudley ME, Wunderlich JR, Yang JC, et al. Adoptive cell transfer therapy following non-myeloablative but lymphodepleting chemotherapy for the treatment of patients with refractory metastatic melanoma. J Clin Oncol. 2005;23:2346–57.
6. Dudley ME, Yang JC, Sherry R, et al. Adoptive cell therapy for patients with metastatic melanoma: evaluation of intensive myeloablative chemoradiation preparative regimens. J Clin Oncol. 2008;26: 5233–9.
7. Aksentijevich I, Galon J, Soares M, et al. The tumor-necrosis-factor receptor-associated periodic syndrome: new mutations in TNFRSF1A, ancestral

origins, genotype-phenotype studies and evidence for further genetic heterogeneity of periodic fevers. Am J Hum Genet. 2001;69:301–14.
8. Chen KG, Valencia JC, Gillet JP, Hearing VJ, Gottesman MM. Involvement of ABC transporters in melanogenesis and the development of multidrug resistance of melanoma. Pigment Cell Melanoma Res. 2009;22:740–9.
9. Di Tomaso T, Mazzoleni S, Wang E, et al. Immunobiological characterization of cancer stem cells isolated from glioblastoma patients. Clin Cancer Res. 2010;16:800–13.
10. Odoux C, Fohrer H, Hoppo T, et al. A stochastic model for cancer stem cell origin in metastatic colon cancer. Cancer Res. 2008;68:6932–41.
11. Lagasse E. Cancer stem cells with genetic instability: the best vehicle with the best engine for cancer. Gene Ther. 2008;15:136–42.
12. Shackleton M. Normal stem cells and cancer stem cells: similar and different. Semin Cancer Biol. 2010;20:85–92.
13. Goodell MA, Brose K, Paradis G, Conner AS, Mulligan RC. Isolation and functional properties of murine hematopoietic stem cells that are replicating in vivo. J Exp Med. 1996;183:1797–806.
14. Lapidot T, Sirard C, Vormoor J, et al. A cell initiating human acute myeloid leukaemia after transplantation into SCID mice. Nature. 1994;367:645–8.
15. Bonnet D, Dick JE. Human acute myeloid leukemia is organized as a hierarchy that originates from a primitive hematopoietic cell. Nat Med. 1997;3:730–7.
16. Al Hajj M, Wicha MS, Benito-Hernandez A, Morrison SJ, Clarke MF. Prospective identification of tumorigenic breast cancer cells. Proc Natl Acad Sci USA. 2003;100:3983–8.
17. Krivtsov AV, Twomey D, Feng Z, et al. Transformation from committed progenitor to leukaemia stem cell initiated by MLL-AF9. Nature. 2006;442:818–22.
18. Deshpande AJ, Cusan M, Rawat VP, et al. Acute myeloid leukemia is propagated by a leukemic stem cell with lymphoid characteristics in a mouse model of CALM/AF10-positive leukemia. Cancer Cell. 2006;10:363–74.
19. Somervaille TC, Cleary ML. Identification and characterization of leukemia stem cells in murine MLL-AF9 acute myeloid leukemia. Cancer Cell. 2006;10:257–68.
20. Hemmati HD, Nakano I, Lazareff JA, et al. Cancerous stem cells can arise from pediatric brain tumors. Proc Natl Acad Sci USA. 2003;100:15178–83.
21. Hermann PC, Huber SL, Herrler T, et al. Distinct populations of cancer stem cells determine tumor growth and metastatic activity in human pancreatic cancer. Cell Stem Cell. 2007;1:313–23.
22. Singh SK, Hawkins C, Clarke ID, et al. Identification of human brain tumour initiating cells. Nature. 2004;432:396–401.
23. O'Brien CA, Pollett A, Gallinger S, Dick JE. A human colon cancer cell capable of initiating tumour growth in immunodeficient mice. Nature. 2007;445:106–10.
24. Ricci-Vitiani L, Lombardi DG, Pilozzi E, et al. Identification and expansion of human colon-cancer-initiating cells. Nature. 2007;445:111–5.
25. Schatton T, Murphy GF, Frank NY, et al. Identification of cells initiating human melanomas. Nature. 2008;451:345–9.
26. Dalerba P, Dylla SJ, Park IK, et al. Phenotypic characterization of human colorectal cancer stem cells. Proc Natl Acad Sci USA. 2007;104:10158–63.
27. Prince ME, Sivanandan R, Kaczorowski A, et al. Identification of a subpopulation of cells with cancer stem cell properties in head and neck squamous cell carcinoma. Proc Natl Acad Sci USA. 2007;104:973–8.
28. Kim CF, Jackson EL, Woolfenden AE, et al. Identification of bronchioalveolar stem cells in normal lung and lung cancer. Cell. 2005;121:823–35.
29. Yang ZF, Ho DW, Ng MN, et al. Significance of CD90+ cancer stem cells in human liver cancer. Cancer Cell. 2008;13:153–66.
30. Kawabata Y, Hirokawa M, Komatsuda A, Sawada K. Clinical applications of CD34+ cell-selected peripheral blood stem cells. Ther Apher Dial. 2003;7:298–304.
31. Helgason GV, Young GA, Holyoake TL. Targeting chronic myeloid leukemia stem cells. Curr Hematol Malig Rep. 2010;5:81–7.
32. Wu Y, Wu PY. CD133 as a marker for cancer stem cells: progresses and concerns. Stem Cells Dev. 2009;18:1127–34.
33. Ferrandina G, Petrillo M, Bonanno G, Scambia G. Targeting CD133 antigen in cancer. Expert Opin Ther Targets. 2009;13:823–37.
34. Lin T, Islam O, Heese K. ABC transporters, neural stem cells and neurogenesis—a different perspective. Cell Res. 2006;16:857–71.
35. Hadnagy A, Gaboury L, Beaulieu R, Balicki D. SP analysis may be used to identify cancer stem cell populations. Exp Cell Res. 2006;312:3701–10.
36. Perego M, Tortoreto M, Tragni G, et al. Heterogeneous phenotype of human melanoma cells with in vitro and in vivo features of tumor-initiating cells. J Invest Dermatol. 2010;130:1877–86.
37. Dey D, Saxena M, Paranjape AN, et al. Phenotypic and functional characterization of human mammary stem/progenitor cells in long term culture. PLoS One. 2009;4:e5329.
38. Fang D, Nguyen TK, Leishear K, et al. A tumorigenic subpopulation with stem cell properties in melanomas. Cancer Res. 2005;65:9328–37.
39. Baaten G, Voogd AC, Wagstaff J. A systematic review of the relation between interleukin-2 schedule and outcome in patients with metastatic renal cell cancer. Eur J Cancer. 2004;40:1127–44.
40. Baguley BC. Tumor stem cell niches: a new functional framework for the action of anticancer drugs. Recent Patents Anticancer Drug Discov. 2006;1:121–7.
41. Voog J, Jones DL. Stem cells and the niche: a dynamic duo. Cell Stem Cell. 2010;6:103–15.

42. LaBarge MA. The difficulty of targeting cancer stem cell niches. Clin Cancer Res. 2010;16:3121–9.
43. Orimo A, Gupta PB, Sgroi DC, et al. Stromal fibroblasts present in invasive human breast carcinomas promote tumor growth and angiogenesis through elevated SDF-1/CXCL12 secretion. Cell. 2005;121: 335–48.
44. Visvader JE, Lindeman GJ. Cancer stem cells in solid tumours: accumulating evidence and unresolved questions. Nat Rev Cancer. 2008;8:755–68.
45. Shackleton M, Quintana E. Progress in understanding melanoma propagation. Mol Oncol. 2010;4:451–7.
46. Dewanji A, Goddard MJ, Krewski D, Moolgavkar SH. Two stage model for carcinogenesis: number and size distributions of premalignant clones in longitudinal studies. Math Biosci. 1999;155:1–12.
47. Roschke AV, Tonon G, Gehlhaus KS, et al. Karyotypic complexity of the NCI-60 drug-screening panel. Cancer Res. 2003;63:8634–47.
48. Osawa M, Egawa G, Mak SS, et al. Molecular characterization of melanocyte stem cells in their niche. Development. 2005;132:5589–99.
49. Shinin V, Gayraud-Morel B, Gomes D, Tajbakhsh S. Asymmetric division and cosegregation of template DNA strands in adult muscle satellite cells. Nat Cell Biol. 2006;8:677–87.
50. Nishimura EK, Jordan SA, Oshima H, et al. Dominant role of the niche in melanocyte stem-cell fate determination. Nature. 2002;416:854–60.
51. Roesch A, Fukunaga-Kalabis M, Schmidt EC, et al. A temporarily distinct subpopulation of slow-cycling melanoma cells is required for continuous tumor growth. Cell. 2010;141:583–94.
52. Nishimura EK, Granter SR, Fisher DE. Mechanisms of hair graying: incomplete melanocyte stem cell maintenance in the niche. Science. 2005;307:720–4.
53. Grichnik JM. Melanoma, nevogenesis, and stem cell biology. J Invest Dermatol. 2008;128:2365–80.
54. Chudnovsky Y, Adams AE, Robbins PB, Lin Q, Khavari PA. Use of human tissue to assess the oncogenic activity of melanoma-associated mutations. Nat Genet. 2005;37:745–9.
55. Tsao H, Goel V, Wu H, Yang G, Haluska FG. Genetic interaction between NRAS and BRAF mutations and PTEN/MMAC1 inactivation in melanoma. J Invest Dermatol. 2004;122:337–41.
56. Grichnik JM, Burch JA, Schulteis RD, et al. Melanoma, a tumor based on a mutant stem cell? J Invest Dermatol. 2006;126:142–53.
57. Klonisch T, Wiechec E, Hombach-Klonisch S, et al. Cancer stem cell markers in common cancers—therapeutic implications. Trends Mol Med. 2008;14:450–60.
58. Huntly BJ, Shigematsu H, Deguchi K, et al. MOZ-TIF2, but not BCR-ABL, confers properties of leukemic stem cells to committed murine hematopoietic progenitors. Cancer Cell. 2004;6:587–96.
59. Zhang M, Behbod F, Atkinson RL, et al. Identification of tumor-initiating cells in a p53-null mouse model of breast cancer. Cancer Res. 2008;68:4674–82.
60. Real C, Glavieux-Pardanaud C, Le Douarin NM, Dupin E. Clonally cultured differentiated pigment cells can dedifferentiate and generate multipotent progenitors with self-renewing potential. Dev Biol. 2006;300:656–69.
61. Herlyn M, Thurin J, Balaban G, et al. Characteristics of cultured human melanocytes isolated from different stages of tumor progression. Cancer Res. 1985;45:5670–6.
62. Herlyn M, Clark WH, Rodeck U, Mancianti ML, Jambrosic J, Koprowski H. Biology of tumor progression in human melanocytes. Lab Invest. 1987;56:461–74.
63. Wang E, Voiculescu S, Le Poole IC, et al. Clonal persistence and evolution during a decade of recurrent melanoma. J Invest Dermatol. 2006;126:1372–7.
64. Sabatino M, Zhao Y, Voiculescu S, et al. Conservation of a core of genetic alterations over a decade of recurrent melanoma supports the melanoma stem cell hypothesis. Cancer Res. 2008;68:222–31.
65. Takahashi K, Yamanaka S. Induction of pluripotent stem cells from mouse embryonic and adult fibroblast cultures by defined factors. Cell. 2006;126:663–76.
66. Okada M, Oka M, Yoneda Y. Effective culture conditions for the induction of pluripotent stem cells. Biochim Biophys Acta. 2010;1800(9):956–63.
67. Okita K, Ichisaka T, Yamanaka S. Generation of germline-competent induced pluripotent stem cells. Nature. 2007;448:313–7.
68. Maherali N, Sridharan R, Xie W, et al. Directly reprogrammed fibroblasts show global epigenetic remodeling and widespread tissue contribution. Cell Stem Cell. 2007;1:55–70.
69. Wernig M, Meissner A, Foreman R, et al. In vitro reprogramming of fibroblasts into a pluripotent ES-cell-like state. Nature. 2007;448:318–24.
70. Yu J, Vodyanik MA, Smuga-Otto K, et al. Induced pluripotent stem cell lines derived from human somatic cells. Science. 2007;318:1917–20.
71. Lowry WE, Richter L, Yachechko R, et al. Generation of human induced pluripotent stem cells from dermal fibroblasts. Proc Natl Acad Sci USA. 2008;105:2883–8.
72. Huangfu D, Osafune K, Maehr R, et al. Induction of pluripotent stem cells from primary human fibroblasts with only Oct4 and Sox2. Nat Biotechnol. 2008;26:1269–75.
73. Shackleton M, Vaillant F, Simpson KJ, et al. Generation of a functional mammary gland from a single stem cell. Nature. 2006;439:84–8.
74. Boiko AD, Razorenova OV, Van de Rijn M, et al. Human melanoma-initiating cells express neural crest nerve growth factor receptor CD271. Nature. 2010;466:133–7.
75. Na YR, Seok SH, Kim DJ, et al. Isolation and characterization of spheroid cells from human malignant melanoma cell line WM-266-4. Tumour Biol. 2009; 30:300–9.
76. Monzani E, Facchetti F, Galmozzi E, et al. Melanoma contains CD133 and ABCG2 positive cells with

enhanced tumourigenic potential. Eur J Cancer. 2007;43:935–46.
77. Mizrak D, Brittan M, Alison MR. CD133: molecule of the moment. J Pathol. 2008;214:3–9.
78. Klein WM, Wu BP, Zhao S, Wu H, Klein-Szanto AJ, Tahan SR. Increased expression of stem cell markers in malignant melanoma. Mod Pathol. 2007;20:102–7.
79. Keshet GI, Goldstein I, Itzhaki O, et al. MDR1 expression identifies human melanoma stem cells. Biochem Biophys Res Commun. 2008;368:930–6.
80. Quintana E, Shackleton M, Sabel MS, Fullen DR, Johnson TM, Morrison SJ. Efficient tumour formation by single human melanoma cells. Nature. 2008;456:593–8.
81. Quintana E, Shackleton M, Foster HR, et al. Phenotypic heterogeneity among tumorigenic melanoma cells from patients that is reversible and not hierarchically organized. Cancer Cell. 2010;18:510–23.
82. Bittner M, Meltzer P, Chen Y, et al. Molecular classification of cutaneous malignant melanoma by gene expression: shifting from a countinuous spectrum to distinct biologic entities. Nature. 2000;406:536–840.
83. Hendrix MJ, Seftor EA, Seftor RE, Kasemeier-Kulesa J, Kulesa PM, Postovit LM. Reprogramming metastatic tumour cells with embryonic microenvironments. Nat Rev Cancer. 2007;7:246–55.
84. Pinner S, Jordan P, Sharrock K, et al. Intravital imaging reveals transient changes in pigment production and Brn2 expression during metastatic melanoma dissemination. Cancer Res. 2009;69:7969–77.
85. Held MA, Curley DP, Dankort D, McMahon M, Muthusamy V, Bosenberg MW. Characterization of melanoma cells capable of propagating tumors from a single cell. Cancer Res. 2010;70:388–97.
86. Lee JT, Herlyn M. Microenvironmental influences in melanoma progression. J Cell Biochem. 2007;101: 862–72.
87. Kaplan RN, Riba RD, Zacharoulis S, et al. VEGFR1-positive haematopoietic bone marrow progenitors initiate the pre-metastatic niche. Nature. 2005;438: 820–7.
88. Wang E, Ngalame Y, Panelli MC, et al. Peritoneal and sub-peritoneal stroma may facilitate regional spread of ovarian cancer. Clin Cancer Res. 2005;11: 113–22.
89. Karnoub AE, Dash AB, Vo AP, et al. Mesenchymal stem cells within tumour stroma promote breast cancer metastasis. Nature. 2007;449:557–63.
90. Alphonso A, Alahari SK. Stromal cells and integrins: conforming to the needs of the tumor microenvironment. Neoplasia. 2009;11:1264–71.
91. Hendrix MJ, Seftor EA, Hess AR, Seftor RE. Vasculogenic mimicry and tumour-cell plasticity: lessons from melanoma. Nat Rev Cancer. 2003;3: 411–21.
92. Husemann Y, Geigl JB, Schubert F, et al. Systemic spread is an early step in breast cancer. Cancer Cell. 2008;13:58–68.
93. Szakacs G, Paterson JK, Ludwig JA, Booth-Genthe C, Gottesman MM. Targeting multidrug resistance in cancer. Nat Rev Drug Discov. 2006;5:219–34.
94. Yilmaz OH, Valdez R, Theisen BK, et al. Pten dependence distinguishes haematopoietic stem cells from leukaemia-initiating cells. Nature. 2006;441: 475–82.
95. Rossi DJ, Weissman IL. Pten, tumorigenesis, and stem cell self-renewal. Cell. 2006;125:229–31.
96. Hassane DC, Guzman ML, Corbett C, et al. Discovery of agents that eradicate leukemia stem cells using an in silico screen of public gene expression data. Blood. 2008;111:5654–62.
97. Schatton T, Schutte U, Frank NY, et al. Modulation of T-cell activation by malignant melanoma initiating cells. Cancer Res. 2010;70:697–708.
98. Sabatino M, Stroncek DF, Klein H, Marincola FM, Wang E. Stem cells in melanoma development. Cancer Lett. 2009;279:119–25.
99. Wicha MS, Liu S, Dontu G. Cancer stem cells: an old idea—a paradigm shift. Cancer Res. 2006; 66:1883–90.
100. Clarke MF, Dick JE, Dirks PB, et al. Cancer stem cells—perspectives on current status and future directions: AACR Workshop on cancer stem cells. Cancer Res. 2006;66:9339–44.
101. Greijer AE, van der Groep P, Kemming D, et al. Up-regulation of gene expression by hypoxia is mediated predominantly by hypoxia-inducible factor 1 (HIF-1). J Pathol. 2005;206:291–304.
102. Kelly PN, Dakic A, Adams JM, Nutt SL, Strasser A. Tumor growth need not be driven by rare cancer stem cells. Science. 2007;317:337.
103. Ascierto PA, Kirkwood JM. Adjuvant therapy of melanoma with interferon: lessons of the past decade. J Transl Med. 2008;6:62.
104. Ascierto PA, Streicher HZ, Sznol M. Melanoma: a model for testing new agents in combination therapies. J Transl Med. 2010;8:38.
105. Costa FF, Le BK, Brodin B. Concise review: cancer/testis antigens, stem cells, and cancer. Stem Cells. 2007;25:707–11.
106. Robbins PF, el-Gamil M, Li YF, et al. A mutated beta-catenin gene encodes a melanoma-specific antigen recognized by tumor infiltrating lymphocytes. J Exp Med. 1996;183:1185–92.
107. Lennerz V, Fatho M, Gentilini C, et al. The response of autologous T cells to a human melanoma is dominated by mutated neoantigens. Proc Natl Acad Sci USA. 2005;102:16013–8.
108. Al-Hajj M. Cancer stem cells and oncology therapeutics. Curr Opin Oncol. 2007;19:61–4.

Surgical Management of Melanoma: Concept of Field Cancerization and Molecular Evaluation of Tissue Margins

Amanda Phelps and Michael J. Murphy

The concept of field cancerization, first proposed by Slaughter in 1953, describes a process whereby cells in a particular tissue or organ are sequentially transformed by multiple cumulative genetic and epigenetic alterations, such that a clonal expansion of pre-neoplastic genetically-altered, but morphologically normal-appearing cells is present, prior to the development of overt malignancy [1]. Additional genomic aberrations are required for cancer development, but these precursor cells may persist with the malignant cells of a tumor [1].

The recent application of molecular technologies to the examination of perilesional and more distant adjacent normal skin samples has demonstrated many of the genotypic aberrations found in cancer [2, 3]. These defects are the earliest changes of oncogenesis that occur in a stepwise, cumulative fashion culminating in metastatic cancer via initiation, promotion, selection, and clonal expansion. Moreover, these findings implicate two distinct levels of field cancerization (1) molecular progression where microscopically normal cells accumulate genomic damage; and (2) phenotypic progression denoted by evolution of microscopically normal skin to precursors to in situ cancer that can be followed by invasion and, ultimately, metastatic disease [2, 3]. In this model, the cutaneous field develops a "tumor stem cell", which acquires a growth advantage and exhibits a "mutator phenotype" (i.e., genomic instability) that enables it to expand beyond its microscopically defined stem cell niche, form diverse clonal fields, and accrue further genetic alterations that eventuate into invasive cancer [2, 3]. Genomic instability is manifested as single base mutations, gain or loss of whole or partial chromosomes, amplification of oncogenes, mismatch repair gene defects, and/or epigenetic alterations including hypermethylation of promoter regions of key tumor suppressor genes [2, 3].

The skin is the most suitable organ to investigate the mechanisms and potential clinical utility of field cancerization—due to its contiguous nature, accessibility, and ease of removing wide tissue margins. The study of field cancerization in the skin may have a role in (1) the assessment of tumor risk; (2) the detection of early neoplasia; (3) the study of tumor pathogenesis and progression; and (4) the accurate delineation of "true" tumor margins (i.e., overt tumor and surrounding "field cells"), and as a consequence, the planning of appropriate surgical treatment.

The standard treatment of primary melanoma is wide excision with a defined margin of clinically uninvolved skin, in an effort to reduce the risk of local recurrence. It is the presence of occult field cells peripheral to a tumor which explains

A. Phelps, B.A. (✉)
Central Connecticut State University,
New Britain, CT, USA
e-mail: mnder410@comcast.net

M.J. Murphy, M.D.
Department of Dermatology, University
of Connecticut Health Center, Farmington, CT, USA

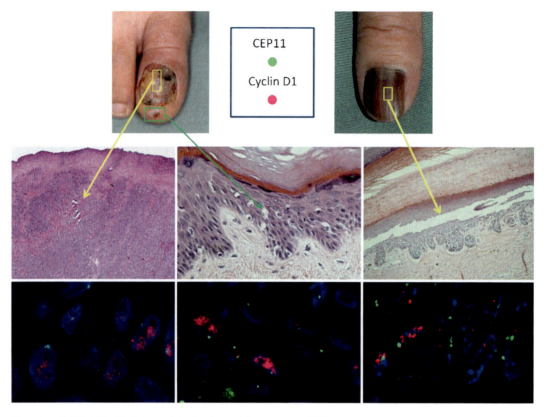

Fig. 18.1 CCND1 (Cyclin D1) amplification in acral lentiginous melanoma (ALM). Fluorescence in situ hybridization (FISH) demonstrating CCND1 (11q13) amplification in an invasive ALM (*left panels*) and an adjacent in situ macular lesion (*middle panels*). An additional case of ALM in situ with CCND1 amplification is shown (*right panels*). CCND1 probe, *red signal*; chromosome 11 centromeric probe/CEP11, *green signal* (From Murphy [2]. Reprinted with permission from Springer, Copyright© 2011. Original figure courtesy of Dr. Minoru Takata, Department of Dermatology, Okayama University Postgraduate School of Medical, Dentistry and Pharmaceutical Sciences, Okayama, Japan)

the efficacy of wide excisions in reducing local recurrences in patients with melanoma [4]. At present, standardized excision recommendations are based on Breslow thickness (i.e., 0.5-cm margins for melanoma in situ, 1-cm margins for invasive melanoma of <2 mm, and 2-cm margins for invasive melanoma of >2 mm) [5]. These guidelines are supported by subsequent histopathological assessment of the microscopic distance between the excision specimen margins and any residual melanocytes which are cytologically atypical, abnormally distributed, and/or increased in number [5]. However, studies have noted that the frequency of local, regional, or distant metastases is not affected by the margins of excision in some patients with melanoma [6]. The development of such melanoma recurrences following recommended excision guidelines could be due to (1) false-negative microscopic review of the excision specimen (due to different tissue processing techniques, pathologist experience, etc.); or (2) intraepidermal pre-neoplastic or frankly neoplastic melanocytes (i.e., melanocytic field cancerization), which cannot be readily identified by current routine histopathological methods, present at or peripheral to the excision site.

The recent use of fluorescence in situ hybridization (FISH) analysis to determine the presence of overt residual disease and/or field cells in acral lentiginous melanoma (ALM) is a potentially exciting application of a molecular test to guide management and control local recurrence of this disease (Fig. 18.1). Recent studies have demonstrated frequent amplifications of regions on chromosomes 5p15, 22q11–13 and 11q13 (site of CCND1) in ALM [4, 5, 7, 8]. Interestingly, in 84% of cases studied, copy number increases of 11q13 and 5p15 have also been identified in the melanocytic cells of histopathologically normal epidermis at varying distances from the overt ALM tumor margins (mean: 6.1 mm for melanoma in situ; 4.5 mm for invasive melanoma) [5]. However, the extent of these latter findings does not appear to correlate with either the Breslow thickness or diameter of the ALM [5]. Both (1) the pattern of aberrations (i.e., stable or progressive increase in gene amplification levels from field cells to in situ to invasive components) and (2) the asymmetric distribution of field cells support the acquirement of additional oncogenic aberrations for progression to frank malignancy [5]. According to the concept of field cancerization, these morphologically normal, but genetically aberrant melanocytes would represent a latent progression phase/early melanoma in situ (supported by gene profiling studies), which precedes a stage of uncontrolled melanocyte proliferation within the epidermis [5, 7, 8]. The results of these FISH studies suggest that the current recommendations for excision margins based on the Breslow thickness are suboptimal for a subset of melanomas [6]. The routine clinical use of FISH technology to detect field cells in melanoma could help determine the appropriate surgical margins required to minimize the risk of tumor recurrence. At present, this technique is only applicable to those melanomas with frequent gene amplifications (i.e., ALM and mucosal subtypes).

A number of studies have investigated the use of additional technologies, such as immunohistochemistry (IHC), for margin analysis in melanomas [5, 9, 10]. Protein expression in excision specimens has been evaluated using antibodies directed against cyclin D1 and melanocyte-differentiation markers, such as MART-1, HMB-45, S-100 and Mel-5 [5, 9, 10]. Of note, HMB-45 (an antibody directed against a melanosomal antigen) has been reported in overt in situ and invasive ALM, but can also be identified in field cell areas of these tumors (in up to 56% of cases) [5, 10]. However, HMB-45 is a marker of melanocytic differentiation, and not genetic instability *per se*, and therefore its ability to reliably distinguish between benign, premalignant or overtly malignant individual melanocytes in the epidermis is questionable. Levels of cyclin D1 protein have also been found to increase from the periphery towards the in situ and invasive portions of ALM [5]. However, the use of IHC analysis for this marker to delineate the extent of the field area in ALM has also been questioned, as cyclin D1 protein expression has not been identified in all field cells that show FISH-detected increased copy numbers of 11q13 [5].

Pathologists often identify changes designated as "atypical melanocytic hyperplasia" (AMH) adjacent to melanomas in tissue sections [11]. However, histopathological and immunohistochemical criteria to distinguish AMH from otherwise benign sun-damaged melanocytes are not fully defined (i.e., such as the number of atypical melanocytes per high-power field/number of keratinocytes). Using loss of heterozygosity (LOH) analysis, Pashaei et al. [11] found increasingly higher defects in the hOGG1 gene progressing from AMH to adjacent melanoma in situ (60% vs. 80%). hOGG1 is an important gene for repair of free radical-induced DNA damage [11]. The authors suggested that AMH could represent an early morphologically-evident stage in melanoma development, and that its presence at the resection margins of melanoma warrants appropriate treatment or close clinical follow-up.

Other studies have found aneusomy of chromosome 7 and mitochondrial DNA (mtDNA) mutations/deletions in perilesional "normal" skin surrounding melanomas [2, 3, 12–14]. The peritumoral skin of melanoma may harbor expanded mtDNA-mutant melanocytes, analogous to the p53 clones seen adjacent to non-melanoma skin cancers [2, 3].

In the future, the tailoring of surgical management, in order to ensure removal of both overt melanoma and its field cells, could be based on the results of molecular diagnostic tests, and may be particularly useful at those cutaneous sites where function or cosmetic outcome are impacted by current margin guidelines.

References

1. Dakubo GD, Jakupciak JP, Birch-Machin MA, et al. Clinical implications and utility of field cancerization. Cancer Cell Int. 2007;7:2.
2. Murphy M. Molecular determination of tissue margins, clonal origin and histogenesis of skin cancers. In: Murphy MJ, editor. Molecular diagnostics in dermatology and dermatopathology. New York: Springer; 2011.
3. Carlson JA, Murphy M, Slominski A, Wilson VL. Evidence of skin field cancerization. In: Dabuko GD, editor. Field cancerization: basic science and clinical applications. New York: Nova; 2011.
4. Bastian BC, Kashani-Sabet M, Hamm H, et al. Gene amplifications characterize acral melanoma and permit the detection of occult tumor cells in the surrounding skin. Cancer Res. 2000;60:1968–73.
5. North JP, Kageshita T, Pinkel D, et al. Distribution and significance of occult intraepidermal tumor cells surrounding primary melanoma. J Invest Dermatol. 2008;128:2024–30.
6. Hinshaw M. Use of genetic tools to control tumor margins in melanoma. Arch Dermatol. 2009;145:475–7.
7. Takata M, Murata H, Saida T. Molecular pathogenesis of malignant melanoma: a different perspective from the studies of melanocytic nevus and acral melanoma. Pigment Cell Melanoma Res. 2010;23:64–71.
8. Takata M, Saida T. Early cancers of the skin: clinical, histopathological, and molecular characteristics. Int J Clin Oncol. 2005;10:391–7.
9. Whalen J, Leone D. Mohs micrographic surgery for the treatment of malignant melanoma. Clin Dermatol. 2009;27:597–602.
10. Griego RD, Zitelli JA. Mohs micrographic surgery using HMB-45 for a recurrent acral melanoma. Dermatol Surg. 1998;24:1003–6.
11. Pashaei S, Li L, Zhang H, Spencer HJ, et al. Concordant loss of heterozygosity of DNA repair gene, hOGG1, in melanoma in situ and atypical melanocytic hyperplasia. J Cutan Pathol. 2008;35:525–31.
12. Udart M, Utikal J, Krähn GM, Peter RU. Chromosome 7 aneusomy. A marker for metastatic melanoma? Expression of the epidermal growth factor receptor gene and chromosome 7 aneusomy in nevi, primary malignant melanomas and metastases. Neoplasia. 2001;3:245–54.
13. Hubbard K, Steinberg ML, Hill H, et al. Mitochondrial DNA deletions in skin from melanoma patients. Ethn Dis. 2008;18(2 Suppl 2):S2-38–43.
14. Steinberg ML, Hubbard K, Utti C, et al. Patterns of persistent DNA damage associated with sun exposure and the glutathione S-transferase M1 genotype in melanoma patients. Photochem Photobiol. 2009;85:379–86.

Chemotherapy for Melanoma

19

Hedwig Stanisz, Thomas Vogt, and Knuth Rass

Introduction

When detected in its early stages, melanoma is a curable disease in the vast majority of patients. Once metastases occur, the prognosis of this disease worsens dramatically. Metastasis localization and tumor burden are critical determinants of survival. In 2008, an estimated 8,420 deaths due to metastatic melanoma were reported in the United States [1]. For distant metastatic disease, the overall 10-year survival rate is less than 10% and median survival of these patients ranges between 6 and 9 months [2].

Although surgery and radiotherapy are important therapeutic approaches for metastatic melanoma, chemotherapy is indispensable, especially in cases where complete resection of metastases cannot be achieved [2, 3]. There are several chemotherapeutic agents that are applied as single-agent substances, combined chemotherapies (polychemotherapy), and biochemotherapies (combination of cytotoxic and immunomodulatory agents). The objective response (OR) rates for single-agent therapies range between 5% and 20%. Combined chemotherapies and biochemotherapies are able to clearly improve OR rates at the expense of enhanced toxicities and impaired quality of life, but unfortunately without prolonging overall survival [4–9]. In a small minority of patients, systemic therapy induces durable remissions [2]. However, due to the poor response rates, especially in achieving durable complete remissions, chemotherapy for melanoma is considered palliative rather than curative. The preservation of quality of life and minimization of tumor-associated symptoms should be the focus of all therapeutic strategies, taking into consideration the expected benefit and potential side effects associated with any specific therapeutic approach [3].

In this chapter, we will first give an overview of tumor biology, outline general mechanisms of action of cytostatic therapy, and discuss the several chemotherapeutic agents used in the treatment of melanoma, including combined chemotherapies and biochemotherapies. We will then describe the mechanisms involved in chemoresistance of melanoma, and conclude with an outlook on the efforts to enhance the efficacy of systemic antitumor therapy in metastatic melanoma [10–12].

Tumor Biology

Cell Cycle and Effects of Chemotherapeutic Agents

Based on decades of experience, it is well established that fast-growing tumors (i.e., Hodgkin lymphoma, testicular cancer) are sensitive to the

H. Stanisz, M.D. (✉) • T. Vogt, M.D. • K. Rass, M.D.
Department of Dermatology, Venereology and Allergology, University Hospital of the Saarland, Homburg/Saar, Germany
e-mail: hedwigstanisz@yahoo.de

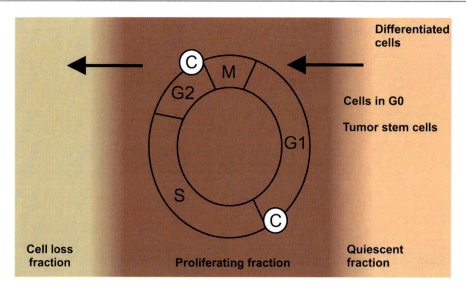

Fig. 19.1 Schematic illustration of the cell cycle. Chemotherapeutic agents show phase-specific (S-phase: DNA synthesis; M-Phase: mitosis) or phase-unspecific (throughout the cell cycle) mechanisms of action. *C* cell cycle check-points

action of cytostatic agents. Such tumors may have a doubling time of a few days and can be cured by chemotherapy. Other tumors with a doubling time of a month or more cannot be eradicated by such treatment [13]. These findings highlight the fact that an understanding of tumor kinetics is crucial for selection of cytostatic therapy. In almost every tumor, several distinct cell populations can be identified. These can be divided into the proliferating cell, the quiescent stem cell-like cell, and the differentiated cell fractions (Fig. 19.1). Differentiated cells have lost their ability to proliferate. Quiescent cells are in the G0 phase, but can enter the proliferating population following activation. The G1 phase prepares cells for the following S phase (the longest phase of the cell cycle), in which DNA synthesis and replication occur. In the G2 phase, which follows the S phase, accurate replication of DNA is determined. If necessary, mistakes are repaired by the cellular DNA repair machinery. The following M phase is characterized by mitosis formation (division of the nucleus and genetic information) and cell division.

Within this cell cycle, two check-points are incorporated: one between the G1 and S phases and another between the G2 and M phases. These cell cycle check-points are necessary to ensure that all processes pertaining to DNA synthesis and replication are correct [14]. If the cell is unable to repair DNA, the cell cycle is arrested and the cell undergoes apoptosis (programmed cell death). The tumor suppressor protein p53 plays a crucial role in cell cycle regulation and apoptosis induction. In many tumors, mutations of TP53 are responsible for uncontrolled proliferation. In melanoma, mutations of TP53 and other cell cycle regulating genes, such as CDKN2A (p16), p19, and CDK4 may be found, particularly in advanced stages of the disease.

Chemotherapeutic agents act predominantly on the proliferating cell fraction in tumors. This explains why fast-growing tumors with a large proliferating cell fraction are more sensitive to cytotoxic drugs than their slow-growing counterparts. The most vulnerable cell cycle phases are the S and M phases, whereas quiescent cells are essentially insensitive to cytostatic drugs.

Chemotherapeutic agents can be divided in two distinct groups, depending on their mode of action in the different phases of the cell cycle. Phase-specific agents exert their effects in a distinct phase of the cell cycle. Antimetabolites (methotrexate, gemcitabine) and DNA intercalating agents (anthracyclines) act in the S phase by inhibiting DNA synthesis, while mitosis inhibitors (vinca alkaloids, taxanes) act on cells in the late G2 and M phases. Phase-unspecific agents (alkylating agents, platinum derivatives) are effective during the entire cell cycle with pronounced effects on proliferating cells. All cytostatic agents have in common the destruction of cells via apoptosis induction. Therefore, apoptosis resistance (i.e., through inactivating mutations of proapoptotic genes [TP53] or upregulation of antiapoptotic pathways [Bcl-2], either acquired by tumor cells or pre-existing in tumor precursor cells) impairs the efficacy of chemotherapeutic agents [10, 12].

Kinetics of Tumor Growth and the Fractional Cell Kill Hypothesis

The interactions between tumor kinetics and cytostatic effects over time are mathematically described by growth curves. These curves are useful to study disease course and provide an approach toward improved cancer therapy. Tumor growth is based on three main criteria: (1) the time required to complete the cell cycle, (2) the proportion of proliferating cells, and (3) the cell loss fraction (Fig. 19.1). The proliferating cell fraction typically exceeds the cell loss fraction, with the relationship between both remaining constant over time. As a consequence, exponential tumor growth kinetics can be assumed. However, in most tumors, growth is not exponential at all times. It is observed that the proliferative fraction gets relatively smaller over time, while the cell loss fraction is increased. Hence, with increasing tumor burden, the growth curve reaches a plateau phase (Fig. 19.2). This phenomenon has been explained by insufficient vascularization of growing tumors. However, other hypotheses suggest an important relationship between tumor cells and the tumor environment, thereby implicating autocrine and paracrine growth factor interactions [10].

Incorporating the effects of cytostatic agents into the mathematical curve of exponentially growing tumors reveals that specific doses of

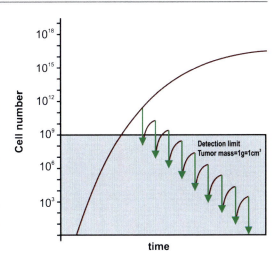

Fig. 19.2 Fractional cell kill hypothesis. Chemotherapy (*green arrows*) eliminates a constant fraction (~99.9%) of tumor cells (*red curve*). In this example, the tumor consists of 10^{11} cells at the beginning of chemotherapy. Following the first administration of the cytostatic agent, $0.1\% = 10^8$ cells remain alive. The surviving tumor cell population grows exponentially to 10^{10} cells before the next drug administration, which again eliminates 99.9% of cells and so on. Based on this model, at least six further cycles of chemotherapy are required to eradicate the tumor. Clinical detection threshold = ~10^9 cells

these drugs result in the destruction of a constant number of malignant cells (fractional cell kill hypothesis) (Fig. 19.2) [15–17]. Due to this constant dose-effect relationship, the absolute number of eliminated cells is dependent on tumor burden, whereas the actual percentage of these cells always remains the same. Hence, several cycles of chemotherapy are required to ensure tumor elimination. Treatment should theoretically be continued, even when tumor mass falls below the threshold for clinical detectability (around 1 g or ~10^9 cells) and evidence of clinical complete remission is achieved.

Chemotherapeutic Agents for Melanoma

Several chemotherapeutic agents are used in the treatment of melanoma as either single agents or in combination regimens with other chemotherapeutic or immunomodulatory substances.

Table 19.1 Overview of chemotherapeutic substance groups (agents frequently used in the treatment of melanoma are underlined)

Alkylating agents (Phase unspecific, cell cycle active)	Antimetabolites (Phase specific, S-Phase)
Nitrogen mustards	*Folate antagonists*
Cyclophosphamide	Methotrexate
Chlorambucil	*Pyrimidine antimetabolites*
Melphalan	Fluorouracil
Triazenes, hydrazines and related compounds	Gemcitabine
Dacarbazine	*Purine antimetabolites*
Temozolomide	Fludarabine
Nitrosureas	Pentostatin
Carmustine (BCNU)	Azathioprine
Lomustine (CCNU)	
Fotemustine	
Platinum-Compounds	
Cisplatin (CDDP)	
Carboplatin	
Alkyl sulfonates and bismethanesulfonates	
Busulfan	
Treosulfan	

Plant alkaloids and other plant-derived substances (Phase specific, M-Phase)	Antibiotics and related substances (Phase specific, S-Phase)
Vinca Alkaloids	*Anthracyclines*
Vindesine	Doxorubicin
Vincristine	*Bleomycines*
Vinblastine	Bleomycin
Taxanes	
Paclitaxel	
Docetaxel	
Topoisomerase inhibitors	
Topotecan	
Iridotecan	
Etoposide	

The most important cytotoxic drugs, their modes of actions, and characteristic side effects are described in the following sections and summarized in Table 19.1.

Single-Agent Chemotherapy

Dacarbazine

As the first approved cytotoxic agent for treatment of melanoma in the 1970s, Dacarbazine (*D*imethyl-1-*t*riazeno-*i*midazole-4-*c*arboxamide: DTIC) is considered to be a reference substance in melanoma chemotherapy. DTIC is a triazene derivative. Following intravenous administration, it requires oxidative demethylation in the liver by a microsomal P450 enzyme to become its active metabolite MTIC (*M*ethyl-1-*t*riazeno-*i*midazole-4-*c*arboxamide). It exerts its antitumoral effects by alkylation and methylation of nucleic acids (DNA and RNA) [18, 19]. DTIC is associated with rather moderate toxicity. Nausea is one of the major side effects, although myelosuppression (leucopenia, neutropenia) and flu-like symptoms can also be observed. As a rare fatal event, sudden hepatic vein thrombosis (Budd-Chiari syndrome) has been reported with DTIC therapy. DTIC is also associated with photosensitivity and must be administered in light-protected settings. The typical dosage is

Table 19.2 Palliative single agent chemotherapies used in the treatment of metastatic melanoma: treatment regimens and reported objective response (OR) rates

Cytotoxic drug	Substance class Mode of action	Treatment schedule	OR
Dacarbazine	*Triazenes* Alkylation and methylation of nucleic acids	250 mg/m² i.v. d1-5, q3w or q4w 800–1,200 mg/m² i.v. d1, q3w or q4w	5–23%
Temozolomide	*Triazenes* Alkylation and methylation of nucleic acids	150–200 mg/m² p.o. d1-5, q4w	14–21%
Fotemustine	*Nitrosoureas* Alkylation of nucleic acids and proteins	100 mg/m² i.v. d1,8,15 (induction) after 5 w rest: d1, q3w (maintenance)	7–25%
Vindesine	*Vinca alkaloids* Microtubule disruption	3 mg/m² i.v. weekly	~14%
Paclitaxel	*Taxanes* Microtubule disruption	80 mg/m² i.v. d1,8,15, q4w 250 mg/m² i.v. (24 h) d1, q3w	0–14%
Docetaxel	*Taxanes* Microtubule disruption	100 mg/m² i.v. d1, q3w	6–13%
Carboplatin	*Platinum drugs* DNA and protein cross-linking	400 mg/m² i.v. d1, q4w	11–19%

150–250 mg/m²/d for 5 consecutive days or a single dose of 800–1200 mg/m² repeated every 3–4 weeks (Table 19.2). The latter schedule is more convenient for the patient and demonstrates comparable clinical outcomes as the other dosage schedule. DTIC is considered the standard for controlled randomized trials that evaluate novel therapies in melanoma [20].

The OR rates in recent phase III studies with stringent tumor response evaluation were 5–12%, with a low frequency of complete remissions [21]. Responses are seldom durable, and the 6-year patient survival is <2% [22]. Nevertheless, in a minority of patients, particularly those with AJCC stage M1a or M1b disease, effective disease control can be achieved. In its three decades of use, DTIC monochemotherapy has never been evaluated in controlled trials versus placebo; therefore, there is a lack of evidence concerning overall survival benefit. To date, no other cytotoxic drug or chemotherapy-based combination regimen has been proven superior to DTIC for treatment of metastatic melanoma. Resistance to DTIC may be due to the induction of DNA repair enzymes (i.e., O6-methylguanine-DNA Methyltransferase: MGMT) [23].

Temozolomide

Temozolomide (TMZ) is a DTIC-related compound. It exerts its antitumoral effects by alkylation and methylation of nucleic acids (RNA and DNA, preferentially in the O6-guanine position). TMZ has been approved for the treatment of primary brain tumors, emphasizing its ability to penetrate the blood–brain barrier, in contrast to DTIC. Furthermore, TMZ does not require active metabolization, converting spontaneously to its active metabolite MTIC. It is orally administered, making it more comfortable for patients [24, 25].

The side effects associated with TMZ are comparable to those of DTIC, but with more pronounced thrombocytopenia. To date, Budd-Chiari syndrome has not been reported. The typical dosage of TMZ is 150–200 mg/m², depending on first- or second-line treatment, for 5 days repeated every 4 weeks (Table 19.2) [4]. The OR rates, time to progression, overall and progression-free survival with TMZ are comparable to those for

DTIC in melanoma patients who are free of brain metastases [4, 26]. In patients with brain metastases, TMZ may be a useful alternative to DTIC. However, as TMZ has not been shown to be superior to DTIC, it is currently not approved for the treatment of melanoma by the FDA or European authorities.

Similar to DTIC, TMZ resistance mechanisms are predominantly MGMT-driven. It has been shown that the activity of this repair enzyme is decreased in peripheral blood mononuclear cells within 4 h of TMZ administration; an effect which remains stable for the first 24 h [23]. As a result of this finding, it has been suggested that a prolonged escalated daily dose of TMZ may increase the chemosensitivity of malignant cells in brain tumors and melanoma [27]. Unfortunately, several different extended TMZ treatment schedules, evaluated in phase II and III studies in melanoma (i.e., 75 mg/m²/d for 6 weeks followed by a 2- to 4-week break; EORTC trial 18032: 150 mg/m²/d, 7 days on/off), did not demonstrate any impact on antitumor activity, especially when randomized against DTIC [26, 27].

Fotemustine

Fotemustine is an alkylating agent from the group of nitrosoureas, which degrades spontaneously under physiological conditions generating electrophilic species that are responsible for DNA and RNA alkylation. The generation of isocyanates as by-products explains its toxicity. Fotemustine is administered intravenously, but as a result of its high lipophilicity, it easily penetrates the blood–brain barrier [28].

The antitumoral activity of fotemustine is considered comparable to that of DTIC; although, there are studies which report some advantages concerning overall survival and time to development of brain metastases with fotemustine therapy [29–32]. Compared to DTIC, fotemustine is associated with higher myelotoxicity, particularly severe thrombocytopenia. Fotemustine is administered intravenously at a dosage of 100 mg/m², with induction (d1, d8, d15) and maintenance (three times weekly from week 8) phases (Table 19.2).

A particular indication for fotemustine therapy is metastatic uveal melanoma. As a result of a lack of lymphatic drainage in the retina, the common site for metastasis of this tumor is the liver. Patients with uveal melanoma and diffuse liver metastases can be effectively treated with catheter-guided intra-arterial fotemustine administration, with OR rates of 36–40% and a median overall survival of 15 months [33, 34]. However, to date, fotemustine is only approved in a few European countries for the treatment of metastatic melanoma.

Vindesine

Vindesine is a vinca alkaloid that inhibits microtubular assembly by specifically binding to the cytoskeletal protein tubulin [35]. Impaired polymerization of microtubules leads to a disruption of mitotic spindles and metaphase arrest, resulting in apoptosis. As microtubules are involved in a wide variety of cellular functions (in addition to mitosis), including motility, mechanical cell stability and intracellular transport processes, many side effects can result from its cytostatic action [36, 37].

Vindesine is administered intravenously and shows no significant penetration of the blood–brain barrier. Neurotoxicity, encompassing peripheral and even autonomic neuropathy, can be seen. Myelosuppression and myalgia may also occur, although alopecia is rather moderate. The typical dosage of vindesine is 3 mg/m² every 14 days. Based on phase I and II studies, the efficacy of vindesine is comparable to that of DTIC; although, phase III trials in the palliative setting have not been undertaken (Table 19.2) [38]. Vindesine is commonly used in combination chemotherapy regimens (CVD, see below).

Paclitaxel

Paclitaxel is a taxane that specifically binds to tubulin, stabilizing the microtubules through inhibition of microtubular disassembly. This results in a perturbation of cellular processes as tubulin assembly and disassembly are necessary for normal cellular function [39].

Paclitaxel is administered intravenously and shows no significant penetration of the blood–brain barrier. Neurotoxicity and myelosuppression are described. Its co-solvent substance cremophor EL may induce hypersensitivity and even anaphylactic reactions in 2–4% of cases, requiring careful monitoring of patients, especially during the initial drug administration. Prophylactic corticosteroid and antihistamine administration is recommended (i.e., dexamethasone 20 mg, clemastine 2 mg, and ranitidine 50 mg i.v. 30 min before paclitaxel administration) [40, 41]. Paclitaxel is also known to cause cardiac arrhythmia and profound alopecia, in addition to onycholysis.

The typical dosage of paclitaxel is 80–100 mg/m^2 on days 1, 8 and 15, every 4 weeks (Table 19.2). Phase III studies using paclitaxel as single-agent therapy are unavailable. However, based on the response rates seen in phase I and II studies, its efficacy is not superior to that of DTIC [42–44]. In melanoma patients, paclitaxel has been reported to be more effective in combination regimens and is commonly used with platinum derivatives [45].

Recently, an albumin-bound nanoparticle form of Cremophor-free paclitaxel (Abraxane, ABI-002) was tested as single-agent therapy in a phase II study of metastatic melanoma. The drug was well-tolerated, and demonstrated an improved OR rate of 21.6% with a median overall survival of 12.1 months in chemo-naive patients, but with only minor effects in pretreated patients (OR rate 2.7%, median overall survival 9.6 months) [46].

Cisplatin and Carboplatin

Cisplatin and Carboplatin are platinum derivatives, which act via DNA and protein crosslinking. They are activated non-enzymatically in cells to reactive platinum complexes. As the aquo-platinum-complexes are highly nucleophilic, they react preferentially with guanine N7 and adenine. The activation process of carboplatin is much slower than that of cisplatin.

Cisplatin is administered intravenously and does not penetrate the blood–brain barrier. Nephrotoxicity, neurotoxicity, ototoxicity, and both short-term and prolonged nausea are described. Because of its associated nephrotoxicity, cisplatin should be administered with appropriate hydration and osmotic diuresis. In a recent study, a combination of enhanced-dose cisplatin with the cytoprotective thiol form of amifostine (WR-2721) revealed no benefit with regard to toxicity or antitumoral effects in patients with melanoma [47]. Results with cisplatin as single-agent therapy for metastatic melanoma are poor. It is now typically used in combination chemotherapy regimens (CVD, see below).

Carboplatin is also administered intravenously, although its possible penetration through the blood–brain barrier is not fully determined. Side effects are similar, but milder than those seen with cisplatin. Efficacy and side effects of carboplatin correlate with renal clearance of the drug, which is dependant on the glomerular filtration rate (GFR). As the GFR differs in each patient, irrespective of body surface area, the carboplatin dosage is calculated according to the Calvert Formula [total dose (mg) = (target AUC) x (GFR + 25), where AUC = target area under the concentration versus time curve in mg/mL min]. Typical carboplatin doses range between AUCs of 5–7.5 mg/ml/min, every 3–4 weeks (Tables 19.2 and 19.3).

Response rates of 11–19% were observed in early phase II studies of metastatic melanoma, in which carboplatin was not administered in AUC-defined doses (400 mg/m^2 i.v. every 4 weeks) [48–50]. However, phase III studies with carboplatin as single-agent therapy for melanoma have not been undertaken. Carboplatin is commonly used with taxanes in combination chemotherapy regimens [45].

Combination Chemotherapy

The modest efficacy of single-agent chemotherapy resulted in attempts to improve antitumor activity by combining several agents. Initial single-institution studies suggested increased response rates and survival outcomes using combination chemotherapy. At first, two-agent regimens were used, in which DTIC was combined with one of the previously described drugs. Response rates of 10–20% were observed, but no real evidence for a superior response compared to single-agent therapy with DTIC could be found. Subsequently, combinations with three or four agents were studied.

Table 19.3 Palliative combination chemotherapies used in the treatment of metastatic melanoma: treatment regimens and reported objective response (OR) rates

Drug	Treatment schedule	OR
CVD	DTIC 450 mg/m² i.v. d1+8 or 250 mg/m² i.v. d1-5 Vindesine 3 mg/m² i.v. d1+8 Cisplatin 50 mg/m² i.v. d1+8, 100 mg/m² i.v. d1 q3w or q4w	24–45%
CP	Paclitaxel 175–225 mg/m² i.v. d1 Carboplatin AUC 6–7.5 i.v. d1 q3w	10–24%
BHD	BCNU 150 mg/m² i.v. d1 odd cycles Hydroxyurea 1,500 mg/m² p.o. d1-5 DTIC 150 mg/m² i.v. d1-5 q4w	13–30%
BOLD	Bleomycin 15 mg i.v. d1+4 Vincristine 1 mg/m² i.v. d1+5 CCNU 80 mg/m² p.o. d1 DTIC 200 mg/m² i.v. d1-5 q4w–q6w	22–40%
DBCT	DTIC 220 mg/m² i.v. d1-3 BCNU 150 mg/m² i.v. d1 odd cycles Cisplatin 25 mg/m² i.v. d1-3 Tamoxifen 2×10 mg p.o./d q3w or q4w	19–54%
Treosulfan/ Gemcitabine (uveal melanoma)	Treosulfan 5 g/m² i.v. d1 Gemcitabine 1 g/m² i.v. d1 q3w or q4w or 3.5 g/m² i.v. d1 and d8 1 g/m² i.v. d1 and d8 q3w	28.6%

Frequent polychemotherapies used in the treatment of metastatic melanoma are the CVD-, BHD-, BOLD- and DBCT-regimens (Table 19.3). The CVD (cisplatin, vindesine/vinblastine, DTIC) and Dartmouth (DBCT) (DTIC, carmustine (BCNU), cisplatin and tamoxifen) regimens are the most investigated in this setting. Phase II studies of the latter drug combinations have shown significantly higher OR rates: up to 40% and 54%, respectively (Table 19.3) [51, 52]. However, phase III studies comparing those polychemotherapies to DTIC did not reveal significant benefit with regard to overall survival [20, 53]. Paclitaxel with carboplatin is another combination regimen recently studied in melanoma patients [45, 54]. In an ongoing phase III study, evaluating the multikinase inhibitor sorafenib in pretreated metastatic melanoma patients, paclitaxel and carboplatin combination chemotherapy resulted in an OR rate of only 11%, but a remarkable median progression free-survival of 4 months [55]. Unfortunately, none of these combination chemotherapies has been shown to improve overall survival compared to single-agent DTIC. Using chemosensitivity testing, combination therapy with gemcitabine and treosulfan was found to generate antitumor activity and response rates up to 28.6% in metastatic uveal melanoma (Table 19.3) [56].

Combination chemotherapies are more likely to be accompanied by adverse events and cumulative toxicities that impair quality of life. Therefore, the selection of a specific treatment regimen should be carefully weighed against a patient's performance status and life expectancy. For patients with metastatic melanoma, combination chemotherapies might be indicated in those situations where an efficient tumor response is required (tumor-associated symptoms, high tumor burden, etc.), following failure of monochemotherapy.

Table 19.4 Palliative biochemotherapies used in the treatment of metastatic melanoma: treatment regimens and reported objective response (OR) rates

Drug	Treatment schedule	OR
Interferon alpha	9–18 MU/m² s.c. tiw, continuously	13–25%
Interleukin-2 (IL-2)	6 MU/kg i.v. every 8 h d1-5 and d15-19 each up to 14 consecutive doses q6w–q12w	16–21.6%
DTIC (or TMZ) + IFN alpha	DTIC 850 mg/m² i.v. d1 (or TMZ) 150 mg/m² p.o. d1-5 IFN-α2a/b 3 MU/m² d1-5 s.c., w1 IFN-α2a/b 5 MU/m² tiw s.c., w2-4, q4w	14–28%
Vindesine + IFN alpha	Vindesine 3 mg/m² i.v. d1 IFN-α2a/b 5 MU/m² d1-5 s.c., 3x/w q2w	24%
"Legha"	DTIC 800 mg/m² i.v. d1 Vinblastine 1.5 mg/m² i.v. d1-4 Cisplatin 20 mg/m² i.v. d1-4 IL-2 9 MU/m² i.v. d1-4 IFN-α2a/b 9 MU s.c. d1-5,7,9,11,13 q3w	48%

Biochemotherapy

Melanoma has been shown to be susceptible to agents that modulate the immune system. Accordingly, cytokines were introduced for the systemic adjuvant and palliative treatment of this disease. Interleukin-2 (IL-2) and Interferon (IFN) alpha are widely investigated as either a single-agent approach or in combination with cytostatic agents (biochemotherapy, BCT) [57–59].

IL-2 is a lymphokine that is known to stimulate T-cell proliferation and immune response, augment natural killer (NK)-cell proliferation and cytotoxicity, and trigger cytokine release (IFN gamma, tumor necrosis factor [TNF]) from activated lymphocytes. In 1998, high-dose IL-2 was approved by the FDA for the treatment of metastatic melanoma. As a single-agent regimen, IL-2 is administered at doses between 6 and 7.2 MU/kg every 8 h on days 1–5 and 15–19 (Table 19.4).

IFN alpha shows moderate antitumor activity in metastatic melanoma when used as single-agent therapy. As a consequence, it has been primarily investigated in combination chemotherapeutic regimens. In several studies, combined high-dose IL-2, IFN alpha and cytostatic therapy (BCT) was associated with high response rates (up to 50%) and even durable complete remissions [59–61]. However, a recent meta-analysis of 18 trials comparing BCT with chemotherapy confirmed that while tumor response and time to disease progression were significantly better for BCT, these benefits did not translate into significantly better overall survival [62]. As cytokine therapy is associated with considerable toxicity, including rhabdomyolysis (high-dose IFN alpha), sepsis, myocardial infarction, and capillary leak syndrome (high-dose IL-2), with treatment-related deaths in individual cases, the use of BCT is dependent on excellent patient performance status. Predictive markers to identify those melanoma patients who would benefit from BCT are urgently needed, but currently not available. Therefore, BCT may be useful in isolated cases, but is not generally recommended as first-line treatment for metastatic melanoma.

Adjuvant Chemotherapy

In the 1980s and 1990s, cytostatic agents began to be tested in the adjuvant setting. Initially, positive results with adjuvant vindesine treatment were reported in a non-randomized study.

However, these were not reproducible in a randomized, observation-controlled trial by the German DeCOG [63]. Data on adjuvant BCT, using DTIC and IFN alpha, are conflicting [64, 65]. Larger randomized trials and a recent meta-analysis have not shown any benefit with adjuvant chemotherapy, while the use of cytostatic drugs clearly enhances morbidity [66]. Therefore, adjuvant chemotherapy is not currently recommended outside of clinical trials.

Locoregional Chemotherapy

Locoregional administration of cytostatic agents and cytokines (IL-2), either intra-arterially or intralesionally, is a useful means of treating cutaneous or subcutaneous metastases in melanoma. Isolated hyperthermic limb perfusion has been shown to be an effective approach when the disease is localized to a distal extremity [67]. A novel method to treat skin and soft-tissue melanoma metastases is electroporation, combined with systemic or intralesional chemotherapy (electrochemotherapy) [68]. With regard to isolated liver metastasis (i.e., from primary uveal melanoma), intra-arterial chemotherapy via the common hepatic artery, isolated hepatic perfusion, or transarterial chemoembolization (TACE) may be feasible treatment options [34, 69].

Isolated Hyperthermic Limb Perfusion

Using isolated limb perfusion (ILP), cytostatic drugs can be administered intra-arterially at much higher doses without the potential for enhanced toxicity. Melphalan is the agent mostly commonly used in this setting, showing optimal efficacy if administered at a temperature of 42°C (hyperthermic). For bulky disease, melphalan may be combined with TNF alpha, in an effort to enhance antitumor response. ILP was initially established as an adjuvant treatment option for melanoma in the 1960s and 1970s. However, in a recent randomized multicenter adjuvant trial, ILP failed to show any benefit with regard to time to distant metastasis or overall survival compared with observation [70]. In contrast, ILP is a very effective palliative treatment option for control of unresectable locoregional metastasis on the extremities, with high response rates (up to 70%) and reductions in recurrent in-transit metastasis [67, 71].

Electrochemotherapy

Electrochemotherapy (ECT) is another option for treatment of unresectable bulky metastases of the skin and superficial subcutaneous tissue, particularly in the setting of melanoma, sarcoma, breast and head and neck cancer. This treatment consists of intravenous or intralesional administration of a chemotherapeutic agent (bleomycin or cisplatin), followed by the application of electrical impulses to the metastases in order to increase drug uptake by tumor cells (Fig. 19.3). The treatment can result in painful muscle contractions and is typically administered under general anesthesia. In a prospective multicenter study, OR rates of up to 85% and complete responses of up to 73% were observed for the above tumor entities [72]. However, any effect on overall survival, which would not be expected due to the local mode of action of ECT, has not been investigated to date. ECT is a useful treatment in the palliative setting, in order to combat tumor-associated symptoms, achieve locoregional disease control, and potentially improve quality of life [68, 72, 73].

Hepatic Intra-Arterial Chemotherapy and Transarterial Chemoembolization (TACE)

Isolated liver metastases occur frequently in patients with primary uveal melanoma. Systemic chemotherapy has been shown to be widely ineffective in this setting, with the exception of treosulfan and gemcitabine [56]. Therefore, local chemotherapy, involving intra-arterial intrahepatic cytotoxic drug administration, may be a useful treatment modality. Fotemustine is the most commonly used agent. Response rates of 30–40%, median overall survival of 15 months, and occasional complete remissions have been reported for metastases from ocular and primary cutaneous melanoma [33, 34, 74]. Catheter dislocations and occasional severe thrombocytopenia are treatment limitations.

In cases that are refractory to systemic and local chemotherapy, liver metastases may also be treated by selectively administered transarterial chemoembolization (TACE), using fotemustine or cisplatin combined with starch microspheres and intermittent oily substrates (Lipiodol). Single-center experiences and a small number of case reports have demonstrated some clinical benefit, with an overall survival of up to 6 months in pretreated patients with liver metastasis from uveal melanoma [69, 75]. Controlled randomized studies have not been undertaken.

Chemoresistance

Several factors can contribute to impaired efficacy of chemotherapeutic agents. Toxicity can influence optimal dosing and/or drugs may not reach sufficient concentrations in particular body compartments because of pharmacokinetic characteristics. In addition, tumors may become resistant to the cytostatic effects of a chemotherapeutic agent. Therapeutic "pressure" can lead to the selection of cells that contain mutations of

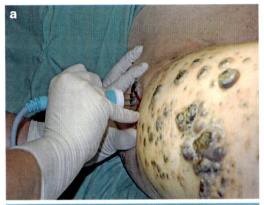

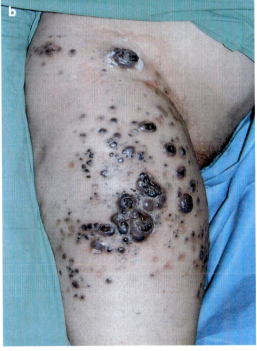

Fig. 19.3 A 46-year-old female patient with advanced melanoma and predominantly locoregional metastases to her right thigh and groin area [Stage IV; pT4b pN3 M1c (AJCC 2009)]. (**a**) Treatment with electrochemotherapy (ECT) 8 min after i.v. administration of 30 mg bleomycin (15 mg/m²). Clinical signs (**b**) before and (**c**) 3 weeks after ECT, with evidence of partial remission

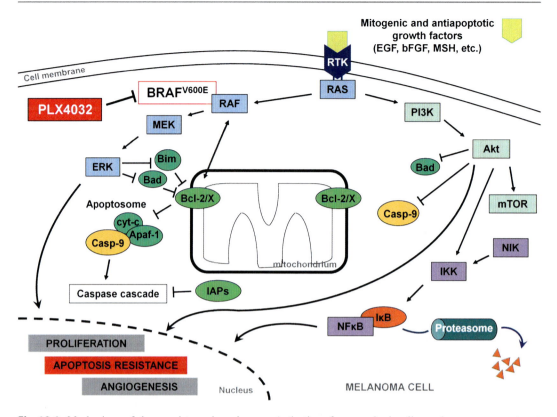

Fig. 19.4 Mechanisms of chemoresistance in melanoma. Activation of oncogenic signaling pathways may counteract drug-mediated apoptosis

genes related to chemosusceptibility. With a mutation rate of one per 10^4–10^8 cell divisions, the probability for initial chemoresistance is much lower for small tumors compared to their larger counterparts [76–79]. Specific cellular mechanisms leading to chemoresistance include (1) mutations which hamper the cellular influx of cytostatic drugs (i.e., carrier proteins) and (2) upregulation of proteins which augment their cellular efflux [multi-drug resistance proteins and other ABC (ATP-binding cassette) transporters: ABCC2 (MRP2), Ral-binding protein 1 (RALBP1)] [80–82]. Furthermore, a chemotherapeutic agent may be inactivated by specific enzymes, repair enzymes can antagonize cytostatic-induced DNA damage (i.e., MGMT in DTIC- and TMZ-induced DNA alkylation), and/or drug targets may be altered (i.e., mutated tubulin proteins—targets for vinca alkaloids and taxanes).

In normal skin melanocytes, physiological resistance to apoptosis ("programmed cell death") protects against ultraviolet radiation (UVR)-induced damage. In contrast to keratinocytes which become apoptotic via a p53-dependent pathway, melanocytes are stimulated to produce melanin by UVR exposure. In melanocytes, resistance to apoptosis results from intracellular upregulation of antiapoptotic proteins (i.e., Bcl-2) and DNA repair mechanisms via endocrine and paracrine signals (melanocortins, endothelin-1) [83, 84]. For melanoma, the most important mechanisms for chemoresistance appear to be related to specific antiapoptotic features of tumor cells. As cytostatic agents promote apoptosis, mechanisms that inhibit cell death are likely to play a crucial role in chemoresistance [85]. Mechanisms counteracting apoptosis in melanoma cells are the mitogen-activated protein kinase (MAPK), phosphoinositol-3-kinase (PI3K), and nuclear factor-kappa B (NF-kB) pathways (Fig. 19.4) [12, 86–88]. The selective inhibition of these pathways (i.e., "targeted therapy") is currently regarded as one of the most promising approaches to overcome therapeutic resistance in metastatic melanoma. The effects of chemotherapeutic drugs might be improved if administered in parallel or sequentially with targeted agents. One of these promising agents is PLX4032, a selective BRAF^{V600E} inhibitor, which showed an OR rate of 70% and a progression-free survival of 7 months in a recent phase I study of metastatic melanoma [89]. A phase III trial comparing PLX4032 with DTIC therapy is currently in progress.

An ongoing phase III study by the German DeCOG is evaluating chemosensitivity-directed cytostatic treatment. The chemosensitivity index of a patient's tumor is calculated using a luciferase-based *in vitro* luminometric assay. Patients are then randomized to the most sensitive chemotherapeutic drug combination or DTIC as control group. A prior phase II study demonstrated a significant median overall survival benefit of 14.6 months in chemosensitive melanoma patients versus 7.4 months in the drug-resistant group [90].

Overcoming Chemoresistance by Stroma-Targeted Combinations of Biomodulating Agents

The tissue microenvironment is crucial for tumor survival and growth. Consequently, drugs directed against the tumor stroma represent a promising molecular-targeted approach in oncology.

Stroma-targeted strategies appear to have some major advantages compared with established chemotherapeutic agents. Acquired drug resistance might be delayed, since the stroma is genetically more stable than respective tumor cells. As stroma-targeted drugs are administered at lower does, toxic side effects are usually milder than those due to conventional chemotherapies. However, the aims of a stroma-targeted approach are often the control/stabilization of disease and prolongation of progression-free survival rather than the achievement of high response rates, which is very different to many established high-dose chemotherapy schedules.

The endothelial cell is an important component of the tumor stroma. Tumors cannot grow beyond a critical size (about 100–200 μm) or metastasize to other organs without adequate nutritional support through a vascular network. Angiogenesis has therefore been identified as a hallmark of cancer. Metabolic stress (hypoglycemia, low pH, low pO2), infiltrating inflammatory cells, genetic mutations (activation of oncogenes or inhibition of tumor suppressor genes that regulate the transcription of angiogenic factors), and other mechanisms can shift the highly sensitive balance between pro- and antiangiogenic factors and promote tumor angiogenesis.

A number of drugs, originally developed for the management of metabolic and rheumatological disorders, have demonstrated antitumor effects. This activity is mediated by the inhibition of angiogenesis and attenuation of tumor-associated inflammation, thereby modulating the tumor stroma and making the tissue environment less permissive and supportive for the tumor itself. Drugs with antiangiogenic activity, such as PPARγ agonists, COX-2 inhibitors, thalidomide, and mTOR (mammalian target of rapamycin) antagonists, have been evaluated in clinical trials with very promising results [91–93]. Furthermore, it has been found that low-dose continuous administration of conventional chemotherapeutic drugs, referred to as "metronomic" chemotherapy, specifically targets endothelial cells within tumors. Therefore, metronomic scheduling of conventional cytostatic agents is regarded as an effective component of broader antiangiogenic therapy. In a recent randomized phase II trial in second-line advanced melanoma patients, the addition of antiangiogenic drugs to metronomic chemotherapy was found to significantly enhance progression-free survival, with a trend toward improved overall survival (18.8 vs. 8.2 months), compared with metronomic chemotherapy alone [94].

Concluding Remarks

Besides surgical resection of localized metastases, chemotherapy is the most important pillar of current palliative melanoma treatment approaches. Unfortunately, the antitumor effects of chemotherapeutic agents are limited and confined to transient tumor responses in the majority of patients. With more than 30 years of use, DTIC remains the reference chemotherapeutic agent for treatment of metastatic melanoma. No other cytostatic drug or combination regimen has demonstrated a better overall survival advantage. Therefore, an urgent need exists to both discover novel biomarkers of disease and develop novel therapeutic strategies, so that individualized melanoma therapy can be realized. A number of different approaches are currently under investigation—agents targeting melanoma signaling pathways, angiogenesis, apoptosis and immune escape. The use of novel strategies may complement established chemotherapeutic approaches and finally improve the prognosis of patients with metastatic melanoma.

References

1. Jemal A, Siegel R, Ward E, et al. Cancer statistics, 2008. CA Cancer J Clin. 2008;58:71–96.
2. Garbe C, Eigentler TK. Diagnosis and treatment of cutaneous melanoma: state of the art 2006. Melanoma Res. 2007;17:117–27.
3. Garbe C, Hauschild A, Volkenandt M, et al. Evidence and interdisciplinary consensus-based German guidelines: surgical treatment and radiotherapy of melanoma. Melanoma Res. 2008;18:61–7.
4. Middleton MR, Grob JJ, Aaronson N, et al. Randomized phase III study of temozolomide versus dacarbazine in the treatment of patients with advanced metastatic malignant melanoma. J Clin Oncol. 2000;18:158–66.
5. Schadendorf D. Is there a standard for the palliative treatment of melanoma? Onkologie. 2002;25:74–6.
6. Eigentler TK, Caroli UM, Radny P, et al. Palliative therapy of disseminated malignant melanoma: a systematic review of 41 randomised clinical trials. Lancet Oncol. 2003;4:748–59.
7. Rass K, Tadler D, Tilgen W. Therapy of malignant melanoma. First-, second-, and pathogenesis-oriented third-line therapies. Hautarzt. 2006;57: 773–84.
8. Nashan D, Müller ML, Grabbe S, et al. Systemic therapy of disseminated malignant melanoma: an evidence-based overview of the state-of-the-art in daily routine. J Eur Acad Dermatol Venereol. 2007; 21:1305–18.
9. Rass K, Tilgen W. Treatment of melanoma and non-melanoma skin cancer. Adv Exp Med Biol. 2008;624:296–318.
10. Morton DL, Essner R, Kirkwood JM, Wollmann RC. Malignant melanoma in cancer medicine, vol. 1. 6th ed. Hamilton: BC Decker; 2003 [Chapter 122].
11. Rass K, Diefenbacher M, Tilgen W. Experimental treatment of malignant melanoma and its rationale. Hautarzt. 2008;59:475–83.
12. Rass K, Hassel JC. Chemotherapeutics, chemoresistance and the management of melanoma. G Ital Dermatol Venereol. 2009;144:61–78.
13. Shackney SE, McCormack GW, Cuchural Jr GJ. Growth rate patterns of solid tumors and their relation to responsiveness to therapy: an analytical review. Ann Intern Med. 1978;89:107–21.
14. Hartwell LH, Weinert TA. Checkpoints: controls that ensure the order of cell cycle events. Science. 1989; 246:629–34.
15. Skipper HE. The effects of chemotherapy on the kinetics of leukemic cell behavior. Cancer Res. 1965; 25:1544–50.
16. Skipper HE. Laboratory models: some historical perspective. Cancer Treat Rep. 1986;70:3–7.
17. Wilcox WS, Griswold DP, Laster Jr WR, et al. Experimental evaluation of potenital anticancer agents. XVII. Kinetics of growth and regression after treatment of certain solid tumors. Cancer Chemother Rep 1. 1965;47:27–39.
18. Vaughan K, Tang Y, Llanos G, et al. Studies of the mode of action of antitumor triazenes and triazines. 6. 1-Aryl-3-(hydroxymethyl)-3-methyltriazenes: synthesis, chemistry, and antitumor properties. J Med Chem. 1984;27:357–63.
19. Farina P, Benfenati E, Reginato R, et al. Metabolism of the anticancer agent 1-(4-acetylphenyl)-3,3-dimethyltriazene. Biomed Mass Spectrom. 1983;10: 485–8.
20. Eggermont AMM, Kirkwood JM. Re-evaluating the role of dacarbazine in metastatic melanoma: what have we learned in 30 years? Eur J Cancer. 2004;40: 1825–36.
21. Lui P, Cashin R, Machado M, et al. Treatments for metastatic melanoma: synthesis of evidence from randomized trials. Cancer Treat Rev. 2007;33:665–80.
22. Hill II GJ, Krementz ET, Hill HZ. Dimethyl triazeno imidazole carboxamide and combination therapy for melanoma. IV. Late results after complete response to chemotherapy (Central Oncology Group Protocols 7130, 7131, and 7131A). Cancer. 1984;53:1299–305.
23. Lee SM, Thatcher N, Margison GP. O^6-Alkylguanine-DNA alkyltransferase depletion and regeneration in human peripheral lymphocytes following dacarbazine and fotemustine. Cancer Res. 1991;51:619–23.
24. Denny BJ, Wheelhouse RT, Stevens MF, et al. NMR and molecular modeling investigation of the mechanism of activation of the antitumor drug temozolomide and its interaction with DNA. Biochemistry. 1994;33:9045–51.
25. Lowe PR, Sansom CE, Schwalbe CH, et al. Antitumor imidazotetrazines. 25. Crystal structure of 8-carbamoyl-3-methylimidazo[5,1-d]-1,2,3,5-tetrazin-4(3H)-one (temozolomide) and structural comparisons with the

related drugs mitozolomide and DTIC. J Med Chem. 1992;35:3377–82.
26. Patel P, Suciu S, Mortier L. Extended schedule, escalated dose temozolomide versus dacarbazine in stage IV malignant melanoma: final results of the randomised phase III study EORTC 18032. 33rd European Society of Medical Oncology (ESMO) Congress; 2008.
27. Neyns B, Tosoni A, Hwu WJ, Reardon DA. Dose-dense temozolomide regimens: antitumor activity, toxicity, and immunomodulatory effects. Cancer. 2010;116:2868–77.
28. Khayat D, Giroux B, Berille J, et al. Fotemustine in the treatment of brain primary tumors and metastases. Cancer Invest. 1994;12:414–20.
29. Avril MF, Aamdal S, Grob JJ, et al. Fotemustine compared with dacarbazine in patients with disseminated malignant melanoma: a phase III study. J Clin Oncol. 2004;22:1118–25.
30. Jacquillat C, Khayat D, Banzet P, et al. Final report of the French multicenter phase II study of the nitrosourea fotemustine in 153 evaluable patients with disseminated malignant melanoma including patients with cerebral metastases. Cancer. 1990;66:1873–8.
31. Calabresi F, Aapro M, Becquart D, et al. Multicenter phase II trial of the single agent fotemustine in patients with advanced malignant melanoma. Ann Oncol. 1991;2:377–8.
32. Kleeberg UR, Engel E, Israels P, et al. Palliative therapy of melanoma patients with fotemustine. Inverse relationship between tumor load and treatment effectiveness. A multicentre phase II trial of the EORTC-Melanoma cooperative group (MCG). Melanoma Res. 1995;5:195–200.
33. Leyvraz S, Spataro V, Bauer J, et al. Treatment of ocular melanoma metastatic to the liver by hepatic arterial chemotherapy. J Clin Oncol. 1997;15:2589–95.
34. Peters S, Voelter V, Zografos L, et al. Intra-arterial hepatic fotemustine for the treatment of liver metastases from uveal melanoma: experience in 101 patients. Ann Oncol. 2006;17:578–83.
35. Bensch KG, Marantz R, Wisniewski H, Shelanski M. Induction in vitro of microtubular crystals by vinca alkaloids. Science. 1969;165:495–6.
36. Chan SY, Worth R, Ochs S. Block of axoplasmic transport in vitro by vinca alkaloids. J Neurobiol 1980;11:251–64.
37. Green LS, Donoso JA, Heller-Bettinger IE, Samson FE. Axonal transport disturbances in vincristine-induced peripheral neuropathy. Ann Neurol. 1977;1:255–62.
38. Quagliana JM, Stephens RL, Baker LH, Costanzi JJ. Vindesine in patients with metastatic malignant melanoma: a Southwest Oncology Group study. J Clin Oncol. 1984;2:316–9.
39. Gelmon K. The taxoids: paclitaxel and docetaxel. Lancet. 1994;344:1267–72.
40. Zidan J, Hussein O, Abzah A, et al. Oral premedication for the prevention of hypersensitivity reactions to paclitaxel. Med Oncol. 2008;25:274–8.
41. Kloover JS, den Bakker MA, Gelderblom H, van Meerbeeck JP. Fatal outcome of a hypersensitivity reaction to paclitaxel: a critical review of premedication regimens. Br J Cancer. 2004;90:304–5.
42. Wiernik PH, Einzig AI. Taxol in malignant melanoma. J Natl Cancer Inst Monogr. 1993;15:185–7.
43. Einzig AI, Hochster H, Wiernik PH, et al. A phase II study of taxol in patients with malignant melanoma. Invest New Drugs. 1991;9:59–64.
44. Nathan FE, Berd D, Sato T, et al. Paclitaxel and tamoxifen. An active regimen for patients with metastatic melanoma. Cancer. 2000;88:79–87.
45. Rao RD, Holtan SG, Ingle JN, et al. Combination of paclitaxel and carboplatin as second-line therapy for patients with metastatic melanoma. Cancer. 2006;106:375–82.
46. Hersh EM, O'Day SJ, Ribas A, et al. A phase 2 clinical trial of nab-paclitaxel in previously treated and chemotherapy-naive patients with metastatic melanoma. Cancer. 2010;116:155–63.
47. Glover D, Ibrahim J, Kirkwood J, et al. Phase II randomized trial of cisplatin and WR-2721 versus cisplatin alone for metastatic melanoma: an Eastern Cooperative Oncology Group Study (E1686). Melanoma Res. 2003;13:619–26.
48. Casper ES, Bajorin D. Phase II trial of carboplatin in patients with advanced melanoma. Invest New Drugs. 1990;8:187–90.
49. Chang A, Hunt M, Parkinson DR, et al. Phase II trial of carboplatin in patients with metastatic malignant melanoma. A report from the Eastern Cooperative Oncology Group. Am J Clin Oncol. 1993;16:152–5.
50. Evans LM, Casper ES, Rosenbluth R. Phase II trial of carboplatin in advanced malignant melanoma. Cancer Treat Rep. 1987;71:171–2.
51. Lattanzi SC, Tosteson T, Chertoff J, et al. Dacarbazine, cisplatin and carmustine, with or without tamoxifen, for metastatic melanoma: 5-year follow-up. Melanoma Res. 1995;5:365–9.
52. Legha SS, Ring S, Papadopoulos N, et al. A prospective evaluation of a triple-drug regimen containing cisplatin, vinblastine, and dacarbazine (CVD) for metastatic melanoma. Cancer. 1989;64:2024–9.
53. Chapman PB, Einhorn LH, Meyers ML, et al. Phase III multicenter randomized trial of the Dartmouth regimen versus dacarbazine in patients with metastatic melanoma. J Clin Oncol. 1999;17:2745–51.
54. Hodi FS, Soiffer RJ, Clark J, et al. Phase II study of paclitaxel and carboplatin for malignant melanoma. Am J Clin Oncol. 2002;25:283–6.
55. Hauschild A, Agarwala SS, Trefzer U, et al. Results of a phase III, randomized, placebo-controlled study of sorafenib in combination with carboplatin and paclitaxel as second-line treatment in patients with unresectable stage III or stage IV melanoma. J Clin Oncol. 2009;27:2823–30.
56. Pföhler C, Cree IA, Ugurel S, et al. Treosulfan and gemcitabine in metastatic uveal melanoma patients: results of a multicenter feasibility study. Anticancer Drugs. 2003;14:337–40.

57. Atkins MB, Lotze MT, Dutcher JP, et al. High-dose recombinant interleukin 2 therapy for patients with metastatic melanoma: analysis of 270 patients treated between 1985 and 1993. J Clin Oncol. 1999;17: 2105–16.
58. Creagan ET, Dalton RJ, Ahmann DL, et al. Randomized, surgical adjuvant clinical trial of recombinant interferon alfa-2a in selected patients with malignant melanoma. J Clin Oncol. 1995;13: 2776–83.
59. Flaherty LE, Robinson W, Redman BG, et al. A phase II study of dacarbazine and cisplatin in combination with outpatient administered interleukin-2 in metastatic malignant melanoma. Cancer. 1993;71:3520–5.
60. Atkins MB, O'Boyle KR, Sosman JA, et al. Multiinstitutional phase II trial of intensive combination chemoimmunotherapy for metastatic melanoma. J Clin Oncol. 1994;12:1553–60.
61. Legha SS, Ring S, Eton O, et al. Development of a biochemotherapy regimen with concurrent administration of cisplatin, vinblastine, dacarbazine, interferon alfa, and interleukin-2 for patients with metastatic melanoma. J Clin Oncol. 1998;16:1752–9.
62. Ives NJ, Stowe RL, Lorigan P, Wheatley K. Chemotherapy compared with biochemotherapy for the treatment of metastatic melanoma: a meta-analysis of 18 trials involving 2,621 patients. J Clin Oncol. 2007;25:5426–34.
63. Eigentler TK, Radny P, Hauschild A, et al. Adjuvant treatment with vindesine in comparison to observation alone in patients with metastasized melanoma after complete metastasectomy: a randomized multicenter trial of the German Dermatologic Cooperative Oncology Group. Melanoma Res. 2008;18:353–8.
64. Garbe C, Radny P, Linse R, et al. Adjuvant low-dose interferon α2a with or without dacarbazine compared with surgery alone: a prospective-randomized phase III DeCOG trial in melanoma patients with regional lymph node metastasis. Ann Oncol. 2008;19:1195–201.
65. Stadler R, Luger T, Bieber T, et al. Long-term survival benefit after adjuvant treatment of cutaneous melanoma with dacarbazine and low dose natural interferon alpha: a controlled, randomised multicentre trial. Acta Oncol. 2006;45:389–99.
66. Verma S, Quirt I, McCready D, et al. Systematic review of systemic adjuvant therapy for patients at high risk for recurrent melanoma. Cancer. 2006;106: 1431–42.
67. Noorda EM, Vrouenraets BC, Nieweg OE, et al. Isolated limb perfusion: what is the evidence for its use? Ann Surg Oncol. 2004;11:837–45.
68. Byrne CM, Thompson JF, Johnston H, et al. Treatment of metastatic melanoma using electroporation therapy with bleomycin (electrochemotherapy). Melanoma Res. 2005;15:45–51.
69. Schuster R, Lindner M, Wacker F, et al. Transarterial chemoembolization of liver metastases from uveal melanoma after failure of systemic therapy: toxicity and outcome. Melanoma Res. 2010;20:191–6.
70. Koops HS, Vaglini M, Suciu S, et al. Prophylactic isolated limb perfusion for localized, high-risk limb melanoma: results of a multicenter randomized phase III trial. J Clin Oncol. 1998;16:2906–12.
71. Cornett WR, McCall LM, Petersen RP, et al. Randomized multicenter trial of hyperthermic isolated limb perfusion with melphalan alone compared with melphalan plus tumor necrosis factor: American College of Surgeons Oncology Group Trial Z0020. J Clin Oncol. 2006;24:4196–201.
72. Marty M, Sersa G, Garbay JR, et al. Electrochemotherapy—an easy, highly effective and safe treatment of cutaneous and subcutaneous metastases: results of ESOPE (European Standard Operating Procedures of Electrochemotherapy) study. Eur J Cancer, Suppl. 2006;4:3–13.
73. Campana LG, Mocellin S, Basso M, et al. Bleomycin-based electrochemotherapy: clinical outcome from a single institution's experience with 52 patients. Ann Surg Oncol. 2009;16:191–9.
74. Siegel R, Hauschild A, Kettelhack C, et al. Hepatic arterial Fotemustine chemotherapy in patients with liver metastases from cutaneous melanoma is as effective as in ocular melanoma. Eur J Surg Oncol. 2007;33: 627–32.
75. Sunderkötter C, Eickelmann M, Köhler M, et al. Remission of extensive intrahepatic metastasis by C-arm computed tomography guides chemoembolization in uveal melanoma. J Dtsch Dermatol Ges. 2010;8:525–8.
76. Goldie JH, Coldman AJ. Genetic instability in the development of drug resistance. Semin Oncol. 1985;12:222–30.
77. Coldman AJ, Goldie JH. Variation in growth parameters and their effect on the acquisition of drug resistance. Prog Clin Biol Res. 1986;223:103–11.
78. Coldman AJ, Goldie JH. A stochastic model for the origin and treatment of tumors containing drug-resistant cells. Bull Math Biol. 1986;48:279–92.
79. Kendal WS, Frost P. Metastatic potential and spontaneous mutation rates: studies with two murine cell lines and their recently induced metastatic variants. Cancer Res. 1986;46:6131–5.
80. Goldenberg GJ, Vanstone CL, Israels LG, et al. Evidence for a transport carrier of nitrogen mustard in nitrogen mustard-sensitive and -resistant L5178Y lymphoblasts. Cancer Res. 1970;30:2285–91.
81. Endicott JA, Ling V. The biochemistry of P-glycoprotein-mediated multidrug resistance. Annu Rev Biochem. 1989;58:137–71.
82. La Porta CA. Drug resistance in melanoma: new perspectives. Curr Med Chem. 2007;14:387–91.
83. Kadekaro AL, Wakamatsu K, Ito S, Abdel-Malek ZA. Cutaneous photoprotection and melanoma susceptibility: reaching beyond melanin content to the frontiers of DNA repair. Front Biosci. 2006;11:2157–73.
84. Leiter U, Schmid RM, Kaskel P, et al. Antiapoptotic bcl-2 and bcl-xL in advanced malignant melanoma. Arch Dermatol Res. 2000;292:225–32.

85. Campioni M, Santini D, Tonini G, et al. Role of Apaf-1, a key regulator of apoptosis, in melanoma progression and chemoresistance. Exp Dermatol. 2005;14:811–8.
86. Davies H, Bignell GR, Cox C, et al. Mutations of the BRAF gene in human cancer. Nature. 2002;417: 949–54.
87. Blanco-Aparicio C, Renner O, Leal JF, Carnero A. PTEN, more than the AKT pathway. Carcinogenesis. 2007;28:1379–86.
88. Haluska F, Pemberton T, Ibrahim N, Kalinsky K. The RTK/RAS/BRAF/PI3K pathways in melanoma: biology, small molecule inhibitors, and potential applications. Semin Oncol. 2007;34:546–54.
89. Smalley KS. PLX-4032, a small-molecule B-Raf inhibitor for the potential treatment of malignant melanoma. Curr Opin Investig Drugs. 2010;11:699–706.
90. Ugurel S, Schadendorf D, Pföhler C, et al. In vitro drug sensitivity predicts response and survival after individualized sensitivity-directed chemotherapy in metastatic melanoma: a multicenter phase II trial of the Dermatologic Cooperative Oncology Group. Clin Cancer Res. 2006;12:5454–63.
91. Hafner C, Reichle A, Vogt T. New indications for established drugs: combined tumor-stroma-targeted cancer therapy with PPARγ-agonists, Cox-2 inhibitors, mTOR Antagonists and metronomic chemotherapy. Curr Cancer Drug Targets. 2005;5: 393–419.
92. Reichle A, Bross K, Vogt T, et al. Pioglitazone and rofecoxib combined with angiostatic sceduling of trofosfamide in far advanced malignant melanomas and soft tissue sarcomas. Cancer. 2004;101:2247–56.
93. Vogt T, Hafner C, Bross K, et al. Antiangiogenetic therapy with pioglitazone, rofecoxib, and metronomic trofosfamide in patients with advanced malignant vascular tumors. Cancer. 2003;98:2251–6.
94. Reichle A, Vogt T, Coras B, et al. Targeted combined anti-inflammatory and angiostatic therapy in advanced melanoma: a randomized phase II trial. Melanoma Res. 2007;17:360–4.

Molecular-Targeted Therapy for Melanoma

Alessia E. Russo, Ylenia Bevelacqua, Andrea Marconi, Andrea Veronesi, and Massimo Libra

Introduction

In its early stages, melanoma can be surgically cured, leading to 5-year survival rates exceeding 90% [1]. However, metastatic melanoma is refractory to current therapies and has a very poor prognosis, with a median survival rate of only ~6 months [2].

Numerous studies have shown that the mitogen-activated protein kinase (MAPK; RAS/RAF/MEK/ERK) and the phosphoinositide 3-kinase/AKT pathways are upregulated in the majority of human melanomas, with alterations of signaling through both pathways playing key roles in melanoma proliferation, progression and survival [3,4]. Mutations of microphthalmia-associated transcription factor (MITF), KIT and cyclin-dependent kinases (CDKs) have also been proposed to contribute to melanoma development [5–8]. Several pharmacologic inhibitors that target various effectors of these pathways continue to be developed. Most agents are still being evaluated in preclinical studies, although some have already reached phase III evaluation.

However, despite encouraging preclinical findings, early clinical trials with these drugs as single agents have been largely disappointing. A possible explanation for the lack of effective single-agent therapies is functional redundancy between the numerous signaling pathways embedded within complex networks that influence each other's activity. Therefore, melanoma researchers now point to the need to simultaneously target several pathways in order to control melanoma growth, invasion and survival.

In addition, failure of single-agent targeted therapy could also be due to melanoma heterogeneity. Melanomas can be effectively subtyped based on distinct mutational profiles. Therefore, in order to maximize the probability of success in future targeted therapy trials, it will be necessary to "genetically pre-select" patients so that appropriate drugs can be matched to the genetic lesions that drive each individual's tumor.

Activating Mutations Within the RAS/RAF/MEK/ERK Pathway

The RAS/RAF/MEK/ERK pathway, also known as the MAPK (mitogen-activated protein kinase) pathway, is a signal transduction cascade relaying extracellular signals from the plasma membrane to the nucleus via an ordered series of consecutive phosphorylation events [9]. In response to a variety of cellular stimuli, including growth factor-mediated activation of receptor tyrosine kinases (RTKs),

A.E. Russo, M.D. (✉) • Y. Bevelacqua, M.D.
• A. Marconi, M.D. • M. Libra, M.D., Ph.D.
Department of Biomedical Sciences,
University of Catania, Catania, Italy
e-mail: alessierikarusso@hotmail.it

A. Veronesi, M.D.
Division of Medical Oncology C,
National Cancer Institute, IRCCS, Aviano, Italy

RAS assumes an activated, GTP-bound state, leading to recruitment of RAF from the cytosol to the cell membrane where it becomes activated, likely via a Src-family tyrosine kinase [10–12]. Activated RAF causes the phosphorylation and activation of MAPK extracellular signal-regulated kinases 1 and 2 (MEK1/MEK2), which in turn phosphorylate and activate extracellular signal-regulated kinases 1 and 2 (ERK1/ERK2) at specific Thr and Tyr residues [13–15]. Activated ERK translocates to the nucleus and phosphorylates several nuclear transcription factors (i.e., Elk-1, Myc, CREB, and Fos) which bind promoters of many genes, including growth factor and cytokine genes that are important for stimulating the cellular proliferation, differentiation, and survival of multiple cell types [16–36].

Dysregulation of the RAS/RAF/MEK/ERK pathway plays an important role in melanoma cell proliferation and survival, with ERK being constitutively activated in up to 90% of melanomas [37]. ERK hyperphosphorylation most commonly results from mutations of the NRAS (15–30%) and particularly BRAF (50–70%) genes [38,39]. The NRAS aberration often represents a substitution of leucine for glutamine at residue 61; this change impairs GTP hydrolysis and maintains the protein in a state of constitutive activation [40]. Mutations in other RAS isoforms are rare in melanoma, suggesting context-dependent activity for specific RAS isoforms [41].

The most frequent BRAF mutation, which accounts for more than 90% of BRAF alterations in melanoma, results in a glutamic acid for valine substitution at codon 600 (Val600Glu; $BRAF^{V600E}$) [38]. This mutation introduces a conformational change in protein structure, with glutamic acid acting as a phosphomimetic between the Thr^{598} and Ser^{601} phosphorylation sites, leading to constitutive activation of the protein and a large increase in basal kinase activity [42]. The resulting hyperactivity of the MAPK pathway promotes tumor development [38,43,44]. $BRAF^{V600E}$ also promotes vascular development by stimulating autocrine vascular endothelial growth factor (VEGF) secretion [45]. Mutations in ARAF and CRAF have not been found in this tumor. Likely, this pattern of mutations is due to the different mechanisms of activation for the three RAF genes: BRAF requires one genetic mutation for oncogenic activation, while ARAF and CRAF require two mutations [46,47].

Interestingly, genetic alterations in NRAS and BRAF rarely coexist in melanoma [38,48,49], suggesting that either mutant BRAF or NRAS is able to activate the MEK-ERK pathway. The RAF/MEK/ERK and PI3K/AKT pathways, in addition to the gene alterations that activate these pathways, in melanoma are outlined in Fig. 20.1.

RAF Inhibitors

Sorafenib was the first BRAF inhibitor to be clinically available. It is an oral multi-kinase inhibitor that decreases activity of RAF, VEGFR-1, -2 and -3, PDGFR, Flt-3, p38, c-KIT, and FGFR-1 [50], thereby inhibiting both tumor cell growth and angiogenesis [45,51,52]. Sorafenib inhibits the growth of melanoma xenografts in mice [46]. However, it has little or no antitumor activity in advanced melanoma patients as a single agent [53]. The reasons for sorafenib failure in clinical trials are not clear. Perhaps, it is unable to reach a concentration sufficient to inhibit BRAF, or proliferation of melanoma cells may be driven by alternative signaling pathways upon RAF/MEK/ERK signaling blockade [53]. To improve sorafenib efficacy in the therapy of melanoma, it has been used in combination with standard chemotherapeutic drugs. Preliminary results from studies combining sorafenib with carboplatin and paclitaxel have been encouraging [54]. However, phase III trials have shown that this combination failed to improve progression-free survival of patients with advanced melanoma [54].

Sorafenib has also been combined with dacarbazine (DTIC) [55,56]. In a randomized, double-blind, placebo-controlled multicenter study, improvements in progression-free survival and time to progression were observed with the addition of sorafenib to dacarbazine [56]. However, these findings did not translate into an improvement in overall survival [56].

Recently, it was reported that sorafenib activates glycogen synthase kinase-3beta (GSK-3beta) in melanoma cell lines [57]. Constitutive

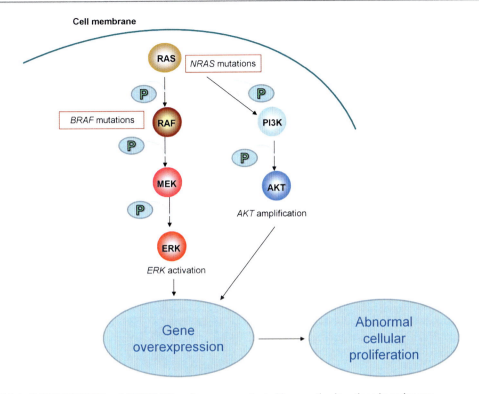

Fig. 20.1 RAF/MEK/ERK and PI3K/AKT pathways are activated by genetic alterations in melanoma

activation of this kinase correlates with a marked increase in basal levels of Bcl-2 and Bcl-xL, and decreased antitumor efficacy of sorafenib. Therefore, sorafenib given in conjunction with targeted therapies against glycogen synthase kinase-3beta or antiapoptotic Bcl-2 family members may prove useful [57,58].

The limited activity of sorafenib in tumors with mutant BRAF has prompted the evaluation of more specific BRAF inhibitors, such as RAF-265 and PLX4032, in phase I–III clinical trials in melanoma subjects (http://clinicaltrials.gov).

MEK Inhibitors

It has been demonstrated that melanoma cell lines with mutant BRAF are more sensitive to MEK inhibition than melanoma cell lines harboring oncogenic RAS [59]. In BRAF-mutant tumors, MEK inhibition results in downregulation of cyclin D1, upregulation of p27, hypophosphorylation of retinoblastoma protein (Rb), and growth arrest in G_1. MEK inhibition also induces differentiation and senescence of BRAF-mutant cells and apoptosis in some, but not all, $BRAF^{V600E}$-mutant models [59–61]. Two MEK inhibitors are currently being tested in clinical trials: PD0325901 and AZD6244.

Phase I trials with PD0325901 have reported clinical activity in melanoma, with two patients demonstrating partial responses and eight patients having stable disease that lasted 3–7 months [62–64]. However, the ocular toxicities associated with PD0325901 have halted its further evaluation. AZD6244 was tested in a randomized phase II trial of 200 patients with stage IV melanoma. Patients were randomized to AZD6244 or temozolomide, but recently reported findings indicate that there was no significant difference in progression-free survival between both arms [65]. However, AZD6244 monotherapy was noted to result in lasting remissions, particularly in patients with documented BRAF mutations.

Dysregulation of the PI3K/AKT Pathway

In response to activated growth factor receptors, the phosphoinositide-3-OH kinase (PI3K) phosphorylates phosphatidylinositol-4,5-biphosphate (PIP2) to phosphatidylinositol-3,4,5-triphosphate (PIP3), leading to activation of the major downstream effector of the PI3K pathway, AKT [66]. Once activated, AKT phosphorylates further downstream cellular proteins that promote cell proliferation and survival [66–68]. The lipid phosphatase PTEN negatively regulates this cascade through dephosphorylation of PIP3 [68].

Recent studies have revealed aberrant regulation of PI3K signaling in a high proportion of melanomas. Indeed, PTEN is deleted and the downstream AKT gene is amplified in ~45% of tumors [69,70]. Both of these genetic alterations result in overexpression of AKT3 [70], an isoform of AKT. Increased phospho-AKT expression in melanoma is associated with tumor progression and lower survival rates [71,72]. Oncogenic RAS can also bind and activate PI3K, resulting in increased AKT activity [73]. These data suggest that loss of PTEN and oncogenic activation of RAS are largely equivalent with regard to their ability to increase oncogenic signaling through the PI3K pathway [74]. This hypothesis is supported by the finding that PTEN somatic mutations are seen in melanomas harboring mutations in BRAF, but not NRAS [75]. This is consistent with the ability of NRAS to activate both the PI3K and MAPK cascades, so that in the presence of oncogenic NRAS, additional mutations in BRAF and PTEN are unnecessary [1,72]. In recent studies of genomic alterations in primary melanomas, tumors with BRAF mutations had fewer copies of PTEN than those with NRAS mutations, suggesting that dual activation of the PI3K and MAPK pathways are important events in melanoma development [72,76]. The effects of PTEN deletion on PI3K/AKT and RAF/MEK/ERK activation in melanoma are outlined in Fig. 20.2.

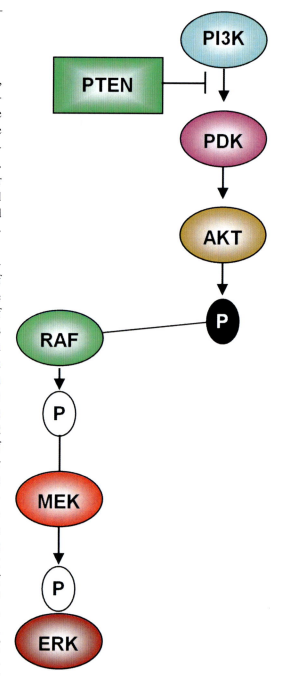

Fig. 20.2 Effects of PTEN deletion on PI3K/AKT and RAF/MEK/ERK activation in melanoma. Upregulation of the RAF/MEK/ERK cascade by PTEN deletion and AKT hyperactivation results in the continuous proliferation, rather than differentiation, of melanocytic cells

Combined Inhibition of MAPK and mTOR Signaling

Temsirolimus and everolimus, which target the PI3K/AKT pathway, have shown minimal activity as single agents in melanoma [77,78]. They target mTOR, a serine/threonine kinase downstream of AKT, which modulates protein synthesis, cell cycle progression, and angiogenesis [79]. Since mTOR is a cytosolic protein expressed by all tissues, these inhibitors do not show high specificity with regard to melanoma cell targeting [58]. Furthermore, it has been determined that the mTOR pathway has a complicated feedback loop that involves suppression of AKT. Hence, mTOR inhibitors could potentially activate AKT in some cells [80].

Given the cooperation between the MAPK and PI3K pathways in melanoma cell proliferation and survival [75], parallel inhibition of targets in both pathways may result in synergistic inhibition of melanoma cell growth. Several studies have demonstrated the feasibility of this new therapeutic approach [71,81–86]. In particular, combining nanoliposomes containing ceramide (a lipid-based AKT inhibitor) with sorafenib has been shown to decrease tumor development through enhanced effects on the signaling cascades [85]. Simultaneously targeting the MAPK pathway with sorafenib and the PI3K/AKT pathway with rapamycin was also reported to inhibit growth, induce cell death, and suppress invasive potential of melanoma cells [86].

However, no study has described complete regression of melanoma tumors with the use of PI3K and MAPK inhibitors, indicating that other targets or drug combinations will need to be identified and validated.

PI3K Inhibitors in Combination with Chemotherapeutic Agents

Recent studies suggest that anticancer agents can trigger prosurvival events that attenuate their therapeutic efficacy. In particular, cisplatin has been shown to induce activation of the AKT pathway and to attenuate cisplatin-induced apoptosis in several human cancer cell lines [87,88]. The MAPK signaling pathway also appears to play a role in chemoresistance [89]. Sinnberg et al. [90] investigated the effects of the AKT pathway inhibitors LY294002, wortmannin, and rapamycin, and the MAPK pathway inhibitors sorafenib, U0126, and PD98059, on chemosensitivity of melanoma cells to cisplatin and temozolomide. The AKT pathway inhibitors significantly increased the growth inhibitory effects of cisplatin and temozolomide, whereas the MAPK pathway inhibitors did not enhance chemosensitivity. Moreover, combinations of the PI3K inhibitor LY294002 or the mTOR inhibitor rapamycin with the chemotherapeutics cisplatin or temozolomide significantly induced apoptosis of melanoma cells in monolayer culture and completely suppressed invasive tumor growth of melanoma cells in organotypic culture. These effects were associated with nearly complete abolishment of the antiapoptotic Bcl-2 family protein Mcl-1. A recently opened phase II study of everolimus in combination with temozolomide in patients with unresectable stage IV melanoma will provide insight into this potential chemosensitization strategy.

Resistance of Melanoma to Drug-Induced Apoptosis

It has been shown that melanoma cells have low levels of spontaneous apoptosis *in vivo* compared with other tumor cell types, and are relatively resistant to drug-induced apoptosis *in vitro* [1,91]. As most chemotherapeutic drugs function by inducing apoptosis in malignant cells, resistance to apoptosis is thought to be the main cause of treatment failure in melanoma [91].

Dysregulation of the intrinsic (mitochondrial-dependent) apoptotic pathway forms the basis for resistance to chemotherapy-induced apoptosis in melanoma [92–98]. The p53/Bcl-2 signaling network is one of the most important regulators of cell apoptosis; the Bcl-2 superfamily includes proapoptotic (BAX, BAK, BAD, BID, Bim, NOXA, and PUMA) and antiapoptotic (Bcl-2, Bcl-xL, Mcl-1, Bcl-w, and A1) members. In response to irreversible DNA damage, p53 becomes activated and induces the expression of proapoptotic members of the Bcl-2 family. These effectors promote mitochondrial membrane permeabilization and release of cytochrome c, which binds to Apaf-1 and leads to the activation of effector caspases that result in apoptosis [99].

The loss of p53 function allows cells that have suffered DNA damage to survive and divide, propagating pro-cancerous mutations; however, unlike many other chemoresistant cancers, melanomas harbor a very low frequency of p53 mutations [100–103]. Therefore, other components of the p53 pathway, either upstream or downstream of p53 are likely defective in melanoma. It has been shown that aberrant methylation leads to loss of Apaf-1 expression, rendering cells unable to execute the normal apoptotic response following p53 activation [58,95]. Decreased levels of Apaf-1 correlate with advanced disease and chemoresistance in melanoma [58,104].

High levels of Bcl-2 expression have been demonstrated in both melanoma and benign melanocytes [91,105]. Recent evidence suggests that mutant BRAF and CRAF signaling may lead to ERK-dependent [106] and ERK-independent prosurvival signals by directly engaging Bcl-2 family members [107].

Alterations in other members of the Bcl-2 family are also found to be involved in melanoma progression and chemoresistance. Several studies have reported that resistance to a variety of both traditional and targeted chemotherapeutic agents is largely mediated by Mcl-1 overexpression [58,108–114]. Unlike other antiapoptotic Bcl-2 family members, Mcl-1 suppresses apoptosis induced by BAK, but not BAX [115]. Mcl-1 also has the unique property of rapid steady-state turnover due to proteasomal degradation [58,115]. Thus, in the presence of chemotherapeutics that inhibit proteasome function, such as bortezomib, Mcl-1 can accumulate and result in decreased sensitivity to these agents [58,111].

Apoptosis Signaling Inhibitors

The first targeted therapy against Bcl-2 was oblimersen (OBL), an antisense oligonucleotide that binds to native Bcl-2 mRNA leading to its degradation. OBL improves the chemosensitivity of human melanoma tumors grown in severe combined immunodeficient (SCID) mice [116]. In a large randomized phase III trial, patients with advanced melanoma received either DTIC or DTIC and OBL [117]. The DTIC plus OBL-containing regimen improved median overall survival compared to patients treated with DTIC alone (9.0 vs. 7.8 months); however, the difference between both groups was not significant ($p=0.077$). Conversely, a subgroup analysis revealed significant improvement in overall survival in patients with normal baseline Lactate Dehydrogenase (LDH). These findings suggest that serum LDH can be used to identify patients who are unlikely to benefit from oblimersen-dacarbazine treatment, and support the use of LDH as a key stratification factor in future randomized trials.

Other inhibitors of Bcl-2 family members have been developed and are currently entering clinical trials. Two of these are ABT-737 and the orally available analogue ABT-263, which mimic the BH domain and tightly bind to Bcl-2, Bcl-xL, and Bcl-w. Both molecules have demonstrated promising activity alone and in combination with cytotoxic and other targeted therapies in preclinical studies [118,119].

Novel Therapeutic Targets in Melanoma

Our understanding of melanoma biology has increased substantially with the availability of genomic technologies. The Sanger Center (http://www.sanger.ac.uk/) maintains a catalogue of all mutations reported in cancer. Currently, there are over 600 genes which have been shown to be altered in melanoma. The number of putative melanoma oncogenes and melanoma tumor suppressor genes (TSGs) continues to grow at a rapid pace and their identification has the potential to promote development of novel, more effective targeted therapies. Molecular-targeted therapies for melanoma used in recent clinical trials are summarized in Table 20.1. Currently, CRAF, c-KIT, MITF, and CDKs seem to be promising targets in melanoma patients.

Table 20.1 Molecular-targeted therapy for melanoma

Agent	Function	Target(s)	Reference
Sorafenib	Multi-kinase inhibitor	RAF, VEGFR-1, -2 and -3, PDGFR, Flt-3, p38, c-KIT, and FGFR-1	[53–58,85,86]
RAF-265	Multi-kinase inhibitor	Mutant BRAF, VEGFR-2	[http://clinicaltrials.gov]
PLX4032	Selective kinase inhibitor	Mutant BRAF	[http://clinicaltrials.gov]
PD0325901	Selective kinase inhibitor	MEK	[62–64]
AZD6244	Selective kinase inhibitor	MEK	[65]
Sirolimus	PI3K/AKT pathway inhibitor	mTOR	[86]
Temsirolimus	PI3K/AKT pathway inhibitor	mTOR	[77,84]
Everolimus	PI3K/AKT pathway inhibitor	mTOR	[78]
Oblimersen	Antisense oligonucleotide	Bcl-2	[117]
ABT-263	BH domain-mimetic	Bcl-2, Bcl-xL, and Bcl-w	[118,119]
Imatinib	RTK inhibitor	c-KIT	[120,121]
Dasatinib	RTK inhibitor	c-KIT	[122]
SNS-032	Multi-CDK inhibitor	CDK2, −7, and −9	[123]

C-KIT or CRAF Signaling-Driven Melanoma Subsets

The recent publication of studies showing the presence of KIT mutation or amplification in acral and mucosal melanomas has evoked interest in c-KIT signaling as a therapeutic target [6,124–127]. C-KIT is a receptor tyrosine kinase that triggers many downstream events, including activation of the MAPK and PI3K pathways [128,129]. The validity of c-KIT as a therapeutic target in melanoma was recently shown by two clinical case reports, in which melanoma patients with activating mutations in KIT showed remarkable responses to the c-KIT inhibitor imatinib [120,121]. Imatinib binds the ATP-binding site of (inactive conformation) c-KIT [130]. Therefore, mutations that stabilize the active conformation of c-KIT will be resistant to imatinib therapy. Dasatinib, a second generation c-KIT inhibitor, may be more relevant as it binds both the active and inactive conformations of c-KIT [122]. On the basis of these data, multiple phase II investigations with imatinib or dasatinib, alone or in combination with other agents, have been initiated.

CRAF has also been proposed as a suitable therapeutic target for subgroups of melanoma presenting with defined characteristics. In RAS-mutant melanoma cells, it is CRAF and not BRAF which activates MEK [131]. In normal melanocytes, activation of the MAPK pathway only proceeds via BRAF, as constitutive protein kinase A (PKA) activity leads to the phosphorylation and inactivation of CRAF. In contrast, for melanomas with NRAS mutations, the cyclic AMP/PKA system is dysregulated, so that PKA no longer suppresses CRAF, allowing CRAF-mediated MAPK activation to occur [131].

Although most studies have focused on the BRAF^{V600E} mutation, at least 70 other BRAF mutations have been identified [42]. Many of these show reduced BRAF kinase activity relative to the V600E mutant form; however, they are able to activate the MAPK pathway by directly binding to CRAF, leading to its phosphorylation and transactivation [42].

In addition, it has recently been reported that elevated CRAF expression mediates resistance to BRAF inhibitors in BRAF^{V600E} melanoma cells [132]. Thus, it is likely that CRAF is a valid therapeutic target in (1) subgroups of melanomas with activating NRAS mutations, (2) those with low-activity mutations in BRAF, or (3) those that become resistant to BRAF inhibitors.

A limited number of drugs targeting CRAF have been developed and tested in preclinical studies. RAF antisense oligonucleotides have shown promising results in preclinical studies, but were disappointing in later clinical studies in which no benefit was seen [133–138]. The failure of antisense treatment could be due to poor selection of study patients (i.e., based on CRAF tumor expression levels). Sorafenib is a potent CRAF inhibitor [50], but it is not CRAF-specific and involves multiple targets and mechanisms. Studies are underway to assess combinations of CRAF inhibitors with other small molecule inhibitors, such as Bcl-2 inhibitors and MEK inhibitors.

Inactivation of Both MITF and BRAF^{V600E} Significantly Inhibit Melanoma Growth

The link between microphthalmia-associated transcription factor (MITF) and melanoma development is complex. MITF acts as a master regulator of melanocyte development, function and survival [139,140], and plays a double role of inducer/repressor of cellular proliferation [141]. High levels of MITF expression lead to G_1 cell cycle arrest and differentiation, through induction of the cyclin-dependent kinase inhibitors p16^{INK4a} and p21^{Cip} [142,143], whereas very low, or null, expression levels predispose to apoptosis [1]. Only intermediate levels promote cell proliferation. Therefore, it is thought that melanoma cells have developed strategies to maintain MITF levels in the range compatible with tumorigenesis. It has been shown that constitutive ERK activity, stimulated by BRAF^{V600E} in melanoma cells, is associated with ubiquitin-dependent MITF degradation [144]. Nevertheless, continued expression of MITF is necessary for proliferation and survival of melanoma cells, as a function of CDK2 and Bcl-2 gene regulation [145,146]. Furthermore, BRAF mutation is associated with MITF amplification in 10–15% of melanomas [5]. However, other mechanisms likely counteract ERK-dependent proteasomal degradation of MITF, since MITF amplification occurs in only a minority of melanomas in which BRAF and NRAS genes are mutated. MITF is a downstream target of β-catenin, a key effector of the Wnt signaling pathway, which stimulates growth of melanoma cells [147]. Thus, an alternative mechanism of MITF recovery could involve stabilizing mutations in β-catenin leading to induction of MITF [58,148,149]. Another mechanism could involve mutant BRAF. It has recently been shown that oncogenic BRAF controls MITF on two levels.

It downregulates the protein by stimulating its degradation, but then counteracts this by increasing MITF expression through the transcription factor BRN2 [150].

To clarify the therapeutic role of MITF as a molecular target in human melanoma, Kido et al. [151] evaluated its effect on cell proliferation in a panel of human melanoma cell lines which expressed different levels of MITF. It was observed that both MITF depletion and overexpression significantly suppressed proliferation. However, half of the melanoma cell lines were relatively resistant to MITF depletion. Therefore, in an effort to enhance the anti-proliferative effect of MITF downregulation, the authors combined shRNA-mediated MITF depletion with BRAF^{V600E} inactivation. This resulted in a significant inhibition of melanoma growth, even in those cell lines resistant to MITF depletion. These data suggest simultaneous inhibition of MITF and MAPK signaling may be an attractive strategy for melanoma treatment.

Cell Cycle Changes in Melanoma

The p16^{INK4a}-Rb pathway is a critical gatekeeper for cell cycle progression. In the CDK4/6-mediated phophosphorylated state, Rb drives cells towards G_1/S-phase transition, while in the hypophosphorylated state, Rb binds and represses the E2F transcription factor and prevents the progression through S-phase [152]. p16^{INK4a} retards the cell cycle and inhibits the cyclin D/CDK4 complex, thereby preventing the latter from phosphorylating Rb [153].

The exit of cells from the cell cycle is a physiological process. Indeed, normal somatic cells have a finite lifespan, and following a defined number of divisions, they exit from the cell cycle and enter a state of senescence [1,154]. Senescence also occurs in response to oncogenic stresses, thereby acting as a cellular protection mechanism against cancer formation [155,156]. It has been shown that abnormally high activation of the MAPK pathway can inhibit cellular growth in a wide variety of both normal cells and cancer cells by promoting cellular senescence [157,158].

Notably, BRAF^{V600E} was recently found to induce p16^{INK4a} expression and senescence in primary human melanocytes *in vitro* [157,159]. Therefore, senescence can only be overcome if the p16^{INK4a}-Rb pathway is not fully engaged (such as when p16^{INK4a} is inactivated) [8,160]. It has been reported that germline mutations in CDKN2A (site of p16^{INK4a}) are linked to familial melanoma susceptibility [161–163]. Somatic mutations of CDKN2A are also found in many sporadic melanomas [7,164]. p16^{INK4a} is inactivated by deletions, point mutations, and promoter methylation [165,166], or through transcriptional silencing via overexpression of the transcriptional suppressor, inhibitor of differentiation 1 (ID1) [167]. Given that p16^{INK4a} requires direct interaction with the cyclin-CDK complex in order to inhibit its protein kinase activity, changes in CDK4 that render it resistant to p16^{INK4a} mimic those associated with p16^{INK4a} loss [149]. In fact, somatic and germline mutations in CDK4 have been detected in melanoma cell lines [168] and familial melanomas [169], respectively.

Molecular-targeted therapeutic approaches aimed at restoration of cell cycle control in melanoma are actively being explored. Because restoration of lost tumor suppressor function (i.e., p16^{INK4a}) is difficult, major efforts have been directed at targeting CDKs (the catalytically active downstream components). Unfortunately, the initial studies of early CDK inhibitors, including a single-agent phase II study of flavopiridol (inhibitor of CDK1/2/4/6), as well as a single-agent phase II study of UCN-01 (7-hydroxystaurosporine), a CDK2 and protein kinase C inhibitor, have not been promising [73]. Recently, PD-0332991, an orally bioavailable, highly selective and potent CDK4/6 inhibitor, demonstrated G$_1$ arrest in Rb-positive tumor cells and significant tumor regression or growth delay in murine xenografts [170,171]. Another novel small molecule inhibitor, SCH 727965, potently inhibits CDK2, in addition to CDK1/5/7/9 [172]. Treatment with SCH 727965 inhibited DNA synthesis and caused cell cycle arrest and apoptosis *in vitro*. In tumor xenograft models, treatment resulted in tumor growth inhibition and regression, which was enhanced by combination with cytotoxics. Other promising agents that target multiple CDKs and are under early clinical investigation include SNS-032 (BMS-387032), which inhibits CDK2/7/9 [123]; AG-024322, which targets CDK1/2/4 [173]; and ZK 304709, a multi-targeted inhibitor of CDK1/2/4/7/9, VEGFR-1, -2, and -3, and PDGFR-β [174].

Conclusions

A better understanding of the molecular pathways responsible for melanoma progression has led to the development of novel targeted therapies for this devastating disease. Currently, a whole array of molecular-targeted agents against BRAF signaling, MEK signaling and mTOR are undergoing clinical evaluation. Interestingly, the inhibition of one pathway can result in the upregulation of other related or redundant pathways. Therefore, the simultaneous targeting of several pathways may be required for disease control and improved patient survival. Moreover, the "genetic pre-selection" of melanoma patients for targeted therapy trials will likely enhance results and improve clinical outcomes.

References

1. Gray-Schopfer V, Wellbrock C, Marais R. Melanoma biology and new targeted therapy. Nature. 2007;445: 851–7.
2. Miller AJ, Mihm Jr MC. Melanoma. N Engl J Med. 2006;355:51–65.
3. Smalley KS. A pivotal role for ERK in the oncogenic behaviour of malignant melanoma? Int J Cancer. 2003;104:527–33.
4. Dhawan P, Singh AB, Ellis DL, Richmond A. Constitutive activation of Akt/protein kinase B in melanoma leads to up-regulation of nuclear factor-κB and tumor progression. Cancer Res. 2002;62: 7335–42.
5. Garraway LA, Widlund HR, Rubin MA, et al. Integrative genomic analyses identify MITF as a lineage survival oncogene amplified in malignant melanoma. Nature. 2005;436:117–22.
6. Curtin JA, Busam K, Pinkel D, Bastian BC. Somatic activation of KIT in distinct subtypes of melanoma. J Clin Oncol. 2006;24:4340–6.
7. Bartkova J, Lukas J, Guldberg P, et al. The p16-cyclin D/Cdk4-pRb pathway as a functional unit frequently

altered in melanoma pathogenesis. Cancer Res. 1996;56:5475–83.
8. Bachmann IM, Straume O, Akslen LA. Altered expression of cell cycle regulators cyclin D1, p14, p16, CDK4 and Rb in nodular melanomas. Int J Oncol. 2004;25:1559–65.
9. Garnett MJ, Marais R. Guilty as charged: B-RAF is a human oncogene. Cancer Cell. 2004;6:313–9.
10. Minden A, Lin A, McMahon M, et al. Differential activation of ERK and JNK mitogen-activated protein kinases by Raf-1 and MEKK. Science. 1994; 266:1719–23.
11. Lange-Carter CA, Johnson GL. Ras-dependent growth factor regulation of MEK kinase in PC12 cells. Science. 1994;265:1458–61.
12. Marais R, Light Y, Paterson HF, Marshall CJ. Ras recruits Raf-1 to the plasma membrane for activation by tyrosine phosphorylation. EMBO J. 1995;14: 3136–45.
13. Marais R, Light Y, Paterson HF, Mason CS, Marshall CJ. Differential regulation of Raf-1, A-Raf, and B-Raf by oncogenic ras and tyrosine kinases. J Biol Chem. 1997;272:4378–83.
14. Mason CS, Springer CJ, Cooper RG, Superti-Furga G, Marshall CJ, Marais R. Serine and tyrosine phosphorylations cooperate in Raf-1, but not B-Raf activation. EMBO J. 1999;18:2137–48.
15. Xu S, Robbins D, Frost J, Dang A, Lange-Carter C, Cobb MH. MEKK1 phosphorylates MEK1 and MEK2 but does not cause activation of mitogen-activated protein kinase. Proc Natl Acad Sci USA. 1995;92:6808–12.
16. Deng T, Karin M. c-Fos transcriptional activity stimulated by H-Ras-activated protein kinase distinct from JNK and ERK. Nature. 1994;371:171–5.
17. Davis RJ. Transcriptional regulation by MAP kinases. Mol Reprod Dev. 1995;42:459–67.
18. Robinson MJ, Stippec SA, Goldsmith E, White MA, Cobb MH. A constitutively active and nuclear form of the MAP kinase ERK2 is sufficient for neurite outgrowth and cell transformation. Curr Biol. 1998;8:1141–50.
19. Aplin AE, Stewart SA, Assoian RK, Juliano RL. Integrin-mediated adhesion regulates ERK nuclear translocation and phosphorylation of Elk-1. J Cell Biol. 2001;153:273–82.
20. McCubrey JA, May WS, Duronio V, Mufson A. Serine/threonine phosphorylation in cytokine signal transduction. Leukemia. 2000;14:9–21.
21. Tresini M, Lorenzini A, Frisoni L, Allen RG, Cristofalo VJ. Lack of Elk-1 phosphorylation and dysregulation of the extracellular regulated kinase signaling pathway in senescent human fibroblast. Exp Cell Res. 2001;269:287–300.
22. Eblen ST, Catling AD, Assanah MC, Weber MJ. Biochemical and biological functions of the N-terminal, noncatalytic domain of extracellular signal-regulated kinase 2. Mol Cell Biol. 2001;21: 249–59.
23. Adachi T, Kar S, Wang M, Carr BI. Transient and sustained ERK phosphorylation and nuclear translocation in growth control. J Cell Physiol. 2002;192: 151–9.
24. Wang CY, Bassuk AG, Boise LH, Thompson CB, Bravo R, Leiden JM. Activation of the granulocyte-macrophage colony-stimulating factor promoter in T cells requires cooperative binding of Elf-1 and AP-1 transcription factors. Mol Cell Biol. 1994;14:1153–9.
25. Thomas RS, Tymms MJ, McKinlay LH, Shannon MF, Seth A, Kola I. ETS1, NFkappaB and AP1 synergistically transactivate the human GM-CSF promoter. Oncogene. 1997;14:2845–55.
26. Ponti C, Gibellini D, Boin F, et al. Role of CREB transcription factor in c-fos activation in natural killer cells. Eur J Immunol. 2002;32:3358–65.
27. Fry TJ, Mackall CL. Interleukin-7: from bench to clinic. Blood. 2002;99:3892–904.
28. Deng X, Kornblau SM, Ruvolo PP, May Jr WS. Regulation of Bcl2 phosphorylation and potential significance for leukemic cell chemoresistance. J Natl Cancer Inst Monogr. 2001;28:30–7.
29. Carter BZ, Milella M, Tsao T, et al. Regulation and targeting of antiapoptotic XIAP in acute myeloid leukemia. Leukemia. 2003;17:2081–9.
30. Jia W, Yu C, Rahmani M, et al. Synergistic antileukemic interactions between 17-AAG and UCN-01 involve interruption of RAF/MEK- and AKT-related pathways. Blood. 2003;102:1824–32.
31. Troppmair J, Rapp UR. Raf and the road to cell survival: a tale of bad spells, ring bearers and detours. Biochem Pharmacol. 2003;66:1341–5.
32. Harada H, Quearry B, Ruiz-Vela A, Korsmeyer SJ. Survival factor-induced extracellular signal-regulated kinase phosphorylates BIM, inhibiting its association with BAX and proapoptotic activity. Proc Natl Acad Sci USA. 2004;101:15313–7.
33. Marani M, Hancock D, Lopes R, Tenev T, Downward J, Lemoine NR. Role of Bim in the survival pathway induced by Raf in epithelial cells. Oncogene. 2004;23:2431–41.
34. Ley R, Balmanno K, Hadfield K, Weston C, Cook SJ. Activation of the ERK1/2 signaling pathway promotes phosphorylation and proteasome-dependent degradation of the BH3-only protein, Bim. J Biol Chem. 2003;278:18811–6.
35. Weston CR, Balmanno K, Chalmers C. Activation of ERK1/2 by deltaRaf-1:ER* represses Bim expression independently of the JNK or PI3K pathways. Oncogene. 2003;22:1281–93.
36. Domina AM, Vrana JA, Gregory MA, Hann SR, Craig RW. MCL1 is phosphorylated in the PEST region and stabilized upon ERK activation in viable cells, and at additional sites with cytotoxic okadaic acid or taxol. Oncogene. 2004;23:5301–15.
37. Cohen C, Zavala-Pompa A, Sequeira JH, et al. Mitogen-actived protein kinase activation is an early event in melanoma progression. Clin Cancer Res. 2002;8:3728–33.

38. Davies H, Bignell GR, Cox C, et al. Mutations of the BRAF gene in human cancer. Nature. 2002;417: 949–54.
39. Libra M, Malaponte G, Navolanic PM, et al. Analysis of BRAF mutation in primary and metastatic melanoma. Cell Cycle. 2005;4:1382–4.
40. Dahl C, Guldberg P. The genome and epigenome of malignant melanoma. APMIS. 2007;115:1161–76.
41. Whitwam T, Vanbrocklin MW, Russo ME, et al. Differential oncogenic potential of activated RAS isoforms in melanocytes. Oncogene. 2007;26:4563–70.
42. Wan PT, Garnett MJ, Roe SM, et al. Mechanism of activation of the RAF-ERK signaling pathway by oncogenic mutations of B-RAF. Cell. 2004;116: 855–67.
43. Tuveson DA, Weber BL, Herlyn M. BRAF as a potential therapeutic target in melanoma and other malignancies. Cancer Cell. 2003;4:95–8.
44. Hoeflich KP, Eby MT, Forrest WF, et al. Regulation of ERK3/MAPK6 expression by BRAF. Int J Oncol. 2006;29:839–49.
45. Sharma A, Trivedi NR, Zimmerman MA, Tuveson DA, Smith CD, Robertson GP. Mutant V599EB-Raf regulates growth and vascular development of malignant melanoma tumors. Cancer Res. 2005;65: 2412–21.
46. Pritchard CA, Samuels ML, Bosch E, McMahon M. Conditionally oncogenic forms of the A-Raf and B-Raf protein kinases display different biological and biochemical properties in NIH 3T3 cells. Mol Cell Biol. 1995;15:6430–42.
47. Emuss V, Garnett M, Mason C, Marais R. Mutations of C-RAF are rare in human cancer because C-RAF has a low basal kinase activity compared with B-RAF. Cancer Res. 2005;65:9719–26.
48. Christensen C, Guldberg P. Growth factors rescue cutaneous melanoma cells from apoptosis induced by knock-down of mutated (V600E) BRAF. Oncogene. 2005;24:6292–302.
49. Goel VK, Lazar AJ, Warneke CL, Redston MS, Haluska FG. Examination of mutations in BRAF, NRAS, and PTEN in primary cutaneous melanoma. J Invest Dermatol. 2006;126:154–60.
50. Wilhelm SM, Carter C, Tang L, et al. BAY 43-9006 exhibits broad spectrum oral antitumor activity and targets the RAF/MEK/ERK pathway and receptor tyrosine kinases involved in tumor progression and angiogenesis. Cancer Res. 2004;64:7099–109.
51. Liu L, Cao Y, Chen C, et al. Sorafenib blocks the RAF/MEK/ERK pathway, inhibits tumor angiogenesis, and induces tumor cell apoptosis in hepatocellular carcinoma model PLC/PRF/5. Cancer Res. 2006;66:11851–8.
52. Kim S, Yazici YD, Calzada G, et al. Sorafenib inhibits the angiogenesis and growth of orthotopic anaplastic thyroid carcinoma xenografts in nude mice. Mol Cancer Ther. 2007;6:1785–92.
53. Eisen T, Ahmad T, Flaherty KT, et al. Sorafenib in advanced melanoma: a phase II randomised discontinuation trial analysis. Br J Cancer. 2006;95:581–6.
54. Flaherty KT. Chemotherapy and targeted therapy combinations in advanced melanoma. Clin Cancer Res. 2006;12:2366–70.
55. Eisen T, Marais R, Affolter A, et al. An open-label phase II study of sorafenib and dacarbazine as first-line therapy in patients with advanced melanoma. J Clin Oncol. 2007;25:8529.
56. McDermott DF, Sosman JA, Gonzalez R, et al. Double-blind randomized phase II study of the combination of sorafenib and dacarbazine in patients with advanced melanoma: a report from the 11715 study group. J Clin Oncol. 2008;26:2178–85.
57. Panka DJ, Cho DC, Atkins MB, Mier JW. GSK-3beta inhibition enhances sorafenib-induced apoptosis in melanoma cell lines. J Biol Chem. 2008;283: 726–32.
58. Hocker TL, Singh MK, Tsao H. Melanoma genetics and therapeutic approaches in the 21st century: moving from the benchside to the bedside. J Invest Dermatol. 2008;128:2575–95.
59. Solit DB, Garraway LA, Pratilas CA, et al. BRAF mutation predicts sensitivity to MEK inhibition. Nature. 2006;439:358–62.
60. Solit DB, Santos E, Pratilas CA, et al. 3'-deoxy-3'-[18F]fluorothymidine positron emission tomography is a sensitive method for imaging the response of BRAF-dependent tumors to MEK inhibition. Cancer Res. 2007;67:11463–9.
61. Halilovic E, Solit DB. Therapeutic strategies for inhibiting oncogenic BRAF signaling. Curr Opin Pharmacol. 2008;8:419–26.
62. Wang D, Boerner SA, Winkler JD, et al. Clinical experience of MEK inhibitors in cancer therapy. Biochim Biophys Acta. 2007;1773:1248–55.
63. Menon SS, Whitfield LR, Sadis SS, et al. Pharmacokinetics (PK) and pharmacodynamics (PD) of PD 0325901, a second generation MEK inhibitor after multiple oral doses of PD 0325901 to advanced cancer patients. J Clin Oncol. 2005;23: 3066.
64. Lorusso PM, Krishnamurthi S, Rinehart J, et al. A phase I-II clinical study of a second generation oral MEK inhibitor, PD 0325901 in patients with advanced cancer. J Clin Oncol. 2005;23:3011.
65. Dummer R, Robert C, Chapman PB, et al. AZD6244 (ARRY-142886) vs temozolomide (TMZ) in patients (pts) with advanced melanoma: an open-label, randomized, multicenter, phase II study. J Clin Oncol. 2008;26:9033.
66. Robertson GP. Functional and therapeutic significance of akt deregulation in malignant melanoma. Cancer Metastasis Rev. 2005;24:273–85.
67. Cully M, You H, Levine AJ, Mak TW. Beyond PTEN mutations: the PI3K pathway as an integrator of multiple inputs during tumorigenesis. Nat Rev Cancer. 2006;6:184–92.
68. Hennessy BT, Smith DL, Ram PT, Lu Y, Mills GB. Exploiting the PI3K/AKT pathway for cancer drug discovery. Nat Rev Drug Discov. 2005;4: 988–1004.

69. Zhou XP, Gimm O, Hampel H, Niemann T, Walker MJ, Eng C. Epigenetic PTEN silencing in malignant melanomas without PTEN mutation. Am J Pathol. 2000;157:1123–8.
70. Stahl JM, Sharma A, Cheung M, et al. Deregulated Akt3 activity promotes development of malignant melanoma. Cancer Res. 2004;64:7002–10.
71. Meier F, Schittek B, Busch S, et al. The RAS/RAF/MEK/ERK and PI3K/AKT signaling pathways present molecular targets for the effective treatment of advanced melanoma. Front Biosci. 2005;10:2986–3001.
72. Fecher LA, Cummings SD, Keefe MJ, Alani RM. Toward a molecular classification of melanoma. J Clin Oncol. 2007;25:1606–20.
73. Sekulic A, Haluska Jr P, Miller AJ, et al. Malignant melanoma in the 21st century: the emerging molecular landscape. Mayo Clin Proc. 2008;83:825–46.
74. Tsao H, Zhang X, Fowlkes K, Haluska FG. Relative reciprocity of NRAS and PTEN/MMAC1 alterations in cutaneous melanoma cell lines. Cancer Res. 2000;60:1800–4.
75. Tsao H, Goel V, Wu H, Yang G, Haluska FG. Genetic interaction between NRAS and BRAF mutations and PTEN/MMAC1 inactivation in melanoma. J Invest Dermatol. 2004;122:337–41.
76. Curtin JA, Fridlyand J, Kageshita T, et al. Distinct sets of genetic alterations in melanoma. N Engl J Med. 2005;353:2135–47.
77. Margolin K, Longmate J, Baratta T, et al. CCI-779 in metastatic melanoma: a phase II trial of the California Cancer Consortium. Cancer. 2005;104:1045–8.
78. Rao RD, Allred JB, Windschitl HE, et al. N0377: results of NCCTG phase II trial of the mTOR inhibitor RAD-001 in metastatic melanoma. J Clin Oncol. 2007;25:8530.
79. Granville CA, Memmott RM, Gills JJ, Dennis PA. Handicapping the race to develop inhibitors of the phosphoinositide 3-kinase/Akt/mammalian target of rapamycin pathway. Clin Cancer Res. 2006;12:679–89.
80. McCubrey JA, Milella M, Tafuri A, et al. Targeting the Raf/MEK/ERK pathway with small-molecule inhibitors. Curr Opin Investig Drugs. 2008;9:614–30.
81. Cheung M, Sharma A, Madhunapantula SV, Robertson GP. Akt3 and mutant V600E B-Raf cooperate to promote early melanoma development. Cancer Res. 2008;68:3429–39.
82. Krasilnikov M, Ivanov VN, Dong J, Ronai Z. ERK and PI3K negatively regulate STAT-transcriptional activities in human melanoma cells: implications towards sensitization to apoptosis. Oncogene. 2003;22:4092–101.
83. Lopez-Bergami P, Fitchman B, Ronai Z. Understanding signaling cascades in melanoma. Photochem Photobiol. 2008;84:289–306.
84. Smalley KS, Flaherty KT. Integrating BRAF/MEK inhibitors into combination therapy for melanoma. Br J Cancer. 2009;100:431–5.
85. Tran MA, Smith CD, Kester M, Robertson GP. Combining nanoliposomal ceramide with sorafenib synergistically inhibits melanoma and breast cancer cell survival to decrease tumor development. Clin Cancer Res. 2008;14:3571–81.
86. Lasithiotakis KG, Sinnberg TW, Schittek B, et al. Combined inhibition of MAPK and mTOR signaling inhibits growth, induces cell death, and abrogates invasive growth of melanoma cells. J Invest Dermatol. 2008;128:2013–23.
87. Belyanskaya LL, Hopkins-Donaldson S, Kurtz S, et al. Cisplatin activates Akt in small cell lung cancer cells and attenuates apoptosis by survivin upregulation. Int J Cancer. 2005;117:755–63.
88. Ohta T, Ohmichi M, Hayasaka T, et al. Inhibition of phosphatidylinositol 3-kinase increases efficacy of cisplatin in in vivo ovarian cancer models. Endocrinology. 2006;147:1761–9.
89. Kolch W. Ras/Raf signalling and emerging pharmacotherapeutic targets. Expert Opin Pharmacother. 2002;3:709–18.
90. Sinnberg T, Lasithiotakis K, Niessner H, et al. Inhibition of PI3K-AKT-mTOR signaling sensitizes melanoma cells to cisplatin and temozolomide. J Invest Dermatol. 2008;129:1500–15.
91. Soengas MS, Lowe SW. Apoptosis and melanoma chemoresistance. Oncogene. 2003;22:3138–51.
92. Borner C, Schlagbauer Wadl H, Fellay I, Selzer E, Polterauer P, Jansen B. Mutated N-ras upregulates Bcl-2 in human melanoma in vitro and in SCID mice. Melanoma Res. 1999;9:347–50.
93. Jansen B, Wacheck V, Heere-Ress E, et al. Chemosensitisation of malignant melanoma by BCL2 antisense therapy. Lancet. 2000;356:1728–33.
94. Helmbach H, Rossmann E, Kern MA, Schadendorf D. Drug-resistance in human melanoma. Int J Cancer. 2001;93:617–22.
95. Soengas MS, Capodieci P, Polsky D, et al. Inactivation of the apoptosis effector Apaf-1 in malignant melanoma. Nature. 2001;409:207–11.
96. Heere-Ress E, Thallinger C, Lucas T, et al. Bcl-X(L) is a chemoresistance factor in human melanoma cells that can be inhibited by antisense therapy. Int J Cancer. 2002;99:29–34.
97. Thallinger C, Wolschek MF, Wacheck V. Mcl-1 antisense therapy chemosensitizes human melanoma in a SCID mouse xenotransplantation model. J Invest Dermatol. 2003;120:1081–6.
98. Galluzzi L, Larochette N, Zamzami N, Kroemer G. Mitochondria as therapeutic targets for cancer chemotherapy. Oncogene. 2006;25:4812–30.
99. Hengartner MO. The biochemistry of apoptosis. Nature. 2000;407:770–6.
100. Albino AP, Vidal MJ, McNutt NS, et al. Mutation and expression of the p53 gene in human malignant melanoma. Melanoma Res. 1994;4:35–45.
101. Barnhill RL, Castresana JS, Rubio MP, et al. p53 expression in cutaneous malignant melanoma: an immunohistochemical study of 87 cases of primary, recurrent, and metastatic melanoma. Mod Pathol. 1994;7:533–5.

102. Lubbe J, Reichel M, Burg G, Kleihues P. Absence of p53 gene mutations in cutaneous melanoma. J Invest Dermatol. 1994;102:819–21.
103. Petitjean A, Mathe E, Kato S, et al. Impact of mutant p53 functional properties on TP53 mutation patterns and tumor phenotype: lessons from recent developments in the IARC TP53 database. Hum Mutat. 2007;28:622–9.
104. Mustika R, Budiyanto A, Nishigori C, Ichihashi M, Ueda M. Decreased expression of Apaf-1 with progression of melanoma. Pigment Cell Res. 2005;18:59–62.
105. Selzer E, Schlagbauer-Wadl H, Okamoto I, Pehamberger H, Potter R, Jansen B. Expression of Bcl-2 family members in human melanocytes, in melanoma metastases and in melanoma cell lines. Melanoma Res. 1998;8:197–203.
106. Sheridan C, Brumatti G, Martin SJ. Oncogenic B-RafV600E inhibits apoptosis and promotes ERK-dependent inactivation of Bad and Bim. J Biol Chem. 2008;283:22128–35.
107. Smalley KS, Xiao M, Villanueva J, et al. CRAF inhibition induces apoptosis in melanoma cells with non-V600E BRAF mutations. Oncogene. 2009;28:85–94.
108. Fernandez Y, Verhaegen M, Miller TP, et al. Differential regulation of noxa in normal melanocytes and melanoma cells by proteasome inhibition: therapeutic implications. Cancer Res. 2005;65:6294–304.
109. Qin JZ, Xin H, Sitailo LA, Denning MF, Nickoloff BJ. Enhanced killing of melanoma cells by simultaneously targeting Mcl-1 and NOXA. Cancer Res. 2006;66:9636–45.
110. Verhaegen M, Bauer JA, Martin de la Vega C, et al. A novel BH3 mimetic reveals a mitogen-activated protein kinase-dependent mechanism of melanoma cell death controlled by p53 and reactive oxygen species. Cancer Res. 2006;66:11348–59.
111. Nguyen M, Marcellus RC, Roulston A, et al. Small molecule obatoclax (GX15-070) antagonizes MCL-1 and overcomes MCL-1-mediated resistance to apoptosis. Proc Natl Acad Sci USA. 2007;104:19512–7.
112. Wang YF, Jiang CC, Kiejda KA, Gillespie S, Zhang XD, Hersey P. Apoptosis induction in human melanoma cells by inhibition of MEK is caspase-independent and mediated by the Bcl-2 family members PUMA, Bim, and Mcl-1. Clin Cancer Res. 2007;13:4934–42.
113. Wolter KG, Verhaegen M, Fernandez Y, et al. Therapeutic window for melanoma treatment provided by selective effects of the proteasome on Bcl-2 proteins. Cell Death Differ. 2007;14:1605–16.
114. Chetoui N, Sylla K, Gagnon-Houde JV, et al. Downregulation of mcl-1 by small interfering RNA sensitizes resistant melanoma cells to fas-mediated apoptosis. Mol Cancer Res. 2008;6:42–52.
115. Nijhawan D, Fang M, Traer E, et al. Elimination of Mcl-1 is required for the initiation of apoptosis following ultraviolet irradiation. Genes Dev. 2003;17:1475–86.
116. Jansen B, Schlagbauer-Wadl H, Brown BD, et al. Bcl-2 antisense therapy chemosensitizes human melanoma in SCID mice. Nat Med. 1998;4:232–4.
117. Bedikian AY, Millward M, Pehamberger H, et al. Bcl-2 antisense (oblimersen sodium) plus dacarbazine in patients with advanced melanoma: the Oblimersen Melanoma Study Group. J Clin Oncol. 2006;24:4738–45.
118. Cragg MS, Jansen ES, Cook M, Harris C, Strasser A, Scott CL. Treatment of B-RAF mutant human tumor cells with a MEK inhibitor requires Bim and is enhanced by a BH3 mimetic. J Clin Invest. 2008;118:3651–9.
119. Miller LA, Goldstein NB, Johannes WU, et al. BH3 mimetic ABT-737 and a proteasome inhibitor synergistically kill melanomas through Noxa-dependent apoptosis. J Invest Dermatol. 2009;129:964–71.
120. Lutzky J, Bauer J, Bastian BC. Dose-dependent, complete response to imatinib of a metastatic mucosal melanoma with a K642E KIT mutation. Pigment Cell Melanoma Res. 2008;21:492–3.
121. Hodi FS, Friedlander P, Corless CL, et al. Major response to imatinib mesylate in KIT-mutated melanoma. J Clin Oncol. 2008;26:2046–51.
122. Schittenhelm MM, Shiraga S, Schroeder A, et al. Dasatinib (BMS-354825), a dual SRC/ABL kinase inhibitor, inhibits the kinase activity of wild-type, juxtamembrane, and activation loop mutant KIT isoforms associated with human malignancies. Cancer Res. 2006;66:473–81.
123. Heath EI, Bible K, Martell RE, et al. A phase 1 study of SNS-032 (formerly BMS-387032), a potent inhibitor of cyclin-dependent kinases 2, 7 and 9 administered as a single oral dose and weekly infusion in patients with metastatic refractory solid tumors. Invest New Drugs. 2008;26:59–65.
124. Antonescu CR, Busam KJ, Francone TD, et al. L576P kit mutation in anal melanomas correlates with kit protein expression and is sensitive to specific kinase inhibition. Int J Cancer. 2007;121:257–64.
125. Beadling C, Jacobson-Dunlop E, Hodi FS, et al. KIT gene mutations and copy number in melanoma subtypes. Clin Cancer Res. 2008;14:6821–8.
126. Rivera RS, Nagatsuka H, Gunduz M, et al. C-kit protein expression correlated with activating mutations in KIT gene in oral mucosal melanoma. Virchows Arch. 2008;452:27–32.
127. Satzger I, Schaefer T, Kuettler U, et al. Analysis of c-KIT expression and KIT gene mutation in human mucosal melanomas. Br J Cancer. 2008;99:2065–9.
128. Roskoski Jr R. Structure and regulation of Kit protein-tyrosine kinase—the stem cell factor receptor. Biochem Biophys Res Commun. 2005;338:1307–15.
129. Grichnik JM. Kit and melanocyte migration. J Invest Dermatol. 2006;126:945–7.
130. Buchdunger E, Cioffi CL, Law N, et al. Abl protein-tyrosine kinase inhibitor STI571 inhibits in vitro signal transduction mediated by c-kit and platelet-derived growth factor receptors. J Pharmacol Exp Ther. 2000;295:139–45.

131. Dumaz N, Hayward R, Martin J, et al. In melanoma, RAS mutations are accompanied by switching signaling from BRAF to CRAF and disrupted cyclic AMP signaling. Cancer Res. 2006;66:9483–91.
132. Montagut C, Sharma SV, Shioda T, et al. Elevated CRAF as a potential mechanism of acquired resistance to BRAF inhibition in melanoma. Cancer Res. 2008;68:4853–61.
133. Stevenson JP, Yao KS, Gallagher M, et al. Phase I clinical/pharmacokinetic and pharmacodynamic trial of the c-raf-1 antisense oligonucleotide ISIS 5132 (CGP 69846A). J Clin Oncol. 1999;17:2227–36.
134. Cunningham CC, Holmlund JT, Schiller JH, et al. A phase I trial of c-Raf kinase antisense oligonucleotide ISIS 5132 administered as a continuous intravenous infusion in patients with advanced cancer. Clin Cancer Res. 2000;6:1626–31.
135. Coudert B, Anthoney A, Fiedler W, et al. Phase II trial with ISIS 5132 in patients with small-cell (SCLC) and non-small cell (NSCLC) lung cancer. A European Organization for Research and Treatment of Cancer (EORTC) Early Clinical Studies Group report. Eur J Cancer. 2001;37:2194–8.
136. Cripps MC, Figueredo AT, Oza AM, et al. Phase II randomized study of ISIS 3521 and ISIS 5132 in patients with locally advanced or metastatic colorectal cancer: a National Cancer Institute of Canada clinical trials group study. Clin Cancer Res. 2002;8:2188–92.
137. Dritschilo A, Huang CH, Rudin CM, et al. Phase I study of liposome-encapsulated c-raf antisense oligodeoxyribonucleotide infusion in combination with radiation therapy in patients with advanced malignancies. Clin Cancer Res. 2006;12:1251–9.
138. Rudin CM, Marshall JL, Huang CH, et al. Delivery of a liposomal c-raf-1 antisense oligonucleotide by weekly bolus dosing in patients with advanced solid tumors: a phase I study. Clin Cancer Res. 2004;10:7244–51.
139. Widlund HR, Fisher DE. Microphthalamia-associated transcription factor: a critical regulator of pigment cell development and survival. Oncogene. 2003;22:3035–41.
140. Levy C, Khaled M, Fisher DE. MITF: master regulator of melanocyte development and melanoma oncogene. Trends Mol Med. 2006;12:406–14.
141. Denat L, Larue L, et al. Malignant melanoma and the role of the paradoxal protein Microphthalmia transcription factor. Bull Cancer. 2007;94:81–92.
142. Loercher AE, Tank EM, Delston RB, Harbour JW. MITF links differentiation with cell cycle arrest in melanocytes by transcriptional activation of INK4A. J Cell Biol. 2005;168:35–40.
143. Carreira S, Goodall J, Aksan I, et al. Mitf cooperates with Rb1 and activates p21Cip1 expression to regulate cell cycle progression. Nature. 2005;433:764–9.
144. Wellbrock C, Marais R. Elevated expression of MITF counteracts B-RAF stimulated melanocyte and melanoma cell proliferation. J Cell Biol. 2005;170:703–8.
145. Du J, Widlund HR, Horstmann MA, et al. Critical role of CDK2 for melanoma growth linked to its melanocyte-specific transcriptional regulation by MITF. Cancer Cell. 2004;6:565–76.
146. McGill GG, Horstmann M, Widlund HR, et al. Bcl2 regulation by the melanocyte master regulator Mitf modulates lineage survival and melanoma cell viability. Cell. 2002;109:707–18.
147. Widlund HR, Horstmann MA, Price ER, et al. Betacatenin-induced melanoma growth requires the downstream target Microphthalmia-associated transcription factor. J Cell Biol. 2002;158:1079–87.
148. Rubinfeld B, Robbins P, El-Gamil M, Albert I, Porfiri E, Polakis P. Stabilization of beta-catenin by genetic defects in melanoma cell lines. Science. 1997;275:1790–2.
149. Rimm DL, Caca K, Hu G, Harrison FB, Fearon ER. Frequent nuclear/cytoplasmic localization of beta-catenin without exon 3 mutations in malignant melanoma. Am J Pathol. 1999;154:325–9.
150. Wellbrock C, Rana S, Paterson H, Pickersgill H, Brummelkamp T, Marais R. Oncogenic BRAF regulates melanoma proliferation through the lineage specific factor MITF. PLoS One. 2008;3:2734.
151. Kido K, Sumimoto H, Asada S, et al. Simultaneous suppression of MITF and BRAF V600E enhanced inhibition of melanoma cell proliferation. Cancer Sci. 2009;100:1863–9.
152. Harbour JW, Dean DC. The Rb/E2F pathway: expanding roles and emerging paradigms. Genes Dev. 2000;14:2393–409.
153. Serrano M, Hannon GJ, Beach D. A new regulatory motif in cell-cycle control causing specific inhibition of cyclin D/CDK4. Nature. 1993;366:704–7.
154. Bennett DC. Human melanocyte senescence and melanoma susceptibility genes. Oncogene. 2003;22:3063–9.
155. Mooi WJ, Peeper DS. Oncogene-induced cell senescence—halting on the road to cancer. N Engl J Med. 2006;355:1037–46.
156. Bartkova J, Rezaei N, Liontos M, et al. Oncogene-induced senescence is part of the tumorigenesis barrier imposed by DNA damage checkpoints. Nature. 2006;444:633–7.
157. Michaloglou C, Vredeveld LC, Soengas MS, et al. BRAFE600-associated senescence-like cell cycle arrest of human naevi. Nature. 2005;436:720–4.
158. Madhunapantula SV, Robertson GP. Is B-Raf a good therapeutic target for melanoma and other malignancies? Cancer Res. 2008;68:5–8.
159. Gray-Schopfer VC, Cheong SC, Chong H, et al. Cellular senescence in naevi and immortalisation in melanoma: a role for p16? Br J Cancer. 2006;95:496–505.
160. Haferkamp S, Becker TM, Scurr LL, Kefford RF, Rizos H. p16INK4a-induced senescence is disabled by melanoma-associated mutations. Aging Cell. 2008;7:733–45.
161. Hussussian CJ, Struewing JP, Goldstein AM, et al. Germline p16 mutations in familial melanoma. Nat Genet. 1994;8:15–21.

162. Eliason MJ, Larson AA, Florell SR, et al. Population-based prevalence of CDKN2A mutations in Utah melanoma families. J Invest Dermatol. 2006;126: 660–6.
163. Goldstein AM, Chan M, Harland M, et al. Features associated with germline CDKN2A mutations: a GenoMEL study of melanoma-prone families from three continents. J Med Genet. 2007;44:99–106.
164. Walker GJ, Flores JF, Glendening JM, Lin AH, Markl ID, Fountain JW. Virtually 100% of melanoma cell lines harbor alterations at the DNA level within CDKN2A, CDKN2B, or one of their downstream targets. Genes Chromosomes Cancer. 1998; 22:157–63.
165. Sharpless E, Chin L. The INK4a/ARF locus and melanoma. Oncogene. 2003;22:3092–8.
166. Zhang H, Rosdahl I. Deletion in p16INK4a and loss of p16 expression in human skin primary and metastatic melanoma cells. Int J Oncol. 2004;24:331–5.
167. Polsky D, Young AZ, Busam KJ, Alani RM. The transcriptional repressor of p16/Ink4a, Id1, is up-regulated in early melanomas. Cancer Res. 2001;61: 6008–11.
168. Tsao H, Benoit E, Sober AJ, Thiele C, Haluska FG. Novel mutations in the p16/CDKN2A binding region of the cyclin-dependent kinase-4 gene. Cancer Res. 1998;58:109–13.
169. Zuo L, Weger J, Yang Q, et al. Germline mutations in the p16INK4a binding domain of CDK4 in familial melanoma. Nat Genet. 1996;12:97–9.
170. Fry DW, Harvey PJ, Keller PR, et al. Specific inhibition of cyclin-dependent kinase 4/6 by PD 0332991 and associated antitumor activity in human tumor xenografts. Mol Cancer Ther. 2004;3:1427–38.
171. Toogood PL, Harvey PJ, Repine JT, et al. Discovery of a potent and selective inhibitor of cyclin-dependent kinase 4/6. J Med Chem. 2005;48:2388–406.
172. Dickson MA, Schwartz GK. Development of cell-cycle inhibitors for cancer therapy. Curr Oncol. 2009;16:36–43.
173. Brown AP, Courtney CL, Criswell KA, et al. Toxicity and toxicokinetics of the cyclin-dependent kinase inhibitor AG-024322 in cynomolgus monkeys following intravenous infusion. Cancer Chemother Pharmacol. 2008;62:1091–101.
174. Siemeister G, Luecking U, Wagner C, Detjen K, McCoy C, Bosslet K. Molecular and pharmacodynamic characteristics of the novel multi-target tumor growth inhibitor ZK 304709. Biomed Pharmacother. 2006;60:269–72.

Anti-Angiogenesis Therapy for Melanoma

Roberta Ferraldeschi and Paul Lorigan

Abbreviations List

ATP	Adenosine triphosphate
Ang	Angiopoietins
CBDCA	Carboplatin
CR	Complete response
DTIC	Dacarbazine
DFS	Disease-free survival
EPC	Endothelial progenitor cells
EGF	Epidermal growth factor
EGFR	Epidermal growth factor receptor
FGF	Fibroblast growth factor
FGFR	Fibroblast growth factor receptor
IMiDs	Immunomodulatory drugs
IFN	Interferon
IL	Interleukin
mTOR	Mammalian target of rapamycin
MTD	Maximum tolerated dose
MS	Median survival
PTX	Paclitaxel
PR	Partial response
PS	Performance status
PLGF	Placenta growth factor
PDGFR	Platelet-derived growth factor receptor
PD	Progressive disease
PFS	Progression-free survival
OS	Overall survival
RTKs	Receptor tyrosine kinases
RR	Response rate
SD	Stable disease
TTP	Time to progression
VEGF	Vascular endothelial growth factor
VEGFR	Vascular endothelial growth factor receptor
TMZ	Temozolimide
TGF	Transforming growth factor
TNF	Tumor necrosis factor

Angiogenesis in Melanoma

Angiogenesis is a necessary condition for tumor growth and dissemination [1]. The ability of tumor cells to induce angiogenesis occurs through a multistep process—the 'angiogenic switch' [2, 3]. The vascular endothelial growth factor (VEGF) family of growth factors and receptors (VEGFR) are key regulators of this process [4, 5]. The VEGF family includes six structurally related glycoproteins referred to as VEGF-A, VEGF-B, VEGF-C, VEGF-D, VEGF-E, and placental growth factor (PLGF). VEGF acts through specific binding to three different cell membrane receptors belonging to the superfamily of receptor tyrosine kinases (RTKs): VEGFR-1 (Flt-1), VEGFR-2 (Flk1/KDR) and VEGFR-3 (Flt-4) [5, 6]. Ligand–receptor interaction induces activation of the tyrosine kinase domain of VEGFR, which leads to subsequent activation of multiple intracellular signaling transduction pathways (Fig. 21.1). The activation of

R. Ferraldeschi, M.D. • P. Lorigan, M.D. (✉)
Department of Medical Oncology,
The Christie Hospital NHS Foundation Trust,
Withington, Manchester, United Kingdom
e-mail: paul.lorigan@christie.nhs.uk

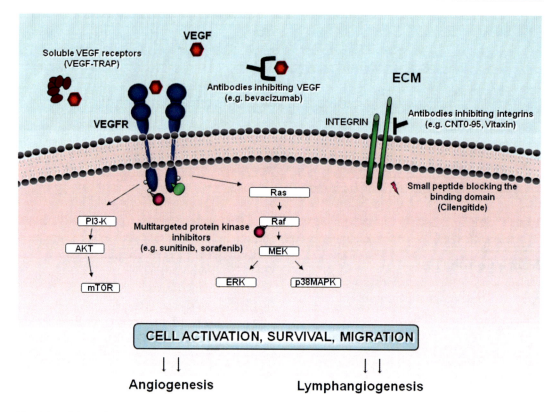

Fig. 21.1 Schematic representation of targets of anti-angiogenic therapy. *ECM* extracellular matrix, *VEGF* vascular endothelial growth factor, *VEGFR* vascular endothelial growth factor receptor

these pathways results in endothelial cell survival, mitogenesis, migration, differentiation, vascular permeability, vasodilatation, and mobilization of endothelial progenitor cells (EPC) from the bone marrow into the peripheral circulation [7, 8]. In addition, many other molecules can serve as pro-angiogenic factors, including fibroblast growth factors (FGF), transforming growth factors (TGF), tumor necrosis factor alpha (TNFα), angiogenin, and interleukin-8 (IL-8) [9].

The angiopoietins (Ang) act in concert with VEGF to control the later stages of the angiogenic cascade related to vessel assembly, maturation, and quiescence [10]. Ang-1 and Ang-2 have been identified as agonistic and antagonistic ligands, respectively, of the vascular receptor tyrosine kinase Tie2/Tek [11, 12]. Ang-1 acts as an endothelial cell survival factor, leading to vessel stabilization and maturation [11]. Constitutive Ang-1/Tie2 signaling is required to maintain the quiescent phenotype of vascular endothelium. Ang-2 acts as a context-specific antagonist of Ang-1/Tie2 signaling. As such, it destabilizes the quiescent endothelial cell phenotype, induces permeability and leads to dissociation of cell-cell contacts in cultured endothelial cells [13]. Ang-2 has also been reported to be capable of acting as an agonist of Tie2 [14]. Interestingly, Nasarre and colleagues demonstrated that Ang-2 effects tumor growth only during early stages of tumor development ($<0.2–0.4$ cm^3) [15].

An increasing number of studies on the molecular basis of angiogenesis are disclosing novel signaling pathways involved in the blood vessel formation process. These include extracellular signaling pathways such as Notch, ephrin/Eph receptor, roundabout/slit, and netrin/UNC (uncoordinated) receptor families, as well as intracellular proteins such as hedgehog and sprouty [16]. Intercellular signaling via Dll4 (Delta-like 4),

Jagged-1 and Notch1 has recently emerged as a key regulator of endothelial cell differentiation and specification during formation of a functional vascular network [17, 18]. Multiple connections between the VEGFR system and the Dll4/Notch signaling pathway have been described, indicating the existence of intricate regulatory feedback loops that play a critical role in proper vascular formation [17, 19].

Cultured melanoma cell lines and melanoma cells derived from primary tumors and metastases have been shown to produce a plethora of cytokines and growth factors, such as TGF-β (beta), IL-1, IL-6, VEGF, PDGF, and IL-8 [20–24]. These factors may have autocrine and/or paracrine effects resulting in tumor growth and invasion. In addition, they may stimulate endothelial cell proliferation, migration, and angiogenesis [25]. In melanoma, the transition from radial to vertical growth phase has been found to be accompanied by induction of VEGF expression and angiogenesis [26, 27]. There are reports that VEGF expression is associated with progression of melanoma [28], and evidence that links expression of angiogenic serum factors VEGF, FGF-b, and IL-8 with prognosis in melanoma patients [29]. Mouawad and colleagues reported that pre-treatment median soluble VEGF-A, VEGF-C and VEGFR-3 levels were significantly higher in melanoma patients [30]. In addition, elevated levels of serum VEGFR-1 were found to exert a significantly adverse impact on both disease-free survival (DFS) and overall survival (OS), while serum VEGFR-3 levels correlated with response [30]. Moreover, the presence of high circulating TGF-β1 and VEGFR-1 in metastatic melanoma patients have been correlated with tumor burden [31]. However, studies have shown that VEGF is expressed in only ~30% of primary melanomas, with increased expression levels in metastases [32]; hence, other angiogenic factors may play important roles in melanoma. Circulating soluble Ang-2 has been identified as a potential biomarker of melanoma progression and metastasis, correlating with tumor load and OS [33]. Analysis of serum samples during the transition from stage III to stage IV identified an increase in soluble Ang-2 of up to 400% [33].

The process of tumor angiogenesis is remarkably complex and depends on interaction between tumor, stromal, endothelial and bone marrow-derived cells. Integrins are a family of at least 24 cell surface heterodimeric glycoproteins, consisting of α (alpha) and β (beta) subunits noncovalently bound, and involved in cell-cell and cell-matrix interactions. Integrins mediate cellular processes such as cell adhesion and migration that are essential not only for embryonic development and tissue regeneration, but also for tumor development, invasion and metastasis in a variety of human cancers, including melanoma [34]. During melanoma development, changes in integrin expression, intracellular control of integrin functions, and signaling through integrin-associated pathways might impact the ability of tumor cells to interact with their environment, and enable melanoma cells to convert from a sessile, stationary phenotype to a migratory and invasive one [34]. Integrin expression also plays an important role in tumor angiogenesis and lymphangiogenesis. Select integrins promote endothelial cell migration and survival during these processes, whereas other integrins are associated with myeloid cell trafficking to tumors [35].

Clinical Experience with Angiogenesis-Targeting Agents in Melanoma

An understanding of the molecular changes underlying angiogenesis-dependent tumor growth has led to the identification of various potential targets for therapeutic intervention. Numerous anti-angiogenic agents are presently used in clinical trials or are being developed for treatment of melanoma. Most of these novel anti-angiogenic drugs currently being evaluated are (1) monoclonal antibodies or soluble forms of receptors designed to bind and neutralize growth factors, (2) small molecules designed to inhibit growth factor-receptor interaction or protein kinase activity of components of the VEGF signaling pathway, and (3) molecules that target the extracellular matrix or receptors for extracellular matrix (Tables 21.1–21.4 and

Table 21.1 Selected anti-angiogenic agents under development in melanoma

Anti-angiogenic drugs	Target	Clinical development
VEGF-blocking agents		
Bevacizumab	VEGF	Phase III
Aflibercept (VEGF Trap)	VEGF	Phase II
Multi-target protein kinase inhibitors		
Semaxanib	VEGFR, c-Kit	Phase II
Axitinib	VEGFR, PDGFR, c-Kit	Phase II
Cediranib	VEGFR, PDGFR, c-Kit	Phase II
Sunitinib	VEGFR, PDGFR, c-Kit, Flt-3	Phase II
Pazopanib	VEGFR, PDGFR, c-Kit	Phase II
Dovitinib	VEGFR, FGFR, PDGFR, c-Kit	Phase II
Sorafenib	VEGFR, Raf, PDGFR, c-Kit, RET, Flt-3	Phase III
Vatalanib	VEGFR, PDGFR, c-Kit	Phase II
Drugs targeting integrins		
Cilengitide	Integrin $\alpha v\beta 3$ and $\alpha v\beta 5$	Phase II
Vitaxin	Integrin $\alpha v\beta 3$	Phase II
CNTO95	Integrin αv	Phase II
Volociximab	Integrin $\alpha v\beta 1$	Phase II
Etaracizumab	Integrin $\alpha v\beta 3$ and $\alpha v\beta 5$	Phase II
Anti-angiogenic and immunomodulatory		
Thalidomide	Multiple mechanisms of action	Phase II
Lenalidomide	Multiple mechanisms of action	Phase III

VEGFR vascular endothelial growth factor receptor, *VEGF* vascular endothelial growth factor, *PDGFR* platelet-derived growth factor receptor, *FGFR* fibroblast growth factor receptor

Table 21.2 Phase II trials of bevacizumab in combination with IFNα (alpha), chemotherapy or biological agents in unresectable stages III and IV melanoma

Author	Study design	Treatment	n	Main results
Varker et al. [44]	Randomized Phase II	Bev with or without low-dose IFNα 2b	32	The addition of low-dose IFN had no effect on RR; eight patients had prolonged disease stabilization (24–146 weeks)
Vihinen et al. [45][a]	Phase II	Bev + low-dose IFNα (alfa) 2a and DTIC	24	RR 17%
Perez et al. [46]	Phase II	Bev + CBDCA and weekly PTX	53	PR 17%; SD 50%; median PFS 6 months; median OS 12 months
Boasberg et al. [47][a]	Phase II	Bev + nab-paclitaxel	41	PFS 6.25 months
González-Cao et al. [48]	Phase II	Bev + weekly PTX	12	RR 16%; SD 58.3%; median DFS 3.7 months; median OS 7.8 months
Von Moos et al. [49][a]	Phase II	Bev + TMZ	62	RR 26%; SD 44%
Wyman et al. [50][a]	Phase II	Bev + Erlotinib	29	RR 9%; SD lasting > 6 months 22%
Peyton et al. [51][a]	Phase II	Bev + Everolimus	56	PR 4%; SD 68%
O'Day et al. [52][a]	Randomized placebo-controlled Phase II	PTX and CBDCA with or without Bev	214	RR higher in Bev arm (26.4% versus 16.4%); OS longer in Bev arm (12.3 versus 9.2 months, HR 0.79, $P=0.19$); PFS longer in Bev arm (5.6 versus 4.2 months, HR 0.78, $P=0.14$)

Bev bevacizumab, *CBDCA* carboplatin, *DFS* disease-free survival, *DTIC* dacarbazine, *IFN* interferon, *nab-paclitaxel* nanoparticle albumin-bound paclitaxel, *OS* overall survival, *PFS* progression-free survival, *PR* partial response, *PTX* paclitaxel, *RR* response rate, *SD* stable disease, *TMZ* temozolimide
[a]Abstract only

Table 21.3 Phase II trials of sorafenib in combination with chemotherapy in unresectable stages III and IV melanoma

Author	Study design	Treatment	n	Main results
Flaherty et al. [58][a]	Phase I-II	Sorafenib plus CBDCA and PTX	35	PR 31%; SD 54%
Eisen et al. [61][a]	Phase II	Sorafenib plus DTIC	83	Median PFS 14 weeks; PR 10%; SD 41%
McDermott et al. [63]	Double-Blind Randomized Phase II	DTIC with either placebo or sorafenib	101	PFS longer in sorafenib arm (21.1 versus 11.7 weeks, HR 0.66, $P=0.068$) TTP significantly longer in sorafenib arm (21.1 versus 11.7 weeks, HR 0.61, $P=0.039$) OS longer in placebo arm (51.3 versus 45.6 weeks, HR 1.022, $P=0.927$)
Amaravadi et al. [64]	Four-arm Phase II trial	Sorafenib plus extended dose TMZ or standard dose TMZ	167	PR between 15% and 24% in patients without prior history of TMZ No significant difference in efficacy outcomes between extended versus standard dosing of TMZ

CBDCA carboplatin, *DFS* disease-free survival, *DTIC* dacarbazine, *OS* overall survival, *PFS* progression-free survival, *PR* partial response, *PTX* paclitaxel, *RR* response rate, *SD* stable disease, *TTP* time to progression, *TMZ* temozolimide
[a]Abstract only

Table 21.4 Randomized, double-blind trials that have tested anti-angiogenic drugs in relapsed or refractory metastatic melanoma

Author	Treatment	n	RR%	P value	TTP (months)	P value	Median survival (months)	P value
Hauschild et al. [36]	Placebo + CP versus Sorafenib + CP	135 135	11 12	1.0	17.9 wks (PFS) 17.4 wks (PFS)	0.49	42 wks 42 wks	0.92
Glaspy et al. [37]	Lenalidomide 25 mg versus Lenalidomide 5 mg	146 148	5.5 3.4	0.38	2.2 1.9	0.24	6.8 7.2	0.71
Eisen et al. [38]	Lenalidomide 25 mg versus Placebo	152 154	5.3 5.8	0.82	2.1 3.0	0.19	5.9 7.4	0.19

RR response rate, *CP* carboplatin + paclitaxel, *PFS* progression-free survival, *TTP* time to progression, *wks* weeks

Fig. 21.1). The majority of the data in this area have not matured fully and are mostly published in abstract form.

VEGF-Blocking Agents

Blockade of the VEGF pathway has been achieved by many different approaches, including antibodies targeting VEGF or its receptors, soluble decoy receptors that prevent VEGF from binding to its normal receptors (VEGF-trap), and small molecule inhibitors of the tyrosine kinase activity of VEGFR.

Bevacizumab is a recombinant humanized monoclonal antibody that prevents VEGF-A from binding to its receptors [39]. It is reported to be effective for treatment of various advanced cancers [40–43], and has been tested in several phase II trials in patients with metastatic melanoma in combination with IFNα (IFNalpha), chemotherapy or biological agents (Table 21.2) [44–51]. An ongoing phase II, multicenter, randomized, placebo-controlled trial (BEAM) is estimating the efficacy and safety of bevacizumab when combined with carboplatin and paclitaxel in previously untreated advanced melanoma. Two hundred and fourteen subjects were randomized to receive these drugs in a 2:1 fashion. Preliminary results were presented at the ESMO Congress in 2009 [52]. At a median follow-up of 17.5 months, results showed a trending benefit with the addition of bevacizumab for progression-free survival (PFS) (5.6 versus 4.2 months, HR 0.78, $p=0.14$) and OS (median of 12.3 versus 9.2 months, HR 0.79, $p=0.19$), with 1-year survival of 53% versus 39%. Response rate (RR) was also higher in the bevacizumab arm (26.4% versus 16.4%). Bevacizumab-related safety events were in line with observations from other disease-based clinical studies using similar chemotherapy. Interestingly, subgroup analysis suggested a survival benefit in patients with performance status 0 (PS0), M1c disease and elevated serum LDH, indicating that anti-angiogenic therapy may be more beneficial in late stage melanoma. A number of other studies evaluating bevacizumab in combination with chemotherapy and other targeted agents are ongoing. A randomized, multicenter phase III trial (AVAST-M) comparing bevacizumab as adjuvant therapy versus standard observation in high-risk melanoma patients following complete resection is underway in the UK. The translational component of this trial could also potentially identify biomarkers of minimal residual disease, predictive markers for bevacizumab response, and markers of disease relapse.

Aflibercept is a high-affinity anti-VEGF compound, engineered by combining domains from VEGFR-2 and VEGFR-1. VEGF Trap, functioning as a soluble decoy receptor, binds to pro-angiogenic VEGF, thereby preventing VEGF from binding to respective cell receptors. Single agent aflibercept is currently being evaluated in a phase II trial in individuals with recurrent stage III and stage IV melanoma. Eight of the first 21 patients enrolled had at least 4 months of PFS [53].

Multi-Target Protein Kinase Inhibitors

Protein kinases play important roles in regulating most cellular functions, including proliferation/cell cycle, cell metabolism, survival/apoptosis, DNA damage repair, cell motility, response to the microenvironment, and angiogenesis. Several means of targeting these enzymes therapeutically, such as with antibodies or small molecules that block kinase-substrate interaction or inhibit an enzyme's adenosine triphosphate (ATP) binding site, have been developed.

Dysregulated signaling via the mitogen-activated protein kinase (MAPK) pathway is associated with the development of solid tumors [54]. BRAF somatic mutations have been identified in about 60% of cases of melanoma [55]. Sorafenib is an oral multikinase inhibitor that was originally developed because of its inhibitory effects on Raf. However, its anti-angiogenic properties through the inhibition of VEGFR-1, -2, and -3, and platelet-derived growth factor receptor (PDGFR)-α (alpha) and -β (beta), in addition to Raf kinases, may be relevant to its antitumor effects [56]. Early studies showed a favourable safety profile, but little activity for single agent sorafenib in melanoma [57]. However, a combination phase I/II study of carboplatin and paclitaxel with escalating doses of sorafenib reported an extremely encouraging 85% disease control rate [58]. Of interest, there was no correlation between BRAF mutational status and treatment responses in patients with melanoma [59]. These promising results have led to the conduct of two randomized phase III trials comparing sorafenib, carboplatin, and paclitaxel with carboplatin and paclitaxel alone. One phase III trial was initiated by the Eastern Cooperative Oncology Group (Intergroup Trial E2603), in which 824 patients were enrolled and randomized to carboplatin and paclitaxel with either placebo or sorafenib. However, this trial was stopped early after an interim analysis found that further study conduct was futile with regard to achieving the primary end point of significantly improved OS. Final results are still pending. A similar, but smaller phase III trial (PRISM) was conducted to compare the same regimens as second-line treatment in patients with advanced melanoma [36]. Two hundred and seventy patients were randomized. No improvement in PFS (17.9 weeks for the placebo-containing arm and 17.4 weeks for the sorafenib-containing arm) or RR (11% versus 12%) was seen. The study was not powered for survival. The reasons for the negative findings of this trial as compared with the promising results of the phase I/II expansion study with the same regimen are unclear. The PFS was significantly better than would be expected for patients receiving first-line therapy, indicating that those individuals fit enough to have second-line therapy for melanoma are probably a self-selecting group with better prognosis.

The results observed with the combination of sorafenib and DTIC were similar [60, 61] (Table 21.3). The rationale for this drug combination is that DTIC treatment has been demonstrated to regulate IL-8 and VEGF protein expression in melanoma cells [62]. A randomized, double-blind, placebo-controlled phase II study of DTIC with either placebo or sorafenib in 101 chemotherapy-naïve advanced melanoma patients confirmed an improvement in PFS in favor of the sorafenib arm (median, 21.1 versus 11.7 weeks). There were statistically significant improvements in PFS rates at 6 and 9 months, and in time to progression (TTP) in favor of the sorafenib plus DTIC arm. However, no difference in survival was observed, with a trend toward a benefit for the DTIC plus placebo arm (median, 51.3 versus 45.6 weeks) [63]. An alternative attractive approach would be a completely oral combination regimen. In a complex randomized phase II study of TMZ and sorafenib, advanced melanoma patients received either extended dose TMZ or standard dose TMZ days 1–5, with sorafenib in each case. Separate cohorts were available for patients who had either brain metastases or prior TMZ. TMZ plus sorafenib was well tolerated and showed antitumor activity (partial response [PR] rate between 15% and 24%) in melanoma patients without prior history of TMZ therapy. There was no significant difference in efficacy outcomes between extended versus standard dosing of TMZ [64]. In addition, no significant association between BRAF mutational status and RR or PFS in patients treated with TMZ and sorafenib was reported.

Axitinib is an oral, potent and selective tyrosine kinase inhibitor of VEGFR-1, -2 and -3, that is in clinical development for multiple tumor types, and which has demonstrated single-agent activity in melanoma [65]. In a phase II study, axitinib demonstrated a 15.6% RR with response duration ranging from 2.3 to more than 10.2 months. Interestingly, unplanned subgroup analysis showed benefit for patients developing hypertension. The relationship between blood pressure and OS was also explored retrospectively across six separate phase II axitinib studies. An association between hypertension and longer OS was reported in this retrospective analysis across multiple tumor types [66].

Semaxanib is a potent inhibitor of VEGFR-2 and c-Kit, which has exhibited modest single-agent activity in melanoma patients [67]. A phase II study evaluated the combination of semaxanib and thalidomide in patients with metastatic melanoma who had failed at least one prior therapy. Of ten patients evaluable for response, one complete response (CR) lasting 20 months and one PR lasting 12 months were observed. Additionally, four patients had stable disease (SD) lasting from 2 to 10 months [68].

Pazopanib, cediranib, sunitinib and valatinib are other multi-target tyrosine kinases inhibitors either planned for or currently under evaluation in phase II studies in advanced melanoma.

More recently, compounds that act through the complex inhibition of multiple kinase targets have been reported and may exhibit improved clinical efficacy. A series of potent, orally efficacious 4-amino-3-benzimidazol-2-ylhydroquinolin-2-one analogues as inhibitors of VEGF, PDGF, and FGF RTKs have been developed [69]. Compounds in this class, such as dovitinib lactate, are reversible ATP-competitive potent inhibitors of VEGFR-2, FGFR-1, and PDGFR-β (PDGFR-beta). Initial data from a phase I study in metastatic melanoma patients demonstrated that dovitinib is safe and well tolerated at doses below 500 mg/day. Dovitinib has shown preliminary biological activity that tended to correlate with disease control. Twenty additional patients will be enrolled at the maximum tolerated dose (MTD) to confirm these preliminary findings [70].

Anti-Angiogenic and Immunomodulatory Drugs

Thalidomide is an orally bioavailable agent with multiple mechanisms of action, including anti-angiogenesis activity, that has been used successfully in the treatment of multiple myeloma [71]. The activity of thalidomide in solid tumors is less evident, but the most promising results have been reported in Kaposi's sarcoma and renal cell cancer [72]. Thalidomide inhibits vasculogenic mimicry channels and mosaic vessel formation in melanoma, through the regulation of vasculogenic factors [73]. It can also induce necrosis of melanoma cells, possibly via the NF-κB signaling pathway [73]. Immunomodulatory effects may include blockade of NF-κB activation through suppression of IκB kinase activity [74], alterations of CD8+ and CD4+ T-cell function, stimulation of IL-2 and IFN-γ (IFNgamma) production, and inhibition of other cytokines such as IL-6 and IL-12 [75]. Although single-agent phase II studies reported mixed results in patients with advanced melanoma [76–78], the combination of thalidomide with TMZ demonstrated antitumor activity [79–81]. A randomized phase II study compared TMZ administered every 8 h or daily in combination with either IFNα-2b or thalidomide in 181 patients [79]. A response or disease stabilization was seen in 25% of patients receiving the TMZ plus thalidomide combination, with a median survival of 7.3 months [79]. This combination was well tolerated, with any toxicity attributable to thalidomide being manageable. A single-institution phase II trial combining TMZ with thalidomide reported a RR of 32% and a median survival time of 9.5 months [80]. The same group published a phase II study which demonstrated that this drug combination was an active oral regimen in patients with brain metastases from melanoma [81]. However, many patients did not complete a full treatment cycle because of adverse events, which included CNS hemorrhage, deep vein thrombosis or pulmonary embolism, and severe rash. Given the poor prognosis and limited treatment options available, together with these preliminary data, the Cancer and Leukemia Group B (CALGB) initiated a multicenter phase II trial with combined extended dose TMZ and thalidomide in patients with melanoma and brain metastases. The trial was closed to accrual due to an unexpected high rate of thromboembolic adverse events [82]. The Cytokine Working Group conducted a phase II trial to test the efficacy of a regimen including TMZ, thalidomide, and whole brain radiation therapy (WBRT) in patients with brain metastases from melanoma [83]. Thirty nine patients received treatment, with three exhibiting response (RR 7.6%). Grade 3–4 side effects included deep venous thrombosis, pulmonary embolism, and CNS events. Eighteen (45%) patients required hospital admission for side effects. More recently, the Southwest Oncology Group (SWOG) conducted a multicenter phase II trial to better define the clinical efficacy of thalidomide and TMZ in patients with metastatic melanoma [84]. Sixty four patients were enrolled. This drug combination did not appear to have a clinical benefit that exceeded DTIC alone. The 6-month PFS was 15%, the 1-year OS was 35%, and the RR was 13%, all partial. One treatment-related death occurred from myocardial infarction, and three other grade 4 events arose, including pulmonary embolism, neutropenia, and CNS ischemia. There was no significant correlation between biomarkers and PFS or OS. Another SWOG protocol evaluated IFNα-2b (IFNalpha-2b) plus thalidomide [85]. Grade 3 treatment-related adverse events arose in 14 of 26 enrolled patients. Because of concern for patient safety, the study was permanently closed. No treatment responses were seen in the 22 evaluable patients. Thalidomide had been the subject of extensive off-label administration in melanoma, but data do not support continuation of its use in this setting.

A class of thalidomide analogues, called immunomodulatory drugs (IMiDs), have recently been developed in order to optimize certain thalidomide properties including its anticancer activity, and minimize much of the drug's toxicity [86]. Lenalidomide is a potent analogue of thalidomide that enhances T-cell stimulation, and has shown single-agent activity in refractory melanoma [87]. A phase II/III trial (MEL-001) comparing the efficacy and safety of two daily doses of lenalidomide (5 mg versus 25 mg) in the treatment of stage IV refractory metastatic melanoma showed no significant RR or PFS differences with either dose, and an acceptable safety profile for lenalidomide at each dose [37]. However, another phase II/III study (MEL-002), comparing lenalidomide monotherapy with placebo, concluded that treatment with lenalidomide (25 mg) had no benefit in RR, TTP, or OS in patients with previously treated metastatic melanoma [38]. Preliminary results of a phase I/II study of lenalidomide in combination with DTIC has established the dose for phase II testing [88].

Drugs Targeting Integrins

The integrin family plays important roles during tumor angiogenesis. Both monoclonal antibodies directed against αv (alphav) integrins and low-molecular-mass peptides blocking αv (alphav) or vitronectin receptors have been developed.

Vitaxin is a humanized monoclonal antibody targeting the αvβ3 (alphavbeta3) integrin, which is highly expressed on both activated endothelial cells and tumor cells, but is not present on resting endothelial cells and most normal organ systems, making it a suitable target for anti-angiogenic cancer therapy [89]. An open-label phase II study randomized 112 metastatic melanoma patients to receive vitaxin with or without DTIC. While vitaxin alone showed no objective responses, the median survival was longer in this group (11.8 versus 9.3 months) [90].

CNTO-95 is a fully human monoclonal antibody against αv (alphav) integrins, which has shown activity in metastatic melanoma [91, 92]. Interim results of a randomized phase II study of CNTO-95 alone, or in combination with DTIC, in 129 patients with stage IV metastatic melanoma have shown a trend toward improvement in PFS for DTIC plus CNTO-95 when compared with DTIC plus placebo (median, 75 versus 54 days) [92].

Volociximab is a high-affinity chimeric monoclonal antibody that specifically binds to α5β1 (alpha5beta1) integrin. Integrin α5β1 (alpha-5beta1), the principal fibronectin receptor, is an important survival factor and possible anti-melanoma target, as it plays a key role in angiogenesis [93, 94]. The combination of volociximab with DTIC was evaluated in a multicenter, open-label, pilot phase II study of 40 patients with metastatic melanoma. Fifteen patients experienced serious adverse events, two of which were possibly related to volociximab, including hypertension and deep vein thrombosis. Best overall response at 8 weeks was SD in 16 of 30 patients evaluable for efficacy, while 14 patients had progressive disease (PD) [95]. More recently, preliminary data on 19 patients from a multicenter, two-stage phase II study of volociximab in patients with relapsed metastatic melanoma have been presented. Weekly volociximab was well tolerated, but demonstrated insufficient clinical activity to proceed to the second stage of the trial [96].

Cilengitide is a cyclic Arg-Gly-Asp peptide that blocks the binding domain on αvβ3 (alphav-beta3) integrin. A phase II study showed minimal single-agent activity in melanoma [97]. However, cilengitide and TMZ exerted synergistic antiproliferative effects against melanoma and endothelial cells *in vitro* [98].

Key Challenges of Anti-Angiogenic Cancer Therapy

Effectively targeting the complex pathways involved in angiogenesis as a therapeutic strategy in the treatment of cancer is an ambitious undertaking, but one which has shown significant clinical benefit in patients with colorectal cancer, breast cancer, non-small cell lung cancer and renal cell cancer. Nevertheless, our fundamental understanding of how these drugs work is poor, and we are increasingly appreciating the challenges that this approach poses. Key issues are why all patients do not respond to anti-angiogenic treatment and why some patients develop resistance to this treatment? Although resistance to VEGF pathway-targeted therapy may be mediated in large part by intrinsic or acquired characteristics of the tumor cells, the vascular microenvironment can also be involved in mediating eventual tumor relapse and regrowth [99]. Furthermore, the timing of intervention and the context in which it is given may be clinically important. Ebos and colleagues showed that short-term (7-day) pretreatment with VEGF RTK inhibitors in mice, prior to intravenous inoculation of human tumor cells or immediately after removal of a primary tumor, "conditioned" them to more aggressive metastasis with decreased survival [100]. Another group reported that angiogenesis inhibitors targeting the VEGF pathway had antitumor effects, but concomitantly elicited tumor adaptation and progression to stages of greater malignancy, with heightened invasiveness and in some cases increased lymphatic and distant metastasis. Increased invasiveness was also seen following genetic ablation of the VEGF-A gene in both models, substantiating the results of pharmacological inhibitor studies [101]. An increasing number of preclinical investigations have disclosed novel pathways implicated in the blood vessel formation process, including angiopoietins, neuropilins and Notch, which might contribute to the inherent refractoriness and/or escape of tumors from VEGF-targeted therapy. Further studies on these molecular mechanisms and their interconnections with the VEGF pathway may provide new approaches in anti-angiogenic therapy [102].

The activity of anti-angiogenic drugs may be dose- and/or schedule-dependent. Compounds that inhibit tumor growth and angiogenesis at high concentrations might stimulate tumor growth at lower levels [103]. In most clinical trials, $\alpha v \beta 3$ inhibitors were administered as infusions of short duration twice weekly. Under these circumstances, plasma drug concentrations fall to nanomolar levels between administration sessions as a consequence of drug metabolism. Reynolds and colleagues recently showed nanomolar concentrations of cilengitide can actually enhance the growth of tumors in vivo by promoting VEGF-mediated angiogenesis [103].

Drugs active against metastatic disease will not necessarily work in the adjuvant setting (i.e., potential differential efficacies of treatments at different stages of tumor progression can exist). Currently, there are more than 40 adjuvant clinical trials underway involving multiple VEGF pathway inhibitors in numerous cancer types. With respect to bevacizumab, one such trial was completed in 2009. In a phase III study, postoperative colorectal patients with stage II–III disease were treated with adjuvant bevacizumab plus chemotherapy [104]. The results showed no benefit in DFS at 3-years after therapy initiation. There was a transient benefit in DFS during the 1-year interval in which bevacizumab was utilized, but this benefit gradually disappeared over time. The potential application of anti-angiogenic strategies in the adjuvant setting is of particular interest in melanoma. A recent analysis of two large studies on adjuvant IFN therapy indicated that ulceration is a determinant of IFN sensitivity [105], and that increasing tumor vascularity is highly correlated with ulceration [106]. However, recent findings from the BEAM study indicated a survival benefit with addition of bevacizumab in patients with PS0, M1c disease and elevated serum LDH, suggesting that anti-VEGF targeted therapy might be more beneficial in late stage melanoma [52].

A new generation of trials is evaluating whether simultaneous inhibition of multiple targets through the use of novel multi-targeting drugs can overcome tumor resistance. However, it is more likely that combinations of anti-angiogenic agents with chemotherapy and/or other targeted therapy will be needed to subvert signaling redundancies and produce significant clinical benefit. To date, combinations of targeted agents have shown mixed results in early phase studies, which have been limited by overlapping, on-target toxicity [107].

Taken together, these preclinical and clinical observations have important implications with respect to optimal dose and schedule of therapy in the adjuvant/neoadjuvant setting.

Finally, several clinical and methodological questions need to be addressed. The advent of agents that have different molecular targets and involve new mechanisms of action may necessitate new methodological approaches in clinical development, particularly in relation to clinical trial end-points [108–110]. It would be desirable to have reliable biomarkers that select patients who are most likely to benefit from angiogenesis-targeting therapy, and that optimize scheduling, dosing and choices of drugs for combination therapies. Currently, no validated biomarkers of either angiogenesis or anti-angiogenesis are available for routine clinical use. However, a number of systemic, circulating, tissue and imaging biomarkers are emerging and need to be prospectively validated [111].

Conclusions

Clinical trials evaluating the role of anti-angiogenic strategies are less advanced in melanoma than in other tumor types. A large number of early phase clinical trials have been completed, and showed promising results in some cases. However, data from two phase III studies did not show the desired improvement in survival with the addition of sorafenib to carboplatin and paclitaxel. More encouraging results have been observed with the addition of bevacizumab to the same chemotherapy regimen.

In the coming years, results from ongoing phase III trials will both clarify the role of angiogenesis-targeting agents in the treatment of melanoma and influence future development of anti-angiogenic strategies. Despite some setbacks, angiogenesis remains a very promising therapeutic target, and researchers are exploring new agents and approaches to maximize the effects of anti-angiogenic therapy.

References

1. Folkman J. Tumor angiogenesis: therapeutic implications. N Engl J Med. 1971;285:1182–6.
2. Folkman J. What is the evidence that tumors are angiogenesis dependent? J Natl Cancer Inst. 1990;82:4–6.
3. Folkman J. Seminars in medicine of the Beth Israel Hospital, Boston. Clinical applications of research on angiogenesis. N Engl J Med. 1995;333:1757–63.
4. Ferrara N. Vascular endothelial growth factor: basic science and clinical progress. Endocr Rev. 2004;25:581–611.
5. Ferrara N, Gerber HP, LeCouter J. The biology of VEGF and its receptors. Nat Med. 2003;9:669–76.
6. Cross MJ, Dixelius J, Matsumoto T, Claesson-Welsh L. VEGF-receptor signal transduction. Trends Biochem Sci. 2003;28:488–94.
7. Shibuya M, Claesson-Welsh L. Signal transduction by VEGF receptors in regulation of angiogenesis and lymphangiogenesis. Exp Cell Res. 2006;312:549–60.
8. Rafii S, Lyden D, Benezra R, et al. Vascular and haematopoietic stem cells: novel targets for anti-angiogenesis therapy? Nat Rev Cancer. 2002;2:826–35.
9. Carmeliet P, Jain RK. Angiogenesis in cancer and other diseases. Nature. 2000;407:249–57.
10. Pfaff D, Fiedler U, Augustin HG. Emerging roles of the angiopoietin-tie and the ephrin-Eph systems as regulators of cell trafficking. J Leukoc Biol. 2006;80:719–26.
11. Suri C, Jones PF, Patan S, et al. Requisite role of angiopoietin-1, a ligand for the TIE2 receptor, during embryonic angiogenesis. Cell. 1996;87:1171–80.
12. Maisonpierre PC, Suri C, Jones PF, et al. Angiopoietin-2, a natural antagonist for Tie2 that disrupts in vivo angiogenesis. Science. 1997;277:55–60.
13. Scharpfenecker M, Fiedler U, Reiss Y, Augustin HG. The Tie-2 ligand angiopoietin-2 destabilizes quiescent endothelium through an internal autocrine loop mechanism. J Cell Sci. 2005;118:771–80.
14. Teichert-Kuliszewska K, Maisonpierre PC, Jones N, et al. Biological action of angiopoietin-2 in a fibrin matrix model of angiogenesis is associated with activation of Tie2. Cardiovasc Res. 2001;49:659–70.
15. Nasarre P, Thomas M, Kruse K, et al. Host-derived angiopoietin-2 affects early stages of tumor development and vessel maturation but is dispensable for later stages of tumor growth. Cancer Res. 2009;69:1324–33.
16. Cristofaro B, Emanueli C. Possible novel targets for therapeutic angiogenesis. Curr Opin Pharmacol. 2009;9:102–8.
17. Jakobsson L, Bentley K, Gerhardt H. VEGFRs and Notch: a dynamic collaboration in vascular patterning. Biochem Soc Trans. 2009;37:1233–6.
18. Dufraine J, Funahashi Y, Kitajewski J. Notch signaling regulates tumor angiogenesis by diverse mechanisms. Oncogene. 2008;1(27):5132–7.
19. Thurston G, Kitajewski J. VEGF and Delta-Notch: interacting signalling pathways in tumour angiogenesis. Br J Cancer. 2008;99:1204–9.
20. Ciotti P, Rainero ML, Nicolo G, et al. Cytokine expression in human primary and metastatic melanoma cells: analysis in fresh bioptic specimens. Melanoma Res. 1995;5:41–7.
21. Mattei S, Colombo MP, Melani C, et al. Expression of cytokine/growth factors and their receptors in human melanoma and melanocytes. Int J Cancer. 1994;56:853–7.
22. Westphal JR, Van't Hullenaar R, Peek R, et al. Angiogenic balance in human melanoma: expression of VEGF, bFGF, IL-8, PDGF and angiostatin in relation to vascular density of xenografts in vivo. Int J Cancer. 2000;86:768–76.
23. Rodeck U, Melber K, Kath R, et al. Constitutive expression of multiple growth factor genes by melanoma cells but not normal melanocytes. J Invest Dermatol. 1991;97:20–6.
24. Graeven U, Fiedler W, Karpinski S, et al. Melanoma-associated expression of vascular endothelial growth factor and its receptors FLT-1 and KDR. J Cancer Res Clin Oncol. 1999;125:621–9.
25. Lazar-Molnar E, Hegyesi H, Toth S, et al. Autocrine and paracrine regulation by cytokines and growth factors in melanoma. Cytokine. 2000;12:547–54.
26. Erhard H, Rietveld FJ, van Altena MC, et al. Transition of horizontal to vertical growth phase melanoma is accompanied by induction of vascular endothelial growth factor expression and angiogenesis. Melanoma Res. 1997;7 Suppl 2:S19–26.
27. Marcoval J, Moreno A, Graells J, et al. Angiogenesis and malignant melanoma. Angiogenesis is related to the development of vertical (tumorigenic) growth phase. J Cutan Pathol. 1997;24:212–8.
28. Brychtova S, Bezdekova M, Brychta T, et al. The role of vascular endothelial growth factors and their

receptors in malignant melanomas. Neoplasma. 2008;55:273–9.
29. Ugurel S, Rappl G, Tilgen W, et al. Increased serum concentration of angiogenic factors in malignant melanoma patients correlates with tumor progression and survival. J Clin Oncol. 2001;19:577–83.
30. Mouawad R, Soubrane C, Khayat D. Prognostic relevance of pretreatment soluble vascular endothelial growth factors (A,C,D) and their receptors (R1, R2, and R3) in advanced melanoma patients. J Clin Oncol. 2007;25(18S) [abstr 8540].
31. Spano J, Mouawad R, Vignot S, et al. Role of circulating angiogenin TGF-β1, VEGF-R1, and VEGF-R2 in metastatic malignant melanoma patients. J Clin Oncol. 2009;27(15s) [abstr 9048].
32. Salven P, Heikkila P, Joensuu H. Enhanced expression of vascular endothelial growth factor in metastatic melanoma. Br J Cancer. 1997;76:930–4.
33. Helfrich I, Edler L, Sucker A, et al. Angiopoietin-2 levels are associated with disease progression in metastatic malignant melanoma. Clin Cancer Res. 2009;15:1384–92.
34. Kuphal S, Bauer R, Bosserhoff AK. Integrin signaling in malignant melanoma. Cancer Metastasis Rev. 2005;24:195–222.
35. Avraamides CJ, Garmy-Susini B, Varner JA. Integrins in angiogenesis and lymphangiogenesis. Nat Rev Cancer. 2008;8:604–17.
36. Hauschild A, Agarwala SS, Trefzer U, et al. Results of a phase III, randomized, placebo-controlled study of sorafenib in combination with carboplatin and paclitaxel as second-line treatment in patients with unresectable stage III or stage IV melanoma. J Clin Oncol. 2009;27:2823–30.
37. Glaspy J, Atkins MB, Richards JM, et al. Results of a multicenter, randomized, double-blind, dose-evaluating phase 2/3 study of lenalidomide in the treatment of metastatic malignant melanoma. Cancer. 2009;115:5228–36.
38. Eisen T, Trefzer U, Hamilton A, et al. Results of a multicenter, randomized, double-blind phase 2/3 study of lenalidomide in the treatment of pretreated relapsed or refractory metastatic malignant melanoma. Cancer. 2010;116:146–54.
39. Ferrara N, Hillan KJ, Novotny W. Bevacizumab (Avastin), a humanized anti-VEGF monoclonal antibody for cancer therapy. Biochem Biophys Res Commun. 2005;333:328–35.
40. Miller K, Wang M, Gralow J, et al. Paclitaxel plus bevacizumab versus paclitaxel alone for metastatic breast cancer. N Engl J Med. 2007;357:2666–76.
41. Hurwitz H, Fehrenbacher L, Novotny W, et al. Bevacizumab plus irinotecan, fluorouracil, and leucovorin for metastatic colorectal cancer. N Engl J Med. 2004;350:2335–42.
42. Sandler A, Gray R, Perry MC, et al. Paclitaxel-carboplatin alone or with bevacizumab for non-small-cell lung cancer. N Engl J Med. 2006;355:2542–50.
43. Escudier B, Pluzanska A, Koralewski P, et al. Bevacizumab plus interferon alfa-2a for treatment of metastatic renal cell carcinoma: a randomised, double-blind phase III trial. Lancet. 2007;370: 2103–11.
44. Varker A, Biber J, Kefauver C, et al. A randomized phase 2 trial of bevacizumab with or without daily low-dose interferon alfa-2b in metastatic malignant melanoma. Ann Surg Oncol. 2007;14:2367–76.
45. Vihinen P, Hernberg M, Vuoristo M, Tyynela K, Laukka M, Pyrhonen S. A Phase II trial of bevacizumab(bev) with dacarbazine (DTIC) and daily low-dose interferon-alfa-2a (IFN-alfa-2a) as first line treatment in metastatic melanoma. Perspectives in Melanoma XII. 2–4 Oct 2008. Scheveningen/The Hague, The Netherlandsr. Poster Abstr P-009.
46. Perez DG, Suman VJ, Fitch TR, et al. Phase 2 trial of carboplatin, weekly paclitaxel, and biweekly bevacizumab in patients with unresectable stage IV melanoma: a North Central Cancer Treatment Group study, N047A. Cancer. 2009;115:119–27.
47. Boasberg P, Cruickshank S, Hamid O, et al. Nab-paclitaxel and bevacizumab as first-line therapy in patients with unresectable stage III and IV melanoma. J Clin Oncol. 2009;27(15s) [abstr 9061].
48. González-Cao M, Viteri S, Díaz-Lagares A, et al. Preliminary results of the combination of bevacizumab and weekly paclitaxel in advanced melanoma. Oncology. 2008;74:12–6.
49. Von Moos R, Seifert B, Ochsenbein A, et al. Temozolomide combined with bevacizumab in metastatic melanoma. A multicenter phase II trial (SAKK 50/07). ECCO 15 and 34th ESMO Multidisciplinary Congress. 20–24 Sept 2009. Berlin, Germany. Abstr 24LBA.
50. Wyman K, Spigel D, Puzanov I, et al. A multicenter phase II study of erlotinib and bevacizumab in patients with metastatic melanoma sites. J Clin Oncol. 2007;25(18S) [abstr 8539].
51. Peyton JD, Spigel DR, Burris HA, et al. Phase II trial of bevacizumab and everolimus in the treatment of patients with metastatic melanoma: preliminary results. J Clin Oncol. 2009;27(15s) [abstr 9027].
52. O'Day SJ, Kim KB, Sosman JA, et al. BEAM: a randomized phase II study evaluating the activity of BEvacizumab in combination with carboplatin plus paclitaxel in patients with previously untreated Advanced Melanoma. In: Proceedings of ECCO 15 and 34th ESMO multidisciplinary congress. Berlin, Germany. 20–24 Sept 2009. Abstract 23LBA.
53. Tarhini AA, Christensen S, Frankel P, et al. Phase II study of aflibercept (VEGF trap) in recurrent inoperable stage III or stage IV melanoma of cutaneous or ocular origin. J Clin Oncol. 2009;27(15s) [abstr 9028].
54. Hilger RA, Scheulen ME, Strumberg D. The Ras-Raf-MEK-ERK pathway in the treatment of cancer. Onkologie. 2002;25:511–8.
55. Davies H, Bignell GR, Cox C, et al. Mutations of the BRAF gene in human cancer. Nature. 2002;417: 949–54.

56. Wilhelm SM, Carter C, Tang L, et al. BAY43-9006 exhibits broad spectrum oral antitumor activity and targets the RAF/MEK/ERK pathway and receptor tyrosine kinases involved in tumor progression and angiogenesis. Cancer Res. 2004;64:7099–109.
57. Eisen T, Ahmad T, Flaherty KT, et al. Sorafenib in advanced melanoma: a phase II randomised discontinuation trial analysis. Br J Cancer. 2006;95:581–6.
58. Flaherty KT, Brose M, Schucter L, et al. Phase I/II trial of BAY 43–9006, carboplatin (C) and paclitaxel (P) demonstrates preliminary antitumor activity in the expansion cohort of patients with metastatic melanoma. J Clin Oncol. 2004;22(14S) [abstr 7507].
59. Flaherty KT, Schiller J, Schuchter LM, et al. A phase I trial of the oral, multikinase inhibitor sorafenib in combination with carboplatin and paclitaxel. Clin Cancer Res. 2008;14:4836–42.
60. Eisen T, Ahmad T, Gore ME, et al. Phase I trial of BAY 43–9006 (sorafenib) combined with dacarbazine (DTIC) in metastatic melanoma patients. J Clin Oncol. 2005;23(16S) [abstr 7508].
61. Eisen T, Marais R, Affolter A, et al. An open-label phase II study of sorafenib and dacarbazine as first-line therapy in patients with advanced melanoma. J Clin Oncol. 2007;25(18S) [abstr 8529].
62. Lev DC, Ruiz M, Mills L, et al. Dacarbazine causes transcriptional up-regulation of interleukin 8 and vascular endothelial growth factor in melanoma cells: a possible escape mechanism from chemotherapy. Mol Cancer Ther. 2003;2:753–63.
63. McDermott DF, Sosman JA, Gonzalez R, et al. Double-blind randomized phase II study of the combination of sorafenib and dacarbazine in patients with advanced melanoma: a report from the 11715 study group. J Clin Oncol. 2008;26:2178–85.
64. Amaravadi RK, Schuchter LM, McDermott DF, et al. Phase II trial of temozolomide and sorafenib in advanced melanoma patients with or without brain metastases. Clin Cancer Res. 2009;15:7711–8.
65. Fruehauf JP, Lutzky J, McDermott DF. Axitinib (AG-013736) in patients with metastatic melanoma: a phase II study. J Clin Oncol. 2008;26(15S) [abstr 9006].
66. Rini BI, Schiller JH, Fruehauf JP, et al. Association of diastolic blood pressure (dBP)>90 mmHg with overall survival (OS) in patients treated with axitinib (AG- 013736). J Clin Oncol. 2008;26(15S) [abstr 3543].
67. Peterson AC, Swiger S, Stadler WM, et al. Phase II study of the Flk-1 tyrosine kinase inhibitor SU5416 in advanced melanoma. Clin Cancer Res. 2004;10:4048–54.
68. Mita MM, Rowinsky EK, Forero L, et al. A phase II, pharmacokinetic, and biologic study of semaxanib and thalidomide in patients with metastatic melanoma. Cancer Chemother Pharmacol. 2007;59:165–74.
69. Renhowe PA, Pecchi S, Shafer CM, et al. Design, structure-activity relationships and in vivo characterization of 4-Amino-3-benzimidazol-2-ylhydroquinolin-2-ones: a novel class of receptor tyrosine kinase inhibitors. J Med Chem. 2009;52:278–92.
70. Kim KB, Saro J, Moschos SS, et al. A phase I dose finding and biomarker study of TKI258 (dovitinib lactate) in patients with advanced melanoma. J Clin Oncol. 2008;26(15S) [abstr 9026].
71. Rajkumar SV, Blood E, Vesole D, et al. Phase III clinical trial of thalidomide plus dexamethasone compared with dexamethasone alone in newly diagnosed multiple myeloma: a clinical trial coordinated by the Eastern cooperative oncology group. J Clin Oncol. 2006;24:431–6.
72. Bamias A, Dimopoulos MA. Thalidomide and immunomodulatory drugs in the treatment of cancer. Export Opin Invest Drugs. 2005;14:45–55.
73. Zhang S, Li M, Gu Y, et al. Thalidomide influences growth and vasculogenic mimicry channel formation in melanoma. J Exp Clin Cancer Res. 2008;27:60.
74. Keifer JA, Guttridge DC, Ashburner BP, et al. Inhibition of NF-kappa B activity by thalidomide through suppression of IkappaB kinase activity. J Biol Chem. 2001;276:22382–7.
75. Marriott JB, Clarke IA, Dredge K, et al. Thalidomide and its analogues have distinct and opposing effects on TNF-α and TNFR2 during costimulation of both CD4(+) and CD8(+) T cells. Clin Exp Immunol. 2002;130:75–84.
76. Eisen T, Boshoff C, Mak I, et al. Continuous low dose thalidomide: a phase II study in advanced melanoma, renal cell, ovarian and breast cancer. Br J Cancer. 2000;82:812–7.
77. Reiriz AB, Richter MF, Fernandes S, et al. Phase II study of thalidomide in patients with metastatic malignant melanoma. Melanoma Res. 2004;14:527–31.
78. Pawlak WZ, Legha SS. Phase II study of thalidomide in patients with metastatic malignant melanoma. Melanoma Res. 2004;14:57–62.
79. Danson S, Lorigan P, Arance A, et al. A randomised study of temozolomide (TMZ) alone, with interferon (TMZ-IFN) or with thalidomide (TMZ-THAL) in metastatic malignant melanoma (MMM). J Clin Oncol. 2003;21:2551–7.
80. Hwu WJ, Krown SE, Menell JH, et al. Phase II study of temozolomide plus thalidomide for the treatment of metastatic melanoma. J Clin Oncol. 2003;21:3351–6.
81. Hwu WJ, Lis E, Menell JH, et al. Temozolomide plus thalidomide in patients with brain metastases from melanoma: a phase II study. Cancer. 2005;103:2590–7.
82. Krown SE, Niedzwiecki D, Hwu WJ, et al. Phase II study of temozolomide and thalidomide in patients with metastatic melanoma in the brain: high rate of thromboembolic events (CALGB 500102). Cancer. 2006;107:1883–90.
83. Atkins MB, Sosman JA, Agarwala S, et al. Temozolomide, thalidomide, and whole brain radiation therapy for patients with brain metastasis from metastatic melanoma: a phase II cytokine working group study. Cancer. 2008;113:2139–45.
84. Clark JI, Moon J, Hutchins LF, et al. Phase 2 trial of combination thalidomide plus temozolomide in patients with metastatic malignant melanoma: southwest oncology group S0508. Cancer. 2010;116:424–31.

85. Hutchins LF, Moon J, Clark JI, et al. Evaluation of interferon alpha-2B and thalidomide in patients with disseminated malignant melanoma, phase 2, SWOG 0026. Cancer. 2007;110:2269–75.
86. Bartlett JB, Dredge K, Dalgleish AG. The evolution of thalidomide and its IMiD derivatives as anticancer agents. Nat Rev Cancer. 2004;4:314–22.
87. Bartlett JB, Michael A, Clarke IA, et al. Phase I study to determine the safety, tolerability and immunostimulatory activity of thalidomide analogue CC-5013 in patients with metastatic malignant melanoma and other advanced cancers. Br J Cancer. 2004;90:955–61.
88. Bedikian A, Kim K, Papadopoulos N, et al. Preliminary results from a phase II study of the combination of lenalidomide and DTIC in patients with metastatic malignant melanoma previously untreated with systemic chemotherapy. J Clin Oncol. 2007; 25(18S) [abstr 8533].
89. Cai W, Chen X. Anti-angiogenic cancer therapy based on integrin avh3 antagonism. Anti-Cancer Agents Med Chem. 2006;6:407–28.
90. Hersey P, Sosman J, O'Day S, et al. A phase II, randomized, open-label study evaluating the antitumor activity of MEDI-522, a humanized monoclonal antibody directed against the human alpha v beta 3 (avb3) integrin, ± dacarbazine (DTIC) in patients with metastatic melanoma (MM). J Clin Oncol. 2005;23(16S) [abstr 7507].
91. Mullamitha S, Ton C, Parker G, et al. Phase I evaluation of a fully human anti-alphav integrin monoclonal antibody (CNTO 95) in patients with advanced solid tumours. Clin Cancer Res. 2007;13:2128–35.
92. Loquai C, Pavlick A, Lawson D, et al. Randomized phase II study of the safety and efficacy of a human anti-αv integrin monoclonal antibody (CNTO 95) alone and in combination with dacarbazine in patients with stage IV metastatic melanoma: 12-month results. J Clin Oncol. 2009;27(15s) [abstr 9029].
93. Kim S, Bell K, Mousa SA, et al. Regulation of angiogenesis in vivo by ligation of integrin a5h1 with the central cell-binding domain of fibronectin. Am J Pathol. 2000;156:1345–62.
94. Qian F, Zhang ZC, Wu XF, et al. Interaction between integrin a(5) and fibronectin is required for metastasis of B16F10 melanoma cells. Biochem Biophys Res Commun. 2005;333:1269–75.
95. Cranmer L, Bedikian AY, Ribas A, et al. Phase II study of volociximab (M200), an $\alpha5\beta1$ anti-integrin antibody in metastatic melanoma. J Clin Oncol. 2006;24(18S) [abstr 8011].
96. Barton J. A multicenter phase II study of volociximab in patients with relapsed metastatic melanoma. J Clin Oncol. 2008;26(15S) [abstr 9051].
97. Kim KB, Diwan AH, Papadopoulos NE, et al. A randomized phase II study of EMD 121974 in patients (pts) with metastatic melanoma (MM). J Clin Oncol. 2007;25(18S) [abstr 8548].
98. Tentori L, Dorio AS, Muzi A, et al. The integrin antagonist cilengitide increases the antitumor activity of temozolomide against malignant melanoma. Oncol Rep. 2008;19:1039–43.
99. Ebos JM, Lee CR, Kerbel RS. Tumor and host-mediated pathways of resistance and disease progression in response to antiangiogenic therapy. Clin Cancer Res. 2009;15:5020–5.
100. Ebos JM, Lee CR, Cruz-Munoz W, et al. Accelerated metastasis after short-term treatment with a potent inhibitor of tumor angiogenesis. Cancer Cell. 2009; 15:232–9.
101. Pàez-Ribes M, Allen E, Hudock J, et al. Antiangiogenic therapy elicits malignant progression of tumors to increased local invasion and distant metastasis. Cancer Cell. 2009;15:220–31.
102. Carmeliet P, De Smet F, Loges S, Mazzone M. Branching morphogenesis and antiangiogenesis candidates: tip cells lead the way. Nat Rev Clin Oncol. 2009;6:315–26.
103. Reynolds AR, Hart IR, Watson AR, et al. Stimulation of tumor growth and angiogenesis by low concentrations of RGD-mimetic integrin inhibitors. Nat Med. 2009;15:392–400.
104. Wolmark N, Yothers G, O'Connel MJ, et al. A phase III trial comparing mFOLFOX6 to mFOLFOX6 plus bevacizumab in stage II or III carcinoma of the colon: results of NSABP protocol C-08. J Clin Oncol. 2009;27(18S) [abstr LBA4].
105. Eggermont AM, Suciu S, Testori A, et al. Ulceration of primary melanoma and responsiveness to adjuvant interferon therapy: analysis of the adjuvant trials EORTC18952 and EORTC18991 in 2,644 patients. J Clin Oncol. 2009;27(15S) [abstr 9007].
106. Kashani-Sabet M, Sagebiel RW, Ferreira CM, et al. Tumor vascularity in the prognostic assessment of primary cutaneous melanoma. J Clin Oncol. 2002;20: 1826–31.
107. Sosman JA, Flaherty KT, Atkins MB, et al. Updated results of phase I trial of sorafenib (S) and bevacizumab (B) in patients with metastatic renal cell cancer (mRCC). J Clin Oncol. 2008;26(15S) [abstr 5011].
108. Booth CM, Calvert AH, Giaccone G, et al. Design and conduct of phase II studies of targeted anticancer therapy: recommendations from the task force on methodology for the development of innovative cancer therapies (MDICT). Eur J Cancer. 2008;44: 25–9.
109. Booth CM, Calvert AH, Giaccone G, et al. Endpoints and other considerations in phase I studies of targeted anticancer therapy: recommendations from the task force on methodology for the development of innovative cancer therapies (MDICT). Eur J Cancer. 2008;44:19–24.
110. Kummar S, Doroshow JH, Tomaszewski JE, et al. On behalf of the task force on methodology for the development of innovative cancer therapies (MDICT). Phase 0 clinical trials: recommendations from the task force on methodology for the development of innovative cancer therapies. Eur J Cancer. 2009;45:741–6.
111. Duda DG, Ancukiewicz M, Jain RK. Biomarkers of antiangiogenic therapy: how do we move from candidate biomarkers to valid biomarkers? J Clin Oncol. 2010;28:183–5.

Immunological Biomarkers and Immunotherapy for Melanoma

Jochen T. Schaefer

Advanced melanoma is an aggressive disease. It is among the most immunogenic of all tumors and many of the lessons learned in cancer immunology have involved the study of melanoma. Clinical regression of both benign and malignant melanocytic neoplasms lends further support for the potential powerful effect of the immune system targeting these neoplasms. However, only a subset of patients shows a favorable response to immune-based therapeutic interventions. Therefore, the identification of biomarkers that may assist in identifying patients who are likely to respond to immunotherapy would be a tremendous improvement with respect to the risk/benefit ratio, patient safety and cost. Gene expression profiling has been used to identify patients with a favorable tumor microenvironment; that is, by detecting activated T-cells in the tumor and cytokines promoting T-cell trafficking to the tumor [1]. This profiling procedure could lead to improved clinical responses to immunotherapy.

J.T. Schaefer, M.D. (✉)
Department of Dermatology,
University of Connecticut Health Center,
Farmington, CT, USA
e-mail: schaefer@uchc.edu

Proof of Principle That Immunotherapy in Patients with Melanoma is Effective

1. Cytokine-based therapies, such as interleukin (IL)-2, enhance the function of cytotoxic T-cells (CTLs) with clinical responses seen in 15% of patients, and durable, complete responses in up to 5% of cases [2].
2. The number of responders to immunotherapy is higher in the group of patients who develop early signs of autoimmunity, such as vitiligo and thyroiditis [3, 4]. The presence of antithyroglobulin, antinuclear and anticardiolipin antibodies seems to be a reasonable index for autoimmunity. Clinical manifestations of autoimmunity in the absence of the above antibodies are exceptionally rare. Overall, response rates for the two United States Food and Drug Administration (FDA)-approved therapies for metastatic melanoma, IL-2 and dacarbazine, are 12–15% [5].
3. Several vaccine-based therapeutic approaches have been shown to increase the immune response. Although some studies demonstrated slightly improved survival rates, the success rates have so far been rather humbling with clinical responses being observed in only 15–20% of patients [6, 7].

Several avenues of immune therapy for melanoma are currently under investigation including (1) melanoma vaccine therapy, (2) heat shock protein therapy, (3) adoptive T-cell transfer therapy, (4) cytokine therapy, (5) administration of activating antibodies, (6) biochemotherapy, and (7) nonspecific immune adjuvants.

Details of Current Immunotherapeutic Approaches in Melanoma

Basic Physiology of the Immune Response

Antigens are processed and then presented to naïve T-cells by antigen-presenting cells (APCs). This maneuver requires the interaction of a particular antigen via the major histocompatibility complex (MHC) with the specific T-cell receptor (TCR) on the naïve T-cell. However, this interaction in itself does not lead to a stable immune response, which includes the proliferation of a specific T-cell clone and the generation of memory T-cells. Additional so-called co-stimulatory signals are required, which can be generally divided into the tumor necrosis factor receptor (TNFR) and immunoglobulin (Ig) superfamilies. To enhance T-cell activation, one approach includes the use of monoclonal antibodies (mAb), such as CD28, 4-1BB and OX40, to trigger co-stimulatory signals. Antibodies can also be used to enhance antigen presentation by triggering CD40 on APCs. Anti-CTLA-4 antibodies can target the CTLA-4 receptor located on the surface of T-cells and block the signal that is triggered by physiologic binding of its ligand. Physiologic engagement of CTLA-4 would inhibit CD28 signaling, which is the most important co-stimulatory molecule. Therefore, CTLA-4 blockade ensures uninhibited interaction between CD28 and its ligands B7.1 (CD80) and B7.2 (CD86). Last, but not least, anti-CD25 antibodies can be used to neutralize the effects of regulatory T-cells (Tregs), also increasing the net immune response. In the absence of mandatory co-stimulatory factors, anergy (T-cell unresponsiveness) may result.

Successful immunotherapy of cancer is multifactorial and requires fully functional T-cells (both cytotoxic CD8+ and helper CD4+ subsets). In order to mount an effective response, several components must be satisfied including responsiveness of T-cells to antigen presentation (including proliferation to the antigenic stimuli), T-cell survival, T-cell homing to the tumor microenvironment, powerful T-cell effector functions and, ultimately, the mounting of an immunological memory response [8–10]. Therefore, all of these components must be addressed in order to optimize the efficacy of any immune-based therapy.

Melanoma Vaccine Therapy

The overarching principle of all cancer vaccine therapy is the immune recognition of antigens expressed by the tumor. Immune responses have been frequently observed using vaccine-based strategies. However, clinical responses only occurred in 15–20% of patients [6, 7]. Over the past three to four decades, a plethora of approaches have been tested. These have included whole-cell and lysed-cell vaccines, peptide/protein-based vaccines, dendritic cell-based vaccines, DNA-based vaccines, and vaccines using viral vectors for antigen delivery.

Whole-Cell and Lysed-Cell Vaccines

Allogenic and autologous whole tumor cells have been tested as potential immunotherapy. In theory, the abundance of antigens presented with this preparation should create powerful anti-tumor responses. However, an early phase II clinical trial using the whole cell vaccine Melacine, in combination with interferon (IFN)-alpha-2b, showed similar relapse-free survival and overall survival when compared with the IFN-alpha-2b arm alone [11]. The limitations of whole-cell/lysed-cell preparations may be due to angiogenic and immune-suppressant factors in the vaccine mixture.

Peptide/Protein-Based Vaccines

Antigenic peptides are either injected intra- or subcutaneously, as emulsions with an adjuvant, such as incomplete Freud's adjuvant (IFA). Of note, incomplete Freud's adjuvant has been given the appellation "incomplete" as it is devoid of dried and inactivated mycobacteria, which are part of the original ("complete") formulation. Clinically durable responses using peptide vaccines have so far been largely marginal. However, small successes have been observed. For instance, vaccination with the synthetic modified peptide gp100:209–217, which was modified to enhance the peptide's affinity for HLA-A2 molecules, increased its immunogenicity both in vitro and in vivo [12]. In another approach, the addition of tetanus helper peptide to the vaccine adjuvant resulted in helper T-cell responses in 79% of patients and an overall patient survival of 75% at 4.7 years follow-up [13]. In the adjuvant setting, administration of multiple peptides has been tested and found to be safe and immunogenic. The most immunogenic antigens, among 12 melanocyte differentiation and cancer testis proteins tested, are tyrosinase, gp100, MAGE-A1 and MAGE-A10 [14].

Improved progression-free survival has been documented in a phase III clinical trial comparing peptide vaccine (gp100) and IL-2 versus IL-2 therapy alone [15]. Therefore, there is enthusiasm to continue efforts to improve peptide vaccine therapy by optimizing antigen combinations and adjuvants. The addition of toll-like receptor (TLR) agonists has shown promising results [16, 17].

A recent study examined the composition of immune cell infiltrates at vaccination sites subject to repeated intradermal and subcutaneous vaccination with a multipeptide vaccine, with or without the addition of an incomplete Freud's adjuvant (IFA)—Montanide ISO51. The multipeptide/IFA combination induced a Th2-dominant microenvironment, which was reversed with repeated vaccination. However, repeat vaccination also increased FoxP3+ T-cells and eosinophils, therefore creating a less favorable milieu [18]. These data suggest opportunities to optimize vaccine regimens and potential endpoints for monitoring the effects of novel adjuvants.

Dendritic Cell-Based Vaccines

Dendritic cells (DCs) are crucial for the *de novo* activation of antigen-specific T-cell responses. Therefore, large efforts have been made to take advantage of DCs' antigen-presenting capabilities. For example, DCs have been loaded with either mRNA encoding the desired antigen or the antigen itself. Alternatively, DCs have also been loaded with full tumor cell lysates in an attempt to increase the antigenic repertoire. However, clinical response rates have been rather disappointing and only rarely resulted in stable disease regression [19]. One trial even concluded that there was no clinical benefit of peptide-pulsed DC therapy when compared to dacarbazine (DTIC) treatment [20]. The effectiveness of this strategy may be associated with (1) the maturation state of the aforementioned manipulated DCs once they are released *in vivo* and (2) the immune suppressive effects of Tregs [21]. It has also been postulated that melanomas may secrete factors inhibiting DC function [22, 23].

Viral Vectors and Plasmid Vaccines

Delivery of immunogenic antigens using a viral vector has been attempted with some success. However, immunodominance of viral antigens competing with the target antigens is problematic. In addition, high titers of neutralizing antibodies to adenoviral vectors have been detected, which may explain the low efficacy of this approach. Therefore, a modification of the vector concept using naked plasmid DNA is currently being explored. For example, the use of Allovectin-7, a plasmid DNA which encodes for HLA-B7 and beta-2 microglobulin, may induce a local inflammatory response within the tumor parenchyma [24].

Heat Shock Protein (HSP) Therapy

Heat shock proteins chaperone intracellular antigenic peptides and are capable of inducing dendritic cell maturation and activation of immune effector cells (CD8+ and CD4+ T-cells and NK-cells). Vaccination with autologous HSPPC-97 (vitespan) induces clinical and tumor-specific T-cell responses in a significant minority of patients [25]. This response could not be enhanced with IFN-alpha or granulocyte-macrophage colony-stimulating factor (GM-CSF) [26]. A recent phase III clinical trial found no difference in overall survival between vitespan and physician's choice of treatment, which included dacarbazine, temozolomide, IL-2 or complete tumor resection [27].

Adoptive T-Cell Transfer Therapy

Adoptive T-cell transfer therapy (ACT) is based on the concept of autologous tumor reactive *ex vivo* lymphocytes. These lymphocytes are either extracted from tumor (tumor infiltrating lymphocytes, TILs) or from peripheral blood. The expanded reactive T-cell clone is then administered as a peripheral infusion. This approach requires lymphodepleting, non-myeloablative chemotherapy (cyclophosphamide and fludarabine) or radiotherapy (12 Gy of total body irradiation) before cell transfer. The rationale for lymphodepletion is threefold: first, it reduces the population of Tregs; second, it increases the availability of cytokines, such as IL-7 and IL-15, required for a powerful reactive T-cell response; and lastly, it engages toll-like receptors (TLRs) on antigen-presenting cells (APCs) which further enhances the cytotoxic T-cell attack [28]. Clinical response rates of 50–70% have been attained using adoptive transfer therapy.

Modifications of ACT therapy have evolved, motivated by the striking clinical responses. Since lymphocyte isolation and *in vitro* expansion of T-cells is both labor- and cost-intensive, additional avenues have been sought. Peripheral T-cells can be reprogrammed to target any desired antigen, which can be accomplished by the genetic transfer of antigen-specific TCRs. These receptors can be human leukocyte antigen (HLA) restricted, heterodimeric TCRs or chimeric antigen receptors. The latter usually recognize native cell surface antigens. Using gene transfer of TCR genes via retroviruses, some responses were reported in a pilot clinical trial [29]. However, this modification will need refinement since the approach has been challenged by the mispairing of TCR chains and the fact that transduced TCRs may not successfully compete against the overwhelming amount of endogenous TCRs [30, 31].

Genetically-modified lymphocytes (GMLs) expressing the cancer germline gene MAGE-A3 were used for treatment in another pilot clinical trial. Ten patients with advanced melanoma were treated with GMLs. Anti-MAGE-A3 lymphocytes were elicited and found in the tumor microenvironment in a subset of patients [32].

Cytokine Therapy

IL-2, IL-12 and IFN-alpha have been used alone and in combination with varied success. In fact, twenty one phase III clinical trials have been carried out testing several combinations of IFN-alpha and IL-2 with mono- or combination therapy [33]. Additional combinations with GM-CSF, tumor necrosis factor (TNF)-alpha or IL-1, IL-4, IL-6, IL-12, IL-18 and IFN-gamma did not improve clinical outcome. Although the number of clinical responses increased, so did the number of adverse events (toxicity) and, unfortunately, overall survival was not improved. IL-2 therapy leads to increased lysis by CTLs and NK-cells, even in the absence of HLA class I restriction. IFN-alpha has multiple anticancer effects. These include antiproliferative/pro-apoptotic effects, anti-angiogenic effects and modulation of both the innate and adaptive immune responses.

Administration of Activating Antibodies

Physiologically, T-cells possess a family of immune-suppressive receptors which counter balance immune effector cell activation and serve to stabilize the immune response. These receptors include cytotoxic T lymphocyte antigen-4 (CTLA-4) and PD-1. CTLA-4 blockade with neutralizing antibodies disables these immune-suppressive receptors and enhances T-cell function and proliferation. The proportion of responders to CTLA-4 therapy is much higher in patients who also experience immune-related adverse events, such as dermatitis and colitis [34, 35], a phenomenon also encountered in other immune-based therapies. The latter are in large part successfully managed with corticosteroids. Dose-escalation studies have shown an improved response rate with higher doses. For example, doses of 10 mg/kg of ipilimumab, a CTLA-4-blocking antibody, have led to long-term survival benefit in at least one third of melanoma patients tested [36]. In addition to ipilimumab, a newer agent that also targets CTLA-4, tremelimumab, is now available. Tremelimumab has so far demonstrated lower response rates than ipilimumab. However, the dose-escalation tested with tremelimumab may not have been aggressive enough.

Additional immunomodulatory monoclonal antibodies include PD-1 antibodies, CD40 agonist mAbs and toll-like receptor agonists.

PD-1 Antibodies

A recent phase I clinical study of single-agent anti-PD-1 (MDX-1106) concluded that blockade of the PD-1 immune checkpoint is well tolerated and associated with antitumor activity. Testing of combination therapy, including vaccines, targeted therapies and/or other checkpoint inhibitors, is now warranted [37].

CD40 Agonist mAbs

CD40 is a member of the tumor necrosis factor (TNF) receptor superfamily and is expressed by antigen-presenting cells (APCs), B-lymphocytes and monocytes. CD40 is also expressed by 30–70% of primary solid human tumors, including melanoma. The natural ligand for CD40 is CD154. This ligand is primarily expressed on activated T-lymphocytes. CD40 engagement enhances both the immune response of APCs and direct cytotoxic effects on tumor cells. In an early phase I trial, use of the CD40 agonist CP-870,893 resulted in objective tumor responses in 27% of melanoma patients [38]. Of note, CD40 antibodies have recently been shown to trigger antitumor activity in a macrophage-dependent and T-cell-independent manner in pancreatic carcinoma [39]. This finding highlights the significance of the cancer micro environment.

Toll-Like Receptor Agonists

Toll-like receptors (TLRs) are signaling molecules on the surface of DCs, which upon engagement enhance DC activation and heighten antitumor immune responses. In a phase II trial of patients with metastatic melanoma, activation of TLR-9 using PF-3512676 (formerly CpG 7909) resulted in partial responses in 10% of patients [40]. Furthermore, TLR-7/8 agonists have been shown to exert multiple immunomodulatory effects including: stimulation of maturation, activation and migration of critical effector cells; increased cytokine production by dendritic cells (IFN-alpha, IL-12 and TNF-alpha); up-regulation of co-stimulatory molecules (CD80 and CD86), skewing the immune response towards the Th1 phenotype; and enhanced tumor cell lysis [41–43]. TLR-7/8 agonists also directly activate both B- and T-cells. Current studies investigating the role of TLR agonists as part of the adjuvant emulsion in cancer vaccine therapy are underway.

Biochemotherapy

Chemotherapy induces cellular disruption and release of antigens. When combined with IL-2 triggered enhanced immune recognition and effector cell function, improved immune responses to released tumor antigens is expected. Several phase III clinical trials have demonstrated mixed results and meta-analyses showed no improvement of overall survival.

Nonspecific Immune Adjuvants

Nonspecific immune adjuvants, such as levamisole, *Corynebacterium parvum*, or Bacille Calmette Guerin (BCG), have been tested in randomized trials in the adjuvant setting and shown to reduce the risk of tumor recurrence [44, 45].

Immune-Evasion Strategies

Tumors develop a rather diverse, and often rapid, armamentarium of strategies to evade immunological attacks that are stimulated by immunotherapy. Several factors within the tumor microenvironment can negatively affect the immune response. For instance, neoangiogenesis within the tumor is controlled by regulator of G-protein signaling 5 (Rgs5), which has been identified as a master gene responsible for the generation of abnormal new blood vessels. In a mouse model, loss of Rgs5 results in pericyte maturation and vascular normalization. As a consequence, there is reduced tumor hypoxia and vessel leakiness leading to enhanced influx of immune effector cells into the tumor microenvironment. Markedly prolonged survival of tumor-bearing mice was observed in this study [46].

Overexpression of endothelin B receptor (ETBR) is another factor leading to an adverse milieu for immune cell attack. Increased expression of ETBR tips the endothelin B receptor/ endothelin A receptor ratio. The effects are threefold: firstly, this further promotes tumor neoangiogenesis; secondly, it decreases endothelial expression of ICAM1; and thirdly, it increases generation of endothelial nitric oxide (NO), which decreases transendothelial migration and homing of immune effector cells [47]. Therefore, ETBR and NO antagonists, as well as TNF-alpha, mitigate these negative effects and lead to upregulation of cadherins, integrins and connexins. This combination of effects can lead to increased transendothelial cell migration and T-cell survival [47].

Regulatory T-cells (Tregs) can be present both systemically and locally in the tumor microenvironment [48–53] and suppress the antitumor responses of both CD4+ and CD8+ T-cells [1, 8, 54, 55]. Their number in patients with metastatic melanoma inversely correlates with patient survival [56]. Several strategies to deplete Tregs are currently being investigated. IL-21 has proven to enhance systemic effector and memory CD8+ T-cell responses, and to decrease the accumulation of Tregs in the tumor microenvironment by up to 50% [57]. Inhibition of STAT3 signaling has been found to directly inhibit Tregs in a dose-dependent manner [58]. Finally, CD25-directed immunotoxins were shown in preclinical trials to reduce Treg populations; however, objective tumor responses have not been achieved in humans.

Functional T-cells require a close spatial association between both the T-cell receptor (TCR) and CD8. Loss of co-localization of these protein complexes leads to anergic cytotoxic T-cells (CTLs). This loss, however, can be rescued by *ex vivo* treatment with galectin disaccharide ligands, with recovery of T-cell effector functions [59].

Tumor infiltrating lymphocytes (TILs) have been found to express high levels of the programmed cell death 1 receptor (PD-1), as compared to normal tissue T-cell infiltrates and peripheral blood lymphocytes. PD-1 expression correlated with an exhausted phenotype and impaired effector function [60]. Recently, PD-1 blockade has been shown to lead to immune enhancement via direct augmentation of melanoma antigen-specific CTL proliferation and direct limitation of the inhibitory ability of Tregs [61].

Downregulation of human leukocyte antigen (HLA) class I expression in surgically removed melanoma lesions has been described [62]. Melanomas can produce several immune-dysregulating factors [22]. In addition, downregulation of components belonging to the antigen processing machinery also results in immunosuppressive effects. These antigen processing machinery components are required for MHC class I antigen presentation and include beta2 microglobulin and transport associated with antigen processing (TAP)-1/2 peptide transporters [63–65]. Histone deacetylase inhibitors, such as valproic acid, have been shown to increase the expression of the antigen processing machinery (TAP1, TAP2, LMP2, Tapasin), costimulatory molecules (CD40, CD80) and MHC class I on melanoma cells, thereby enhancing immunogenicity [66].

Infiltration of tumors by myeloid-derived suppressor cells (MDSCs) has also been described. MDSCs have a remarkable ability to suppress T-cell responses [67, 68]. Additional tumor escape mechanisms include suppression of co-stimulatory molecules (i.e., CD40, CD80 and CD86).

The following biomarkers have been proposed and tested for use in the diagnosis and prognostication of primary melanoma:

A biomarker is defined as a marker which can be used as an indicator of a particular disease state or some other biological state of an organism. As such a biomarker may indicate the normal/physiological state, pathologic events or the response to a therapeutic pharmacological intervention. While prognostic biomarkers convey a defined clinical outcome, predictive biomarkers foretell the clinical effect of a specific therapeutic intervention.

1. *C-reactive protein (CRP)* has shown some promise in the prognostication of advanced melanoma. For instance, patients with metastatic melanoma and high serum CRP levels show decreased survival. Furthermore, patients with elevated CRP are likely to respond to treatment with IL-2 [69]. However, CRP appears to be of less value in predicting patient responses to IFN treatment.
2. Elevation of *peripheral blood neutrophil and monocyte counts* have been shown to be associated with a worse prognosis in patients with stage IV melanoma [70]. As a rare event, paraneoplastic granulocytosis has been reported in patients with metastatic melanoma. Increased serum GM-CSF, possibly produced by melanoma tumor cells, may induce peripheral leukocytosis.
3. Responders to IL-2 therapy exhibited increased *absolute lymphocytes counts (ALCs)* compared with non-responders [3]. Patients with low ALCs (less than 1,000 cells/µl) may not benefit from ipilimumab therapy. However, patients with high ALCs showed improved survival.
4. *Human leukocyte antigen (HLA) status* has been linked to the risk of developing melanoma. HLA-DQB*0301 and HLA-DRB*1101 have been associated with increased risk for disease recurrence [71, 72]. Homozygosity of HLA-DR has been linked to tolerance to IL-2 therapy [73].

Additional predictive biomarkers in melanoma patients gauging the probability of successful immune-based therapy:

1. Pre-treatment elevations of *vascular endothelial growth factor (VEGF)* and *fibronectin* have been shown to be negative predictive biomarkers for IL-2 therapy [74].
2. *Germline polymorphisms in host immunoregulatory genes* have been examined in the context of cancer vaccine clinical trials [75]. Both sequencing analysis of specific genes and the examination of large collections of genes by microarray profiling have been performed. As a result, a distinct profile of gene expression has been identified. In essence, this analysis broadly divides metastatic tumors into two groups: patients with or without evidence of a baseline (prior to vaccination) inflammatory tumor microenvironment. Patients likely to respond to melanoma vaccine therapy showed a so-called inflammatory tumor microenvironment prior to treatment, which included the presence of immune effector cells and chemokines. These chemokines are responsible for the locomotion and homing of effector cells to the tumor microenvironment. Therefore, the pre-treatment "inflammatory" status of a tumor may be decisive as to whether a patient will be successful in mounting a strong and durable immune attack following melanoma vaccine treatment. The inflammatory tumor microenvironment seems to play a similar role in other non-vaccine immune-based interventions, such as anti-CTLA-4 directed therapy [76].

Concluding Remarks

As outlined in this chapter, there is proof-of-principle that immune-based therapies can effectively improve outcome in patients with melanoma. However, responses are often limited and do not exceed a 15% response rate threshold. Any future advances in immunotherapy will need to take into consideration several factors, including (1) polymorphisms in immunoregulatory genes of the host; (2) tumor-induced immunosuppression; (3) standardized biomarkers for immune monitoring methods to allow comparison of clinical trials; and (4) development of more accurate diagnostic biomarkers. The Society for Immunotherapy of Cancer (SITC, formerly known as iSBTc) has established a task force in collaboration with the United States FDA to address the development of predictive biomarkers both for monitoring and diagnostic purposes [77].

References

1. Harlin H, Kuna TV, Peterson AC, et al. Tumor progression despite massive influx of activated CD8(+) T cells in a patient with malignant melanoma ascites. Cancer Immunol Immunother. 2009;55: 1185–97.
2. Atkins MB, Lotze MT, Dutcher JP, et al. High-dose recombinant interleukin 2 therapy for patients with metastatic melanoma: analysis of 270 patients treated between 1985 and 1993. J Clin Oncol. 1999;17: 2105–16.
3. Phan GQ, Attia P, Steinberg SM, et al. Factors associated with response to high-dose interleukin-2 in patients with metastatic melanoma. J Clin Oncol. 2001;19:3477–82.
4. Rosenberg SA, White DE. Vitiligo in patients with melanoma: normal tissue antigens can be targets for cancer immunotherapy. J Immunother Emphasis Tumor Immunol. 1996;19:81–4.
5. Tsao H, Atkins MB, Sober AJ. Management of cutaneous melanoma. N Engl J Med. 2004;351: 998–1012.
6. Rosenberg SA, Yang JC, Restifo NP. Cancer immunotherapy: moving beyond current vaccines. Nat Med. 2004;10:909–15.
7. Parmiani G, Castelli C, Dalerba P, et al. Cancer immunotherapy with peptide-based vaccines: what have we achieved? Where are we going? J Natl Cancer Inst. 2002;94:805–18.
8. Appay VV, Jandus C, Voelter V, et al. New generation vaccine induces effective melanoma-specific CD8+ T cells in the circulation but not in the tumour site. J Immunol. 2006;177:1670–8.
9. Klebanoff CA, Gattinoni L, Restifo NP. CD8+ T-cell memory in tumour immunology and immunotherapy. Immunol Rev. 2006;211:214–24.
10. Wherry EJ, Teichgraber V, Becker TC, et al. Lineage relationship and protective immunity of memory CD8 T cell subsets. Nat Immunol. 2003;4:225–34.
11. Mitchell MS, Abrams J, Thompson JA, et al. Randomized trial of an allogeneic melanoma lysate vaccine with low-dose interferon alfa-2b compared with high-dose interferon alfa-2b for resected stage III cutaneous melanoma. J Clin Oncol. 2007;25: 2078–85.
12. Smith 2nd JW, Walker EB, Fox BA, et al. Adjuvant immunization of HLA-A2-positive melanoma patients with a modified gp100 peptide induces peptide-specific CD8+ T-cell responses. J Clin Oncol. 2003; 21:1562–73.
13. Slingluff CL, Yamshchikov G, Neese P. Phase I trial of melanoma vaccine with gp100 280–288 peptide and tetanus helper peptide in adjuvant: immunologic and clinical outcomes. Clin Cancer Res. 2001;7: 3012–24.
14. Slingluff CL, Petroni G, Bullock KA, et al. Immunological results of a phase II randomized trial of multipeptide vaccines for melanoma. Proc Am Soc Clin Oncology. 2004;22(14s):abstract 7503.
15. Schwartzentruber DJ, Lawson DH, Richards JM, et al. gp100 peptide vaccine and interleukin-2 in patients with advanced melanoma. NEJM. 2011;364: 2119–27.
16. Brichard VG, Lejeune D. Cancer immunotherapy targeting tumor-specific antigens: towards a new therapy for minimal residual disease. Expert Opin Biol Ther. 2008;8:951–68.
17. Kruit WH, Suciu S, Dreno B. Immunization with recombinant MAGE-A3 protein combined with adjuvant systems AS15 or AS02B in patients with unresectable and progressive metastatic cutaneous melanoma. J Clin Oncol. 2008;26 (May 20 2008) ASCO Annual Meeting. Abstract 9065.
18. Schaefer JT, Patterson JW, Deacon DH, et al. Dynamic changes in cellular infiltrates with repeated cutaneous vaccination: a histologic and immunophenotypic analysis. J Transl Med. 2010;8:79.
19. Tuettenberg A, Becker C, Huter E, et al. Induction of strong and persistent Melan A/MART-1-specific immune responses by adjuvant dendritic cell-based vaccination of stage II melanoma patients. Int J Cancer. 2006;118:2617–27.
20. Schadendorf D, Ugurel S, Schuler-Thurner B, et al. Dacarbazine (DTIC) versus vaccination with autologous peptide-pulsed dendritic cells (DC) in first-line treatment of patients with metastatic melanoma: a randomized phase III trial of the DC study group of the DeCOG. Ann Oncol. 2006;17:563–70.
21. Min WP, Zhou D, Ichim TE, et al. Inhibitory feedback loop between tolerogenic dendritic cells and regulatory T cells in transplant tolerance. J Immunol. 2003;170:1304–12.
22. Ilkovitch D, Lopez DM. Immune modulation by melanoma-derived factors. Exp Dermatol. 2008;17: 977–85.
23. Kim R, Emi M, Tanabe K. Functional roles of immature dendritic cells in impaired immunity of solid tumor and their targeted strategies for provoking tumor immunity. Clin Exp Immunol. 2006;146:189–96.
24. Bergen M, Chen R, Gonzalez R. Efficacy and safety of HLA-B7/beta-2 microglobulin plasmid DNA/lipid complex (Allovectin-7) in patients with metastatic melanoma. Expert Opin Biol Ther. 2003;3:377–84.
25. Belli F, Testori A, Rivoltini L, et al. Vaccination of metastatic melanoma patients with autologous tumor-derived heat shock protein gp-96 peptide complexes: clinical and immunologic findings. J Clin Oncol. 2002;20:4169–80.
26. Pilla L, Patuzzo R, Rivoltini L, et al. A phase II trial of vaccination with autologous tumor-derived heat-shock protein peptide complexes Gp96, in combination with GM-CSF and interferon-alpha in metastatic melanoma patients. Cancer Immunol Immunother. 2006;55:958–68.
27. Testori A, Richards J, Whitman E, et al. Phase III comparison of vitespan, an autologout tumor-derived heat shock protein gp96 peptide complex vaccine, with physician's choice of treatment for stage IV melanoma: the C-100-21 study group. J Clin Oncol. 2006;26:955–62.

28. Dudley ME, Yang JC, Sherry R, et al. Adoptive cell therapy for patients with metastatic melanoma: evaluation of intensive myeloablative chemoradiation preparative regimens. J Clin Oncol. 2008;26:5233–9.
29. Morgan RA, Dudley ME, Wunderlich JR, et al. Cancer regression in patients after transfer of genetically engineered lymphocytes. Science. 2006;314(5796):126–9.
30. Bendle GM, Haanen JB, Schumacher TN. Preclinical development of T cell receptor gene therapy. Curr Opin Immunol. 2009;21(2):209–14.
31. Heemskerk MH, Hagedoorn RS, van der Hoorn MA, et al. Efficiency of T-cell receptor expression in dual-specific T cells is controlled by the intrinsic qualities of the TCR chains within the TCR-CD3 complex. Blood. 2007;109(1):235–43.
32. Fontana R, Bregni M, Cipponi A, et al. Peripheral blood lymphocytes genetically modified to express the self/tumor antigen MAGE-A3 induce antitumor immune responses in cancer patients. Blood. 2009;113:1651–60.
33. Eggermont AM, Schadendorf D. Melanoma and immunotherapy. Hematol Oncol Clin North Am. 2009;23:547–64. Ix–x.
34. Downey SG, Klapper JA, Smith FO, et al. Prognostic factors related to clinical response in patients with metastatic melanoma treated by CTL-associated antigen-4 blockade. Clin Cancer Res. 2007;13:6681–8.
35. Sanderson K, Scotland R, Lee P, et al. Autoimmunity in a phase I trial of fully human anti-cytotoxic T-lymphocyte antigen-4 monoclonal antibody with multiple melanoma peptides and montanide ISA51 for patients with resected stages III and IV melanoma. J Clin Oncol. 2005;23:741–50.
36. O'Day S, Weber J, Lebbe C, et al. Effect of ipilimumab treatment on 18-month survival: update of patients (pts) with advanced melanoma treated with 10mg/kg ipilimumab in three phase II clinical trials. J Clin Oncol. 2009;27(15s). abstract 9033.
37. Brahmer JR, Drake CG, Wollner I, et al. Phase I study of single-agent anti-programmed death-1 (MDX-1106) in refractory solid tumors: safety, clinical activity, pharmacodynamics and immunologic correlates. J Clin Oncol. 2010;28:3167–75.
38. Vonderheide RH, Flaherty KT, Khalil M, et al. Clinical activity and immune modulation in cancer patients treated with CP-870,893, a novel CD40 agonist monoclonal antibody. J Clin Oncol. 2007;25:876–83.
39. Beatty GL, Chiorean EG, Fishman MP, et al. CD40 agonists alter tumor stroma and show efficacy against pancreatic carcinoma in mice and humans. Science. 2011;25:1612–6.
40. Wagner SN, Pashenkov M, Goess G, et al. TLR-9-targeted CpG immunostimulatory treatment of metastatic melanoma: a phase II trial with CpG 7909 (promune). J Clin Oncol, ASCO. 2004;22(14s). abstract 7513.
41. Lehner M, Morhart P, Stilper A, et al. Efficient chemokine-dependent migration and primary and secondary IL-12 secretion by human dendritic cells stimulated through toll-like receptors. J Immunother. 2007;30:312–22.
42. Birmachu W, Gleason RM, Bulbulian BJ, et al. Transcriptional networks in plamacytoid dendritic cells stimulated with TLR7 agonists. BMC Immunol. 2007;8:26.
43. Stary G, Bangert C, Tauber M, et al. Tumoricidal activity of TLR7/8-activated inflammatory dendritic cells. J Exp Med. 2007;204:1441–51.
44. Parkinson DR. Levamisole as adjuvant therapy for melanoma: quo vadis? J Clin Oncol. 1991;9:716–7.
45. Lipton A, Harvey HA, Balch CM, et al. Corynebacterium parvum versus bacillus Calmette-Guerin adjuvant immunotherapy of stage II malignant melanoma. J Clin Oncol. 1991;9:1151–6.
46. Hamzah J, Jungold M, Kiesssling F, et al. Vascular normalization in Rgs5-deficient tumours promotes immune destruction. Nature. 2008;453(1783):410–4.
47. Kandalaft LE, Facciabene A, Buckanovich RJ, et al. Endothelin B receptor, a new target in cancer immune therapy. Clin Cancer Res. 2009;15:4521–8.
48. Ahmadzadeh M, Felipe-Silva A, Heemskerk B, et al. FoxP3 expression accurately defines the population of intratumoral regulatory T cells that selectively accumulate in metastatic melanoma lesions. Blood. 2008;112:4953–60.
49. Kryczek I, Liu R, Wang G, et al. FoxP3 defines regulatory T cells in human tumor and autoimmune disease. Cancer Res. 2009;69:3995–4000.
50. Nicholaou T, Ebert LM, Davis ID, et al. Regulatory T-cell mediated attenuation of T-cell response to the NY-ESO-1 ISCOMATRIX vaccine in patients with advanced malignant melanoma. Clin Cancer Res. 2009;15:2166–73.
51. Viguier M, Lemaitre F, Verola O, et al. FoxP3 expressing CD4+CD25(high) regulatory T cells are overrepresented in human metastatic melanoma lymph nodes and inhibit the function of infiltrating T cells. J Immunol. 2004;173:1444–53.
52. Wang HY, Lee DA, Peng G, et al. Tumour-specific human CD4+ regulatory T cells and their ligands: implications for immunotherapy. Immunity. 2004;20:107–18.
53. Wang HY, Peng G, Guo Z, et al. Recognition of a new ARTC1 peptide ligand uniquely expressed in tumor cells by antigen-specific CD4+ regulatory T cells. J Immunol. 2005;174:2661–70.
54. Mortarini R, Piris A, Maurichi A, et al. Lack of terminally differentiated tumor-specific CD8+ T cells at tumor site in spite of antitumor immunity to self-antigens in human metastatic melanoma. Cancer Res. 2003;63:2535–45.
55. Zippelius A, Batard P, Rubio-Godoy V, et al. Effector function of human tumour-specific CD8 T cells in melanoma lesions: a state of local functional tolerance. Cancer Res. 2004;64:2865–73.
56. Baumgartner JM, Gonzalez R, Lewis KD, et al. Increased survival from stage IV melanoma associated

with fewer regulatory T cells. J Surg Res. 2008;154(1): 13–20.
57. Kim-Schulze S, Kim HS, Fan Q, et al. Local IL-21 promotes the therapeutic activity of effector T cells by decreasing regulatory T cells within the tumor microenvironment. Mol Ther. 2009;17:380–8.
58. Kong LY, Wei J, Sharma AK, et al. A novel phosphorylated STAT3 inhibitor enhances T cell cytotoxicity against melanoma through inhibition of regulatory T cells. Cancer Immunol Immunother. 2008;58(7): 1023–32.
59. Demotte N, Stroobant V, Courtoy PJ, et al. Restoring the association of the T cell receptor with CD8 reverses anergy in human tumor-infiltrating lymphocytes. Immunity. 2008;28:414–24.
60. Ahmadzadeh M, Johnson LA, Heemskerk B, et al. Tumor antgien-specific CD8 T cells infiltrating the tumor express high levels of PD-1 and are functionally impaired. Blood. 2009;114:1537–44.
61. Wang W, Lau R, Yu D, et al. PD1 blockade reversed the suppression of melanoma antigen-specific CTL by CD3+ CD25(Hi) regulatory T cells. Int Immunol. 2009;21:1065–77.
62. Kageshita T, Ishihara T, Campoli M, Ferrone S. Selective monomorphic and polymorphic HLA class I antigenic determinant loss in surgically removed melanoma lesions. Tissue Antigens. 2005;65:419–28.
63. Chang CC, Ogino T, Mullins DW, et al. Defective human leukocyte antigen class I-associated antigen presentation caused by a novel beta2-microglobulin loss-of-function in melanoma cells. J Biol Chem. 2006;281:18763–73.
64. Chang CC, Campoli M, Restifo NP, et al. Immune selection of hot-spot beta 2-microglobulin gene mutations, HLA-A2 allospecificity loss, and antigen-processing machinery component down-regulation in melanoma cells derived from recurrent metastases following immunotherapy. J Immunol. 2005;174: 1462–71.
65. Dissemond J, Gotte P, Mors J, et al. Association of TAP1 downregulation in human primary melanoma lesions with lack of spontaneous regression. Melanoma Res. 2003;13:253–8.
66. Khan AN, Gregorie CH, Tomasi TB. Histone deacetylase inhibitors induce TAP, LMP, Tapasin genes and MHC class I antigen presentation by melanoma cells. Cancer Immunol Immunother. 2008;57:647–54.
67. Gabrilovich DI, Nagaraj S. Myeloid-derived suppressor cells as regulators of the immune system. Nat Rev Immunol. 2009;9:162–74.
68. Mandruzzato S, Solito S, Falisi E, et al. IL4Ralpha+ myeloid-derived suppressor cell expansion in cancer patients. J Immunol. 2009;182:6562–8.
69. Tartour E, Blay JY, Dorval T, et al. Predictors of clinical responses to interleukin-2-based immunotherapy in melanoma patients: a French multiinstitutional study. J Clin Oncol. 1996;14:1697–703.
70. Schmidt H, Suciu S, Punt CJ, et al. Pretreatment levels of peripheral neutrophils and leukocytes as independent predictors of overall survival in patients with American Joint Committee on Cancer Stage IV Melanoma: results of the EORTC 18951 biochemotherapy trial. J Clin Oncol. 2007;25:1562–9.
71. Lee JE, Lu M, Mansfield PF, et al. Malignant melanoma: relationship of the human leukocyte antigen class II gene DQB1*0301 to disease recurrence in American Joint Committee on Cancer Stage I or II. Cancer. 1996;78(4):758–63.
72. Lee JE, Abdalla J, Porter GA, et al. Presence of the human leukocyte antigen class II gene DRB1*1101 predicts interferon gamma levels and disease recurrence in melanoma patients. Ann Surg Oncol. 2002; 9(6):587–93.
73. Rubin JT, Day R, Duquesnoy R, et al. HLA-DQ1 is associated with clinical response and survival of patients with melanoma who are treated with interleukin-2. Ther Immunol. 1995;2(1):1–6.
74. Sabatino M, Kim-Schulze S, Panellin MC, et al. Serum vascular endothelial growth factor and fibronectin predict clinical response to high-dose interleukin-2 therapy. J Clin Oncol. 2009;27: 2645–52.
75. Gajewski TF, Louahed J, Brichard VG. Gene signature in melanoma associated with clinical activity. Cancer J. 2010;1:399–403.
76. Sullivan RJ, Hoshida Y, Brunet J, et al. A single center experience with high-dose IL-2 treatment for patients with advanced melanoma and pilot investigation of a novel gene expression signature as a predictor of response. J Clin Oncol 2009;27(15s). abstract 9003.
77. Butterfield LH, Isis ML, Fox BA, et al. A systematic approach to biomarker discovery; preamble to "the iSBTc-FDA taskforce on immunotherapy biomarkers". J Transl Med. 2008;6:81.

Diagnostic and Prognostic Biomarkers and Therapeutic Targets in Melanoma: An Overview

Ahmad A. Tarhini and John M. Kirkwood

Introduction

Biomarkers that are of interest in patients with melanoma may relate to the individual host or to the tumor, and may represent molecules or other factors that indicate genetic predisposition, prognosis, clinical course or therapeutic outcome. Biomarkers include clinical covariates, host proteomic/genomic markers and tumor proteomic/genomic markers that allow improved prognostic assessment and/or serve to predict and subclassify patients in relation to their disease and/or its therapy.

Identification of biomarkers that are predictive of therapeutic outcome would enable the better selection of patients, in order to treat only those who are most likely to benefit from therapy, while sparing those at risk from the significant toxicities associated with treatment. Currently, BRAF mutational status leads the way as a well-established therapeutic predictor to BRAF kinase inhibitors designed for this purpose. Of interest, recent information suggests that BRAF mutational status is also a prognostic biomarker in melanoma, with patients who have BRAF-mutant melanomas appearing in one series to exhibit more aggressive disease than those with wild-type tumors. While equally useful predictive biomarkers for other classes of cytotoxic, immunologic, and targeted therapies have not been identified at this time, some progress has been made. In addition, disease prognostic biomarkers may also advance patient management, by enabling the identification of individuals who are most likely to relapse and therefore derive the most benefit from therapy in the adjuvant and advanced disease settings.

This chapter reviews current melanoma biomarkers with prognostic or therapeutic predictive value. While this is a rapidly advancing field with various biomarkers being evaluated on a continuous basis, we will focus on those biomarkers that we consider to be the most well-established and likely to serve as a model or basis for the development of the next generation of biomarkers in melanoma.

Melanoma Staging

Melanoma is a malignant tumor of cutaneous melanocytes that is highly curable when detected early, but also has a dismal prognosis when it advances to inoperable stages. The American Joint Committee on Cancer (AJCC) divides the spectrum of cutaneous melanoma into four stages. In the seventh edition (2010), stages I and II are assigned to primary tumors that are confined to the skin and without regional lymph node involvement [1]. These stages are defined on the basis of histopathological parameters of the primary

A.A. Tarhini, M.D., M.Sc. (✉) • J.M. Kirkwood, M.D.
Department of Medicine/Division of Hematology/
Oncology, UPMC Cancer Pavilion, University
of Pittsburgh Cancer Institute, Pittsburgh, PA, USA
e-mail: tarhiniaa@upmc.edu

tumor that carry significant prognostic value. These include the Breslow thickness (depth) of the tumor and ulceration of the overlying epithelium. In the seventh edition, the prognostic significance of mitotic activity (microscopically defined as mitoses/mm^2) has been recognized as an important primary tumor prognostic factor [1]. The mitotic rate (equal to or greater than 1/mm^2) has now replaced the Clark level of invasion as a primary criterion (in addition to tumor ulceration) for defining the T1b subcategory.

Stage III melanoma comprises a disease with clinical and/or histopathological evidence of regional lymph node involvement, or the presence of in-transit or satellite metastases. Among these patients, the number of tumor-bearing lymph nodes, tumor burden at the time of staging [i.e., microscopic (identified by sentinel lymph node biopsy and completion lymphadenectomy) versus macroscopic], presence or absence of primary tumor ulceration, and thickness of the primary melanoma are the most predictive independent factors for survival [1]. Moreover, there is no lower threshold of tumor burden now taken to define the presence of regional nodal disease. Specifically, nodal tumor deposits less than 0.2 mm in diameter (previously adopted as the threshold for defining nodal metastasis in the AJCC sixth edition) are not ignored in the staging of nodal disease. The consensus that smaller volumes of metastatic tumor are still clinically significant for patients with melanoma differs from understandings held for other solid tumors, such as breast cancer, where the biological consequences of tumor burden are not felt to be significant. The presence of nodal micrometastases can be defined by either hematoxylin and eosin (H&E) or immunohistochemical staining (in the sixth edition, only H&E staining could be used).

Stage IV disease is defined by the presence of distant metastases. In these patients, the site(s) of metastases and elevated serum levels of lactate dehydrogenase (LDH) are used to subclassify the M1 stage into three categories: M1a, M1b, and M1c with varying prognosis [1]. Patients with distant metastasis in the skin, subcutaneous tissue, or distant lymph nodes, and a normal LDH level are classified as M1a and have a better prognosis compared to M1b and M1c. Patients with metastasis to the lung (with or without cutaneous, subcutaneous or nodal metastases) and a normal LDH level are classified as M1b and have an intermediate prognosis. Patients with metastases to any other visceral sites or at any location with an elevated LDH level are classified as M1c and have the worst prognosis [1].

Host Immunity in Primary Melanoma, Regional Nodal Metastases and Advanced Disease

Host immunity to melanoma appears to be important for disease control in both early and advanced disease settings. Spontaneous regression of disease has been reported more frequently in patients with melanoma compared with other solid tumors, suggesting a role for host immunity in the pathobiology of this disease. This concept is indirectly supported by the frequent presence of microscopically evident lymphocytic infiltrates at the primary melanoma site, and associated primary tumor regression features, such as dermal fibrosis and melanophagocytosis. Host cellular immune responses associated with melanoma have potential prognostic and predictive significance. T-cell infiltrates in primary melanoma are reported to be of prognostic value [2]. In addition, T-cell infiltrates within regional nodal metastases predict benefit in patients undergoing neoadjuvant interferon (IFN)-α2b therapy [3–5].

The quality of the host immune response has been shown to differ between early localized and regional or more advanced disease settings. While T helper type 1 (Th1) CD4+ antitumor T-cell function appears to be critical for the induction and maintenance of antitumor cytotoxic T-lymphocyte (CTL) responses *in vivo*, and Th2- or Th3/Tr-type CD4+ T-cell responses may subvert Th1-type cell-mediated immunity yielding a microenvironment that facilitates disease progression, patients with active melanoma (and renal cell carcinoma) have been shown to display strong tumor antigen-specific Th2-type polarization. In contrast, normal donors and patients who are disease-free following therapy demonstrate either weak, mixed Th1-/Th2-type responses or strongly polarized Th1-type responses to the same epitopes [6, 7]. Therefore, host immune tolerance appears to be an impediment to therapy of advanced disease. This may be avoidable in the high-risk setting of operable disease, where host susceptibility to immunologic interventions may be greater, and where IFN-α2b has demonstrated its most significant impact upon melanoma relapse and survival.

Serum Biomarkers of Prognostic and/or Therapeutic Predictive Value in Melanoma

Lactate Dehydrogenase (LDH)

The sixth edition (2002) AJCC staging system for melanoma first recognized the importance of serum LDH as an independent prognostic factor in patients with disseminated disease. Patients with elevated serum LDH and distant metastases at any site have very short survival, and are designated as M1c.

LDH has been shown to have a strong, incremental prognostic value ($p<0.0001$), based on the analysis of a recent phase III trial with oblimersen (GM301; Genesense®, Bcl-2 antisense; $n=771$) [8] and a large EORTC study with biochemotherapy +/− interleukin (IL)-2 (EORTC 18951 Biochemotherapy Trial; $n=365$) [9] in patients with advanced melanoma. Overall, the higher the LDH value at baseline, the shorter the overall survival (OS). Median OS in patients with baseline $LDH<0.8\times$ upper limit of the normal range (ULN) was ±1 year versus <2 months in patients with $LDH>5\times ULN$. Patients with baseline LDH in the range of $0.8-1.1\times ULN$ had a shorter median OS (±9 months) compared to patients with $LDH<0.8\times ULN$. Overall, treatment outcomes were not statistically significant in either study [8, 9]. An interaction between LDH and treatment was observed in the oblimersen study ($p=0.01$): the greatest benefit with oblimersen was achieved in patients with $LDH<0.8\times ULN$ (hazard ratio [HR]=0.64, with 24-month follow-up) [8]. In the EORTC study, no similar interaction was observed, and the trend for an IL-2 advantage was distributed across several LDH categories [9].

S100B

Serum S100B (isoforms S100AB and S100BB) are proteins of the S100 family that have shown promise as prognostic markers for melanoma relapse and mortality risk. S100B is shed by melanoma cells [10], and its level in the peripheral blood has been investigated as a melanoma biomarker [11–13]. Its prognostic potential is supported by many reports in the literature [14–32]. Serum S100B was found to be as reliable as serum LDH with respect to the prediction of clinical outcome in a recent study of 179 AJCC stage III-IV melanoma patients tested at diagnosis. Survival analysis indicated that initially elevated LDH and S100B levels in patients with stage IV disease predict comparably short survival [16]. S100B has been shown to be an independent prognostic factor in melanoma, and valuable for the detection of tumor progression and metastases [19, 20, 33]. The mean serum concentration of S100B protein is reported to be significantly related to the clinical stage of disease, and to have a high sensitivity and specificity for the detection of metastatic deposits [15, 17, 34].

A recent report from our laboratory highlighted that serum S100B level is a prognostic marker for patients with high-risk melanoma [35]. Sera from 691 patients, banked at baseline and subsequently at three additional time-points, were tested by chemiluminescence for S100B in this phase III E1694 trial. Univariate analysis showed baseline $S100B \geq 0.15$ µg/l significantly correlated with OS ($p=0.010$). Cox multivariate analysis was performed, adjusting for significant prognostic factors (ulceration and lymph node status) and treatment. Baseline S100B was found to be a significant prognostic factor for survival ($HR=1.39$; 95% CI, 1.01–1.92; $p=0.043$). S100B values measured at later time-points over 1 year were also demonstrated to be significant prognostic factors for both relapse-free survival (RFS) and OS. Lower S100B values at baseline and during follow-up were associated with longer survival. A changing S100B level from low at baseline to high on follow-up was associated with the worst RFS and OS [35].

Melanoma-Inhibiting Activity (MIA)

MIA is a soluble small protein secreted by melanoma cells that has been found to have growth-inhibiting activities [36]. Like S100B, MIA was shown to be potentially valuable in the monitoring of therapy and the detection of tumor progression in melanoma patients at different stages of disease [37]. Serum MIA levels increase with disease progression and are elevated in 60% and 89.5% of patients with stage III and IV melanoma, respectively [38]. Simultaneous evaluation of MIA and S100B may have added prognostic value. The sensitivity and specificity of S100B and MIA levels have been compared in a study of 96 patients with no evidence of disease (NED) and 86 patients with measurable metastatic melanoma. Abnormal S100B (>0.2 µg/l) and elevated MIA (>14 ng/ml) were found in 1.1% and 3.2% of patients with NED and in 59.3% and 54.6% of patients with metastatic disease (p<0.001). Using both tumor markers simultaneously, the sensitivity increased to 69.8%, with the specificity unchanged at 96.8% [39].

C-Reactive Protein (CRP)

Serum CRP has been shown to be potentially superior to conventional LDH measurement for initial detection of stage IV melanoma. In a prospective study, serum LDH and CRP levels were measured in 91 consecutive melanoma patients progressing to AJCC stage IV disease and 125 patients staying in AJCC stages I, II or III. Comparing distributions of the parameters by median values and quartiles, LDH was not significantly elevated in patients entering AJCC stage IV melanoma (p=0.785), whereas CRP was (p<0.001). Analyzing the sensitivity and specificity jointly by the areas under the receiver operating characteristic curves (ROC-AUC), LDH did not discriminate between the defined groups of patients (AUC=0.491; 95% confidence interval, 0.410, 0.581), whereas CRP did (AUC=0.933; 95% confidence interval, 0.900, 0.966; p<0.001). Upon logistic regression analysis, LDH provided no additional information to CRP. Choosing a cutoff point of 3.0 mg/l, CRP yielded a sensitivity of 76.9% and specificity of 90.4% in diagnosing AJCC stage IV entry [40].

Baseline serum CRP was found to have potential therapeutic predictive value in patients treated with the anti-CTLA4 antibody tremelimumab [41, 42]. CRP was evaluated in 525 patients participating in a randomized phase III study comparing tremelimumab to dacarbazine or temozolomide in patients with unresectable melanoma [41]. In the low baseline CRP group (CRP<1.5×ULN; n=326 [62%]), the HR for survival was 1.48 (95% CI: 1.14, 1.94) favoring tremelimumab, with a median OS of 19.1 months for the tremelimumab arm versus 12.7 months for the chemotherapy arm (p=0.0037). For patients with baseline CRP>1.5×ULN, the HR for survival was 0.86 (95% CI: 0.64, 1.15), favoring the chemotherapy arm. Similar findings were noted in a phase II study testing the combination of tremelimumab and high-dose IFN-α2b (HDI) [42]. In this study, baseline CRP≤2.5×ULN was significantly associated with therapeutic benefit (p=0.049).

Vascular Endothelial Growth Factor (VEGF)

The VEGF family plays a critical role in mediating angiogenesis and lymphangiogenesis, and has an impact on host innate and adaptive immunity [43, 44]. In cancer, in contrast to normal tissues, VEGF is not produced by endothelial cells, but rather by tumor cells and/or the tumor stroma, consistent with a paracrine mode of action [45–47]. Therefore, one might expect elevated serum VEGF levels in patients with high tumor burden. The role of excess VEGF in tumor angiogenesis is well documented, and high circulating levels of VEGF were recently found to be associated with poor prognosis in patients with metastatic melanoma [48]. VEGF has been shown to block the maturation of dendritic cells and inhibit effective priming of T-cell responses [49, 50]. These data support an important role for VEGF in the progression of cancer and evasion of antitumor immunity.

Serum VEGF-A and VEGF-C levels are reported to be elevated in patients with high tumor burden as compared to those with low burden disease [51–53]. Pretreatment sVEGF-C levels are higher in patients who are refractory to biochemotherapy (CDDP, recombinant IL-2 and α-IFN) as compared with responding patients. Following treatment, sVEGF-C was noted to be specifically increased in non-responding patients with high tumor burden. Prior to treatment, sVEGF-A levels were not significantly different between responders and non-responders. However, an increase in VEGF-A levels has been shown to correlate with disease progression following biochemotherapy. In addition, a decrease of serum VEGF-A levels is associated with objective response to treatment, as assessed by WHO criteria.

Recent studies have identified baseline serum VEGF as a marker of immune resistance and predictive for non-response to high-dose IL-2 [54]. A proteomic analysis evaluated the sera of patients ($n=100$, including 48 with predominantly metastatic melanoma and 11 with renal cell carcinoma) who were treated with high-dose IL-2, using a customized, multiplex antibody-targeted protein array platform to survey expression of soluble factors associated with tumor immunobiology. Patients with serum VEGF levels >125 pg/ml or fibronectin levels $>8 \times 10^6$ pg/ml did not respond to IL-2 therapy. Elevated levels of these proteins were also associated with significantly worse OS.

Other Serum Biomarkers

A number of other serum biomarkers have been evaluated in patients with melanoma. These include the tumor-associated antigen 90-immune complex (TA90IC) [25], YKL-40 (a heparin- and chitin-binding lectin secreted by activated neutrophils and macrophages) [55], and the L-DOPA/tyrosine ratio [56].

Induction of Autoimmunity is Associated with the Therapeutic Benefits of Immunotherapy

Paraneoplastic depigmentation among patients with melanoma has been reported to be a sign of favorable prognosis [57–59]. Recent studies of immunotherapy for melanoma, including high-dose IL-2 and anti-CTLA4 blocking antibody, have suggested a correlation between antitumor effects and induced autoimmune phenomena, such as thyroiditis, hypophysitis, enteritis, hepatitis and dermatitis [42, 60–72]. A strong association with prolonged RFS and OS was recently documented among high-risk melanoma patients treated with a modified adjuvant IFN regimen (HeCOG 13A/97), where a strong correlation between favorable clinical outcome and prospectively assessed autoimmune phenomena and/or the appearance of serum autoantibodies was rigorously established [73]. Autoantibodies were detected in 52 (26%) of 200 patients tested. Clinical manifestations of autoimmunity were observed among 15 (7%) patients, including vitiligo-like depigmentation in 11 cases (5%). A total of 113 patients have subsequently relapsed and 82 have died. The median time to progression (TTP) was 27.6 months, with a median survival of 58.6 months. The median TTP for those patients who did not develop clinical or serological evidence of autoimmunity was 15.9 months, while it has not been reached for the 52 patients who developed autoimmunity (106 vs 7; $p<0.0001$). The median survival was 37.5 months for those who were negative for autoimmunity, but has also not been reached for the autoimmune group (80 vs 2, $p<0.001$). In multivariate analysis, the presence of autoimmunity was an independent favorable prognostic marker.

We, at the University of Pittsburgh and Eastern Cooperative Oncology Group (ECOG), have evaluated the E2696 and E1694 trials to better understand the prognostic value of serological evidence of HDI-induced autoimmunity. In E2696, patients with resectable high-risk melanoma were randomized to GM2-KLH/QS–1 (GMK) vaccine plus concurrent HDI, GMK plus sequential HDI, or GMK alone. Sera from 103 patients in E2696 and 691 patients in E1694, banked at baseline and up to three additional time-points, were tested by enzyme-linked immunosorbent assay (ELISA) for the development of five autoantibodies. In E2696, autoantibodies were induced in 17 subjects (25%; $n=69$) receiving HDI and GMK versus two subjects (6%; $n=34$) receiving GMK alone ($p=0.029$). In E1694, 67 subjects (19.3%; $n=347$) who received HDI developed autoantibodies versus only 15 subjects (4.4%; $n=344$) in the vaccine control group ($p<0.001$). In the HDI arms, almost all induced autoantibodies were detected at ≥ 12 weeks after initiation of therapy. A 1-year landmark analysis of E1694 resected stage III patients showed survival advantage associated with HDI-induced autoimmunity that approached statistical significance ($HR=1.54$; $p=0.072$), adjusting for treatment [72].

IFN-α2b-mediated induction of autoimmunity may provide a useful surrogate biomarker of adjuvant therapeutic benefit. Studies of autoimmunity and its genetic determinants could help identify patients most likely to benefit from HDI and other newer immunotherapies, such as the anti-CTLA4 blocking antibodies ipilimumab and tremelimumab.

Primary Tumor Ulceration

A meta-analysis of individual patient data from 13 IFN-α adjuvant trials has suggested that the histopathological presence of primary tumor ulceration predicted therapeutic benefit to IFN [74]. A more recent analysis of the adjuvant trials EORTC 18952 and EORTC 18991 has assessed the predictive value of ulceration in relation to the therapeutic impact of IFN-α on RFS, distant metastases-free survival (DMFS), and OS, according to stage of disease (IIB and III; N1 microscopic nodal and N2 macroscopic nodal disease). Among 2,644 patients randomized in these studies, less than one third ($n=849$) had ulcerated primaries and 1,336 had non-ulcerated primaries, while the ulceration status was unknown for 459 individuals. The estimated reduction or increase in HR (SE %) of pegylated-IFN-α2b versus observation for the ulcerated group versus the non-ulcerated group was −27% (7%) versus −4% (7%) for RFS, −33% (7%) versus +7% (8%) for DMFS, and −31% (7%) versus +11% (8%) for OS. The most profound therapeutic effects were noted in patients with ulcerated and stage IIB/III-N1 tumors. Based on this retrospective analysis, the EORTC 18081 trial has been planned and will compare the benefit of pegylated-IFN-α2b versus observation in patients with ulcerated primaries of Breslow thickness >1 mm and lymph node-negative disease. It is noteworthy that, unlike US cooperative groups, the EORTC does not perform centralized histopathological review for its melanoma trials [1]. Interestingly, the E1684, E1690, and E1694 studies have never shown an association between primary tumor ulceration and response to HDI.

Cytokine Levels in Patients with Melanoma

Melanoma cell lines in culture and cultured melanoma cells derived from primary melanoma and metastatic tumors have demonstrated bFGF, IL-1α, IL-1β, IL-6, VEGF, PDGF, and IL-8 production [75–77]. These factors appear to promote tumor cell growth and increase the capacity of tumor cells to survive. In addition, they have paracrine effects and may stimulate endothelial cell proliferation, migration and angiogenesis, which are important for melanoma growth and metastasis [78]. Increased production of pro-angiogenic and growth factors by both melanoma and stromal cells *in vivo* might result in elevated circulating levels of these factors in the peripheral blood. In fact, numerous studies have demonstrated significantly increased serum IL-6 and IL-8 levels in melanoma patients [75, 79–81]. Elevated levels of IL-6 have been linked to poor prognosis in patients with stage IV melanoma [82–84]. In addition, EGF and IL-1, which modulate the tumor microenvironment and stimulate tumor growth and invasion, have also been reported to be elevated in the sera of patients with melanoma [78, 81]. Elevated levels of IL-10 are associated with advanced stage (III and IV) disease [85]. sIL-2R levels correlate with outcome in patients with melanoma [85]. In addition, serum levels of TNF-α and soluble TNF receptor 55 (sTNFR55) have been shown to have prognostic roles [86].

Baseline pro-inflammatory cytokine levels were reported to predict RFS benefit with HDI in the E1694 trial [87]. The detection of serum biomarkers that are either prognostic of clinical outcome or predictive of response to IFN-α2b has been pursued, utilizing the high-throughput xMAP® multiplex immunobead assay (Luminex Corp.). This technology was employed to simultaneously measure the levels of 29 cytokines, chemokines, angiogenic factors, growth factors and soluble receptors in the sera of 179 patients with high-risk melanoma who participated in the E1694 trial, and 378 healthy age- and gender-matched controls. The 179 melanoma patients were chosen at random from the two trial arms based on disease status (whether the subject had relapsed at <1 year, between 1 and 3 years, or more than 5 years). Of those samples tested, 93 were derived from patients who received GMK vaccination and 86 were derived from patients treated with HDI. The clinical data from the E1694 trial were then matured to a median of 4.6 years of follow-up. The results demonstrated that serum concentrations of IL-1α, IL-1β, IL-6, IL-8, IL-12p40, IL-13, G-CSF, MCP-1, MIP-1α, MIP-1β, IFN-α, TNF-α, EGF, VEGF, and TNFRII were significantly higher among patients with resected high-risk melanoma when compared to healthy controls. Serum levels of immunosuppressive, angiogenic/growth-stimulatory factors (VEGF, EGF, and HGF) were decreased significantly by IFN-α2b therapy, while levels of anti-angiogenic IP-10 and IFN-α were elevated posttreatment. Comparing patients according to relapse outcome, pretreatment levels of the pro-inflammatory cytokines IL-1α, IL-1β, IL-6, and TNF-α, and chemokines MIP-1α and MIP-1β, were significantly higher in sera of patients with longer RFS of >5 years, compared with patients who experienced shorter RFS of less than 1 year.

Biomarkers Associated with Anti-CTLA4 Therapy for Advanced Melanoma

Melanoma tumors can demonstrate spontaneous immune-mediated regression [71, 88–97]. In addition, tumor-specific cytotoxic T-cells and antibodies may be found in the peripheral blood of melanoma patients [71, 88–97]. Therefore, as described previously, immunotherapy could be an effective treatment strategy for individuals with this disease [71, 88–97].

One approach is the enhancement of anti-melanoma immune responses through the optimization of T-cell activation. The latter involves interactions between the T-cell receptor (TCR), the co-stimulatory receptor CD28, and the ligands CD80 and CD86 [71, 88–97]. T-cell inhibition is mediated by the inhibitory receptor, cytotoxic T lymphocyte-associated antigen 4 (CTLA4), a molecule that shares 30% homology with CD28, and is expressed by activated T-cells and T-regulatory cells (Tregs) [88]. CTLA4 binds CD80/CD86 with greater affinity than CD28 does, thereby inhibiting CD28-mediated T-cell activation and IL-2 production [88]. CTLA4 is critical for maintaining immune tolerance to self-antigens, but may also limit host responses to tumor antigens and the efficacy of vaccine therapy. CTLA4 blockade, either alone or in combination with melanoma-specific vaccines, has been explored as a potential strategy to treat advanced-stage melanoma [71, 88–97]. A recent phase III clinical trial found that patients with advanced, previously treated melanoma who received ipilimumab (MDX-010, a monoclonal antibody targeting CTLA4), with or without a gp100 peptide vaccine, showed improved OS compared with those who received gp100 alone [94]. Importantly, this clinical trial was the first randomized study to show an improvement in OS in advanced melanoma, where few treatment options exist [94]. However, not all patients have responded well to CTLA4 blockade, and some have developed severe autoimmune reactions. Of note, the presence of serum antibodies against the cancer-associated antigen, NY-ESO-1, has been found to be associated with efficacy of anti-CTLA4 therapy. In addition, metastatic tumors at different sites in an individual patient can demonstrate distinct immunological signatures and local microenvironmental changes, possibly explaining the variable responses to immunotherapy seen in some patients. Variations in the CTLA4 gene could also influence the response to its inhibition in patients with metastatic melanoma. In a recent study, three single nucleotide polymorphisms (SNPs) in this gene were found to be associated with responses to CTLA4 blockade: proximal promoter SNPs, rs4553808 and rs11571327, and the nonsynonymous SNP rs231775 [89]. A haplotype analysis, that included seven SNPs, suggested that the common haplotype TACCGGG is associated with no response, whereas the haplotype TGCCAGG does predict treatment response. Unfortunately, no specific haplotype or SNP predicts which patients will develop the severe autoimmune reactions triggered by CTLA4 blockade therapy [89]. Other potential immunological approaches in melanoma patients include the use of Toll-like receptor antagonists (i.e., imiquimod) and a HLA-B7/β2-microglobulin gene transfer product [88].

In a pooled analysis of three studies (CA184-007, CA184-008, and CA184-022), and confirmed prospectively in another study testing anti-CTLA4 blockade in metastatic melanoma (CA184-004), higher peripheral blood absolute lymphocyte counts (ALC) were significantly associated with clinical activity [98]. In a smaller analysis of 51 evaluable patients who received ipilimumab at a single institution, ALC also correlated with clinical benefit [99]. Patients with an ALC ≥ 1,000/μl after two ipilimumab doses (week 7) had a significantly improved clinical benefit rate and median OS than those with an ALC < 1,000/μl (51% vs 0%; 11.9 months vs 1.4 months) [99]. In addition to an association with increased ALC, relapse-free survival following ipilimumab treatment also correlates with an increase in IL-17-secreting helper T-cells [100]. In a phase II study of ipilimumab, examining tumor biopsies (comparing pre- and post-ipilimumab effects), clinical activity was associated with high expression of both FOXP3 (p=0.014) and indoleamine 2,3-dioxygenase (IDO) (p=0.012) at baseline, in addition to an increase from baseline of tumor-infiltrating lymphocytes (TILs) (week 4) (p=0.005) [101].

Interesting data has recently emerged showing that hair depigmentation develops alongside durable responses to ipilimumab in patients with metastatic melanoma [102]. In two trials that involved a total of 43 patients, six patients with hair depigmentation following treatment (median 10 months) demonstrated stable disease (SD) or complete remission (CR), ranging from 24 to 36 months. No non-responsive patient demonstrated hair depigmentation, although five patients without hair depigmentation had durable SD, ranging from 24 to 48 months. Hair depigmentation suggests an association between induced autoimmunity and clinical benefit for ipilimumab, and appears to be a potential surrogate biomarker for therapeutic response in some patients. However, it can take some time to evolve, and a link between its presence and drug response is not absolute. Finally, an association between low baseline serum CRP and survival benefit from tremelimumab compared to chemotherapy in patients with advanced melanoma has also been reported [41, 42]. It is possible that a similar association may be found for ipilimumab.

Molecular Biomarkers of Predictive Value for Novel Molecular-Directed Therapies

The BRAF gene encodes a Ras-regulated kinase, which mediates cell growth and is a component of the mitogen-activated protein kinase (MAPK) pathway. Activating mutations in BRAF have been described in two thirds of melanoma tumors in primary culture and in 70% of melanoma cell lines [103]. $BRAF^{V600E}$ is the most common kinase mutation found in melanoma (~50–60% prevalence). Results of phase I-III studies with Vemurafenib (PLX4032), a selective inhibitor of oncogenic $BRAF^{V600E}$, were recently completed and have shown significant antitumor activity, although responses appear to be transient [104, 105]. BRAF mutational status is a predictor of response to this class of specific inhibitors [88, 104].

Mutations and amplifications in the receptor tyrosine kinase KIT have been recently reported in acral melanomas (palms, soles, and subungual sites), mucosal melanomas, and cutaneous melanomas that arise in the setting of chronic sun damage [106]. These categories account for only ~25% of all melanomas in Western countries. However, acral and mucosal melanomas are the most prevalent subtypes in the rest of the world. In a cohort of 102 primary melanomas, KIT gene alterations (defined as mutations or copy number increases) were found in 15/38 (39%) of mucosal melanomas, 10/28 (36%) of acral melanomas, 5/18 (28%) of melanomas on skin with chronic sun-induced damage, and 0/18 (0%) of melanomas on skin without sun-induced damage [106]. Three phase II trials were initiated to examine the role of KIT/PDGFR inhibition (utilizing imatinib mesylate in two studies and dasatinib in the third) in patients with metastatic melanoma, regardless of whether their tumors displayed KIT/PDGFR expression [107–109]. Only modest activity was demonstrated in this unselected population [107–109]. A fourth study with imatinib mesylate enrolled only patients with unresectable melanoma arising from acral, mucosal, and chronic sun-damaged cutaneous sites. Patients were included if their tumors harbored (1) amplifications on chromosome 4q12 (site of KIT) detected by fluorescence in situ hybridization (FISH) or (2) KIT gene mutations (exons 9, 11, 13, 17, or 18) [110]. Of 146 patient tumors screened, 21% (31/146) were characterized by either mutation or amplification of KIT. Among the first 12 patients treated in this ongoing trial, response rate was 33% (4/12) with 2CR (18+ and 37+ weeks), 2PR (partial response), and 6SD. An ECOG study (E2607) is currently testing the role of dasatinib in this selected patient population. Following additional molecular analyses of patients with mucosal, acral, and chronic sun damage-associated melanoma, the incidence of KIT mutation has been found to be substantially lower than originally observed, and may be as low as 10% among mucosal and acral subtypes, with lower mutational frequencies in melanomas associated with chronic sun damage. Thus, it is important to evaluate molecular interventions specifically in terms of the appropriate somatic genomic alterations, and not use clinical and/or histopathological features as guides to the administration of these therapies.

Many treatment-responsive patients ultimately relapse as a result of acquired resistance to selective kinase-targeted therapies. This may be due to a number of factors, including alternative activation of MAPK signaling (CRAF-bypass signaling), other BRAF mutations or amplifications, mutations in RAS genes (HRAS, KRAS, or NRAS), mutations in MEK1, activation of alternative pathways that may drive proliferation and resistance to apoptosis (PI3K-AKT), or upregulation of escape pathways (CMET, KIT, FGFR, and EGFR) [88, 111–117]. As a result of the intrinsic redundancy in the multiple genetic pathways that are activated in melanoma, it is likely that the use of synergistic combinations of mutation-targeted agents will be required to achieve optimal outcomes and overcome potential drug resistance in patients with metastatic disease [88, 111–117]. In addition to MAPK-related mechanisms, other possible therapeutic targets in melanoma include GNAQ, CDK4, ERBB4, and ETV_1, as well as PI3K-AKT, apoptosis, DNA repair, angiogenesis, ubiquitin-proteosome and epigenetic pathways [29, 46–51]. Clinical trials evaluating novel drugs directed against some of these targets are currently in progress [88, 111–116].

References

1. Balch CM, et al. Final version of 2009 AJCC melanoma staging and classification. J Clin Oncol. 2009;27:6199–206.
2. Clemente CG, et al. Prognostic value of tumor infiltrating lymphocytes in the vertical growth phase of primary cutaneous melanoma. Cancer. 1996;77: 1303–10.
3. Hakansson A, et al. Tumour-infiltrating lymphocytes in metastatic malignant melanoma and response to interferon alpha treatment. Br J Cancer. 1996;74: 670–6.
4. Mihm Jr MC, Clemente CG, Cascinelli N. Tumor infiltrating lymphocytes in lymph node melanoma metastases: a histopathologic prognostic indicator and an expression of local immune response. Lab Invest. 1996;74:43–7.

5. Moschos SJ, et al. Neoadjuvant treatment of regional stage IIIB melanoma with high-dose interferon alfa-2b induces objective tumor regression in association with modulation of tumor infiltrating host cellular immune responses. J Clin Oncol. 2006;24:3164–71.
6. Tatsumi T, et al. Disease-associated bias in T helper type 1 (Th1)/Th2 CD4(+) T cell responses against MAGE-6 in HLA-DRB10401(+) patients with renal cell carcinoma or melanoma. J Exp Med. 2002;196:619–28.
7. Tatsumi T, et al. Disease stage variation in CD4+ and CD8+ T-cell reactivity to the receptor tyrosine kinase EphA2 in patients with renal cell carcinoma. Cancer Res. 2003;63:4481–9.
8. Bedikian AY, et al. Bcl-2 antisense (oblimersen sodium) plus dacarbazine in patients with advanced melanoma: the Oblimersen Melanoma Study Group. J Clin Oncol. 2006;24:4738–45.
9. Keilholz U, Bedikian AY, Punt CJA, et al. LDH is a prognostic factor in stage IV melanoma patients (pts) but is a predictive factor only for bcl2 antisense treatment efficacy: re-analysis of GM301 and EORTC18951 randomized trials. In: Proceedings of ASCO. Chicago. 2007.
10. Ghanem G, et al. On the release and half-life of S100B protein in the peripheral blood of melanoma patients. Int J Cancer. 2001;94:586–90.
11. Harpio R, Einarsson R. S100 proteins as cancer biomarkers with focus on S100B in malignant melanoma. Clin Biochem. 2004;37:512–8.
12. Kounalakis N, Goydos JS. Tumor cell and circulating markers in melanoma: diagnosis, prognosis, and management. Curr Oncol Rep. 2005;7:377–82.
13. Salama I, et al. A review of the S100 proteins in cancer. Eur J Surg Oncol. 2008;34:357–64.
14. Domingo-Domenech J, et al. Serum protein s-100 predicts clinical outcome in patients with melanoma treated with adjuvant interferon–comparison with tyrosinase rt-PCR. Oncology. 2005;68:341–9.
15. Andres R, et al. Prognostic value of serum S-100B in malignant melanoma. Tumori. 2004;90:607–10.
16. Banfalvi T, et al. Comparison of prognostic significance of serum 5-S-cysteinyldopa, LDH and S-100B protein in stage III-IV malignant melanoma. Pathol Oncol Res. 2002;8:183–7.
17. Martenson ED, et al. Serum S-100b protein as a prognostic marker in malignant cutaneous melanoma. J Clin Oncol. 2001;19:824–31.
18. Hauschild A, et al. Prognostic significance of serum S100B detection compared with routine blood parameters in advanced metastatic melanoma patients. Melanoma Res. 1999;9:155–61.
19. Hauschild A, et al. Predictive value of serum S100B for monitoring patients with metastatic melanoma during chemotherapy and/or immunotherapy. Br J Dermatol. 1999;140:1065–71.
20. Hauschild A, et al. S100B protein detection in serum is a significant prognostic factor in metastatic melanoma. Oncology. 1999;56:338–44.
21. Bonfrer JM, et al. The luminescence immunoassay S-100: a sensitive test to measure circulating S-100B: its prognostic value in malignant melanoma. Br J Cancer. 1998;77:2210–4.
22. Buer J, et al. Elevated serum levels of S100 and survival in metastatic malignant melanoma. Br J Cancer. 1997;75:1373–6.
23. Cao MG, et al. Melanoma inhibiting activity protein (MIA), beta-2 microglobulin and lactate dehydrogenase (LDH) in metastatic melanoma. Anticancer Res. 2007;27:595–9.
24. Curry BJ, Farrelly M, Hersey P. Evaluation of S-100beta assays for the prediction of recurrence and prognosis in patients with AJCC stage I-III melanoma. Melanoma Res. 1999;9:557–67.
25. Faries MB, et al. A Comparison of 3 tumor markers (MIA, TA90IC, S100B) in stage III melanoma patients. Cancer Invest. 2007;25:285–93.
26. Juergensen A, et al. Comparison of two prognostic markers for malignant melanoma: MIA and S100 beta. Tumour Biol. 2001;22:54–8.
27. Miliotes G, et al. Evaluation of new putative tumor markers for melanoma. Ann Surg Oncol. 1996;3:558–63.
28. Mohammed MQ, et al. Serum S100beta protein as a marker of disease activity in patients with malignant melanoma. Med Oncol. 2001;18:109–20.
29. Rebmann V, et al. Soluble HLA-DR is a potent predictive indicator of disease progression in serum from early-stage melanoma patients. Int J Cancer. 2002;100:580–5.
30. Schultz ES, Diepgen TL, Von Den Driesch P. Clinical and prognostic relevance of serum S-100 beta protein in malignant melanoma. Br J Dermatol. 1998;138:426–30.
31. Smit LH, et al. Normal values of serum S-100B predict prolonged survival for stage IV melanoma patients. Eur J Cancer. 2005;41:386–92.
32. Ugurel S, et al. Tumor type M2 pyruvate kinase (TuM2-PK) as a novel plasma tumor marker in melanoma. Int J Cancer. 2005;117:825–30.
33. Schmitz C, et al. Comparative study on the clinical use of protein S-100B and MIA (melanoma inhibitory activity) in melanoma patients. Anticancer Res. 2000;20:5059–63.
34. Ortiz B, et al. [S100 protein as tumoral marker in melanoma patients. Comparative study with sentinel node biopsy and whole body FDG-PET]. Rev Esp Med Nucl. 2003;22:87–96.
35. Tarhini AA, et al. Prognostic significance of serum S100B protein in high-risk surgically resected melanoma patients participating in intergroup trial ECOG 1694. J Clin Oncol. 2009;27:38–44.
36. Bogdahn U, et al. Autocrine tumor cell growth-inhibiting activities from human malignant melanoma. Cancer Res. 1989;49:5358–63.
37. Djukanovic D, et al. Comparison of S100 protein and MIA protein as serum marker for malignant melanoma. Anticancer Res. 2000;20:2203–7.

38. Bosserhoff AK, et al. Melanoma-inhibiting activity, a novel serum marker for progression of malignant melanoma. Cancer Res. 1997;57:3149–53.
39. Auge JM, et al. S-100beta and MIA in advanced melanoma in relation to prognostic factors. Anticancer Res. 2005;25:1779–82.
40. Deichmann M, et al. Diagnosing melanoma patients entering American Joint Committee on Cancer stage IV, C-reactive protein in serum is superior to lactate dehydrogenase. Br J Cancer. 2004;91:699–702.
41. Marshall M, Ribas A, Huang B. Evaluation of baseline serum C-reactive protein (CRP) and benefit from tremelimumab compared to chemotherapy in first-line melanoma. Proc Am Soc Clin Oncol. 2010;28(15s):2609.
42. Tarhini AA, et al. Phase II evaluation of tremelimumab (Treme) combined with high-dose interferon alpha-2b (HDI) for metastatic melanoma. Proc Am Soc Clin Oncol. 2010;28(15s):8524.
43. Kerbel RS. Tumor angiogenesis. N Engl J Med. 2008;358:2039–49.
44. Folkman J. Tumor angiogenesis: therapeutic implications. N Engl J Med. 1971;285:1182–6.
45. Mehnert J, et al. VEGF, VEGFR1, and VEGFR2 expression in melanoma. Proc Am Soc Clin Oncol. 2007;25(18s):8520.
46. Duff SE, et al. Vascular endothelial growth factors C and D and lymphangiogenesis in gastrointestinal tract malignancy. Br J Cancer. 2003;89:426–30.
47. Paley PJ, et al. Vascular endothelial growth factor expression in early stage ovarian carcinoma. Cancer. 1997;80:98–106.
48. Tas F, et al. Circulating serum levels of angiogenic factors and vascular endothelial growth factor receptors 1 and 2 in melanoma patients. Melanoma Res. 2006;16:405–11.
49. Gabrilovich DI, et al. Production of vascular endothelial growth factor by human tumors inhibits the functional maturation of dendritic cells. Nat Med. 1996;2:1096–103.
50. Ohm JE, et al. VEGF inhibits T-cell development and may contribute to tumor-induced immune suppression. Blood. 2003;101:4878–86.
51. Soubrane C, et al. Changes in circulating VEGF-A levels related to clinical response during biochemotherapy in metastatic malignant melanoma. Proc Am Soc Clin Oncol. 2004;22(14s):7531.
52. Soubrane C, et al. Soluble VEGF-A and lymphangiogenesis in metastatic malignant melanoma patients. Proc Am Soc Clin Oncol. 2006;24(18s):8049.
53. Mouawad R, et al. Relationship of soluble VEGF-C and VEGF-D with clinicopathological parameters in metastatic malignant melanoma patients treated by biochemotherapy. Proc Am Soc Clin Oncol. 2005;23(16s):7540.
54. Sabatino M, et al. Serum vascular endothelial growth factor and fibronectin predict clinical response to high-dose interleukin-2 therapy. J Clin Oncol. 2009;27:2645–52.
55. Schmidt H, et al. Elevated serum level of YKL-40 is an independent prognostic factor for poor survival in patients with metastatic melanoma. Cancer. 2006;106:1130–9.
56. Garnier JP, et al. Clinical value of combined determination of plasma L-DOPA/tyrosine ratio, S100B, MIA and LDH in melanoma. Eur J Cancer. 2007;43:816–21.
57. Nordlund JJ, et al. Vitiligo in patients with metastatic melanoma: a good prognostic sign. J Am Acad Dermatol. 1983;9:689–96.
58. Bystryn JC, et al. Prognostic significance of hypopigmentation in malignant melanoma. Arch Dermatol. 1987;123:1053–5.
59. Schallreuter KU, Levenig C, Berger J. Vitiligo and cutaneous melanoma. A case study. Dermatologica. 1991;183:239–45.
60. Atkins M, et al. Hypothyroidism after treatment with interleukin-2 and lymphokine-activated killer cells. N Engl J Med. 1988;318:1557–63.
61. Weijl NI, et al. Hypothyroidism during immunotherapy with interleukin-2 is associated with antithyroid antibodies and response to treatment. J Clin Oncol. 1993;11:1376–83.
62. Scalzo S, et al. Primary hypothyroidism associated with interleukin-2 and interferon alpha-2 therapy of melanoma and renal carcinoma. Eur J Cancer. 1990;26:1152–6.
63. Krouse RS, Royal RE, Heywood G, et al. Thyroid dysfunction in 281 patients with metastatic melanoma or renal carcinoma treated with interleukin-2 alone. J Immunother Emphasis Tumor Immunol. 1995;18:272–8.
64. Phan GQ, et al. Factors associated with response to high-dose interleukin-2 in patients with metastatic melanoma. J Clin Oncol. 2001;19:3477–82.
65. Becker JC, et al. Antiphospholipid syndrome associated with immunotherapy for patients with melanoma. Cancer. 1994;73:1621–4.
66. Rosenberg SA, White DE. Vitiligo in patients with melanoma: normal tissue antigens can be targets for cancer immunotherapy. J Immunother Emphasis Tumor Immunol. 1996;19:81–4.
67. Franzke A, et al. Autoimmunity resulting from cytokine treatment predicts long-term survival in patients with metastatic renal cell cancer. J Clin Oncol. 1999;17:529–33.
68. Phan GQ, et al. Cancer regression and autoimmunity induced by cytotoxic T lymphocyte-associated antigen 4 blockade in patients with metastatic melanoma. Proc Natl Acad Sci USA. 2003;100:8372–7.
69. Sanderson K, et al. Autoimmunity in a phase I trial of a fully human anti-cytotoxic T-lymphocyte antigen-4 monoclonal antibody with multiple melanoma peptides and Montanide ISA 51 for patients with resected stages III and IV melanoma. J Clin Oncol. 2005;23:741–50.

70. Dranoff G, et al. Vaccination with irradiated tumor cells engineered to secrete murine granulocyte-macrophage colony-stimulating factor stimulates potent, specific, and long-lasting anti-tumor immunity. Proc Natl Acad Sci USA. 1993;90:3539–43.
71. Ribas A, et al. Antitumor activity in melanoma and anti-self responses in a phase I trial with the anti-cytotoxic T lymphocyte-associated antigen 4 monoclonal antibody CP-675,206. J Clin Oncol. 2005;23: 8968–77.
72. Stuckert J, Tahrini AA, Lee S, et al. Interferon alfa-induced autoimmunity in patients with high-risk melanoma participating in ECOG trial E2696. In: Proceedings of AACR. Los Angeles. 2007.
73. Gogas H, et al. Prognostic significance of autoimmunity during treatment of melanoma with interferon. N Engl J Med. 2006;354:709–18.
74. Wheatley K, et al. Interferon-α as adjuvant therapy for melanoma: an individual patient data meta-analysis of randomised trials. In: Proceedings of ASCO Annual Meeting. Chicago, 2007.
75. Ciotti P, et al. Cytokine expression in human primary and metastatic melanoma cells: analysis in fresh bioptic specimens. Melanoma Res. 1995;5(1):41–7.
76. Westphal JR, et al. Angiogenic balance in human melanoma: expression of VEGF, bFGF, IL-8, PDGF and angiostatin in relation to vascular density of xenografts. Int J Cancer. 2000;86:768–76.
77. Ijland SA, et al. Expression of angiogenic and immunosuppressive factors by uveal melanoma cell lines. Melanoma Res. 1999;9:445–50.
78. Lazar-Molnar E, et al. Autocrine and paracrine regulation by cytokines and growth factors in melanoma. Cytokine. 2000;12:547–54.
79. Gorelik E, et al. Multiplexed immunobead-based cytokine profiling for early detection of ovarian cancer. Cancer Epidemiol Biomarkers Prev. 2005;14: 981–7.
80. Colombo MP, et al. Expression of cytokine genes, including IL-6, in human malignant melanoma cell lines. Melanoma Res. 1992;2:181–90.
81. Mattei S, et al. Expression of cytokine/growth factors and their receptors in human melanoma and melanocytes. Int J Cancer. 1994;56:853–7.
82. Tartour E, et al. Serum interleukin 6 and C-reactive protein levels correlate with resistance to IL-2 therapy and poor survival in melanoma patients. Br J Cancer. 1994;69:911–3.
83. Mouawad R, et al. Serum interleukin-6 concentrations as predictive factor of time to progression in metastatic malignant melanoma patients treated by biochemotherapy: a retrospective study. Cytokines Cell Mol Ther. 2002;7:151–6.
84. Soubrane C, Mouawad R, Rixe O, et al. Soluble VEGF and its receptors (1 and 2) in metastatic malignant melanoma patients: relationship with survival. 2005 ASCO annual meeting proceedings. J Clin Oncol. 2005;23:7541.
85. Vuoristo MS, et al. Serum levels of interleukins 2, 6 and 8, soluble interleukin-2 receptor and intercellular adhesion molecule-1 during treatment with interleukin-2 plus interferon-alfa. Immunopharmacol Immunotoxicol. 1996;18:337–54.
86. Ocvirk J, et al. Serum values of tumour necrosis factor-[alpha] and of soluble tumour necrosis factor-R55 in melanoma patients. Melanoma Res. 2000;10: 253–8.
87. Yurkovetsky ZR, et al. Multiplex analysis of serum cytokines in melanoma patients treated with interferon-alpha2b. Clin Cancer Res. 2007;13:2422–8.
88. Ji Z, Flaherty KT, Tsao H. Molecular therapeutic approaches to melanoma. Mol Aspects Med. 2010;31:194–204.
89. Breunis WB, Tarazona-Santos E, Chen R, et al. Influence of cytotoxic T lymphocyte-associated antigen 4 (CTLA4) common polymorphisms on outcome in treatment of melanoma patients with CTLA-4 blockade. J Immunother. 2008;31: 586–90.
90. Fischkoff S, Hersch E, Weber J, et al. Durable responses and long-term progression-free survival observed in a phase II study of mdx-010 alone or in combination with dacarbazine (DTIC) in metastatic melanoma. 2005 ASCO annual meeting proceedings. J Clin Oncol. 2005;23 Suppl 1:7525.
91. Maker AV, Phan GQ, Attia P, et al. Tumor regression and autoimmunity in patients treated with cytotoxic T lymphocyte-associated antigen 4 blockade and interleukin 2: a phase I/II study. Ann Surg Oncol. 2005;12:1005–16.
92. Attia P, Phan GQ, Maker AV, et al. Autoimmunity correlates with tumor regression in patients with metastatic melanoma treated with anti-cytotoxic T-lymphocyte antigen-4. J Clin Oncol. 2005;23: 6043–53.
93. Weber JS, Targan S, Scotland R, et al. Phase II trial of extended dose CTLA-4 antibody ipilimumab (formerly MDX-010) with a multi-peptide vaccine for resected stages IIIC and IV melanoma. 2006 ASCO annual meeting proceedings part I. J Clin Oncol. 2006;24(Suppl):2510.
94. Hodi FS, O'Day SJ, McDermott DF, et al. Improved survival with ipilimumab in patients with metastatic melanoma. N Engl J Med. 2010;363:711–23.
95. Bulanhagui CA, Ribas A, Pavlov D, et al. Phase I clinical trials of ticilimumab: tumor responses are sufficient but not necessary for prolonged survival. J Clin Oncol. 2006;24(461s):8036.
96. Reuben M, Lee BN, Li C, et al. Biologic and immunomodulatory events after CTLA-4 blockade with ticilimumab in patients with advanced malignant melanoma. Cancer. 2006;106:2437–44.
97. Gomez-Navarro J, Sharma A, Bozon VA, et al. Dose and schedule selection for the anti-CTLA4 monoclonal antibody ticilimumab in patients (pts) with metastatic melanoma. J Clin Oncol. 2006;24(460s):8032.
98. Hamid O, et al. Dose effect of ipilimumab in patients with advanced melanoma: results from a phase II, randomized, dose-ranging study. J Clin Oncol. 2008;26:9025. Proc Am Soc Clin Oncol, 2008.

99. Ku GY, Yuan J, Page DB, et al. Single-institution experience with ipilimumab in advanced melanoma patients in the compassionate use setting: lymphocyte count after 2 doses correlates with survival. Cancer. 2010;116:1767–75.
100. Weber J. Ipilimumab: controversies in its development, utility and autoimmune adverse events. Cancer Immunol Immunother. 2009;58:823–30.
101. Hamid O, Chasalow SD, Tsuchihashi Z, et al. Association of baseline and on-study tumor biopsy markers with clinical activity in patients (pts) with advanced melanoma treated with ipilimumab. J Clin Oncol. 2009;27:9008.
102. Pavlick A, et al. Hair depigmentation as an indicator of durable response to CTLA-4 therapy. Proc Am Soc Clin Oncol. 2010;28(15s):8571.
103. Davies H, et al. Mutations of the BRAF gene in human cancer. Nature. 2002;417:949–54.
104. Flaherty KT, Puzanov I, Kim KB, et al. Inhibition of mutated, activated BRAF in metastatic melanoma. N Engl J Med. 2010;363:809–19.
105. Chapman PB, Hauschild A, Robert C, et al. The BRIM-3 study group. Improved survival with Vemurafenib in Melanoma with BRAF V600E mutation. N Engl J Med. 2011;364:2507–16.
106. Curtin JA, et al. Somatic activation of KIT in distinct subtypes of melanoma. J Clin Oncol. 2006;24:4340–6.
107. Wyman K, et al. Multicenter phase II trial of high-dose imatinib mesylate in metastatic melanoma: significant toxicity with no clinical efficacy. Cancer. 2006;106:2005–11.
108. Eton O, et al. Phase II trial of imatinib mesylate (STI-571) in metastatic melanoma (MM). Proc Am Soc Clin Oncol. 2004;22:7528.
109. Kluger HM, et al. A phase II trial of dasatinib in advanced melanoma. Proc Am Soc Clin Oncol. 2009;27(15s):9010.
110. Carvajal R, et al. A phase II study of imatinib mesylate (IM) for patients with advanced melanoma harboring somatic alterations of KIT. Proc Am Soc Clin Oncol. 2009;27(15s):9001.
111. Wellbrock C, Hurlstone A. BRAF as therapeutic target in melanoma. Biochem Pharmacol. 2010;80:561–7.
112. Shepherd C, Puzanov I, Sosman JA. B-RAF inhibitors: an evolving role in the therapy of malignant melanoma. Curr Oncol Rep. 2010;12:146–52.
113. Flaherty KT, Hodi FS, Bastian BC. Mutation-driven drug development in melanoma. Curr Opin Oncol. 2010;22:178–83.
114. Gray-Schopfer V, Wellbrock C, Marais R. Melanoma biology and new targeted therapy. Nature. 2007;445:851–7.
115. Nathanson KL. Using genetics and genomics strategies to personalize therapy for cancer: focus on melanoma. Biochem Pharmacol. 2010;80:755–61.
116. Davies MA, Samuels Y. Analysis of the genome to personalize therapy for melanoma. Oncogene. 2010;29:5545–55.
117. Smalley KSM, Haass NK, Brafford P, et al. Multiple signaling pathways must be targeted to overcome therapeutic resistance in cell lines derived from melanoma metastases. Mol Cancer Ther. 2006;5:1136–44.

Index

A

ABT-263, 270, 271
Acral lentiginous melanoma (ALM), 244, 245
Adjuvant, 255–256
Administration of activating antibodies, 296, 298–299
Adoptive cell therapies, 296, 298
Aflibercept, 284, 286
Age, 49, 50, 59, 60, 62
Akt, 183
Allelic imbalance, 69–70
ALM. *See* Acral lentiginous melanoma
American Joint Committee on Cancer (AJCC), 39–42, 45–46
  guidelines, 177
AMH. *See* Atypical melanocytic hyperplasia
Anatomic location, 49, 50, 58, 62
Angiogenesis, 281–291
Angiogenesis targeting agents, 283–285, 291
Angiopoietin (Ang), 281–283, 290
Angiotropism, 49, 57, 62
Anti-apoptotic proteins, 163
Anti-miR, 136–138
Apoptosis, 267, 269–270, 272, 273
Association with a benign melanocytic nevus, 49, 60
Atypical melanocytic hyperplasia (AMH), 245
Autoimmunity, 309–310, 312
Axitinib, 284, 287
AZD6244, 267, 271

B

Bcl–2, 267, 269–272
Bevacizumab, 284, 285, 286, 290, 291
Biochemotherapy (BCT), 255, 256, 296, 299
Biocomputing, 189
Biomarkers, 1–7, 9–14, 89–105, 189–193, 305–313
Borderline melanocytic lesions, 49, 54, 60
BRAF, 2, 4, 5, 20–24, 26–28, 72–74, 266, 267, 268, 270–273, 305, 312, 313
Breslow thickness, 49–53, 58, 62

C

Cancer stem cell (CSC), 227–238
CCND1, 244, 245
CDK4, 24–25
CDKN2A, 21–27
CDKs. *See* Cyclin-dependent kinases
Cell cycle, 178–180, 185, 247–250
Chemoresistance, 247, 257–259
Chemotherapeutic agent, 3
Chemotherapy, 247–260
CI. *See* Confidence interval
Cilengitide, 284, 289, 290
Circulating exosomes, 134
Circulating miRNAs, 134, 135
Circulating tumor cells (CTC), 195–203
c-KIT, 266, 270–272
Clark anatomic level, 49, 51–52, 62
Clinical characteristics, 9
CLND. *See* Completion lymph node dissection
Clonal evolution, 227–238
c-Met, 183
c-Myc, 183
CNTO–95, 289
Combination chemotherapy (polychemotherapy), 247, 252–255
Comparative genomic hybridization, 70
Completion lymph node dissection (CLND), 210, 214, 216, 217, 220
Confidence interval (CI), 219
CpG methylation, 74
CRAF, 266, 270–272
C-reactive protein (CRP), 308, 312
Cross-sectional profile, 49, 52, 62
CSC. *See* Cancer stem cell
CTC. *See* Circulating tumor cells
CTLA4, 308–312
CTLA–4 receptor, 296
Cyclin D1, 244, 245
Cyclin-dependent kinase inhibitors, 163, 164
Cyclin-dependent kinases (CDKs), 265, 270–273
Cyclins, 163–166, 168
Cytokines, 310–311

Cytokine therapy, 296, 298
Cytologic atypia, 49, 59, 60
Cytologic variation, 49

D

Dasatinib, 271
Deacetylation, 98, 101, 105
Dedifferentiation, 236, 237
Deletions, 146–149, 152–154
Demethylation, 94, 95, 98, 100, 101, 105
Depigmentation, 309, 312
Dermatopathology report, 49, 50, 52, 59, 61, 62
Desmoplasia, 49, 59, 62
Diagnosis, 1, 3, 7
Dicer, 116, 121–123
Distant metastasis (M), 39, 40, 42–43
DNA
    copy number changes, 70, 74
    hypermethylation, 91–94
    hypomethylation, 94–95
    methylation, 91, 92, 94–98, 102, 105
    microarray, 73
Dovitini, 6, 284, 287

E

Efficacy, 247, 249, 252, 253, 256, 257
EGFR, 183
Epigenetics, 69–76, 89–105, 113, 121
Epithelial-to-mesenchymal transition (EMT), 196, 201, 202
Everolimus, 269, 271
Excision margin, 243–245

F

FGFR–1, 183
Field cancerization, 243–245
Field cells, 243–245
Fluorescence in situ hybridization (FISH), 71–72, 244, 245
Formalin-fixed paraffin-embedded (FFPE), 131–133, 190–193

G

GADD. *See* Growth arrest DNA-damage
Gain-of-function mutations, 4
Gene expression, 198–203
Gene expression analysis, 79, 82
Gene therapy, 136–138
Genomics, 189, 190
Growth arrest DNA-damage (GADD), 180
Growth phase, 49, 54–56, 58, 62

H

Hazard ratio, 219
HDM–2. *See* Human double minute–2
Heat shock protein (HSP) therapy, 296–298
Hematoxylin-eosin, 214
Histologic tumor type, 49, 58, 62
Histone modifications, 97, 98, 100–102
Histopathological characteristics, 9, 14
Histopathology, 49, 61
HMB–45, 160–163, 168–171
Host immunity, 306–307
Host inflammatory response, 49, 56, 59 62
HRAS, 72–74
Human double minute–2 (HDM–2), 180

I

Imatinib, 271, 313
Immune biomarkers, 295–301
Immunohistochemistry (IHC), 9, 12, 81, 82, 85, 86, 177–185, 190–193, 210, 245
Immunomagnetic bead capture, 199, 200
Immunomodulatory drugs (IMiDs), 281, 287–288
Immunotherapy, 295–301
Inducible nitric oxide synthase (iNOS), 22, 30–31
Integrins, 283, 284, 289
Interconversion, 227–238
Interferon (IFN)-α2b, 306–311
Interleukin (IL)–2, 307, 309, 311
Ipilimumab, 310, 311, 312

K

Ki–67, 162, 163, 166–171, 179, 180, 181, 183, 185
KIT, 20, 21, 23–24, 26, 313

L

Lactate dehydrogenase (LDH), 13, 14, 306–308
Lenalidomide, 284, 285, 288
Locoregional, 256, 257

M

MAP–2. *See* Microtubule-associated protein–2
MAPK. *See* Mitogen-activated protein kinase
Markers, 227–229, 232–236, 238
MART–1, 160, 161, 169, 171
Mass spectrometry, 189–193
MCAM. *See* Melanoma cell adhesion molecule
Melanin, 150–152
Melanocortin-1-receptor (MC1R), 25, 26
Melanocytic nevi, 160, 161, 163, 167, 170
Melanoma, 1–7, 9–14, 69–76, 89–105, 113–123, 145–155, 159–172, 189–193, 247–260
Melanoma cell adhesion molecule (MCAM), 181, 183
Melanoma-inhibiting activity (MIA), 12, 14, 308
Melanoma metastasis risk, 178, 185
Melanoma prognostication, 177–185
Melanoma-relevant miRNAs, 131
Melanoma stem cell (MSC), 227, 228, 230, 232–238
Messenger RNA, 116
Metallothionein, 181, 183, 185
Metastasis, 116, 118, 120, 195–199, 203, 227, 234, 236, 237, 247, 252, 256, 257

Metastatic, 79, 81, 83–87
MIA. *See* Melanoma-inhibiting activity
MIB–1, 179–181
Micrometastases, 40–42, 45
Microphthalmia-associated transcription
    factor (MITF), 21, 27–28, 161, 162, 169,
    171, 265, 270, 272
microRNA (miRNA), 89, 90, 102–105,
    113–123, 201, 203
  biogenesis, 127–130
  biomarker, 131–136
  classifier, 131, 133
  function, 137, 139
  microarray, 134, 135
  mimetic, 136–138
  profiling, 131–133
Microtubule-associated protein–2 (MAP–2), 180, 181,
    183, 185
Minichromosome maintenance protein, 180, 184
MITF. *See* Microphthalmia-associated transcription factor
Mitochips, 153–155
Mitochondria, 145, 149–150
mitochondrial DNA (mtDNA), 145–155
Mitogen-activated protein kinase (MAPK), 21, 23, 27,
    29, 265, 266, 268, 269, 271, 272, 312, 313
Mitotic index, 179
Mitotic rate, 39–41, 44–46, 49, 51–55
Mitotic rate biomarkers, 179–180
MLPA. *See* Multiplex ligation-dependent probe amplification
MMP–2, 182, 183, 185
Molecular markers, 202
Monoclonal antibody, 283, 285, 289
mRNA, 79–87
MSC. *See* Melanoma stem cell
mTOR, 269, 271, 273
Multicenter selective lymphadenectomy trial, 210
Multimarker, 184
Multiplex ligation-dependent probe amplification
    (MLPA), 71, 74
Multi-target protein kinase inhibitors, 284, 286–287

N
Negative predictive value (NPV), 209, 211, 212, 219
Neurotropic factors, 49
NF-kβ, 22, 26, 29–31
Niche, 230–232, 236, 237
Noncoding RNA, 113
Nonspecific immune adjuvants, 296, 299
Notch, 22, 28, 29
NPV. *See* Negative predictive value
NRAS, 2, 4, 5, 20, 23, 24, 72–74, 266, 268, 271, 272

O
Oblimersen (OBL), 270, 271, 307
Oncogene mutation, 72
Oncogenic miRNA, 137
Osteopontin, 183–185

P
5p15, 245
p53, 163, 165, 166, 168, 170
Parameters, 49–62
Paratumoral epidermal hyperplasia, 49, 60–62
PCNA. *See* Proliferating cell nuclear antigen
PCR. *See* Polymerase chain reaction
PD0325901, 267, 271
PI3K-AKT, 21, 23, 26–27, 29, 266–269, 271
p16^{INK4a}, 182, 183, 272, 273
Plasticity, 227, 231–233, 235–238
PLX4032, 267, 271, 312
Polymerase chain reaction (PCR), 209, 211, 213, 214,
    217–220
Positive predictive value (PPV), 219
Posttranscriptional silencing, 129
Presence or absence of regression, 49
Primary, 79, 81–86
Primary tumor (T), 39–43, 45
Prognosis, 1, 2, 9–12, 14, 85, 86
Prognostic marker, 122
Progression, 79, 81–85, 87, 115–119, 122, 123
Proliferating cell nuclear antigen (PCNA), 163, 166, 180,
    182, 183
Proliferation biomarkers, 179–180
Protein, 189–193
Protein biomarker, 177–185
Proteomics, 189–193
PTEN, 26–27, 183, 268

Q
11q13, 244, 245
Quantitative RT-PCR (qPCR), 199–202

R
Radial growth phase (RGP) melanoma, 82–83
RAF–265, 267, 271
RAS/RAF/MEK/ERK, 265–268
Reactive oxygen species (ROS), 145, 147–152
Recurrence, 243–245
Regional lymph nodes (N)
REMARK criteria, 180, 181, 184, 185
Response rate, 247, 253–256, 259
Retinoblastoma protein (Rb), 267, 272, 273
Risk assessment, 177, 185
RNAi-based therapy, 137
RNA-Induced Silencing Complex (RISC), 116, 118
RNA interference (RNAi), 136–138
RNAi therapeutics, 137, 138
ROS. *See* Reactive oxygen species

S
S100, 160, 161, 169, 171
Satellite and in-transit metastasis, 61, 62
S100β (S100-beta), 12–13, 307–308
Self-renewal, 227–232, 235–237
Semaxanib, 284, 287

Sentinel lymph node (SLN), 209–220
Sentinel lymph node biopsy (SNLB), 209–211, 213
Serum, 12–14
serum-based miRNA biomarkers, 136
Sex, 50, 62
Single-agent, 247, 250–255
siRNA, 136–138
siRNA-based therapeutics, 136
siRNA delivery, 136
Sirolimus, 271
SLN. *See* Sentinel lymph node
SNLB. *See* Sentinel lymph node biopsy
SNS–032, 271, 273
Sorafenib, 266, 267, 269, 271, 272, 284–287, 291
Spitz nevus, 69, 70, 72
Spitz tumors, 160, 166–170
Staging, 1–3, 7, 39–46, 305–307
Stroma-targeted, 259

T

Targeted-melanoma therapy, 136–138
Targeted therapy, 3, 5, 7
Target protectors, 137
Temsirolimus, 269, 271
Thalidomide, 284, 287, 288
Thickness, 39–41, 44, 45
Tissue-based, 189–193
Tissue microarrays (TMAs), 184, 185
TNM, 39, 40, 46
Tremelimumab, 308, 310, 312
Tumorigenesis, 79, 82
Tumor-related DNA, 201, 203
Tumor suppressive miRNA, 137
Tumor vascularity, 49, 55–57, 62
Tumor volume, 49, 52, 62
Tyrosinase, 161, 169, 171

U

Ulceration, 39–41, 44–46, 49–55, 57, 59, 62, 306, 307, 310

V

Vaccine therapy, 295, 297, 299, 301
Vascular endothelial growth factor (VEGF), 183, 212–214, 266, 271, 273, 281–287, 289, 290, 308–311
Vascular invasion, 49, 57, 62
VEGF-trap, 285
Vemurafenib, 312
Vertical growth phase (VGP) melanoma, 82–84
Vitaxin, 284, 289
Volociximab, 284, 289

W

WNT, 28, 29